AF333772

1997
YEAR BOOK OF
OBSTETRICS, GYNECOLOGY, AND WOMEN'S HEALTH

Statement of Purpose

The YEAR BOOK Service

The YEAR BOOK series was devised in 1901 by practicing health professionals who observed that the literature of medicine and related disciplines had become so voluminous that no one individual could read and place in perspective every potential advance in a major specialty. In the final decade of the 20th century, this recognition is more acutely true than it was in 1901.

More than merely a series of books, YEAR BOOK volumes are the tangible results of a unique service designed to accomplish the following:

- to *survey* a wide range of journals of proven value
- to *select* from those journals papers representing significant advances and statements of important clinical principles
- to provide *abstracts* of those articles that are readable, convenient summaries of their key points
- to provide *commentary* about those articles to place them in perspective

These publications grow out of a unique process that calls on the talents of outstanding authorities in clinical and fundamental disciplines, trained literature specialists, and professional writers, all supported by the resources of Mosby, the world's preeminent publisher for the health professions.

The Literature Base

Mosby and its Editors survey more than 1,000 journals published worldwide, covering the full range of the health professions. On an annual basis, the publisher examines usage patterns and polls its expert authorities to add new journals to the literature base and to delete journals that are no longer useful as potential YEAR BOOK sources.

The Literature Survey

The publisher's team of literature specialists, all of whom are trained and experienced health professionals, examines every original, peer-reviewed article in each journal issue. More than 250,000 articles per year are scanned systematically, including title, text, illustrations, tables, and references. Each scan is compared, article by article, to the search strategies that the publisher has developed in consultation with the 270 outside experts who form the pool of YEAR BOOK editors. A given article may be reviewed by any number of editors, from one to a dozen or more, regardless of the discipline for which the paper was originally published. In turn, each editor who receives the article reviews it to determine whether or not the article should be included in the YEAR BOOK. This decision is based on the article's inherent quality, its probable usefulness to readers of that YEAR BOOK, and the editor's goal to represent a balanced picture of a given field in each volume of the YEAR BOOK. In addition, the editor indicates when to include figures and tables from the article to help the YEAR BOOK reader better understand the information.

Of the quarter million articles scanned each year, only 5% are selected for detailed analysis within the YEAR BOOK series, thereby assuring readers of the high value of every selection.

The Abstract

The publisher's abstracting staff is headed by a seasoned medical professional and includes individuals with training in the life sciences, medicine, and other areas, plus extensive experience in writing for the health professions and related industries. Each selected article is assigned to a specific writer on this abstracting staff. The abstracter, guided in many cases by notations supplied by the expert editor, writes a structured, condensed summary designed so that the reader can rapidly acquire the essential information contained in the article.

The Commentary

The YEAR BOOK editorial boards, sometimes assisted by guest commentators, write comments that place each article in perspective for the reader. This provides the reader with the equivalent of a personal consultation with a leading international authority—an opportunity to better understand the value of the article and to benefit from the authority's thought processes in assessing the article.

Additional Editorial Features

The editorial boards of each YEAR BOOK organize the abstracts and comments to provide a logical and satisfying sequence of information. To enhance the organization, editors also provide introductions to sections or individual chapters, comments linking a number of abstracts, citations to additional literature, and other features.

The published YEAR BOOK contains enhanced bibliographic citations for each selected article, including extended listings of multiple authors and identification of author affiliations. Each YEAR BOOK contains a Table of Contents specific to that year's volume. From year to year, the Table of Contents for a given YEAR BOOK will vary depending on developments within the field.

Every YEAR BOOK contains a list of the journals from which papers have been selected. This list represents a subset of the more than 1,000 journals surveyed by the publisher and occasionally reflects a particularly pertinent article from a journal that is not surveyed on a routine basis.

Finally, each volume contains a comprehensive subject index and an index to authors of each selected paper.

The 1997 Year Book Series

Year Book of Allergy, Asthma, and Clinical Immunology: Drs. Rosenwasser, Borish, Gelfand, Leung, Nelson, and Szefler

Year Book of Anesthesiology and Pain Management®: Drs. Tinker, Abram, Chestnut, Roizen, Rothenberg, and Wood

Year Book of Cardiology®: Drs. Schlant, Collins, Gersh, Graham, Kaplan, and Waldo

Year Book of Chiropractic®: Dr. Lawrence

Year Book of Critical Care Medicine®: Drs. Parrillo, Balk, Calvin, Franklin, and Shapiro

Year Book of Dentistry®: Drs. Meskin, Berry, Kennedy, Leinfelder, Roser, Summitt, and Zakariasen

Year Book of Dermatologic Surgery®: Drs. Greenway, Papadopoulos, and Whitaker

Year Book of Dermatology®: Drs. Sober and Fitzpatrick

Year Book of Diagnostic Radiology®: Drs. Federle, Clark, Gross, Dalinka, Maynard, Rebner, Smirniotopolous, and Young

Year Book of Digestive Diseases®: Drs. Greenberger and Moody

Year Book of Drug Therapy®: Drs. Lasagna and Weintraub

Year Book of Emergency Medicine®: Drs. Wagner, Dronen, Davidson, King, Niemann, and Roberts

Year Book of Endocrinology®: Drs. Bagdade, Braverman, Haas, Horton, Kannan, Landsberg, Molitch, Morley, Nathan, Odell, Poehlman, Rogol, and Ryan

Year Book of Family Practice®: Drs. Berg, Bowman, Davidson, Dexter, and Scherger

Year Book of Geriatrics and Gerontology®: Drs. Beck, Burton, Ostwald, Rabins, Reuben, Roth, Shapiro, and Whitehouse

Year Book of Hand Surgery®: Drs. Amadio and Hentz

Year Book of Hematology®: Drs. Spivak, Bell, Ness, Quesenberry, Wiernik, and Blume

Year Book of Infectious Diseases®: Drs. Keusch, Barza, Bennish, Poutsiaka, Skolnik, and Snydman

Year Book of Medicine®: Drs. Klahr, Cline, Petty, Frishman, Greenberger, Malawista, Mandell, and O'Rourke

Year Book of Neonatal and Perinatal Medicine®: Drs. Fanaroff and Klaus

Year Book of Nephrology, Hypertension, and Mineral Metabolism:

Year Book of Neurology and Neurosurgery®: Drs. Bradley and Wilkins

Year Book of Nuclear Medicine®: Drs. Gottschalk, Blaufox, Neumann, Strauss, and Zubal

Year Book of Obstetrics, Gynecology, and Women's Health: Drs. Mishell, Herbst, and Kirschbaum

Year Book of Occupational and Environmental Medicine®: Drs. Emmett, Frank, Gochfeld, and Hessl

Year Book of Oncology®: Drs. Ozols, Cohen, Glatstein, Loehrer, Tallman, and Wiersma

Year Book of Ophthalmology®: Drs. Wilson, Augsburger, Cohen, Eagle, Flanagan, Grossman, Laibson, Maguire, Nelson, Rapuano, Sergott, Spaeth, Tipperman, and Ms. Salmon

Year Book of Orthopedics®: Drs. Sledge, Poss, Cofield, Dobyns, Griffin, Springfield, Swiontkowski, Wiesel, and Wilson

Year Book of Otolaryngology–Head and Neck Surgery®: Drs. Paparella, and Holt

Year Book of Pain®: Drs. Gebhart, Haddox, Jacox, Janjan, Marcus, Rudy, and Shapiro

Year Book of Pathology and Laboratory Medicine: Drs. Mills, Bruns, Gaffey, and Stoler

Year Book of Pediatrics®: Dr. Stockman

Year Book of Plastic, Reconstructive, and Aesthetic Surgery®: Drs. Miller, Cohen, McKinney, Robson, Ruberg, Smith, and Whitaker

Year Book of Podiatric Medicine and Surgery®: Dr. Kominsky

Year Book of Psychiatry and Applied Mental Health®: Drs. Talbott, Ballenger, Breier, Frances, Meltzer, Schowalter, and Tasman

Year Book of Pulmonary Disease®: Dr. Petty

Year Book of Rheumatology®: Drs. Sergent, LeRoy, Meenan, Panush, and Reichlin

Year Book of Sports Medicine®: Drs. Shephard, Drinkwater, Eichner, Torg, Anderson, and Mr. George

Year Book of Surgery®: Drs. Copeland, Bland, Deitch, Eberlein, Howard, Luce, Seeger, Souba, and Sugarbaker

Year Book of Thoracic and Cardiovascular Surgery®: Drs. Ginsberg, Wechsler, and Williams

Year Book of Urology®: Drs. Andriole and Coplin

Year Book of Vascular Surgery®: Dr. Porter

1997

The Year Book of OBSTETRICS, GYNECOLOGY, AND WOMEN'S HEALTH

Editors

Daniel R. Mishell, Jr., M.D.
The Lyle G. McNeile Professor and Chairman, Department of Obstetrics and Gynecology, University of Southern California School of Medicine, Los Angeles, California

Arthur L. Herbst, M.D.
Joseph Bolivar De Lee Distinguished Service Professor and Chairman, University of Chicago, Chicago, Illinois

Thomas H. Kirschbaum, M.D.
Professor, Department of Obstetrics and Gynecology, Albert Einstein College of Medicine, The Bronx, New York

Contributing Editors

Arieh Bergman, M.D.
Clinical Professor, Department of Obstetrics and Gynecology, University of Southern California School of Medicine, Los Angeles, California

William H. Hindle, M.D.
Director, Breast Diagnostic Center, Women's and Children's Hospital; Professor of Clinical Obstetrics and Gynecology, University of Southern California, Los Angeles, California

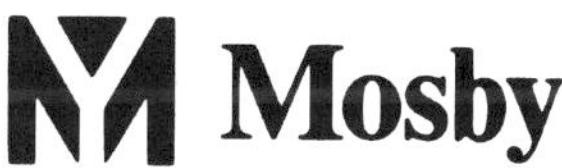

St. Louis Baltimore Boston Carlsbad Chicago Naples New York Philadelphia Portland
London Madrid Mexico City Singapore Sydney Tokyo Toronto Wiesbaden

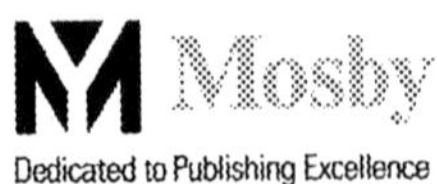
Dedicated to Publishing Excellence

A Times Mirror
Company

Vice President and Publisher, Continuity Publishing: Kenneth H. Killion
Director, Editorial Development: Gretchen C. Murphy
Developmental Editor: Donna Steinhagen
Acquisitions Editor: Linda Sheehan
Illustrations and Permissions Coordinator: Nancy Dunne
Director, Continuity–EDP: Maria Nevinger
Senior Project Manager, Production: Max F. Perez
Project Manager, Editing: Jill C. Waite
Freelance Staff Supervisor: Barbara M. Kelly
Director, Editorial Services: Edith M. Podrazik, B.S.N., R.N.
Information Specialist: Kathleen Moss, R.N.
Circulation Manager: Lynn D. Stevenson

Printed in the United States of America
Composition by Reed Technology and Information Services, Inc.
Printing/binding by Maple-Vail

Mosby–Year Book, Inc.
11830 Westline Industrial Drive
St. Louis, MO 63146

Editorial Office:
Mosby–Year Book, Inc.
161 N. Clark Street
Chicago, IL 60601

International Standard Serial Number: 1090-798X
International Standard Book Number: 0-8151-6019-4

Table of Contents

Journals Represented

Mosby and its editors survey more than 1,000 journals for its abstract and commentary publications. From these journals, the editors select the articles to be abstracted. Journals represented in this YEAR BOOK are listed below.

Acta Cytologica
Acta Obstetricia et Gynecologica Scandinavica
American Journal of Clinical Pathology
American Journal of Epidemiology
American Journal of Hematology
American Journal of Hypertension
American Journal of Kidney Diseases
American Journal of Medicine
American Journal of Obstetrics and Gynecology
American Journal of Perinatology
American Journal of Physiology
American Journal of Public Health
American Journal of Respiratory and Critical Care Medicine
American Journal of Roentgenology
American Journal of Surgery
Annals of Internal Medicine
Annals of Surgical Oncology
Archives of Disease in Childhood
Archives of Family Medicine
Australian and New Zealand Journal of Obstetrics and Gynaecology
Biology of the Neonate
Bone
Breast Journal
British Journal of Haematology
British Journal of Obstetrics and Gynaecology
British Journal of Surgery
British Journal of Urology
British Medical Journal
Cancer
Contraception
European Journal of Cancer
European Journal of Obstetrics, Gynecology and Reproductive Biology
European Journal of Pediatric Surgery
European Journal of Vascular and Endovascular Surgery
Fertility and Sterility
Genitourinary Medicine
Gynecologic Oncology
Gynecologic and Obstetric Investigation
Gynecological Endocrinology
Heart
Human Reproduction
International Journal of Gynaecology and Obstetrics
International Journal of Gynecological Cancer
International Journal of Gynecological Pathology
International Journal of Radiation, Oncology, Biology, and Physics
Journal of Acquired Immune Deficiency Syndromes

Journal of Applied Physiology: Respiratory, Environmental and Exercise
  Physiology
Journal of Assisted Reproduction and Genetics
Journal of Clinical Endocrinology and Metabolism
Journal of Clinical Investigation
Journal of Clinical Microbiology
Journal of Clinical Oncology
Journal of Clinical Pathology
Journal of Clinical Rheumatology
Journal of Clinical Ultrasound
Journal of Family Practice
Journal of Hypertension
Journal of Infectious Diseases
Journal of Laboratory and Clinical Medicine
Journal of Maternal-Fetal Investigation
Journal of Pediatric Surgery
Journal of Pediatrics
Journal of Perinatology
Journal of Psychiatric Research
Journal of Reproductive Medicine
Journal of Urology
Journal of the American College of Surgeons
Journal of the American Geriatrics Society
Journal of the American Medical Association
Journal of the National Cancer Institute
Journal of the North American Menopause Society
Journal of the Royal College of Surgeons of Edinburgh
Lancet
Maturitas
Medical Journal of Australia
Metabolism: Clinical and Experimental
Modern Pathology
New England Journal of Medicine
Obstetrics and Gynecology
Paediatric and Perinatal Epidemiology
Pediatric Neurology
Pediatric Research
Pediatrics
Prenatal Diagnosis
Proceedings of the National Academy of Sciences
Radiology
Radiotherapy and Oncology
Scandinavian Journal of Urology and Nephrology
Ultrasound in Medicine and Biology
Ultrasound in Obstetrics and Gynecology
Western Journal of Medicine
World Journal of Surgery

STANDARD ABBREVIATIONS

The following terms are abbreviated in this edition: acquired immunodeficiency
syndrome (AIDS), cardiopulmonary resuscitation (CPR), central nervous system
(CNS), cerebrospinal fluid (CSF), computed tomography (CT), deoxyribonucleic

acid (DNA), electrocardiography (ECG), health maintenance organization (HMO), human immunodeficiency virus (HIV), intensive care unit (ICU), intramuscular (IM), intravenous (IV), magnetic resonance (MR) imaging (MRI), and ribonucleic acid (RNA).

NOTE

The YEAR BOOK OF OBSTETRICS, GYNECOLOGY, AND WOMEN'S HEALTH is a literature survey service providing abstracts of articles published in the professional literature. Every effort is made to assure the accuracy of the information presented in these pages. Neither the editors nor the publisher of the YEAR BOOK OF OBSTETRICS, GYNECOLOGY, AND WOMEN'S HEALTH can be responsible for errors in the original materials. The editors' comments are their own opinions. Mention of specific products within this publication does not constitute endorsement.

To facilitate the use of the YEAR BOOK OF OBSTETRICS, GYNECOLOGY, AND WOMEN'S HEALTH as a reference tool, all illustrations and tables included in this publication are now identified as they appear in the original article. This change is meant to help the reader recognize that any illustration or table appearing in the YEAR BOOK OF OBSTETRICS, GYNECOLOGY, AND WOMEN'S HEALTH may be only one of many in the original article. For this reason, figure and table numbers will often appear to be out of sequence within the YEAR BOOK OF OBSTETRICS, GYNECOLOGY, AND WOMEN'S HEALTH.

Introduction

The traditional specialty of obstetrics and gynecology was limited to the care of pregnant, parturient, and postpartum women, as well as those with abnormalities of the genital tract. The specialty has now expanded to include the care and maintenance of both reproductive age and post-reproductive age women. Because this YEAR BOOK selects articles dealing with all these areas of women's health care, including breast disease and menopause, the Editorial Board decided to change the title to YEAR BOOK OF OBSTETRICS, GYNECOLOGY, AND WOMEN'S HEALTH. Thus, all clinicians caring for women will find reading this YEAR BOOK useful in providing their patients with the latest information dealing not only with obstetrics and gynecology but also with breast problems, disorders of the urinary tract, postmenopausal hormonal replacement, and other areas of female health care and maintenance.

Throughout the year, the editors of the YEAR BOOK OF OBSTETRICS, GYNECOLOGY, AND WOMEN'S HEALTH continuously review not only the journals relative to the specialty, but also articles published in other medical journals that are relevant to the practice of treating women. The editors then select those articles that have the most pertinent clinical information, and write comments regarding the relevance of the articles for clinical practice. Complete abstracts of the articles are then written and returned to the editor who selected the article for placement in the YEAR BOOK.

By reading these abstracts and comments, the busy clinician will become knowledgeable about the most important articles relating to the area of women's health that have been published in the previous year.

As in the past, Dr. Arthur Herbst has reviewed and selected articles in gynecologic oncology and pelvic surgery. Dr. Tom Kirschbaum thoroughly reviewed the field of maternal fetal medicine. I have reviewed and selected articles in the areas of reproductive endocrinology, infertility, menopause, contraception, and gynecologic infection. Drs. William Hindle and Arieh Bergman are contributing editors for the areas of breast disease and gynecologic urology, respectively.

During the past year, after receiving numerous scientific journals, the authors have selected 336 articles from 92 journals to appear in this volume of the YEAR BOOK.

In addition to the abstracted articles, we have included Dr. Craig Towers' excellent review of hepatitis in pregnancy. The editors believe that reading this volume will enhance each clinicians' knowledge of the specialty. We welcome suggestions to assist our efforts in providing clinically relevant information to our readers.

Daniel R. Mishell, Jr., M.D.

Hepatitis in Pregnancy

CRAIG V. TOWERS, M.D.
Associate Professor in Residence, Department of Obstetrics and Gynecology, University of California, Irvine; Director of Perinatal Services, Long Beach Memorial Women's Hospital, Long Beach, California

General Overview

Viral hepatitis has always been a complex subject that has resulted in confusion, especially in its relationship to pregnancy. Presently, there are five distinct primary viruses that can lead to viral hepatitis, although many other viruses including cytomegalovirus, Epstein-Barr virus, herpesvirus, and coxsackieviruses can also cause a hepatitis-like appearance. The five main viruses have been designated with letters and are hepatitis A, B, C, D, and E.

As an overview, the incidence of viral hepatitis in the pregnant population in the United States is no different from that for the nonpregnant population. In addition, the severity of the illness in this country also does not appear to be affected by the possibility that a woman could be pregnant.[1] One virus (hepatits E) does seem to be more severe in the pregnant population, although this has mainly been seen in populations outside the United States.[2]

Regardless of the viral type, most patients with viral hepatitis are asymptomatic. If symptoms do appear, they often are misdiagnosed as a viral flu syndrome. These symptoms include anorexia, nausea and vomiting, fatigue, myalgias, and low-grade fever. Only the more affected cases develop jaundice with light-colored stools, dark urine, and right upper-quadrant pain consistent with a classic diagnosis of hepatitis. Although rare, severe cases of hepatitis can lead to acute liver failure resulting in coagulopathy delirium and even death.[3]

The preliminary evaluation for hepatitis is relatively simple and involves obtaining liver enzymes (alanine aminotransferase and aspartate aminotransferase) along with a bilirubin level. Most patients with active hepatitis will have elevated liver enzymes and elevated bilirubin levels. Once the patient is noted to have elevated liver enzymes suggestive of hepatitis, confusion sets in when trying to identify the viral types. The patient's blood should then be screened for the presence of acute hepatitis A, acute hepatitis B, and possibly acute hepatitis C. If all of these screening tests are negative, the patient should then be evaluated for atypical viruses such as cytomegalovirus, Epstein-Barr virus, and herpes.

The differential diagnosis for disorders that can affect the liver in pregnancy is shown in Table 1. Table 2 lists the common drugs that have been associated with liver toxicity, although hundreds more probably exist.[4] Hepatitis is the most common cause of jaundice in pregnancy, accounting for about 40% of cases. The main risk to the mother is the potential for acute liver failure developing, as well as transmitting the virus to other family members. The fetal risks are primarily related to an increased risk of premature delivery, in addition to becoming infected with the virus. In

---

TABLE 1.—Differential Diagnosis of Liver Disorders in Pregnancy

Hepatitis—Viral
  Hepatitis A virus (HAV)
  Hepatitis B virus (HBV)
  Non-A, non-B hepatitis/hepatitis C virus (HCV)
  Hepatitis D virus (HDV)
  Hepatitis E virus (HEV)
  Cytomegalovirus (CMV)
  Epstein-Barr virus (EBV)
  Herpesvirus (types I and II)
  Coxsackie B virus
  Mumps virus
Hyperbilirubinemic States
  Gilbert's syndrome
  Dublin-Johnson syndrome
  Rotor syndrome
Intrahepatic Cholestasis of Pregnancy
Drug Reaction/Toxicity (see Table 2)
Hemolysis (e.g., sepsis)
Cholelithiasis/Cholecystitis
Acute Fatty Liver of Pregnancy
Budd-Chiari Syndrome
Liver Involvement With Preeclampsia (HELLP syndrome)
Hyperemesis Gravidarum
Cirrhosis/Chronic Active Hepatitis
Chronic Liver Disorders (e.g., Wilson's disease, hemochromatosis)

---

the United States, the spontaneous abortion rate and stillbirth rate do not appear to be increased compared with the general population. In addition, there have been no confirmed fetal abnormalities related to any of the hepatitis viruses.[1]

TABLE 2.—Drugs Associated With Liver Toxicity

Phenothiazines (chlorpromazine)
Phenytoin
Isoniazide
Halogenated anesthetics
Tetracycline
Methyldopa
Monoamine oxidase inhibitors
Alcohol
Acetaminophen (overdose)
Carbon tetrahydrochloride/hydrocarbons
Industrial solvents and phosphorus
Total parenteral nutrition
Disulfiram
Propylthiouracil
Sulfonamides
Excess vitamin A
Nitrofurantoin
Zidovudine (AZT)
Erythromycin estolate
Captopril

The management of hepatitis in pregnant patients is similar to its management in patients who are not pregnant. Patients with acute hepatitis in pregnancy are at an increased risk for intractable nausea and vomiting developing, with a similar type of symptoms as occurs with hyperemesis gravidarum. These patients may require hospitalization for hydration and treatment of the nausea and vomiting. In addition, patients with fulminant hepatitis and evidence of liver failure will obviously require hospitalization to treat the severe problems that occur with this disorder. However, the overall treatment is supportive care along with expectant management and appropriate immunization of family members and offspring. In addition, drugs that are metabolized by the liver should be avoided if possible.

Hepatitis A

Hepatitis A virus (HAV) is a single-stranded, 27-nm RNA virus that has no viral envelope. It is in the enterovirus subgroup of the picornavirus family.[3] The initial reports on this viral infection were seen in the 1940s, when it was shown that the hepatitis that was epidemic in soldiers during World War II was caused by contaminated drinking water. These publications reported that treatment with γ-globulin and superchlorination of the drinking water could minimize the risk of this infection developing.[5–7]

Transmission of HAV is mainly through the oral-fecal route. Therefore, HAV infection may occur when a person ingests food, water, or shellfish that is contaminated with stool containing the virus. This promotes spread in areas of close contact, e.g., families, military, and institutionalized individuals.[8] In addition, HAV spread is seen in the homosexual male population as well as in day-care centers.[9, 10] This virus has been transmitted through blood products, although only rare reports exist.[11] The parenteral transmission of HAV is extremely rare and can only occur during the short window of viremia, because a chronic carrier state does not exist.

The virus has a relatively short incubation period of approximately 2–7 weeks. The onset of the illness is usually abrupt and resolution usually occurs approximately 2 or 3 weeks later, although some cases may last for up to 6–9 weeks. There is no known chronic carrier state for hepatitis A, and once the disease has completely resolved, the patient is then immune, usually for life.[3]

The best diagnostic procedure for identifying acute hepatitis A is the presence of an IgM antibody.[12] A positive IgG antibody only implies past infection. The IgM antibody usually disappears within 3 or 4 months of the onset of the illness but can last up to 6–10 months. Infection with HAV is very common in the United States, with 40% to 50% of American urban adults being positive for the IgG antibody; however, only 5% of these patients had symptoms.[13]

Figure 1 shows the typical clinical and serologic events that occur with an HAV infection. Hepatitis A is a disease that is usually self-limited unless a fulminant case occurs, resulting in liver failure. Because no chronic form exists for this viral infection, long-term sequelae are thought to be negligible.

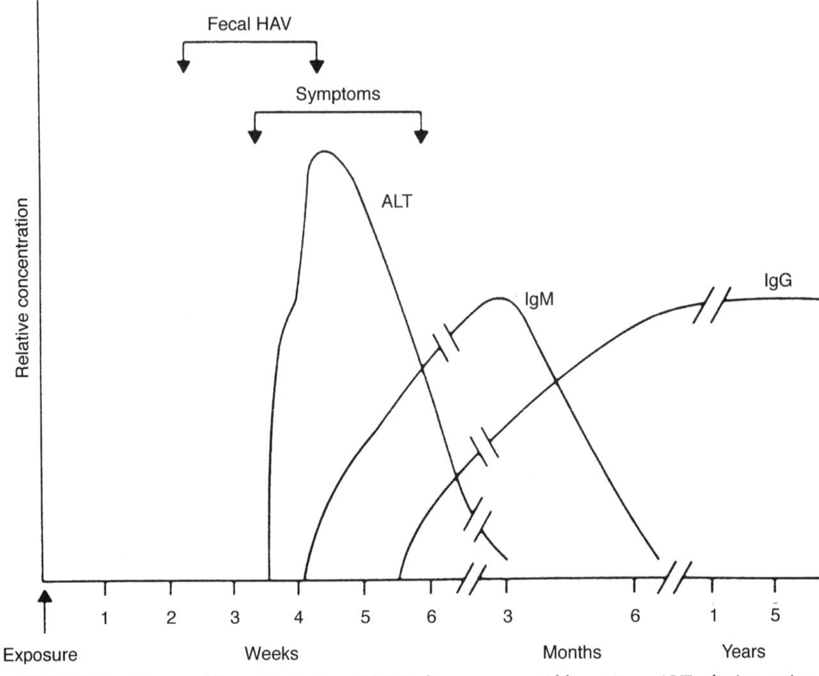

FIGURE 1.—Course of hepatitis A virus (*HAV*) after exposure. *Abbreviation: ALT*, alanine amino-transferase. (From Queenan J (ed): *Management of High Risk Pregnancy*, ed 3. Cambridge, Mass, Blackwell Science, 1994, p 336. Used by permission.)

Traditionally, transmission of the virus from the mother to the neonate was not believed to occur; however, treatment of the newborn was indicated in a mother who had active disease near delivery. Two possible cases of perinatal vertical transmission have been reported.[14, 15]

The treatment for preventing HAV infection is administration of serum immunoglobulin in the dosages indicated in Table 3. It is important to remember that most fecal excretion of the virus occurs before jaundice develops and that infectivity rapidly declines once the jaundice is clinically apparent. Therefore, immunoprophylaxis must occur rapidly for household contacts once the index case has been diagnosed. If the exposure to hepatitis A has been greater than 2 weeks, immunoglobulin is not indicated because it probably would not be effective.[16]

Recently, a formalin-inactivated hepatitis A vaccine has been produced and marketed. Initial studies in children have revealed good results in preventing the illness. In a prospective trial, Werzberger et al. randomly assigned 1,037 children to receive either the hepatitis A vaccine or a placebo. The incidence of hepatitis A was 0 cases per 519 vaccinated children compared with 25 cases of acute hepatitis A per 518 placebo-treated children. In their evaluation, antibody developed in 99.7% of the children studied by 1 month after the vaccination.[17] A second study administered more than 109,000 doses of HAV vaccine, and no serious adverse reactions were reported. The development of antibody after the

TABLE 3.—Centers for Disease Control and Prevention Recommendations for Immunoprophylaxis of Viral Hepatitis

Hepatitis A Virus
  Travel to endemic area
    0.02 cc/kg single injection of immunoglobulin (IG) if fewer than 2 months' stay
    0.06 cc/kg every 5 months for prolonged stay
  Postexposure prophylaxis
    if exposure more than 2 weeks in the past, IG not indicated
    0.02 cc/kg single injection of IG (especially for sexual and household contacts)
  Perinatal exposure
    0.02 cc of IG per kg at birth for the infant and possibly repeat at 1 month
Hepatitis B Virus
  Perinatal exposure
    0.5 cc hepatitis B IG (HBIG) (10 µg) at birth (younger than 12 hours of age) followed by 0.5 cc
      of hepatitis B vaccine* within 7 days of birth (most now give vaccine at same time as HBIG in
      other hip)—the vaccine is repeated at 1 month of age and at 6 months of age
    then check for hepatitis B surface antigen (HBsAg) and antibody to HBsAg (anti-HBsAg) at
      12–15 months of age (presence of HBsAg is treatment failure and the presence of anti-HBsAg
      is treatment success).
  Postexposure prophylaxis against known carrier
    0.06 cc of HBIG per kg, single injection, within 14 days of sexual contact (if sexual contact is to
      be continued, hepatitis B vaccine is an option)
    if percutaneous exposure occurs in someone already vaccinated, check for anti-HBsAg in the
      exposed person; if absent, give 0.06 cc of HBIG per kg, single injection, and give hepatitis B
      vaccine booster (1.0-cc injection of vaccine); if anti-HBsAg is present, the patient is immune
    if the percutaneously exposed person has not been vaccinated, give 0.06 cc of HBIG per kg,
      single injection, with 24 hours and then start the hepatitis B vaccine series (3 doses: initial, at 1
      month, and at 6 months). Another option is to draw blood from the exposed person for anti-
      HBcAg/anti-HBsAg and then give 0.06 cc HBIG per kg, single injection. If the tests are nega-
      tive, give the vaccine series; if positive, the exposed person was already previously exposed and
      the vaccine is not indicated.
  Postexposure prophylaxis from known source with unknown HBsAg testing
    if the source is in the high-risk group, and the exposed person has been vaccinated, test the
      source for HBsAg and the exposed person for anti-HBsAg. If the source is positive and the ex-
      posed is negative for the antibody, give 0.06 cc of HBIG per kg, single injection, and give
      hepatitis B vaccine booster
    if the source is in the high-risk group and the exposed person has not been vaccinated, give 0.06
      cc of HBIG per kg, single injection, and test the source of HBsAg. If positive, continue with
      the vaccine series; if negative, the vaccine can still be instituted for patient protection from
      other reexposures
    if the source is in the low-risk group, and the exposed person has been vaccinated, nothing is
      required.
    if the source is in the low-risk group, and the exposed person has not been vaccinated, the vac-
      cine series can be given.
Hepatitis D Virus
  There is no specific prophylaxis for HDV infection. The best prophylaxis is to prevent infection by
    hepatitis B because HDV cannot exist without hepatitis B's presence.
Non-A, Non-B Hepatitis Virus/Hepatitis C
  Studies on prophylaxis against hepatitis C/non-A, non-B hepatitis have been equivocal. Immunoglo-
    bulin does not appear to prevent the infection from occurring. Some studies, however, suggest
    that the carrier state may be less. Thus, a single dose of IG (0.06 cc/kg) post percutaneous ex-
    posure may be reasonable. In addition, treatment of an exposed infant at delivery may be rea-
    sonable at a dose of 0.5 cc of IG at birth and at 1 month.

*Hepatitis B vaccine doses for an infant and children younger than the age of 10 years are generally 0.5 cc or half the adult dose. The dose for adults and children older than the age of 10 years is generally 1.0 cc. Heptavax comes as a concentration of 20 µg of HBsAg per cc. Recombivax HB is 10 µg of HBsAg per cc, and Engerix-B is a concentration of 20 µg/cc.

initial dose and a second dose at 1 month was 94%, which increased to 99% after a third dose at 12 months.[18]

The future use of the HAV vaccine is uncertain. A good cost-benefit evaluation is necessary to better define the use of this vaccine.

Hepatitis B

Hepatitis B virus (HBV) is a circular DNA virus that is 42 nm in size. It is unique because it is double stranded for two thirds of its length and it contains its own DNA polymerase.[3] The transmission of hepatitis B is primarily through a percutaneous or permucosal route. This virus has a relatively long incubation period of 1–6 months after exposure. In addition, the disease onset is more insidious, but the overall disease state is usually more severe. Presently, there are 200 million carriers in the world. The carrier rate in the United States ranges between 0.1% and 0.8%, depending on the population tested. Eight distinct serotypes exist. These are primarily important when performing epidemiology studies. All HBV particles contain a group-reactive determinant labeled "a" along with two sets of subdeterminants designated "d" or "y" and "w" or "r." The "w" was then found to have four different variants: w_1, w_2, w_3, and w_4. The eight distinct serotypes identified are ayw_1, ayw_2, ayw_3, ayw_4, ayr, adw_2, adw_4, and adr.[3]

Many patients are at increased risk for being chronic carriers of HBV, including those of the following ethnic groups: Asians, Inuits, Pacific Islanders, Haitians, and sub-Saharan Africans. Others at risk include male homosexuals, prostitutes, IV drug users, individuals with multiple tattoos, prior blood transfusion recipients, hemodialysis patients, hemophiliacs or other patients with bleeding disorders, and individuals who work in hospitals or chronic care facilities.[16]

In the general laboratory evaluation, five distinct blood tests exist.[19] These include the hepatitis B surface antigen (HBsAg), antibody to HBsAg (anti-HBsAg), antibody to hepatitis B core antigen (anti-HBcAg), hepatitis B e antigen (HBeAg), and antibody to hepatitis B e antigen (anti-HBeAg). The IgG antibody to the HBcAg develops shortly after infection and usually remains positive for life. Some laboratories also measure an IgM antibody to the core antigen, and this in conjunction with a positive HBsAg is more indicative of an acute HBV infection.[20] In addition, the presence of HBsAg is usually seen shortly after the infection and remains positive until the patient becomes immune (Fig 2). Immunity occurs when an antibody to the HBsAg develops. A subset of the population never produces an antibody to the surface antigen, and these patients become chronic carriers.[21] The presence of an e antigen only signifies active viral replication and a more infectious state. The presence of antibody to the e antigen implies that the patient has a lower infectivity capability but does not exclude the possibility of transmission. A patient who becomes immune to HBV infection will have circulating anti-HBcAg as well as anti-HBsAg antibodies. During a long period, the antibody to the surface antigen may become nondetectable, whereas the presence of the anti-HBcAg usually remains positive. Patients who become chronic carriers will

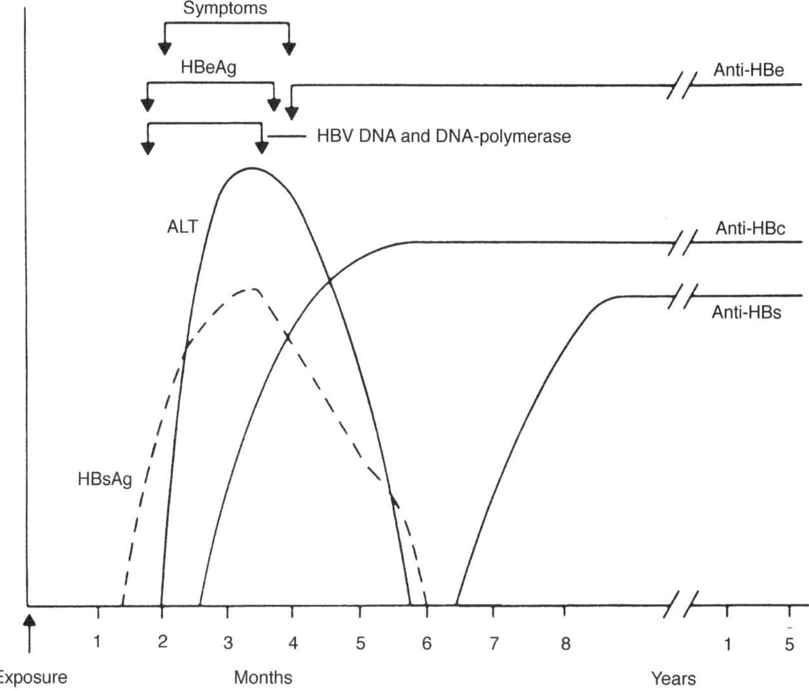

FIGURE 2.—Course of hepatitis B after exposure. *Abbreviations: HBeAg,* hepatitis B virus e antigen; *Anti-HBe,* antibody to hepatitis B virus e antigen; *HBV DNA,* DNA specific for hepatitis B virus; *ALT,* alanine aminotransferase; *Anti-HBc,* antibody to hepatitis B virus core antigen; *Anti-HBs,* antibody to hepatitis B virus surface antigen; *HBsAg,* hepatitis B surface antigen. (From Queenan J [ed]: *Management of High Risk Pregnancy,* ed 3. Cambridge, Mass, Blackwell Science, 1994, p 337. Used by permission.)

also have anti-HBcAg antibodies; however, they never produce the anti-HBsAg antibody. Instead, chronic carriers will continue to have circulating HBsAg. Therefore, a positive IgG anti-HBcAg only denotes that an HBV infection occurred sometime in the past. A breakdown of the potential laboratory results is shown in Table 4 along with an explanation for the laboratory findings.

A chronic carrier state will develop in approximately 10% of infected adults,[16] which can lead to the development of chronic persistent hepatitis, chronic active hepatitis, and/or cirrhosis. In addition, chronic carriers have a 200-fold increased risk for the development of hepatocellular carcinoma.[22, 23] The overall expected outcome of a population of HBV-infected adult patients is shown in Table 5.

Unfortunately, there is no cure for hepatitis B. The only treatment approach is to prevent infection based on immunization. If a person is exposed to the virus through blood or sexual transmission, the treatment requires use of both hepatitis B immunoglobulin (HBIG) in conjunction with the hepatitis B vaccine.[16] If a person wants to prevent infection, the treatment primarily involves administration of the hepatitis B vaccine series (Table 3). The immunogenicity of the hepatitis B vaccine is excellent

TABLE 4.—The Potential Meaning of Various Hepatitis B Blood Test Results

	HBsAg	Anti-HBsAg	Anti-HBcAg	HBeAg	Anti-HBeAg
1.	+	−	−	−	−
2.	+	−	+	+	−
3.	+	−	+	−	+
4.	+	−	+	−	−
5.	−	−	+	−	+/−
6.	−	+	+	−	+/−
7.	−	+	−	−	−
8.	+	+	+	+/−	+/−***

1. Acute HBV infection (very early stages)* or chronic HBV carrier state (with low levels of nondetected anti-HBcAg)
2. Acute HBV infection* or chronic HBV carrier state (that is highly infectious)
3. Acute HBV infection* (later stages) or chronic HBV infection (lower infectious status but still infectious)
4. Acute HBV infection* or chronic HBV infection (without HBeAg or anti-HBeAg)**
5. Window state between the disappearance of HBsAg before the development of anti-HBsAg* or evidence of past HBV infection with a low-level undetected anti-HBsAg
6. Recovery from acute infection or infection in the remote past.
7. Infection in the remote past with a low-level, undetected anti-HBcAg or patient status post hepatitis B vaccination
8. Late acute infection with early detection of antibodies (anti-HBsAg and anti-HBeAg) before the disappearance of the antigens HBsAg and HBeAg or a very rare unusual entity where the HBsAg is 1 serotype and the anti-HBsAg is for a different serotype

*In this setting, an anti-HBcAg IgM might be helpful because a positive IgM denotes recent infection.

**In some patients, HBeAg or anti-HBeAg never develops.

***HBeAg and anti-HBeAg essentially never exist at the same time. However, the ability to detect antibodies has improved so much that this may occur transiently when anti-HBeAg is developing while the HBeAg is disappearing.

with more than 90% of the population having antibody to the HBsAg after the third dose.[24, 25] It is important to note that the site of vaccine injection is significant. Adults should receive an IM injection in the deltoid region. Intradermal injections and gluteal injections have resulted in lower response rates.[26] For infants an injection in the anterolateral thigh is preferable because their deltoid muscles are smaller.

Vertical transmission of HBV from the mother to the neonate is a major concern. Studies show that up to 70% to 90% of neonates can become chronic carriers of the disease if they do not receive appropriate prophylaxis after delivery, especially if they have HBeAg antigens or an acute

TABLE 5.—Long-Term Outcomes of Hepatitis B Infections Assuming 1,000 Infected Individuals

	ADULTS (number)	INFANTS* (number)
Total patients	1,000	1,000
Asymptomatic	750	750
Chronic carriers	75	500
Chronic active hepatitis/cirrhosis/or hepatocellular carcinoma	15–25	125

*Infants delivered of hepatitis B surface antigen (HBsAg)–positive mothers assuming an equal distribution of HBeAg-positive and anti-HBeAg–positive carriers and the infants receiving no immunoprophylaxis post delivery.

infection in the third trimester.[27, 28] It is important to note that even if the HBsAg-positive mother is HBeAg-negative or even if she tests positive for anti-HBeAg, transmission to the neonate can occur and immunoprophylaxis is indicated.[29, 30] A similar long-term outcome of neonatal hepatitis B infection is also seen in Table 5. The transmission from the mother to the infant primarily occurs at birth, caused by exposure to infected maternal blood or vaginal secretions. The recommended treatment of the newborn born to a HBsAg-positive mother involves administering a dose of HBIG followed by the hepatitis B vaccine series (Table 3). If an infant receives this prophylaxis after delivery, the risk that the child will become a chronic carrier falls to 2% to 5%.[31, 32]

Breast-feeding an infant by a mother who is HBsAg-positive is controversial. Hepatitis B surface antigen has been found in breast milk in several studies; however, most of these have not shown an increase in the neonatal infection rate. It is of utmost importance that these infants are adequately treated with HBIG and the full vaccine protocol.[33, 34]

Several studies have evaluated the incidence of HBsAg positivity in the pregnant population. These studies found that only 50% of mothers with HBsAg would be identified if screening was only performed in individuals with risk factors.[35–38] Because of these studies, the Centers for Disease Control and the American College of Obstetricians and Gynecologists have recommended that routine prenatal screening include the HBsAg blood test.[39, 40]

Since the development of the hepatitis B vaccine in 1982, the rate of acute HBV infection in the United States has not changed. Epidemiology studies reveal that approximately 200,000 to 300,000 acute HBV infections occur in the United States each year.[41] Perinatal hepatitis B infections constitute a small proportion of the total picture (approximately 20,000 cases). Research has now shown that there is a significant incidence of child-to-child transmission of this virus.[42] Therefore, the American Academy of Pediatrics and the Centers for Disease Control now recommend that all children receive the hepatitis B vaccine series in the hope that this will prevent future infections and eventually lower the rate of new cases in the United States.[39, 43]

Hepatitis C

In 1989, Choo et al.[44] and Kuo et al.[45] identified an RNA viral strand that was thought to be the cause of non-A, non-B hepatitis. Before this finding, the viral type of non-A, non-B hepatitis was unknown. In addition, the diagnosis of this disease was one of exclusion, ruling out all other known viral causes. Since the discovery of the hepatitis C virus (HCV), several distinct genetic variants have been identified based on different nucleic acid sequence differences.

Presently, six major genotypes exist and each of these have several subtypes (labeled a, b, c, etc.). The most common genotypes in Western Europe and the United States are 1a, 1b, 2a, 2b, and 3a.[46] The HCV has been classified as a separate genus to the flavivirus family. This RNA virus is approximately 9,379 to 9,481 nucleotides long and is 30–38 nm in diameter.[47] Attempts at culture have not shown much success. Therefore, the diagnosis of an HCV infection primarily relies on the detection of antibodies to the virus or identifying the nucleic acid by polymerase chain reaction (PCR). The laboratory workup primarily involves an enzyme-linked immunosorbent assay (ELISA) screening test looking for the presence of antibody to the virus. Currently, most laboratories now use a third-generation anti-HCV ELISA test called ELISA-3.[47] This ELISA test can have a very high incidence of false positive results, especially if used in a low-risk population. Therefore, a positive test is usually confirmed by a more specific test—a recombinant immunoblot assay (RIBA). The RIBA test is also currently a third-generation test called RIBA-3.[47] This is an evaluation of a series of antibodies to HCV antigens that come from more than one region of the virus. The mean period from the onset of an HCV infection to the development of an anti-HCV response is 12 weeks but can take up to 6 months in some cases. Therefore, during an acute episode of hepatitis, the anti-HCV may be negative. In this setting, an HCV-RNA-PCR test can be helpful.[47]

As more information is obtained on HCV, the potential clinical impact of this disease is becoming apparent. Research does show that most posttransfusion hepatitis is caused by hepatitis C.[48, 49] The Centers for Disease Control estimate that 170,000 new cases occur per year in the United States with approximately 85,000 individuals (50%) subsequently having chronic hepatitis from the infection. Chronic hepatitis C is slowly progressive, with cirrhosis developing in up to 20% of infected individuals after 20 years; 10% of these patients progress to hepatocellular carcinoma.[50] The difficulty in evaluating the literature for this virus is that a viral marker antigen that denotes infectivity has not been identified. When hepatitis B is investigated, the presence of the HBsAg denotes the possibility that a person is infectious. A similar antigen marker for hepatitis C does not exist presently. Therefore, research on the potential ramification of this virus is limited to antibody studies and nucleic acid probes.

The risk of HCV transmission between family members or sexual partners seems to be low. In a recent study of more than 1,100 residents in an HCV endemic area of Japan, anti-HCV was detected in 14% of the population.[51] However, the positive rate among sexually active spouses was only 7%, with half of those tested showing different serotypes. In a study by Bresters et al.,[52] all 50 heterosexual partners of HCV-positive individuals were HCV-RNA– and anti-HCV–negative. The median duration of sexual relations was 13 years. Several other studies have also shown a low transmission rate by sexual activity.[53, 54] This low transmission rate through sexual activity may result from a low detection rate of HCV in human secretions (other than blood).[55, 56] Therefore, most HCV transmission in the population seems to stem from blood transmission, with the major risks being transfusion with blood products, IV drug abuse, organ transplantation, or other external sources such as acupuncture. However,

TABLE 6.—Selected Studies on Vertical Transmission of Hepatitis C Virus (HCV): Mother to Infant

Study	Number of Infants Delivered of HCV	Number of Infants Infected	Length of Neonatal Follow-up ($\geq$)	Probable HCV Transmission Rate (%)
Novati et al., 1992	8*	1	10 months	13
Weintrub et al., 1991	9*	4	12 months	44
	34	0	12 months	0
Giovannini et al., 1990	25*	11	12 months	44
Cilla et al., 1992	20*	2	10 months	10
Lam et al., 1993	8	1	12 months	13
	58*	3	12 months	5
Giacchino et al., 1995	31	2	12 months	6
Zanetti et al., 1995	22*	8	12 months	36
	94	0	12 months	0
Total HCV+ HIV+ cases	142*	29		20
Total HCV+ HIV− cases	167	3		2
Overall Combined	309	32		10

*HCV+ and HIV+ patients.

the use of condoms is still recommended for sexual activity with an infected HCV partner because heterosexual HCV transmission is possible.

Vertical transmission of HCV from the mother to the infant does occur during pregnancy. The original study that proved this occurrence was performed in 1981[28] on a group of patients with non-A, non-B hepatitis in pregnancy. There was a 67% transmission rate when the infection occurred in the third trimester. However, the incidence of long-term infections or carrier status was not able to be determined from these older data. Recent studies evaluating the presence of hepatitis C infections through PCR nucleic acid probes and hepatitis C antibodies suggest that the transmission rate ranges between 5% and 50% (Table 6). The information presented in Table 6 is a collection of studies that evaluated infants for 10–12 months or more after delivery.[57–63] The risk of vertical HCV transmission appears to be higher when the mother is also HIV-positive. The data in this table are not inclusive of all studies evaluating this issue. Many others exist along with case reports, but many of these are hampered by short neonatal follow-up or the tests used in evaluation.[64–68]

Many questions are still unanswered in regard to vertical HCV transmission. Is the main risk of transmission transplacental, intrapartum, or after delivery from breast-feeding? Studies show that all infants born to anti-HCV–positive mothers are also anti-HCV–positive, as would be expected, because of passive maternal IgG antibody transfer. Most of these studies document that these infants become anti-HCV–negative within the first 6 months after birth with a few having antibodies redevelop later, suggesting that their infection was through the birth process or after delivery.[59] How long can passively transferred maternal antibody remain in

TABLE 7.—Current Transfusion Risks Per Unit of Blood for Units That Are Negative in the Laboratory According to the American Red Cross

Hepatitis B	1:200,000
Hepatitis C	1:3,000
HIV	1:420,000
Human T-lymphotropic virus I and II	1:50,000

an uninfected neonate? Most infants lose maternal antibody within 6 months: however, there have been reports of its presence up to 12 months and longer.[58] If transmission is mainly intrapartum, does the mode of delivery affect this? Can transmission occur through breast-feeding? Because a viral antigen marker that denotes infectivity does not exist, are all anti-HCV–negative individuals (infants or adults) with a documented HCV exposure uninfected?

In summary, with regard to vertical transmission, all infants are anti-HCV–positive at birth, with most of these clearing a few months after birth. However, active HCV transmission does occur with documented cases confirmed by liver biopsy. Unfortunately, no treatment to prevent this vertical transmission has been successfully identified. Some authorities have suggested that infants born to HCV-positive mothers receive serum immunoglobulin. Unfortunately, the success of this treatment regimen has been less than adequate.

The main area of concern when looking at the impact of hepatitis C is its relation to posttransfusion hepatitis. Previously up to 90% of posttransfusion hepatitis was secondary to HCV. With the addition of anti-HCV testing of donated blood, the risk of posttransfusion hepatitis developing is now about 3 per 10,000 units transfused.[69] This test has markedly decreased the incidence of posttransfusion hepatitis in the United States. Table 7 shows the current risks of transfusion per unit of blood according to the American Red Cross as of February 1995.

Immunoglobulin therapy has been used for years to help prevent or reduce the risk of infections (e.g., serum immunoglobulin, HBIG, varicella zoster immunoglobulin). In addition, anti-D immunoglobulin (Rhogam) has nearly eliminated Rh sensitization in the United States.[70] The safety of these products over the years has been excellent, even though these immunoglobulin products come from pooled plasma where some donors probably carry transmissible infections. Recently, there have been reports of HCV transmission after the administration of some brands of serum immunoglobulin.[71, 72] The frequency of this occurrence is low, but it does underscore the importance of having clear indications for the usage of these products.

Immunoglobulin production starts with a fractionation procedure that effectively removes most, if not all, potentially infectious agents. However, because of the recently reported HCV transmissions, most products (especially those used in the United States) add other steps such as a solvent-detergent treatment or a low pH treatment and pepsin.[73] Therefore, HCV transmission with these products will hopefully be nonexistent in the future.

Presently, there is no available HCV immunoglobulin or vaccine to help in the prevention of this infection. Patients who are already chronically HCV infected may obtain some benefit from interferon-α, although the success rates are mixed.[74, 75] Most reports show a response to treatment while being treated. This response rate varies but on average is about 50%. Unfortunately, nearly half of these patients relapse when treatment is discontinued. It also appears that the risk of relapse may be somewhat affected by the HCV serotype, with the best response occurring in serotype 3 (more than 70% long-term response) and the worst response in serotype 1 (about 30% long-term response rate).[76] The duration of therapy may also be important. A recent study showed that with a 12-month additional therapy arm, the long-term response rate increased.[77] In the event of percutaneous exposure, serum immunoglobulin is recommended (Table 3), although the efficacy of this treatment has not been fully evaluated.

In summary, HCV has rapidly become a difficult, confusing topic with many unanswered questions. Hopefully, an effective immunoglobulin and vaccine for prevention will be developed, as well as a better mechanism to follow potential infectivity.

Hepatitis D

The hepatitis D virus (HDV) or delta agent was discovered in 1977 by Rizzetto et al. in Italy.[78] It was identified within the liver cell of a patient with hepatitis and was distinct from the HBV. The viral particle was found to be a defective RNA virus that was 35–37 nm in diameter and was encapsulated by the HBsAg coating. It is considered defective because it requires a co-infection with hepatitis B to support its replication. It is not seen in the presence of anti-HBsAg or as an infection by itself.[79] Three distinct genotypes have been cloned. Genotype I is the most common and has been found worldwide. Genotype II has been found in Japan and genotype III in Peru and Columbia.[80]

The infection with HDV can develop in three separate ways. It can occur as an acute infection simultaneously with an acute hepatitis B infection; it can occur as an acute infection superimposed on a chronic hepatitis B infection; and a chronic hepatitis D infection can be superimposed on a chronic hepatitis B infection.[81]

The significance of this viral infection is still relatively undefined. However, a combined acute HBV/HDV infection may take on a more fulminant course when compared with an acute HBV infection alone. In addition, in patients who have a chronic HBV/HDV infection, cirrhosis may develop in 70% to 80% of patients, and up to 25% may die of hepatic failure.[82, 83]

The diagnosis of an acute HDV infection involves the detection of the delta antigen in hepatic tissue in conjunction with a positive anti-HDV IgM antibody by ELISA testing. The patient must also be HBsAg-positive. A patient with a chronic HDV infection will have a positive delta antigen on liver biopsy with a positive anti-HDV IgG antibody in the presence of a positive HBsAg.[79, 84]

Vertical transmission of hepatitis D has also been documented; however, the significance of this event is unknown. Very few pregnant women with an ongoing HDV infection have been studied. Therefore, the incidence of transmission and neonatal outcome are poorly understood.[85]

Unfortunately for patients with an active HDV infection, no specific treatment has been found that greatly impacts the disease course. However, because HDV cannot survive without the presence of HBV, immunity to HBV will prevent a superinfection with HDV. In addition, the postdelivery administration of HBIG and hepatitis B vaccine to a neonate whose mother has active HBV/HDV infection should be 95% effective in preventing infection because HDV cannot survive without HBV.

Hepatitis E

The first report on this new virus actually appeared in 1957, when approximately 30,000 cases of hepatitis developed in Delhi, India, in the winter of 1955–1956 after a sewage contamination of the city water.[86] The virus appeared to have an oral-fecal spread and did not have an apparent chronic disease state. The infection was very similar to hepatitis A, but tests were negative. The disease was eventually called epidemic or enterically transmitted non-A, non-B hepatitis.

Most literature on this viral infection comes from epidemics and sporadic cases seen in North Africa, parts of the former Soviet Union, Pakistan, Southeast Asia, China, and Latin America.[87, 88] Very few cases have occurred in the United States. Reported cases of hepatitis E in the United States describe patients who most likely contracted the infection while traveling outside the country and had the illness on return.[89] Between 1984 and 1988, several reports described the detection of virus-like particles by immune electron microscopy in fecal specimens of patients with enterically transmitted non-A, non-B hepatitis.[90–92] In 1989, a report described the detection of viral antigen in liver tissue using an immunofluorescent method.[93]

The isolation of hepatitis E virus (HEV) was eventually reported by Reyes et al. in 1990.[94] It was found to be a single-stranded, nonenveloped RNA virus that was distinct from the other hepatitis viruses. This virus was most closely related to the calcivirus family.

Hepatitis E has a relatively short incubation time of 2–9 weeks with a mean of 40–45 days. The diagnosis of this disease is by clinical presentation in conjunction with positive serology. Usually, hepatitis A, B, and C are ruled out first. An anti-HEV antibody by fluorescent antibody blocking assay or by ELISA can detect IgG and IgM antibodies.[95] A positive IgM antibody is indicative of acute infection, and this antibody usually disappears within 3–6 months. A Western blot assay also now exists.[96]

Based on clinically apparent infections, the highest attack rate seems to occur between the ages of 15 and 40 years, with a mortality rate of about 0.5% to 4% for the nonpregnant population. However, this virus acts differently in the pregnant population, with an attack rate of 10% to 20% and a mortality rate that ranges between 20% and 50%.[2] Whether this increase in severity seen in pregnancy is the result of the pregnancy itself or the poor living conditions and malnutrition in these populations is uncertain.

Presently, no treatment is described for this infection other than supportive care. In the case of pregnancy, the development of fulminant hepatitis needs to be watched for. Vertical transmission of HEV has been reported, although the true incidence is unknown because of the few cases described. Khuroo et al.[97] described 10 women in India who had acute HEV develop in the third trimester. Six of these women had fulminant hepatic failure, and three died (two of which were undelivered). In the evaluation of the eight delivered infants, five (63%) showed strong evidence for transplacental infection with positive cord blood for HEV RNA by PCR (all five), elevated liver enzymes at birth (all five), and positive IgM antibody (three of five). Two of these neonates died and, on autopsy, one showed massive hepatic necrosis. All eight neonates were positive for IgG antibody, as would be expected, because IgG antibodies can cross the placenta. The three surviving infected neonates remained IgG-positive. Two apparently uninfected infants cleared antibody at 3 and 6 months. The final case was still IgG-positive at 6 months.

Many unanswered questions still exist for HEV. During acute infection, is the virus found in other body fluids such as saliva, semen, and vaginal secretions? Can the virus be transmitted sexually or through blood transfusion? A recent study did show that the viremia can be protracted in some patients for up to 45–112 days.[98] In addition, fecal shedding can occur up to 7 weeks, well after clinical and biochemical recovery. These long periods of viremia and viral shedding will make disease prevention more difficult. Immunoglobulin for household contacts is of little or no benefit because significant antibody levels to HEV have not been detected in immunoglobulin. Future treatment will probably require a separate HEV immunoglobulin and vaccine.

References

1. Hieber JP, Dalton D, Shorey J, et al: Hepatitis and pregnancy. *J Pediatr* 91:545–549, 1977.
2. Scharschmidt BF: Hepatitis E: A virus in waiting. *Lancet* 346:519–520, 1995.
3. Friedman LS, Dienstag JL: *Recent Developments in Viral Hepatitis.* St Louis, Year Book, 1986, 313–385.
4. Lee WM: Drug-induced hepatotoxicity. *N Engl J Med* 333:1118–1127, 1995.
5. Neefe JR, Stokes J: An epidemic of infectious hepatitis apparently due to a waterborne agent. *JAMA* 128:1063–1075, 1945.
6. Stokes J, Neefe JR: The prevention and attenuation of infectious hepatitis by gamma globulin. *JAMA* 127:144–145, 1945.
7. Neefe JR, Stokes J, Baty JB, et al: Disinfection of water containing causative agent of infectious (epidemic) hepatitis. *JAMA* 128:1076–1080, 1945.
8. Shapiro CN, Coleman PJ, McQuillan GM, et al: Epidemiology of hepatitis A: Seroepidemiology and risk groups in the USA. *Vaccine* 10:59S–62S, 1992.
9. Gingrich GA, Hadler SC, Elder HA, et al: Serologic investigation of an outbreak of hepatitis A in a rural day-care center. *Am J Public Health* 73:1190–1195, 1983.

10. Hepatitis A among homosexual men—United States, Canada, and Australia: *MMWR* 41:155–164, 1992.

11. Sheretz RJ, Russell BA, Reuman PD: Transmission of hepatitis A by transfusion of blood products. *Arch Intern Med* 144:1579–1580, 1984.

12. Snydman DR, Dienstag JL, Stedt B, et al: Use of IgM–hepatitis A antibody testing. *JAMA* 245:827–830, 1981.

13. Szmuness W, Dienstag JL, Purcell RH, et al: Distribution of antibody to hepatitis A antigen in urban adult populations. *N Engl J Med* 295:755–759, 1976.

14. Watson JC, Fleming DW, Borella AJ, et al: Vertical transmission of hepatitis A resulting in an outbreak in a neonatal intensive care unit. *J Infect Dis* 167:567–571, 1993.

15. Tanaka I, Shima M, Kubota Y, et al: Vertical transmission of hepatitis A virus. *Lancet* 345:397, 1995.

16. Centers for Disease Control: Protection against viral hepatitis. Recommendations of the Immunization Practices Advisory Committee. *MMWR* 39:1S–26S, 1990.

17. Werzberger A, Mensch B, Kuter B, et al: A controlled trial of a formalin-inactivated hepatitis A vaccine in healthy children. *N Engl J Med* 327:453–457, 1992.

18. Innis BL, Snitbhan R, Kunasol P, et al: Protection against hepatitis A by an inactivated vaccine. *JAMA* 271:1328–1334, 1994.

19. Ahtone J, Maynard JE: Laboratory diagnosis of hepatitis B. *JAMA* 249:2067–2069, 1983.

20. Chau KH, Hargie MP, Decker RH, et al: Serodiagnosis of recent hepatitis B infection by IgM class anti-HBc. *Hepatology* 3:142–149, 1983.

21. Hoofnagle JH, Seeff LB, Bales ZB, et al: Type B hepatitis after transfusion with blood containing antibody to hepatitis B core antigen. *N Engl J Med* 298:1379–1383, 1978.

22. Beasley RP. Hwang LY, Lin CC, et al: Hepatocellular carcinoma and hepatitis B virus. *Lancet* 2:1129–1133, 1981.

23. Lohiya GS, Pirkle H, Nguyen H, et al: Hepatocellular carcinoma in hepatitis B surface antigen carriers in eight institutions. *West J Med* 148:426–429, 1988.

24. Krugman S, Holley HP, Davidson M, et al: Immunogenic effect of inactivated hepatitis B vaccine comparison of 20 μg and 40 μg doses. *J Med Virol* 8:119–121, 1981.

25. Francis DP, Handler SC, Thompson SE, et al: Prevention of hepatitis B with vaccine: Report of the CDC multicenter efficacy trial. *Ann Intern Med* 97:362–369, 1982.

26. Wistrom J: Intramuscular vs intradermal hepatitis B vaccination: A 6-year follow-up. *JAMA* 273:1835–1836, 1995.

27. Beasley RP, Trepo C, Stevens CE, et al: The e antigen and vertical transmission of hepatitis B surface antigen. *Am J Epidemol* 105:94–98, 1977.

28. Tong MJ, Thursby M, Rakela J, et al: Studies on the maternal-infant transmission of the viruses which cause acute hepatitis. *Gastroenterology* 80:999–1004, 1981.

29. Sinatra FR, Shah P, Weissman JY, et al: Perinatal transmitted acute icteric hepatitis B in infants born to hepatitis B surface antigen-positive and anti-hepatitis B$_e$-positive carrier mothers. *Pediatrics* 70:557–559, 1992.

30. Tong MJ, Sinatra FR, Thomas DW, et al: Need for immunoprophylaxis in infants born to HBsAg-positive carrier mothers who are HBeAg negative. *J Pediatr* 105:945–947, 1984.

31. Beasley RP, Hwang LY, Lee GCY, et al: Prevention of perinatally transmitted hepatitis B virus infections with hepatitis B immune globulin and hepatitis B vaccine. *Lancet* 2:1099–1102, 1983.

32. Wong VCW, Ip HMH, Reesink HW, et al: Prevention of the HBsAg carrier state in newborn infants of mothers who are chronic carriers of HBsAg and HBeAg by administration of hepatitis-B vaccine and hepatitis-B immunoglobulin. *Lancet* 1:921–926, 1984.

33. Beasley RP, Stevens CE, Shiao I-S, et al: Evidence against breast-feeding as a mechanism for vertical transmission of hepatitis B. *Lancet* 2:740–741, 1975.

34. DeMartino M, Appendino C, Resti M, et al: Should hepatitis B surface antigen positive mothers breast feed? *Arch Dis Child* 60:972–974, 1985.
35. Cruz AC, Frentzen BH, Behnke M: Hepatitis B: A case for prenatal screening of all patients. *Am J Obstet Gynecol* 156:1180–1183, 1987.
36. Summers PR, Biswas MK, Pastorek JG, et al: The pregnant hepatitis B carrier: Evidence favoring comprehensive antepartum screening. *Obstet Gynecol* 69:701–704, 1987.
37. Malecki JM, Guarin O, Hulbert A, et al: Prevalence of hepatitis B surface antigen among women receiving prenatal care at the Palm Beach County Health Department. *Am J Obstet Gynecol* 154:626–662, 1986.
38. Jones MM, Schiff ER, O'Sullivan MJ, et al: Failure of Centers for Disease Control criteria to identify hepatitis B infection in a large municipal obstetrical population. *Ann Intern Med* 107:335–337, 1987.
39. Hepatitis B virus: A comprehensive strategy for eliminating transmission in the United States through universal childhood vaccination. *MMWR* 40(RR 13):1–19, 1991.
40. Guidelines for hepatitis B virus screening and vaccination during pregnancy. ACOG Committee Opinion No 111, May 1992.
41. Alter MJ, Hadler SC, Margolis HS, et al: The changing epidemiology of hepatitis B in the United States: Need for alternative vaccination strategies. *JAMA* 263:1218–1222, 1990.
42. Franks AL, Berg CJ, Kane MA, et al: Hepatitis B virus infection among children born in the United States to southeast Asian refugees. *N Engl J Med* 321:1301–1305, 1989.
43. Universal hepatitis B immunization. Committee on Infectious Diseases. *Pediatrics* 89:795–800, 1992.
44. Choo QL, Kuo G, Weiner AJ, et al: Isolation of a cDNA clone derived from a blood-borne non-A, non-B viral hepatitis genome. *Science* 244:359–362, 1989.
45. Kuo G, Choo QL, Alter HJ, et al: An assay for circulating antibodies to a major etiologic virus of human non-A, non-B hepatitis. *Science* 244:362–364, 1989.
46. Genetic diversity of hepatitis C virus: Implications for pathogenesis, treatment and prevention. Grand round. *Lancet* 345:562–566, 1995.
47. Van der Poel CL, Cuypers HT, Reesink HW: Hepatitis C virus six years on. *Lancet* 344:1475–1479, 1994.
48. Alter HJ, Purcell RH, Shih JW, et al: Detection of antibody to hepatitis C virus in prospectively followed transfusion recipients with acute and chronic non-A, non-B hepatitis. *N Engl J Med* 321:1494–1500, 1989.
49. Aach RD, Stevens CE, Hollinger B, et al: Hepatitis C virus infection in post-transfusion hepatitis. *N Engl J Med* 325:1325–1329, 1991.
50. Alter MJ, Sampliner RE: Hepatitis C. *N Engl J Med* 321:1538–1540, 1989.
51. Nakashima K, Ikematsu H, Hayashi J, et al: Intrafamilial transmission of hepatitis C virus among the population of an endemic area of Japan. *JAMA* 274:1459–1461, 1995.
52. Bresters D, Mauser-Bunschoten EP, Reesink HW, et al: Sexual transmission of hepatitis C virus. *Lancet* 342:210–211, 1993.
53. Osmond DH, Padian NS, Sheppard HW, et al: Risk factors for hepatitis C virus seropositivity in heterosexual couples. *JAMA* 269:361–365, 1993.
54. Brettler DB, Mannucci PM, Gringeri A, et al: The low risk of hepatitis C virus transmission among sexual partners of hepatitis C-infected hemophilic males: An international, multicenter study. *Blood* 80:540–543, 1992.
55. Hsu HH, Wright TL, Luba D, et al: Failure to detect hepatitis C virus genome in human secretions with the polymerase chain reaction. *Hepatology* 14:763–767, 1991.
56. Terada S, Kawanishi K, Katayam K: Minimal hepatitis C infectivity in semen. *Ann Intern Med* 117:171–172, 1992.
57. Novati R, Thiers V, Monforte A, et al: Mother-to-child transmission of hepatitis C virus detected by nested polymerase chain reaction. *J Infect Dis* 165:720–723, 1992.

58. Weintrub PS, Veereman-Wauters G, Cowan MJ, et al: Hepatitis C virus infection in infants whose mothers took street drugs intravenously. *J Pediatr* 119:869–874, 1991.

59. Giovannini M, Tagger A, Ribero ML, et al: Maternal-infant transmission of hepatitis C virus and HIV infections: A possible interaction. *Lancet* 335:1166, 1990.

60. Cilla G, Trallero P, Iturriza M, et al: Maternal-infant transmission of hepatitis C virus infection. *Pediatr Infect Dis J* 11:417, 1992.

61. Lam JPH, McOmish F, Burns SM, et al: Infrequent vertical transmission of hepatitis C virus. *J Infect Dis* 167:572–576, 1993.

62. Giacchino R, Picciotte A, Tasso L, et al: Vertical transmission of hepatitis C. *Lancet* 345:1122–1123, 1995.

63. Zanetti AR, Tanzi E, Paccagnini S, et al: Mother-to-infant transmission of hepatitis C virus. *Lancet* 345:289–291, 1995.

64. Ohto H, Terazawa S, Sasaki N, et al: Transmission of hepatitis C virus from mothers to infants. *N Engl J Med* 330:744–750, 1994.

65. Thaler MM, Park CK, Landers DV, et al: Vertical transmission of hepatitis C virus. *Lancet* 338:17–18, 1991.

66. Wejstal R, Norkrans G: Chronic non-A, non-B hepatitis in pregnancy: Outcome and possible transmission to the offspring. *Scand J Infect Dis* 21:485–490, 1989.

67. Reinus JF, Leikin EL, Alter HJ, et al: Failure to detect vertical transmission of hepatitis C virus. *Ann Intern Med* 117:881–886, 1992.

68. Wejstal R, Widell AN, Mansson AS, et al: Mother-to-infant transmission of hepatitis C virus. *Ann Intern Med* 117:887–890, 1992.

69. Donahue JG, Munoz A, Ness PM, et al: The declining risk of post-transfusion hepatitis C virus infection. *N Engl J Med* 327:369–373, 1992.

70. Prevention of D Isiommunization. ACOG Technical Bulletin No 147, 1990.

71. YU MW, Mason BL, Guo ZP, et al: Hepatitis C transmission associated with intravenous immunoglobulins. *Lancet* 345:1173–1174, 1995.

72. Outbreak of hepatitis C associated with intravenous immunoglobulin administration—United States, October 1993-June 1994. *MMWR* 43:505–509, 1994.

73. Schiff RI: Hepatitis C and immune globulin. *N Engl J Med* 332:1236–1237, 1995.

74. Davis GL, Balart LA, Schiff ER, et al: Treatment of chronic hepatitis C with recombinant interferon alfa: A multicenter randomized, controlled trial. *N Engl J Med* 321:1501–1506, 1989.

75. DiBisceglie AM, Martin P, Kassianides C, et al: Recombinant interferon alfa therapy for chronic hepatitis C: A randomized, double-blind, placebo-controlled trial. *N Engl J Med* 321:1506–1510, 1989.

76. Chemello L, Alberti A, Rose K, et al: Hepatitis C serotype and response to interferon therapy. *N Engl J Med* 330:143, 1994.

77. Poynard T, Bedossa P, Chevallier M, et al: A comparison of three interferon alfa-2b regimens for the long-term treatment of chronic non-A, non-B hepatitis. *N Engl J Med* 332:1457–1462, 1995.

78. Rizzetto M, Canese MG, Arico S, et al: Immunofluorescence detection of a new antigen/antibody system (delta/anti-delta) associated with hepatitis B virus in liver and serum of HBsAg carriers. *Gut* 18:997–1003, 1977.

79. Rizzetto M: The delta agent. *Hepatology* 3:729–737, 1983.

80. Wu JC, Choo KB, Chen CM, et al: Genotyping of hepatitis D virus by restriction-fragment length polymorphism and relation to outcome of hepatitis D. *Lancet* 346:939–941, 1995.

81. Jacobson IM, Dienstag JL, Werner BG, et al: Epidemiology and clinical impact of hepatitis D virus (delta) infection. *Hepatology* 5:188–191, 1985.

82. Shattock AG, Irwin FM, Morgan BM, et al: Increased severity and morbidity of acute hepatitis in drug abusers with simultaneously acquired hepatitis B and hepatitis D virus infections. *BMJ* 290:1377–1380, 1985.

83. Caredda F, Rossi E, Monforte A, et al: Hepatitis B virus-associated coinfection and superinfection with delta agent: Indistinguishable disease with different oucome. *J Infect Dis* 151:925–928, 1985.

84. Farci P, Gerin JL, Aragona M, et al: Diagnostic and prognostic significance of the IgM antibody to the hepatitis delta virus. *JAMA* 255:1443–1446, 1986.

85. Smedile A, Dentico P, Zanetti A, et al: Infection with the delta agent in chronic HBsAg carriers. *Gastroenterology* 81:992–997, 1981.

86. Vashwanathan R: Infectious hepatitis in Delhi (1955-1956): A critical study: Epidemiology. *Indian J Med Res* 45:1S–30S, 1957.

87. Enterically transmitted non-A, non-B hepatitis—Mexico. *MMWR* 36:597–602, 1987.

88. Enterically transmitted non-A, non-B hepatitis—East Africa. *MMWR* 36:241–244, 1987.

89. Hepatitis E among US travelers, 1989-1992. *MMWR* 42:1–4, 1993.

90. Sreenivasan MA, Arankalle VA, Sehgal A, et al: Non-A, non-B epidemic hepatitis: Visualization of virus-like particles in the stool by immune electron microscope. *J Gen Virol* 65:1005–1007, 1984.

91. Arankalle VA, Ticehurst J, Screenivasan MA, et al: Aetiological association of a virus-like particle with enterically transmitted non-A, non-B hepatitis. *Lancet* 1:550–554, 1988.

92. Bradley DW, Krawczynski K, Cook EH, et al: Enterically transmitted non-A, non-B hepatitis: Serial passage of disease in cynomolgus macaques and tamarins and recovery of disease associated 27- to 34-nm viruslike particles. *Proc Natl Acad Sci U S A* 84:6277–6281, 1987.

93. Krawczynski K, Bradley DW: Enterically transmitted non-A, non-B hepatitis: Identification of virus associated antigen in experimentally infected cynomolgus macaques. *J Infect Dis* 159:1042–1049, 1989.

94. Reyes GR, Purdy MA, Kim JP, et al: Isolation of a cDNA from the virus responsible for enterically transmitted non-A, non-B hepatitis. *Science* 24:1335–1339, 1990.

95. Goldsmith R, Yarbough PO, Reyes GR, et al: Enzyme-linked immunosorbent assay for diagnosis of acute sporadic hepatitis E in Egyptian children. *Lancet* 339:328–331, 1992.

96. Favorov MO, Fields HA, Purdy MA, et al: Serologic identification of hepatitis E virus infections in epidemic and endemic settings. *J Med Virol* 36:246–250, 1992.

97. Khuroo MS, Kamili S, Jameel S: Vertical transmission of hepatitis E virus. *Lancet* 345:1025–1026, 1995.

98. Nanda SK, Ansari IH, Acharya SK, et al: Protracted viremia during acute sporadic hepatitis E virus infection. *Gastroenterology* 108:225–230, 1995.

OBSTETRICS

1 Maternal and Fetal Physiology

Glucose Homeostasis During Spontaneous Labor in Normal Human Pregnancy

Maheux PC, Bonin B, Dizazo A, et al (Institut de Recherche Clinique de Montreal; Hôtel-Dieu de Montréal Hosp, Montreal; Univ of Montreal)

J Clin Endocrinol Metab 81:209–215, 1996

1–1

Background.—Many different labor-related changes in the endocrine milieu are recognized, but the factors leading to the onset of labor remain unclear. Plasma glucose concentration is known to increase during normal parturition; however, the accompanying changes in glucose metabolism have not been studied much. In the absence of data on glucose turnover during labor, it is difficult to ascertain the cause of the increase in plasma glucose. Glucose turnover during labor in normal women was studied with the use of a stable isotope technique.

Methods.—Six normal pregnant women underwent isotopic measurements of glucose turnover during various stages of labor: the latent (A1) and active (A2) phases of cervical dilation, fetal expulsion (B), and placental expulsion (C). The same measurements were made in 5 women post partum. The changes occurring in glucose turnover were correlated with the levels of various gestational and nongestational hormones, as well as with free fatty acids and other important substrates.

Results.—During labor, plasma glucose increased from 4.0 mmol/L in phase A1 to 5.5 mmol/L in phase C. Plasma glucose level in the women post partum was 5.7 mmol/L. The mean glucose production during labor was 32.8 μmol/kg·min, compared with 8.2 μmol/kg·min in women post partum, with a similar increase in glucose utilization during labor (Fig 2). Glucose metabolic clearance was 7.5 mL/kg·min during labor, compared with 1.8 mL/kg·min in nonpregnant women. Although plasma insulin level remained stable at about 59 pmol/L from phase A1 through phase B of labor, it increased to 115 pmol/L in phase C. Plasma glucagon was 127 pg/mL during labor vs. 4 pg/mL in women post partum. As labor progressed, plasma cortisol increased from 921 to 2,018 nmol/L, compared

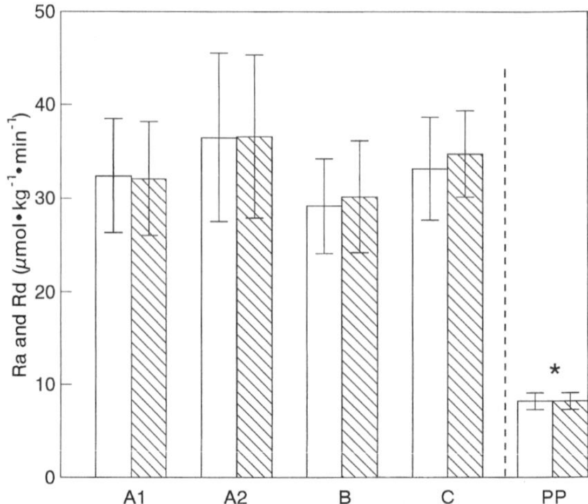

FIGURE 2.—The appearance (R_a) (*open bars*) and disappearance (R_d) (*hatched bars*) during the different phases of labor (*A1, A2, B,* and *C*) and in the postpartum period (*PP*). Data are expressed as the mean ± SEM. *, $P < 0.001–0.002$ compared with the various phases of labor. (Courtesy of Maheux PC, Bonin B, Dizazo A, et al: Glucose homeostasis during spontaneous labor in normal human pregnancy. *J Clin Endocrinol Metab* 81:209–215, 1996; Copyright The Endocrine Society.)

with 645 nmol/L in women post partum. In the laboring women, epinephrine increased from 218 to 1,119 pmol/L and norepinephrine from 1.09 to 3.61 nmol/L.

Conclusions.—Normal labor is associated with an increase in glucose disposal—much of which is insulin independent—and in glucose production. Uterine and skeletal muscle contraction appears to play a major role in regulating glucose utilization during labor. An increase in hepatic glucose production is noted as well, which could be promoted by the documented increases in glucagon, catecholamines, and cortisol.

▶ This is a unique study using tritium-labeled glucose isotopes to evaluate changes imposed on glucose metabolism by the energy requirements of normal active labor. All 10 women were in labor after at least 10 hours of fasting. The glucose rate of appearance (R_a) and disappearance (R_d) were calculated, as was the metabolic clearance rate for glucose (R_d/serum glucose concentration) using steady-state and bolus infusion techniques during labor stages 1 (A1 and A2), 2 (B) and 3 (C), and compared with 5 sets of postpartum measurements. Glucose isotopes were measured by combined mass spectroscopy and gas chromatography. The techniques are well established, although the use of 5 labeled sites in a single glucose isotope introduces a risk of error from the effects of isotope recombinations with labeled or unlabeled glucose molecules.

Both glucose production and disappearance were increased equally during labor and maternal blood glucose concentration increased. Because plasma insulin declined slightly with the third stage of labor, the increased metabolic clearance rate for glucose appeared to be independent of insulin effects and likely arises from direct insulin-independent glucose utilization known to take place in the systemic and uterine muscle mass of laboring women. Augmented hepatic glucose production likely arises from hepatic gluconeogenesis and glycogenolysis driven by the increase in maternal cortisol, epinephrine, and glucagon during labor, although no direct studies of hepatic function were done. Experimental data suggest that fetal glucose transfer is likely decreased during periods of intense muscular activity leading to fetal hypoglycemia,[1] a deficit which is met by increased placental lactate production. Lactate in turn serves as a carbon substrate replacement in fetal metabolism. This work helps make clear why patients with diabetes who are in labor tend toward hypoglycemia and benefit by an infusion of 5–10 g/hr of exogenous glucose—and why insulin resistance as measured by maternal blood glucose concentration tends to decrease so rapidly after the third stage of labor.

T.H. Kirschbaum, M.D.

Reference

1. *Focus & Opinion: Obstetrics and Gynecology* 2(1):103–104, 1996.

The Impact of Gestational Age and Fetal Growth on the Maternal-Fetal Glucose Concentration Difference
Marconi AM, Paolini C, Buscaglia M, et al (Univ of Milano, Italy; Univ of Colorado, Denver)
Obstet Gynecol 87:937–942, 1996
1–2

Background.—Some animal research has demonstrated a significant reduction of umbilical arterial glucose concentration during pregnancy, as reflected in an increased maternal-fetal gradient. However, some research on human pregnancy has shown no relationship between the umbilical venous glucose concentration and gestational age. In these studies, fetal glucose levels appear to be decreased in association with fetal growth restriction (FGR). This study determined whether the human fetus accommodates to the increasing glucose needs of late pregnancy partly by gradual reduction in fetal glucose levels, resulting in an increased maternal-fetal glucose concentration gradient, and whether the association of fetal and maternal glucose levels and their concentration differences vary with the clinical severity of FGR.

Methods.—Seventy-seven women with normal pregnancies and 42 with pregnancies complicated by FGR were studied. Umbilical venous glucose concentrations were measured at the time of fetal blood sampling. A maternal arterialized blood sample was also obtained in 40 women with normal pregnancies and all with FGR pregnancies. Three groups of growth-restricted fetuses were designated, based on fetal heart rate (FHR) recordings and Doppler measures of the umbilical artery pulsatility index

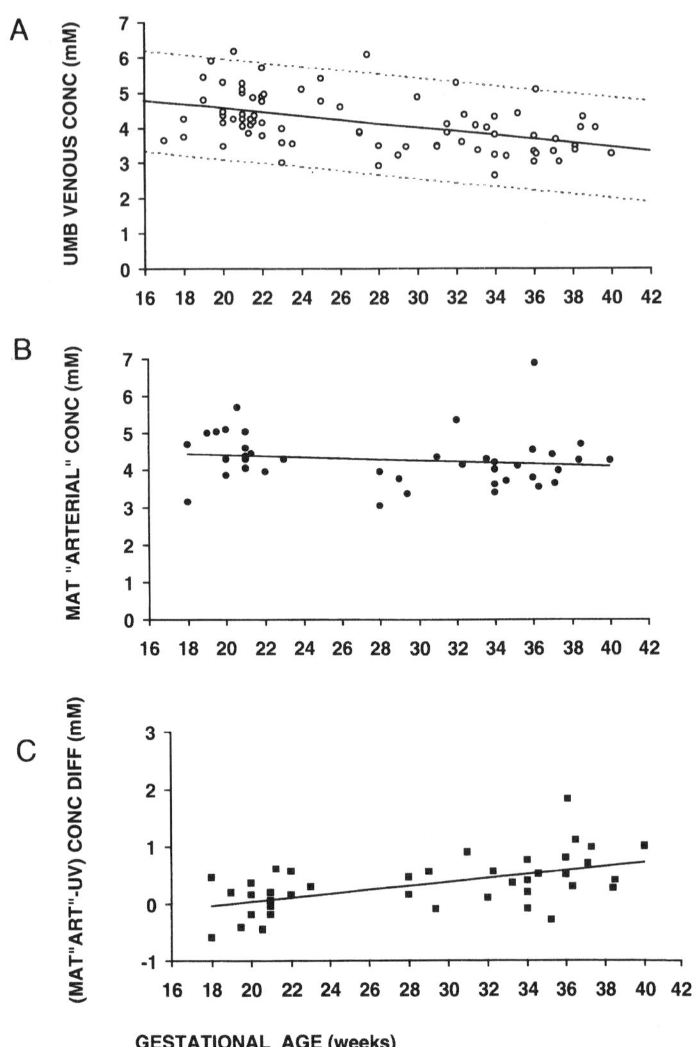

FIGURE 1.—A, umbilical venous glucose concentrations (*UMB VENOUS CONC*) vs. gestational age for appropriate-for-gestational-age pregnancies. *Dashed lines* indicate mean ± 2 standard deviations of fetal glucose concentration during pregnancy, according to the equation: umbilical venous glucose (mmol/L) = 5.66−0.056 gestational age (weeks). **B,** maternal "arterial" glucose concentration (*MAT "ARTERIAL" CONC*) vs. gestational age. **C,** maternal "arterial"-umbilical venous glucose concentration difference (*MAT "ART"-UV CONC DIFF*) vs. gestational age in appropriate-for-gestational-age pregnancies. (Courtesy of Marconi AM, Paolini C, Buscaglia M, et al: The impact of gestational age and fetal growth on the maternal-fetal glucose concentration difference. *Obstet Gynecol* 87:937–942, 1996. Reprinted with permission from The American College of Obstetricians and Gynecologists.)

(PI). Group 1 consisted of 12 fetuses with normal FHR and PI; group 2, 17 with normal FHR and abnormal PI; and group 3, 13 with abnormal FHR and PI.

Findings.—Umbilical venous glucose levels were significantly reduced and maternal-fetal glucose level differences significantly increased in normal pregnancies as gestational age advanced. Fetal and maternal glucose concentrations were also significantly correlated. In pregnancies complicated by FGR, maternal-fetal glucose concentration differences in groups 2 and 3 were significantly greater than those in group 1 and in normal pregnancies (Fig 1).

Conclusion.—Fetal glucose concentration is a function of gestational age and maternal glucose levels. In pregnancies affected by FGR, the maternal-fetal glucose concentration difference is increased, as the fetus accommodates to the restricted placental size and placental glucose transport capacity. This increase depends on the clinical severity of FGR.

▶ Continuing a now long-standing relationship between the University of Colorado's Pediatric Department and the University of Milano, these investigators provide us with some interesting data based on longitudinal crosssectional maternal fetal blood glucose values in normal infants and some biochemical observations in 42 growth-retarded fetuses. In appropriate-forgestational-age infants, their data are consonant with the proposition that as fetuses mature, they increase the maternal-to-fetal glucose gradient across the placenta, thereby increasing the glucose flux and nutrients available to the fetus. But glucose transport from mother to fetus is not by simple diffusion but by facilitated transport, using intramembranous transport proteins that allow transfer rates to exceed those of simple diffusion.[1, 2]

In discussing the importance of the maternal-fetal gradient for glucose, the authors implicitly assume no facilitated diffusion and, at the same time, demonstrate its presence, certainly in the 23% of cases where umbilical vein glucose is greater than maternal arterial glucose concentrations. The clinical independent variables contain some problems as they are defined in contrast to American obstetrical usage. One third of "growth-retarded" fetuses are below the 10th but not the fifth percentile for Italian norms. Criteria for abnormal fetal heart rate include failure of movement accelerations and of beat-to-beat variability which, in nonstress testing, would lead to vibroacoustic stimulation to attempt to disrupt a possible sleep state. The "U"-shaped decelerations which are taken to be late decelerations would likely be called variable decelerations by most American obstetricians. For growth-retarded fetuses, no increase in maternal fetal glucose gradients were seen, except in 13 fetuses with both abnormal FHR and Doppler PIs, and no additional clinical description of those cases is included. The authors fail to consider the evidence for increased placental surface with intrauterine growth retardation cited in the reference above. These interesting data are obtained at the cost of a great deal of work, and they add to what is known about normal mechanisms of glucose transport in the human.

T.H. Kirschbaum, M.D.

References

1. 1995 YEAR BOOK OF OBSTETRICS AND GYNECOLOGY, pp 16–19.
2. 1995 YEAR BOOK OF OBSTETRICS AND GYNECOLOGY, pp 88–90.

Uteroplacental Carbon Substrate Metabolism and O_2 Consumption After Long-Term Hypoglycemia in Pregnant Sheep

Carver TD, Hay WW Jr (Univ of Colorado, Denver)
Am J Physiol 269:299E–308E, 1995   1–3

Background.—The uteroplacental tissues are highly metabolic, consuming as much oxygen (O_2) and twice the glucose and producing 66% as much lactate as the fetus near full-term. Transporting the amino acids used by the fetus for protein synthesis, accretion, and oxidation produces a high-energy requirement in the placenta. It can be presumed then, that changes in placental metabolism could have a profound impact on nutrient substrate transfer to the fetus, fetal nutritional metabolism, and fetal growth. Animal models of maternal hypoglycemia have consistently resulted in fetal growth restriction. The mechanisms involved in fetal growth restriction caused by reduced glucose supply were investigated.

Methods.—Beginning at approximately 70 days' gestation, maternal and fetal hypoglycemia were induced in 6 pregnant ewes with chronic insulin infusions during the second half of gestation, and the effects were compared with 7 normal controls. After 125 days' gestation, indwelling catheters were placed in all study fetuses, and maternal and fetal blood was obtained daily for measurement of glucose concentration. Approximately 10 days later, blood samples were obtained simultaneously from the maternal artery, uterine vein, fetal abdominal aorta, and umbilical vein after infusion into the fetal femoral vein of tritiated water (^3H_2O). The animals were then sacrificed, and the fetus, fetal organs, and placenta were weighed.

Results.—Fetal and placental weight were significantly and proportionally reduced in the hypoglycemic group, compared with the control group. Between 125 and 135 days' gestation, maternal and fetal blood glucose levels and fetal plasma insulin levels were significantly lower in the hypoglycemic group than in the control group; there were no significant differences in fetal concentrations of other substrates between the 2 groups. The absolute uterine net glucose uptake rate was reduced by 48%. Compared with the control group, the hypoglycemic group demonstrated uteroplacental lactate production preferentially directed into the fetal rather than maternal circulation and reduced fetal and uteroplacental consumption of β-hydroxybutyrate and acetoacetate (Fig 3). The maternal O_2 content and uterine O_2 uptake rate were significantly reduced in the hypoglycemic group, whereas there were no significant differences in fetal blood O_2 content or fetal and uteroplacental O_2 consumption rates. Fetal blood had lesser concentrations of amino acids. Glucose infusion inducing

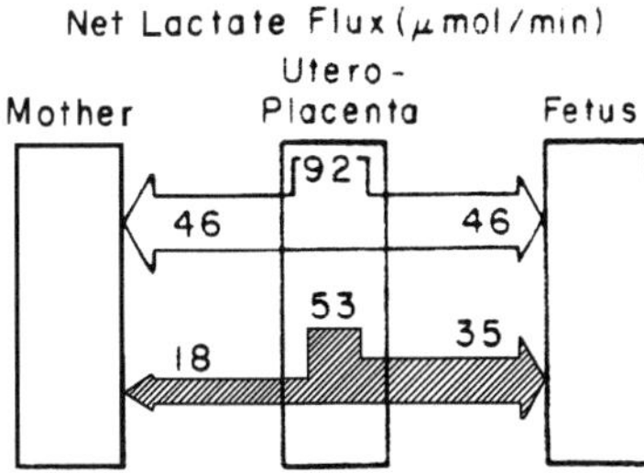

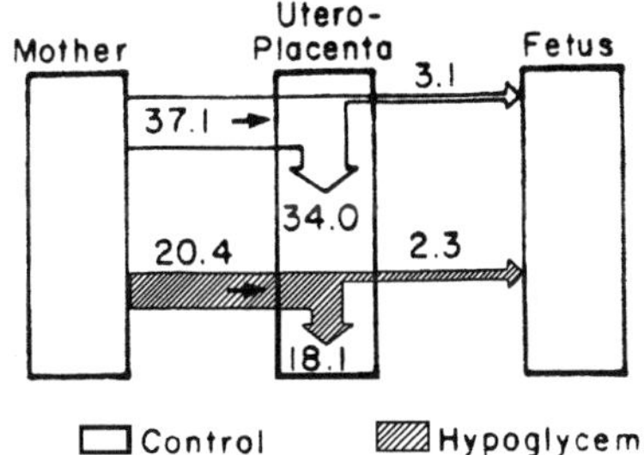

FIGURE 3.—Mean net lactate and ketoacid flux rates between uteroplacenta and maternal circulation and between uteroplacenta and fetal circulation in control and hypoglycemic groups. *Arrows* indicate direction of flux. *Abbreviations:* β-*OHB*, β-hydroxybutyrate; *AcAc*, acetoacetate. (Courtesy of Carver TD, Hay WW Jr: *Am J Physiol* 269:299E-308E, 1995.)

normalized maternal and fetal glucose concentrations resulted in greater placental glucose and O_2 consumption rates in the hypoglycemic group than in the control group.

Conclusions.—In the presence of a reduced glucose supply, the transfer of glucose and other substrates to the fetus is reduced, as these nutrients are diverted to placental consumption. These metabolic adaptations preserve the normal relationships of oxidative and nonoxidative metabolism within the placenta, even though its size is reduced, suggesting placental metabolic autonomy.

▶ Those who use the term "uteroplacental insufficiency" fail to realize the placenta uses a number of transfer mechanisms almost equal in number to the kidney and liver, and to define any one of them as insufficient, one must make the sorts of measurements of blood flow rates and blood contents in both maternal and fetal blood that are made here. Animal preparations are needed, because it is impossible in the intact human to identify reduced placental transport due solely to placental and not to maternal or fetal functional changes. Here, the stressor is chronic maternal insulin infusion for 60 days, sufficient to decrease maternal plasma glucose into the range of 25–30 mg/dL and to reduce fetal and placental weight by 30%. Under those circumstances, the placenta proves to be quite adaptable, maintaining its own rate of glucose uptake and metabolism at the expense of that of the fetus. Maternal lactate concentration is increased, and the placenta appears to produce both lactate and glucose to supplement fetal carbohydrate metabolism in states of need. Metabolism and transfer of ketones are undisturbed. Abrupt restoration to normal maternal glucose concentration leads to very rapid reversion to normal values of fetal concentrations and metabolic fluxes. This beautifully performed study illuminates the important and dynamic role of the placenta where nutrient delivery to the placenta is reduced through external manipulation.

T.H. Kirschbaum, M.D.

"Physiologic" Intracellular Acidosis in Pregnancy

Bardicef O, Bardicef M, Sorokin Y, et al (Wayne State Univ, Detroit)
Am J Obstet Gynecol 173:879–880, 1995   1–4

Purpose.—Although hyperventilation with resultant respiratory alkalosis is common in pregnancy, a compensatory increase in renal bicarbonate excretion and decrease in bicarbonate levels maintain maternal pH at normal levels. If alkalosis was present intracellularly, it would lead to a shift of the oxyhemoglobin dissociation curve and decreased oxygen delivery to the fetus. Acid-base homeostasis in pregnancy was studied by measuring intracellular pH in erythrocytes from pregnant and nonpregnant women.

Methods.—Thirty-three nonpregnant and 22 third-trimester pregnant women were studied. Blood samples were obtained, and intracellular pH in packed cells was measured by phosphorus-31 nuclear magnetic resonance spectroscopic techniques.

Results.—The mean intracellular pH was 7.23 in the pregnant women vs. 7.29 in nonpregnant women. The difference was significant. Intracellular pH did not vary by age, body mass index, or race.

Conclusions.—Pregnant women have lower intracellular pH than do nonpregnant controls. This "physiologic" intracellular acidosis may potentiate oxygen-hemoglobin dissociation and oxygen delivery across the placenta. The exact mechanisms of this effect—possibly including progesterone and other hormonal factors—remain to be determined.

▶ Nuclear MRI spectroscopy using phosphorus-31 allows estimate of cellular phosphocreatine and inorganic phosphorus from which concentrations it is possible, given the chemical shifts of both peaks in the power spectrum, to calculate the intracellular pH appropriate to the ratio of their concentrations. Other approaches are possible as well. It's important that the calculation provides the activity of hydrogen ions, that is, the product of the actual concentration of hydrogen ions and their activity coefficient. The activity coefficient represents the steric hindrance to hydrogen ions in the intracellular environment, comprised largely of intraerythrocytic stromal elements, other molecules of varying charge and volume, and water content. Intraerythrocytic water increases in pregnancy from an average value of

63.8% to nearly 66.5% of total red cell mass. This hydration had the effect of increasing the proton activity coefficient and provides the likely basis for the apparent change in pH that the authors note here.

T.H. Kirschbaum, M.D.

Effect of Altitude on Uterine Artery Blood Flow During Normal Pregnancy

Zamudio S, Palmer SK, Droma T, et al (Univ of Colorado, Denver; Tibet Inst of Med Sciences, Lhasa, People's Republic of China)
J Appl Physiol 79:7–14, 1995   1–5

Objective.—High altitudes and low maternal oxygen transport lead to lower birth weight. To determine whether lower arterial oxygen content or uteroplacental blood flow or both lead to decreased uteroplacental oxygen delivery, blood flow velocity and diameters of uterine, common iliac, and external iliac arteries were compared in women with normal and high blood pressure during pregnancy and post partum.

Methods.—At 35.8 weeks of pregnancy, 16 women who were residents of a low-altitude city were studied, and 6 of them also were studied 15 weeks post partum. Twenty-three women from a high-altitude city were studied at 35.6 weeks of pregnancy, 19 of whom were also studied at 25.8 weeks post partum. Six nonpregnant women were also studied.

Results.—Women from both high- and low-altitude cities had larger uterine artery diameters, blood flow velocities, and blood flow volume during pregnancy. In women living in a high-altitude city, uterine artery diameter was significantly smaller and blood flow velocity was significantly higher during pregnancy, yielding a blood flow volume one third lower at high altitude at week 36. Pregnancy increased diameters of the common iliac and external iliac arteries. At both high and low altitudes, common iliac blood flow velocity increased and external iliac blood flow velocity and volume flow decreased during pregnancy. Arterial oxygen content was higher and uterine artery oxygen flow was a significant 30% lower in women living in high-altitude cities than in those living in low-altitude cities. Birth weight was lower at higher altitudes than at lower altitudes, and birth weight was significantly associated with uterine blood flow velocity but not volume flow at low altitudes.

Conclusion.—A decrease in calculated uterine artery blood flow and decreased uterine artery oxygen flow were associated with lower birth weight at higher altitudes and may contribute to the higher incidence of growth retardation seen at high altitudes.

▶ This group has published several studies bringing Doppler measurements of uterine artery mean flow velocity and vessel diameters to bear on uterine hemodynamics and oxygen delivery as a function of altitude, comparing 5,250 with 10,170 ft above sea level. They conclude that high altitude is associated with less uterine artery dilatation but greater flow velocity, the combination resulting in less uterine bulk blood flow calculated as the product of blood flow velocity and vessel surface area. Despite the greater hematocrit at 10,000 ft, oxygen delivery calculated in that way is about 30% less, possibly explaining the reduced newborn body weight. The problems in that interpretation stem from inferences regarding the conversion of velocity to bulk flow values, the sensitivity of vessel area calculations to the square of coefficients of variability (3% to 5% here), and problems of experimental design. Since vessel diameter and flow calculations could only be made at Denver, all 5 high-altitude Leadville women were in fact studied in that regard in Denver at 5,250 ft. The authors assume no changes resulted in the loss of 5,000 ft of altitude over 3 hours but offer nothing but intuition in support. Means and standard errors for calculated volume flows are not printed but can be read from Figure 1 in the original article; they fail a test of statistical significance for difference using simple T tests since the high-altitude mean values appear to be 200 ± 89 mL/min and at low altitude 310 ± 66 mL/min expressed as means and standard deviations. Only when 2-factor analysis of variance is used to combine data from nonpregnant and pregnant women to consider the effect of altitude do differences appear. When one subtracts calculated uterine artery and external iliac blood flow rates from calculated common iliac blood flow rates for Denver gravidas, there is virtually no blood flow available for other hypogastric artery branches, seemingly a physiologic impossibility. The use of indirect Doppler techniques for estimation of uterine oxygen delivery continues to be too fraught with technical problems and unproven assumptions to be reliable.

T.H. Kirschbaum, M.D.

Renal Artery Doppler Velocimetry in Nonpregnant and Pregnant Women

Kublickas M, Randmaa I, Lunell NO, et al (Huddinge Univ, Sweden)
J Matern Fetal Invest 5:216–221, 1995   1–6

Background.—Color Doppler ultrasonography allows noninvasive, accurate visualization of the renal vasculature and evaluation of changes in intrarenal blood flow velocity. However, the results of previous studies of the effects of pregnancy on renal blood flow velocity indices have been conflicting. The effects of pregnancy on renal artery Doppler blood flow indices were investigated in healthy, normotensive women.

Methods.—Twenty-eight nonpregnant women (median age, 29 years) and 15 pregnant women (median age, 26 years) were studied with an echocardiograph Vingmed CFM 700. Two-dimensional imaging, color flow mapping, and pulsed Doppler examinations of the right kidney were obtained with the women in the left lateral position. Each pregnant woman was studied at least once in each trimester. Cardiac output and blood flow velocities in the segmental renal arteries were measured using a mechanical sector transducer combined with a pulsed Doppler.

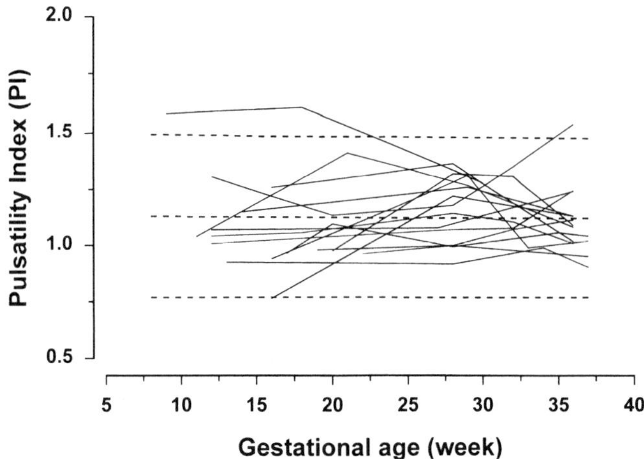

FIGURE 1.—Pulsatility index (*PI*) in 15 normal pregnant women, demonstrating the individual variation throughout the pregnancy (*straight lines*). Linear regression line presented with a 95% prediction interval for individual PI values (*dashed lines*). (Courtesy of Kublickas M, Randman I, Lunell NO, et al: Renal artery Doppler velocimetry in nonpregnant and pregnant women. *J Matern Fetal Invest* 5:216–221, 1995.)

Results.—Although the renal Doppler indices did not change significantly throughout pregnancy (Fig 1), these indices were significantly higher in pregnant than in nonpregnant women. Except for a significant positive correlation between pulsatility index and stroke volume, central hemodynamic parameters and the Doppler indices showed no relationship. The greatest variability found with repeated measurements was in the absolute velocity; the least variability was in the pulsatility index.

Conclusions.—Renal blood flow velocity indices do not change significantly throughout pregnancy, but these indices are higher in pregnant than in nonpregnant women. Results of Doppler renal blood flow assessments in pregnant women should be interpreted with caution—these renal Doppler indices may reflect both renal vascular resistance and kidney perfusion factors related to central hemodynamics.

▶ Although it lacks promise of clinical utility, this is a nice piece of work from the Huddinge Hospital of the Karolinska Institute. Reliable Doppler signals from the maternal renal arteries during pregnancy are very difficult to obtain but apparently even harder to interpret. Doppler velocity signals from pregnant women are elevated as early as 9 weeks of gestation, compared with those from normal renal arteries in nonpregnant individuals. However, individual variability is large, and none of the derived indices reflect the increase in renal blood flow defined by p-aminohippurate measurements through the course of pregnancy to term. Cautious Swedish investigators indicate that the Doppler signals should be interpreted with caution with respect to renal blood flow in pregnancy. More realistically, because these fail to conform with other external measurements of renal blood flow, the Doppler signals appear to be of very questionable value.

T.H. Kirschbaum, M.D.

Fetal Heart Rate and Uterine Contractility During Maternal Exercise at Term

Spinnewijn WEM, Lotgering FK, Struijk PC, et al (Erasmus Univ, Rotterdam, The Netherlands)
Am J Obstet Gynecol 174:43–48, 1996   1–7

Background.—Despite repeated studies, the normal response of the fetal heart rate (FHR) remains uncertain. Problems associated with motion artifacts have precluded measurement of FHRs during exercise per se. Some pregnant women note increased uterine contractility during exercise. The FHR and uterine contractility responses to moderate maternal exercise were assessed with the use of internal monitoring.

Methods.—Thirty healthy women with term pregnancies were admitted for elective induction of labor. Each patient was studied before, during, and after exercising to a heart rate of 140 beats minute on a cycle ergometer. The FHR response was assessed with a scalp electrode and the intrauterine pressure response with a catheter filled with intra-amniotic fluid. Three independent observers classified the FHR tracings according to Fischer et al., as a measure of fetal well-being, and Nijhuis et al., as a measure of behavior. The intrauterine pressure recordings were used to determine the frequency and intensity of contractions.

Results.—All 30 women delivered a healthy baby by the vaginal route. Fischer FHR scores were not significantly different from those before, during, and after exercise. The FHR pattern was A or B—corresponding to a behavioral state of 1F or 2F—85% of the time. Changes in the FHR pattern appeared to be unaffected by maternal exercise. A 5.5-fold increase was found in the frequency of uterine contractions during exercise compared with the pre-exercise period, as well as a fourfold increase in the time-pressure integral. The changes in uterine contractility rapidly normalized after exercise.

Conclusions.—Exercise appears to produce no significant changes in FHR pattern in healthy pregnant women at term. Thus, maternal exercise does not seem to produce fetal distress nor to change the fetal behavior pattern. Exercise does produce a significant increase in uterine contractility, perhaps through a hormonal mechanism or mechanical stimulation. The results cannot be extrapolated to preterm women with an unripe cervix, however.

▶ Thanks to a study group of 30 Rotterdam women, most of them multiparas, we now have direct scalp recordings of the fetal heart in women exercising at term before presentation for elective induction and in normal pregnancy. After fixation of the scalp electrode and insertion of an interuterine pressure catheter and after a 20-minute stabilization period, a cycle ergometer set at 50 W or more was used for exercise sufficient to increase the maternal pulse rate above 140 beats per minute for 20 minutes. Twenty-six women completed the protocol. Fetal heart rate tracings at 3 cm/min were evaluated after Fischer, a German scoring technique that is as reliable as anything used in the United States.

The Nijhuis approach to evaluating fetal behavioral state is based on FHR criteria thought to correlate with ultrasonically viewed wake–sleep activity states and is of less certain interpretability. In only 1 case did FHR patterns interpreted as ominous appear, and in that case the findings vanished after recovery and a normal neonate was delivered 3 hours later. All others behaved normally. An increase in uterine contraction frequency basal and peak systolic pressures and the integral of the pressure time plot over a 20-minute period increased during physical activity. The authors caution that the results are valid only for normal term pregnancies, but this should be enough to convince most of us that exercise in such patients does not cause FHR abnormality.

T.H. Kirschbaum, M.D.

Morphometric Analysis of Gap Junctions in Nonpregnant and Term Pregnant Human Myometrium

Çiray HN, Güner H, Håkansson H, et al (Uppsala Univ, Sweden; Gazi Univ, Ankara, Turkey; Ankara Univ, Turkey)
Acta Obstet Gynecol Scand 74:497–504, 1995   1–8

Background.—Hormonal changes associated with the course of pregnancy influence the myometrium. The events leading to delivery may be achieved primarily by enhanced intercellular communication through gap junctional (GJ) channels. The morphologic differences occurring in human myometrium in different stages and kinds of labor were investigated.

Methods.—Twenty-four pregnant and 10 nonpregnant women, aged 18 to 49 years, were studied. Tissue was obtained from the 2 groups, including pregnant women who were not in labor and women in spontaneous or oxytocin-induced labor. Caveolae, extracellular space, and GJs were quantified.

Findings.—Differences were noted in GJs and in cell growth, accompanied by enlargement of the extracellular space. Gap junctions were found in nonpregnant women, including 1 postmenopausal woman. The frequency and size of GJs gradually increased among groups of pregnant women not in labor, in oxytocin-induced labor, and in spontaneous labor. The increase in junction size was not as great as the increase in number.

Conclusions.—Most often, GJs occur in human myometrial cells during spontaneous labor. This indicates a possible role for these structures in the termination of pregnancy. The effect of oxytocin on the appearance of GJs was negligible, suggesting that the contribution of oxytocin to the establishment of myometrial contractile synchronicity is minor. Because the distribution of caveolae did not differ among groups, they are probably not relevant for the initiation of labor.

▶ Though myometrial cells possess an intrinsic rhythmic contractility and the steroid endocrinology of pregnancy increases their dimensions and available force, the key to productive contractile organization in labor is coordination; the capacity of millions of myometrial cells to contract in simultaneity. Much of that coordination appears to be linked to GJ loci of tight adherence between adjoining smooth muscle cells. There they serve as sites of low resistance to the transfer of ions and action potentials between adjoining cells. Widely distributed among human and animal tissues, they are produced by genes that appear to undergo expression in response to estrogen and result in the production of 43,000-Dalton protein fragments (Connexin-43), which are assembled in groups of 6–8 molecules to form GJs. Assembly is very rapid in rodents, within an hour after the onset of labor, and the disassembly is correspondingly fast.

In this piece of uterine morphometry, the assembly of GJs in labor is demonstrated, but it is surprising that there are fewer GJs, which are generally also smaller in size among women undergoing oxytocin induction compared with those in spontaneous labor. Further, though oxytocin may play a role in releasing calcium ions stored in the endoplasmic reticulum in myometrial cells, thereby increasing muscle contractility, it appears to have no role in the increase in GJ density. Again, here's evidence that oxytocin plays little role in the onset of coordinated contractile of normal labor, howsoever important it may be when released in large amounts by the posterior pituitary in the third stage of labor. This study provides a physical explanation for the occasional failure of oxytocin induction at term.

T.H. Kirschbaum, M.D.

Effect of Corticotropin-Releasing Factor-binding Protein on Prostaglandin Release From Cultured Maternal Decidua and on Contractile Activity of Human Myometrium *In Vitro*
Petraglia F, Benedetto C, Florio P, et al (Universities of Modena, Torino, and Pisa, Italy; Salk Inst, La Jolla, Calif)
J Clin Endocrinol Metab 80:3073–3076, 1995   1–9

Background.—Corticotropin-releasing factor (CRF) is produced by and acts in human placenta and uterine tissues. Recent research suggests that placental tissues produce CRF-binding protein (CRF-BP), a protein blocking CRF-induced pituitary adrenocorticotropic hormone release. The effects of CRF-BP on prostaglandin release and contractile activity of myometrial strips were investigated.

Methods.—Decidual cells were obtained from 5 healthy women undergoing elective cesarean section at 38 to 40 weeks. Primary cultures were prepared, and mechanical and enzymatic cell dispersions were performed. Experiments were conducted 24 to 28 hours after cell planting. Radioim-

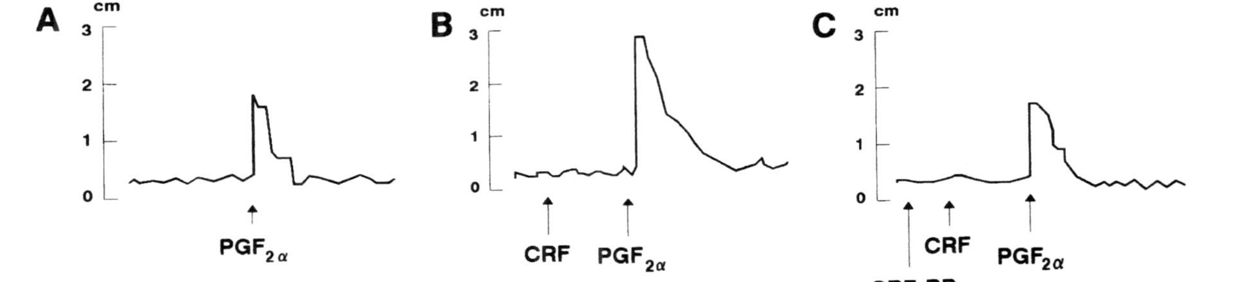

FIGURE 2.—Addition of corticotropin-releasing factor (*CRF*) (10^{-9} mol/L; 40 minutes before) potentiates the prostaglandin F_{2a}-induced (1.4 µmol/L) contractile activity of human myometrial strips in vitro. The preincubation with corticotropin-releasing factor-binding protein (*CRF-BP*) (48 nmol/L; 15 minutes before corticotropin-releasing factor) completely blocks the contractile activity. * $P < 0.01$ vs. prostaglandin F_{2a} and prostaglandin F_{2a}, corticotropin-releasing factor, plus corticotropin-releasing factor-binding protein. (From Petraglia F, Benedetto C, Florio P, et al: Effect of Corticotropin-Releasing Factor-binding Protein on Prostaglandin Release From Cultured Maternal Decidua and on Contractile Activity of Human Myometrium In Vitro. *J Clin Endocrinol Metab* 80:3073-3076, 1995; Copyright The Endocrine Society.)

munoassay was used to measure the prostaglandin E_2 (PGE_2) concentration in cultured medium. Myometrial strips from the upper edge of the uterine incision were also obtained during operative delivery. The strips were dissected free of connective tissue, mounted in a 30-mL 2-chamber organ bath, and connected to a 2-channel isometric smooth muscle transducer.

Findings.—In the presence of CRF, cultured decidual cells significantly increased PGE_2 release. Adding CRF-BP did not affect PGE_2 release significantly. However, it completely reversed the effect of CRF. There was a significant increase in contractile activity when human myometrial strips were incubated in the presence of CRF and $PGF_{2\alpha}$. Preincubation with CRF-BP prevented the increased CRF-induced contractile activity (Fig 2).

Conclusions.—Corticotropin-releasing factor–binding protein can counteract the biological effect of CRF on human pregnancy endometrium and myometrium. This binding protein may be regulatory, playing a role in the local function of uterine tissues during pregnancy.

▶ The role of CRF in reproductive biology continues to expand in the hands of this collaborative research effort between the University of Pisa and the Salk Institute near San Diego. Since last reviewed here,[1] placental CRF has been shown to increase trophoblast cell culture production of adrenocorticotropic (ACTH), to stimulate $PGF_{2\alpha}$ production from decidual cells, to increase myometrial contractility in vitro, and to increase blood flow in perfused placental explants as well as the intact human placenta, acting through nitric oxide production.[2] All of these studies have been carried out in human tissue. This work follows their 1993 demonstration of trophoblast production of CRF-BP, which totally blocks the effect of CRF on placental ACTH production in vitro. Here, using human myometrial strips, they demonstrate that pretreatment with CRF-BP both abolishes the ability of CRF to produce rhythmic uterine contractility and enhances the effect of exogenous $PGF_{2\alpha}$. Since CRF-BP has no effect in the absence of CRF, it's likely that it forms a biologically inactive complex with CRF and speeds its removal from the circulation. Evidence that CRF-BP exists in low levels in preterm labor[3] together with high plasma levels of unbound CRF[4] means this releasing factor–binding protein interaction may play a role in preterm labor and, some think, in preeclampsia as well.

T.H. Kirschbaum, M.D.

References

1. 1995 YEAR BOOK OF OBSTETRICS AND GYNECOLOGY, pp 9–11.
2. Clifton VL, Read MA, Leitch IM, et al: Corticotropin-releasing hormone-induced vasodilation in the human fetal-placental circulation: Involvement of the nitric oxide-cyclic guanosine 3', 5'-monophosphate-mediated pathway. *J Clin Endocrinol Metab* 80:2888–2893, 1995.
3. Perkins AV, Eben F, Wolfe CDA, et al: Plasma measurement of corticotropin-releasing hormone-binding protein in normal and abnormal human pregnancy. *J Endocrinol* 138:149, 1993.

4. Warren WB, Patrick SL, Goland RS: Elevated maternal plasma corticotropin releasing hormone levels in pregnancies complicated by pre-term labour. *Am J Obstet
Gynecol* 166:1198, 1992.

Variability of Continuously Measured Arterial pH and Blood Gas Values in the Near Term Fetal Lamb

Woudstra BR, De Wolf BTHM, Smits TM, et al (Univ Hosp, Groningen, The
Netherlands; Cornell Univ, Ithaca, NY)
Pediatr Res 38:528–532, 1995   1–10

Objective.—Studies in fetal sheep have shown considerable variation in
arterial blood oxygen tension (PaO_2) and oxygen saturation (SaO_2). There
are few quantitative data on arterial pH (pHa) and blood gas variability in

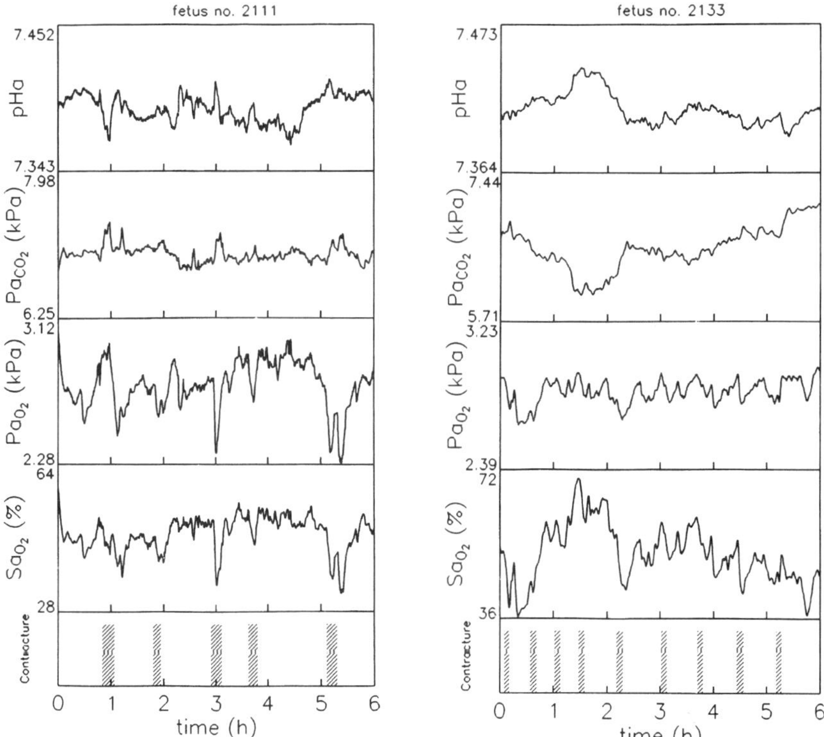

FIGURE 2A, B.—Continuous measurements of arterial blood gas values in 2 of the fetuses, each for
6 hours; signals of pHa, partial pressure of arterial blood carbon dioxide ($PaCo_2$), arterial blood oxygen
tension (Pao_2), oxygen saturation (Sao_2), and uterine contractures (computer-processed uterine electromyogram activity) are shown from **top** to **bottom**. For each quantity, the same calibration of y axis was
used in all experiments. (Courtesy of Woudstra BR, De Wolf BTHM, Smits TM, et al: *Pediatr Res*
38:528–532, 1995.)

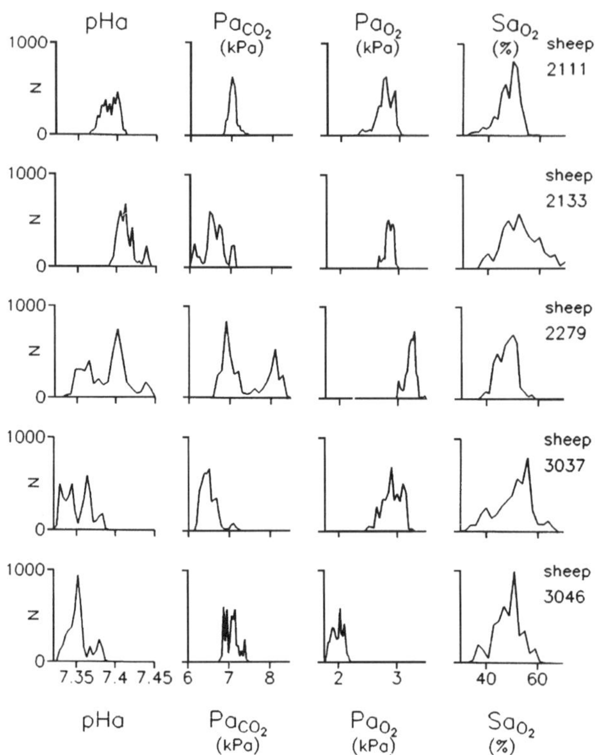

FIGURE 3.—Relative frequency distribution of pHa, partial pressure of arterial blood carbon dioxide (Pa_{CO_2}), arterial blood oxygen tension (Pa_{O_2}), and oxygen saturation (Sa_{O_2}) in the 5 fetal lambs during 6 hours of recording. *Abbreviation: N,* number of samples. (Courtesy of Woudstra BR, De Wolf BTHM, Smits TM, et al: *Pediatr Res* 38:528–532, 1995.)

the fetus. Such information is important to have because umbilical cord blood samples are commonly taken to evaluate the condition of human fetuses. Quantitative data on pHa and blood gas variability during several hours were collected in fetal sheep.

Methods.—A small extracorporeal flow-through cuvette, containing pH and blood gas electrodes and a fiberoptic oximeter probe, was developed to enable continuous measurement of these variables. Carotid artery blood flowed into the cuvette at a constant rate of 2 mL/min before draining into the jugular vein. This system was used to perform 6-hour continuous recordings in 5 chronically instrumented fetal sheep, with gestational ages of 134–137 days. The data were analyzed to quantitatively describe the variability of fetal pHa, partial pressure of arterial blood carbon dioxide ($PaCO_2$), PaO_2, and SaO_2.

Results.—There was wide variation in individual pH and blood gas values, with significant differences in variability between fetuses (Figs 2A and B and 3). Uterine contractions had only a transient effect on fetal arterial blood gas levels, whereas more sustained changes could last as long as 3 hours. Variation coefficients for individual fetuses ranged from 0.1% to 0.4% for pHa, from 1.4% to 7.6% for $PaCO_2$, from 2.5% to 5.5% for PaO_2, and from 3.6% to 7.0% for SaO_2. Values for 5th to 95th percentile intervals ranged from 0.03 to 0.09 for pHa, from 0.3 to 1.6 kPa for $PaCO_2$, from 0.22 to 0.5 kPa for PaO_2, and from 10.5% to 26.0% for SaO_2.

Conclusions.—Significant variations in the arterial blood gas levels of fetal sheep occur during a 6-hour period. This variability is related to uterine contractions and to changes in maternal and fetal activity. It can be reasonably assumed that similar variation occurs in human fetuses. If the changes are of similar magnitude, the clinical value of a single umbilical cord blood sample for measuring pH and blood gas levels may be questionable.

▶ The use of continuous fetal blood gas, pH, and oxyhemoglobin saturation measurements over the past 10 years has demonstrated considerable variability among individuals and in any given individual with time. This is one of the most impressive demonstrations of those observations conducted by a group of expert animal investigators employing great care.

Circulation from the fetal aortic arch returning to the superior vena cava is first accessed through chronic catheter implants, and after 12 days to allow for surgical recovery, a flow-through cuvette is interposed in the circuit with a roller pump ensuring constant flow over the 6 hours during which measurements are recorded. Heparinization is used to prevent clotting. The system allows careful calibration of sensors in vitro before and after studies, and sensor values were collected every 5 seconds over the 6-hour interval. Every 30 minutes, blood samples were withdrawn and checked against independent blood gas instruments to be certain of the absence of drift. Obviously, the work can be done only in experimental studies in animals.

As the frequency distributions of measurements by experimental studies in animals have shown, values differ widely among animals for all measurements. In fetus number 2279, PCO_2 is almost equally often registered at 7 $kPaO_2$ (52.5 mm Hg) and at 8 kPO_2 (60 mm Hg). Similarly, PaO_2 ranges from 15 mm Hg in fetus number 3046 to 22.5 mm Hg in fetus number 3037 as modal values. Figure 2A shows the real-time range of PO_2 from 17.1 to 23.4 mm Hg, with decreases sometimes coincident with low-intensity, nonlabor uterine contractions (contractures) occurring with durations of 3–15 minutes. What all this demonstrates is that cord blood gas values obtained by percutaneous umbilical sampling or after delivery cannot be assumed to represent long-term steady-state measures of fetal respiration without additional evidence.

T.H. Kirschbaum, M.D.

Immunohistochemical Characterization of Placental Nitric Oxide Synthase Expression in Preeclampsia

Ghabour MS, Eis ALW, Brockman DE, et al (Univ of Cincinnati, Ohio; Abbott Labs, Abbott Park, Ill)

Am J Obstet Gynecol 173:687–694, 1995   1–11

Background.—The cause of preeclampsia is unclear, although recent reports have suggested a pathophysiologic role for alterations in the activity of nitric oxide, an endothelial cell–derived vasodilator. In a previous study, positive endothelial nitric oxide synthase immunostaining was found in the endothelium and arteries and veins of the umbilical cord, chorionic plate, and stem villus but not in the endothelium of terminal villous capillaries. Some of the characteristics of the preeclamptic placenta suggest the possibility of decreased trophoblastic endothelial nitric oxide synthase expression. Expression of endothelial nitric oxide synthase was compared in the placenta and umbilical cord of preeclamptic vs. normal pregnancies.

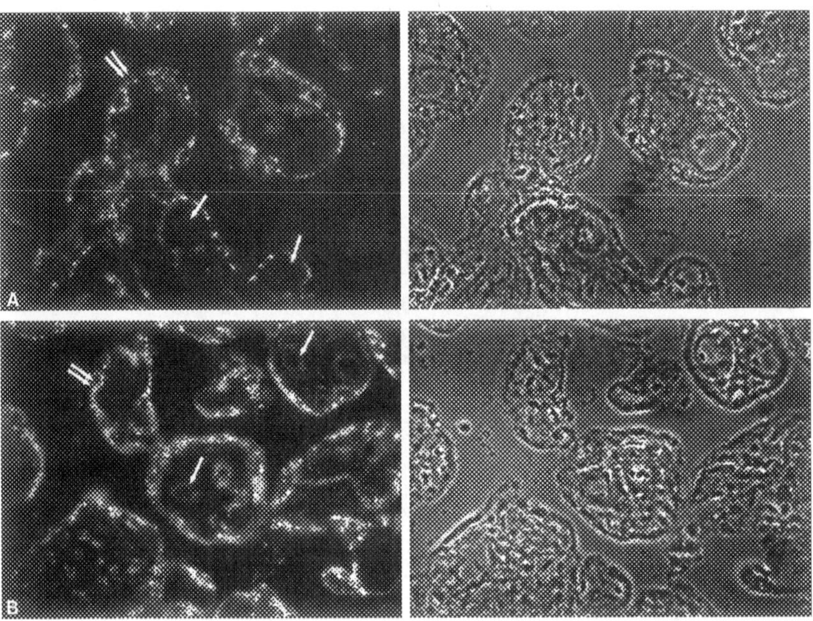

FIGURE 2A and B.—Immunohistochemical localization of endothelial nitric oxide synthase in terminal villi from normal and preeclamptic placentas. Frozen sections from terminal villi (7 µm) were immunostained with antibody against endothelial nitric oxide synthase isoform and fluorescein isothiocyanate–conjugated second antibody. Positive immunostaining is seen in endothelium of terminal vessels (*single arrows*) of preeclamptic (**B**) but not normal (**A**) placenta. Positive staining is seen in syncytiotrophoblast of both placentas (*double arrows*). Each *panel* represents immunofluorescent (**left**) and corresponding phase-contrast (**right**) images; original magnification, ×500. (Courtesy of Ghabour MS, Eis ALW, Brockman DE, et al: *Am J Obstet Gynecol* 173:687–694, 1995.)

Methods.—The placentas and umbilical cords of 3 preeclamptic and 3 normal pregnancies were studied. Pregnancies with possible chorioamnionitis, diabetes mellitus, chromosomal abnormalities, or preexisting maternal hypertension were excluded. The monoclonal endothelial nitric oxide synthase antibody H32 was used for immunostaining of frozen sections of umbilical cords, chorionic plate vessels, and terminal villi.

Results.—The preeclamptic and control groups showed no significant differences in immunostaining of the endothelium of the umbilical cord artery and vein, chorionic plate vessels, and stem villous vessels. However, endothelial nitric oxide synthase immunostaining was observed in the small terminal villous vessels with underlying smooth muscle only in the preeclamptic pregnancies (Figs 2A and B). The syncytiotrophoblast of the preeclamptic placentas showed primarily apical and diffuse immunostaining, compared with a basal and punctate pattern in the normotensive placentas.

Conclusions.—Preeclamptic and normal pregnancies differ in endothelial nitric oxide synthase expression in the terminal villous vessels and in the syncytiotrophoblast. The differences could be caused by vascular changes or damage occurring in the preeclamptic placenta, leading to altered regulation of blood flow in the fetal and placental blood vessels. The differences in placental oxide synthase expression are probably not the primary mediators of preeclampsia.

▶ Nitric oxide (NO) or endothelial-derived relaxation factor *is* produced by endothelial cells as a result of the enzymatic conversion of L-arginine to L-citrulline employing nitric oxide synthase. Diffusing to vascular smooth muscle that adjoins the endothelium, NO increases cyclic guanosine monophosphate, which in turn produces smooth muscle relaxation and vasodilatation. Nitric oxide released into the vessel lumen is almost instantly inactivated by hemoglobin and has its effect only close to its site of production. The distribution and action of this paracrine agent must be investigated in cell culture or tissue media, and this group has previously plotted the distribution of NO synthase in the normal placenta. They find it in the endothelium of the umbilical cord and chorionic plate vessels as well as in the syncytial layer of villus trophoblast. Here, comparison is between normal and preeclamptic third-trimester placentas using a monoclonal antibody specific for the constituitive synthase coupled to a fluorescent-detector antibody. Two differences were noted in preeclamptic placentas compared with the normal. Villus endothelial structures apparently adjoining newly acquired smooth muscle envelopments showed NO synthetase, and the heavy basal deposits of the enzyme in the normal syncytial trophoblast appeared reduced in amount and were located largely apically in trophoblast cells. This work supports the involvement of NO production in preeclampsia, though its precise role can only be conjectured. Perhaps the villus endothelial enzyme is reactive to structural changes resulting from vasoconstriction due to other agents. Perhaps the trophoblastic changes leave the intravillus blood relatively unprotected from the risk of platelet activation and agglutination that NO normally confers. Certainly the role of NO in maintaining low umbilical vessel tone is very important.[1] We will be reading much more about changes in NO metabolism in pathologic pregnancy in the near future.

T.H. Kirschbaum, M.D.

Reference

1. 1995 YEAR BOOK OF OBSTETRICS AND GYNECOLOGY, pp 25–26.

NOS Expression Is Increased in Endothelial Cells Exposed to Plasma From Women With Preeclampsia
Davidge ST, Baker PN, Roberts JM (Univ of Pittsburgh, Pa)
Am J Physiol 269:1106H–1112H, 1995   1–12

Background.—Preeclampsia is a vascular pathology of pregnancy that appears to be caused by endothelial cell functional changes. It has been hypothesized that reduced nitric oxide production by endothelial cells may be responsible for this vascular pathophysiology of preeclampsia. However, endothelial nitric oxide synthase (eNOS) activity was found to increase when endothelial cells were incubated with plasma from women with preeclampsia. The effect of plasma from women with preeclampsia on the transcription and translation of eNOS from cultured epithelial cells was investigated.

Study Group.—Thirty-six nulliparous women were recruited when they were admitted to labor and delivery at Magee-Womens Hospital, Pittsburgh. Half of these women had preeclampsia and half had uncomplicated pregnancies.

Study Design.—Bovine coronary microvascular cells were incubated with plasma from women with preeclampsia and from women with uncomplicated pregnancies. Nitrite production was significantly higher when the plasma was from the preeclampsia group. Immunoblotting suggested that eNOS was significantly increased in cultured endothelial cells exposed to preeclamptic plasma. The level of eNOS messenger RNA was similar in both types of cells. When cells were preincubated with a transcription inhibitor before incubation with plasma, nitrite production was decreased in those cells that had been exposed to the plasma from the women with preeclampsia, so that there was no longer any significant difference between these cells and those incubated with plasma from women with uncomplicated pregnancies.

Conclusions.—When cultured endothelial cells are exposed to plasma from women with preeclampsia, eNOS activity is higher than when these cells are exposed to plasma from women with uncomplicated pregnancies. Factors in the plasma of women with preeclampsia may regulate the expression of eNOS.

▶ Since nitric oxide (NO) is an endothelial cell product that is effective in inducing vasodilatation in vessels adjoining its site of production, and since endothelial injury might be expected to reduce NO production and result in vessel constriction by removing tonic NO production, reduced NO production was a good candidate for a cellular indicator of preeclampsia. Indeed, general inhibition of NO synthesis in pregnant rodents produces a hypertensive pattern resembling in some respects preeclampsia. These Pittsburgh investigators demonstrated that, at least using bovine endothelial cells cultures in vitro, plasma from preeclamptic gravidas increases not decreases NO production by endothelial cells through NO synthetase activity on its arginine precursor. Here the authors illuminate the genetic basis for that increase. They find preeclamptic plasma increases NO synthetase gene transcription and the expression of messenger RNA for the synthetase as promoter sequences of DNA activate RNA polymerase to produce the messenger. Further, translation of messenger RNA by ribosomes, which results in increased synthetase protein, is augmented and is essential to the observed changes in NO activity. There's some hazard in inferring in vivo effects from in vitro studies, but this is further evidence suggesting changes in NO production are not important in the production of the increased peripheral vascular resistance of preeclampsia.

T.H. Kirschbaum, M.D.

2 Maternal Complications in Pregnancy

The Length of the Cervix and the Risk of Spontaneous Premature Delivery

Iams JD, and the National Inst of Child Health and Human Development Maternal Fetal Medicine Unit Network (Ohio State Univ, Columbus; Univ of Alabama, Birmingham; Bowman Gray School of Medicine, Winston-Salem, NC; et al)

N Engl J Med 334:567–572, 1996   2–1

Background.—Previous studies have found a relation between short cervical length as measured by transvaginal ultrasonography and an increased frequency of spontaneous premature delivery. However, the role of the cervix in the pathogenesis of preterm delivery remains controversial. To further examine the relation between cervical length and the risk of preterm delivery, a prospective study was conducted.

Methods.—Transvaginal ultrasonography was performed at 24 weeks' gestation in 2,915 pregnant women attending 10 university-affiliated prenatal clinics; 2,531 of them were available for repeat transvaginal ultrasonography at 28 weeks' gestation. Only women with normal singleton pregnancies were included in the study. Spontaneous preterm delivery was defined as delivery after premature labor or rupture of membranes occurring less than 35 weeks from the last menstrual period.

Results.—Spontaneous preterm delivery occurred in 126 (4.3%) of the women examined at 24 weeks' gestation. The mean cervical length at 24 weeks was 34.0 mm for nulliparous women and 36.1 mm for parous women; the mean cervical length at 28 weeks was 32.6 mm for nulliparous women and 34.5 mm for parous women. Logistic regression analysis revealed that the relative risk of preterm delivery increased as the length of the cervix decreased. The difference in pregnancy duration between women with a cervical length of 25 mm or less and those whose cervical length was more than 25 mm was significant. Furthermore, in a subgroup of 323 women with a previous history of preterm delivery, the duration of the preterm pregnancy correlated with cervical length, as measured by transvaginal ultrasonography during a subsequent pregnancy.

Conclusions.—An inverse relation was found between cervical length during pregnancy, as measured by transvaginal ultrasonography, and the frequency of spontaneous preterm delivery. Transvaginal ultrasonography may prove useful as a screening tool for predicting preterm delivery and selecting candidates for cerclage.

▶ In an elegant study, the product of the Maternal Fetal Medicine Network of the National Institute of Child Health and Human Development, cervical length studied at 2 intervals—between 22 and 24 weeks and 26 to 29 weeks of gestation—was found to be inversely related to the risk of delivery before 35 weeks of pregnancy. Using vaginal ultrasound, it was possible to show that the mean nulliparous cervix was longer than the multiparous cervix at both time intervals, but the mean differences, though statistically significant, were only 2 mm. Similarly, those women whose cervical length was less than the 50th, 25th, or 10th percentile for length at either gestational age had a significantly greater risk of preterm delivery than those above the 75th cervical length percentile. Decreasing cervical length in the interval between the 2 examinations showed a small but statistically significant increased risk of preterm delivery independent of actual cervical length.

However, in a nice demonstration of the difference between statistical significance and clinical utility, the ultrasound measurements of cervical length had little value in predicting preterm labor. Using 5th percentile cervical length to predict preterm labor carried a 74% false positive rate at 24 weeks and an 83% false positive rate at 28 weeks. False negative rates, largely a function of the low 4.3% prevalence of preterm delivery in this group of women with a 16% incidence of previous preterm delivery, were about 4% in all cases. Although a Bishop score equal to or less than 6 with a manual examination of the cervix showed slightly less sensitivity than the ultrasound method, it had a lower false positive rate at both 24 weeks (61%) and 28 weeks (75%). The incidence of funneling of the cervix varied so much among the 5 centers involved as to be useless for predictive purposes. In this case, technology has yielded a set of differences apparently too small to be of clinical usefulness, but it has brought some possible comfort to those of us who still believe in the value of palpating the cervix.

T.H. Kirschbaum, M.D.

Detection of Fetal Fibronectin as a Predictor of Preterm Delivery in High Risk Asymptomatic Pregnancies
Leeson SC, Maresh MJA, Martindale EA, et al (St Mary's Hosp, Manchester, England; Bolton Gen Hosp, England; North Manchester Gen Hosp, England; et al)
Br J Obstet Gynaecol 103:48–53, 1996   2–2

Background.—Preterm delivery is a major source of infant mortality. At best, only 50% of preterm deliveries currently are predicted by previous history of preterm delivery, twin pregnancy, uterine abnormality, low socioeconomic status, or cervical incompetence. Serial vaginal examinations, ultrasound screening for reduced fetal breathing, and screening for recurrent contractions with external tocography have done little to aid predictions of preterm delivery. The aim of this study was to determine whether fetal fibronectin could predict delivery before 37 weeks' gestation among patients at high risk of preterm labor.

Patients and Methods.—Forty-three women at risk of preterm delivery were included in this blind longitudinal study. Sequential high vaginal swabs were obtained every 2 weeks between 24 and 34 weeks of gestation. Fetal fibronectin assays were performed, with positive concentrations defined as equal to or greater than 0.05 µg/mL. Results were analyzed by swab and by patient.

Results.—Sixteen of the 43 women had preterm deliveries, and 27 delivered at term. A complete sequence of 6 swabs was not available in some patients because of missed appointments, poor compliance, and preterm delivery. Differing numbers of swabs therefore were taken at various gestational ages (Fig 1). A total of 168 swabs were assayed. When evaluating prediction of preterm delivery within 14 days of testing, individual fibronectin swabs yielded a sensitivity of 71%, a specificity of 93%, an overall positive predictive value of 31%, and an overall negative predictive value of 99%. The sensitivity of fibronectin swabs in predicting delivery before 37 weeks was 17%, and specificity was 93%, positive predictive value was 50%, and negative predictive value was 73%. Women were considered to have positive results only when final swabs were positive and predicted delivery by 14 days or less. Positive predictive value was 36% and negative predictive value was 97%. Prediction of delivery before 37 weeks in women who had had a positive swab was associated with a sensitivity of 54%, a specificity of 85%, a positive predictive value of 64%, and a negative predictive value of 79%. Women were considered to have positive results when any swab in the sampling sequence was positive. When analyzed by patient, fibronectin swabs did predict delivery within 14 days of testing and before 37 weeks. The best prediction for delivery was within the following 14 days when evaluating the accuracy of predicting delivery from 7 to 28 days after samples were obtained.

Conclusions.—Among women at high risk of preterm delivery, serial fetal fibronectin evaluations performed between 24 and 34 weeks' gesta-

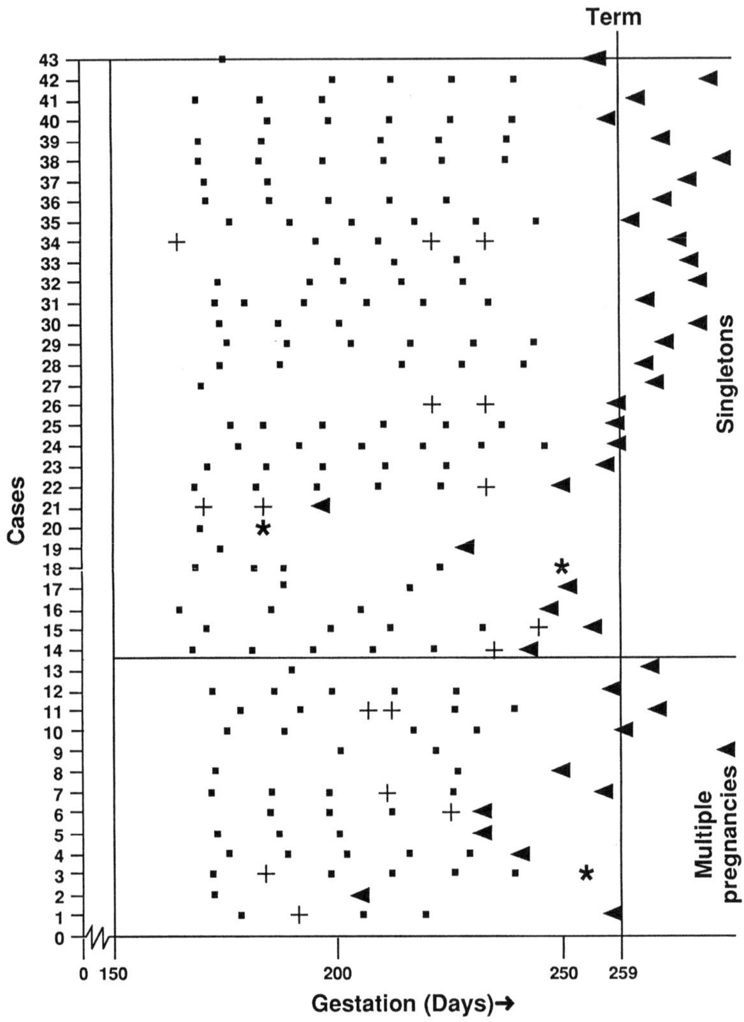

FIGURE 1.—Scattergram to illustrate times of sampling and delivery. *Plus sign*, positive swabs; *solid square*, negative swabs; *triangles*, delivery; *asterisk*, elective preterm delivery. (Courtesy of Leeson SC, Maresh MJA, Martindale EA, et al: Detection of fetal fibronectin as a predictor of preterm delivery in high risk asymptomatic pregnancies. *Br J Obstet Gynaecol* 103:48–53, 1996, Blackwell Science Ltd.)

tion appear to the authors to be a reliable marker for preterm delivery, even among asymptomatic individuals.

▶ This study of the role of cervicovaginal fetal fibronectin determination as a predictor of premature labor in 43 women at risk of preterm delivery by virtue of previous history concludes that the test is of value, but that conclusion is not supported by the data provided. Each patient received roughly 4 determinations over time. Significance testing at each of the 4 testing intervals could not be done because each test was not independent but in fact highly correlated with previous tests in the same women. Put another way, a woman whose fetal fibronectin predicts preterm delivery who delivered within 7 days of the examination would be counted as a success in each of the 4 aggregate time intervals used to draw the authors' conclusions. If this principle of counting successive determinations in each time interval is ignored, the numbers of cases in each interval are insufficient for nonparametric statistical analysis.

Prediction of preterm delivery within 7 days after testing has a false positive rate of 87%. If the test of predictability is delivery within 28 days, the false positive rate drops to 56% at the cost of a 7% false negative rate. The results are similar to Lockwood's discussed here earlier.[1] The high specificity rates here reflect only the low prevalence of preterm delivery, even among women with a 37.5% risk of repeat preterm delivery. If this is the best that can be accomplished with cervicovaginal fetal fibronectin determinations, it is hard to see how it can be recommended for regular use.

T.H. Kirschbaum, M.D.

Reference

1. 1995 Year Book of Obstetrics and Gynecology, pp 66–67.

Reduced Incidence of Preterm Delivery With Metronidazole and Erythromycin in Women With Bacterial Vaginosis
Hauth JC, Goldenberg RL, Andrews WW, et al (Univ of Alabama, Birmingham)
N Engl J Med 333:1732–1736, 1995   2–3

Background.—Bacterial vaginosis approximately doubles the risk of spontaneous preterm delivery. The hypothesis that treatment with antimicrobials during the second trimester would lower the incidence of preterm delivery in women at increased risk of preterm delivery was investigated in a prospective trial.

Methods.—The study group included 624 otherwise healthy women who were at risk of preterm delivery (they had a previous spontaneous preterm delivery or weighed less than 50 kg before pregnancy). Vaginal and cervical cultures and other tests for bacterial vaginosis were done at a mean of 23 weeks' gestation. A 2:1 double-blind randomization was

TABLE 3.—Rates and Risks of Delivery Before 37 Weeks of Gestation Among the Women Assigned to Treatment with Metronidazole and Erythromycin or Placebo

Group of Women	Treatment Group (N = 426)	Placebo Group (N = 190)	P Value	Relative Risk (95% CI)
	no. delivering before 37 wk/total no. (%)			
All studied	110/426 (26)	68/190 (36)	0.01	1.4 (1.1–1.8)
Without bacterial vaginosis	56/254 (22)	26/104 (25)	0.55	1.1 (0.8–1.7)
With bacterial vaginosis	54/172 (31)	42/86 (49)	0.006	1.6 (1.1–2.1)
And previous preterm delivery	47/121 (39)	32/56 (57)	0.02	1.5 (1.1–2.0)
And weight <50 kg before pregnancy	7/51 (14)	10/30 (33)	0.04	2.4 (1.0–5.7)

Note: Eight women were lost to follow-up after randomization.
Abbreviation: CI, confidence interval.
(Courtesy of Hauth JC, Goldenberg RL, Andrews WW, et al: Reduced incidence of preterm delivery with metronidazole and erythromycin in women with bacterial vaginosis. *N Engl J Med* 333:1732–1736, 1995, reprinted by permission of *The New England Journal of Medicine.*)

used—433 women (the treatment group) received metronidazole for 1 week and erythromycin for 2 weeks; 191 women received a placebo. Two to 4 weeks later the tests were repeated. Women with vaginosis then received a second course of metronidazole and erythromycin.

Results.—Significantly fewer of the women in the treatment group (26%) delivered prematurely than women in the placebo group (36%) (Table 3). However, the lower rates of prematurity associated with anti-microbial treatment were only present in the 258 women with bacterial vaginosis (31% delivered prematurely with treatment vs. 49% with placebo; $P = 0.006$). The premature delivery rate was similar in the 358 women without bacterial vaginosis (treatment group, 22%; placebo group, 25%).

Conclusions.—Women with risk factors for premature delivery and bacterial vaginitis are likely to deliver prematurely. Treatment with metronidazole and erythromycin in the second trimester may reduce their risk of premature delivery.

▶ After reading this paper, I am left with lingering questions about the purported benefit in the prevention of preterm labor in this experience compared with the 6 prospective randomized studies using erythromycin with or without ampicillin, which have failed to show any benefit in reducing preterm delivery in women at high risk of threatening preterm labor.[1] Another large prospective NIH-sponsored trial of erythromycin use in treatment of vaginal infection also has failed to show benefit in the prevention of preterm labor.[2, 3]

Perhaps this difference reflects the general excellence in clinical research done by this University of Alabama at Birmingham group. There is strong evidence of an association between bacterial vaginosis and preterm labor, but that does not mean they are causally related. Here the effort is to prove that treating vaginal infection prevents birth before 37 weeks' gestation, adding to the strength and likelihood of a causal relationship between the two. The data suggest that therapy with erythromycin and metronidazole works, but only for women with bacterial vaginosis and not those with other vaginal infections. However, this finding bears exploration by others, and it may be that this drug combination has special merit in this undertaking. Certainly we can ill afford to pass up clues in successful management of this problem in view of our general failure to prevent preterm delivery with existing therapeutics.

However, it is important to note here the relative lack of robustness in the nonparametric statistical inferences used to test for significances of differences in treated and placebo results in Table 3. Remember that if the 95% confidence interval includes a risk ratio of 1.0, the result is not statistically significant. The relative risk values are generally rounded upward—thus, for all studied, 1.38 becomes 1.4; for the subset with bacterial vaginosis, 1.55 becomes 1.6; and for the subset without previous preterm birth, 1.47 becomes 1.5. Although the confidence intervals are also rounded off, note that the lower range of the corresponding 95% confidence interval for these values of relative risk becomes 1.03, 1.05, and 1.02, respectively.

In dealing with confidence ranges so close to unity, it would be essential to express them in 2 decimal places. Although significant in the sense commonly used, it is fair to say that the impact of antibiotic therapy is weak, if present, as shown in these data. Remember that selection of the $P = 0.05$ value means the chances of some or larger differences being derived from the data are 5% in the absence of any real difference in fact. These concerns should lead readers to accept the authors' conclusions with caution.

T.H. Kirschbaum, M.D.

References

1. *Am J Obstet Gynecol* 168:1239, 1993.
2. 1992 Year Book of Obstetrics and Gynecology, pp 78–79.
3. *Focus & Opinion: Obstetrics and Gynecology* 1:416–417, 1995.

Antimicrobial Therapy in Expectant Management of Preterm Premature Rupture of the Membranes
Mercer BM, Arheart KL (Univ of Tennessee, Memphis)
Lancet 346:1271–1279, 1995

2–4

Background.—Isolated case reports suggest that antimicrobial treatment may be effective in preterm premature rupture of the membranes (pPROM) before 37 weeks' gestation. A number of clinical trials have also been done to assess the efficacy of this treatment. To determine the impact of antimicrobial therapy and fetal outcome during expectant management of pPROM, the available prospective clinical trials were reviewed.

Methods.—Three databases were searched: MEDLINE, from 1966 to 1994; Excerpta Medica, from 1972 to 1994; and the Cochrane database of systemic reviews. Unpublished data from a randomized, placebo-controlled clinical trial of ceftizoxime were also reviewed. Studies selected for

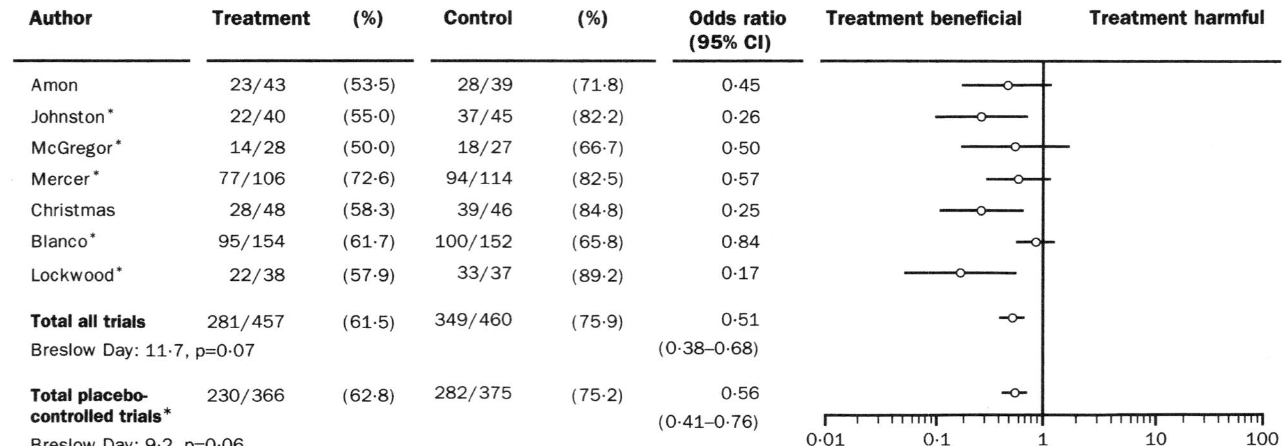

Author	Treatment	(%)	Control	(%)	Odds ratio (95% CI)
Amon	23/43	(53·5)	28/39	(71·8)	0·45
Johnston*	22/40	(55·0)	37/45	(82·2)	0·26
McGregor*	14/28	(50·0)	18/27	(66·7)	0·50
Mercer*	77/106	(72·6)	94/114	(82·5)	0·57
Christmas	28/48	(58·3)	39/46	(84·8)	0·25
Blanco*	95/154	(61·7)	100/152	(65·8)	0·84
Lockwood*	22/38	(57·9)	33/37	(89·2)	0·17
Total all trials	281/457	(61·5)	349/460	(75·9)	0·51 (0·38–0·68)
Breslow Day: 11·7, p=0·07					
Total placebo-controlled trials*	230/366	(62·8)	282/375	(75·2)	0·56 (0·41–0·76)
Breslow Day: 9·2, p=0·06					

FIGURE 1.—Impact on delivery at 7 days of antimicrobial therapy after premature rupture of the membranes. *Abbreviation: Cl,* confidence interval. (Courtesy of Mercer BM, Arheart KL: Antimicrobial therapy in expectant management of preterm premature rupture of the membranes. *Lancet* 346:1271–1279, 1995. © by The Lancet Ltd.)

review were randomized, controlled trials of systemic antimicrobial treatment for prolongation of gestation in nonlaboring women after pPROM.

Data Synthesis.—Antimicrobial treatment after pPROM was associated with a decrease in the number of women delivering within 1 week and in the diagnosis of maternal morbidity, including chorioamnionitis and postpartum infection. In addition, fetal diagnoses of confirmed sepsis, pneumonia, and intraventricular hemorrhage were less common. In a separate analysis of the 6 placebo-controlled trials, the odds of pregnancy prolongation, chorioamnionitis, neonatal sepsis, postpartum infection, positive infant blood cultures, and pneumonia were similar or improved (Fig 1).

Conclusions.—Antimicrobial treatment in the expectant management of pPROM prolongs pregnancy and reduces the diagnosis of maternal and infant morbidity. Additional research should focus on determining optimal antimicrobial therapy, increasing pregnancy prolongation, and enhancing corticosteroid therapy for the induction of pulmonary maturity after pPROM.

▶ Since positive placental culture is regularly strongly related to premature birth, it's reasonable to employ antibiotic therapy prophylactically where premature labor appears truly imminent. Where evidence for impending preterm labor is simply threatened preterm labor, antibiotics do not influence outcome, largely due to the high rate of false diagnosis of labor.[1] However, the diagnosis of premature rupture of membranes can be made unequivocably, and the event is strongly related to premature labor. This review article nicely summarizes the evidence for benefit as it is has been reviewed here earlier.[2-5] Meta-analysis is applied to 13 studies with the assumption that differences among studies with respect to antibiotic regimen, use of steroids and tocolytics will be randomly distributed and not confound the outcomes. Unfortunately, inclusion of data incompletely published in one case[6] complicates the analysis, but that study appears not to support favorable results of antibiotic therapy and has no impact on the overall interpretation of this study. Including only the 6 studies with matched placebo controls, improvement was seen in prolonging latency between rupture of membranes and onset of labor, in reduction of clinical evidence of chorioamnionitis and of confirmed newborn sepsis. Using all studies, including those with unblinded but concurrent controls, antibiotic therapy was associated with a decrease in maternal postpartum infection rate, newborn pneumonia incidence, and occurrence of newborn intraventricular hemorrhage (IVH). Since brain scans were not routinely performed, the benefit in terms of IVH is possibly underreported. No improvement in mortality was seen. Nonetheless, the usefulness of antibiotic therapy in premature preterm rupture of membranes seems well established.

T.H. Kirschbaum, M.D.

References

1. Kirschbaum T: *Am J Obstet Gynecol* 168:1239, 1993.
2. 1990 YEAR BOOK OF OBSTETRICS AND GYNECOLOGY, pp 33–34, 209–210.

3. 1992 Year Book of Obstetrics and Gynecology, pp 117–118.
4. 1993 Year Book of Obstetrics and Gynecology, pp 31–33.
5. 1995 Year Book of Obstetrics and Gynecology, pp 185–186.
6. Blanco J, Iams J, Artal R, et al: Multicenter double-blind prospective random trial of ceftizoxime vs. placebo in women with preterm premature ruptured membranes (pPROM). *Am J Obstet Gynecol* 168:378, 1993.

Antibiotic Treatment in Preterm Premature Rupture of Membranes and Neonatal Morbidity: A Metaanalysis

Egarter C, Leitich H, Karas H, et al (Univ of Vienna)
Am J Obstet Gynecol 174:589–597, 1996   2–5

Background.—Preterm premature rupture of the fetal membranes occurs in a substantial portion of preterm births. Although there is some evidence that infection plays a role in preterm premature rupture of membranes, studies with significant statistical power to demonstrate an effect of antibody treatment are not available. A meta-analysis was done to determine the effects of prophylactic antibiotics on neonatal morbidity.

Methods.—In January 1995, 18 medical databases were searched for literature on preterm premature rupture of fetal membranes and antibiotics. To evaluate the effects of antibiotics alone, studies including tocolytics or corticosteroids were excluded.

Findings.—Seven clinical trials, published between 1989 and 1994, that met the inclusion criteria were found in the databases. These trials included 657 patients. Meta-analysis demonstrated that prophylactic antibiotic therapy significantly reduced the risk of neonatal sepsis and of intraventricular hemorrhage. There was no significant effect of antibiotic therapy on respiratory distress syndrome, necrotizing enterocolitis, or on overall mortality.

Conclusions.—This meta-analysis found that prophylactic antibiotic therapy after preterm premature rupture of membranes significantly reduced the risk of sepsis and intraventricular hemorrhage among newborns. This suggests that antibiotics are useful in the treatment of preterm premature rupture of fetal membranes.

▶ Meta-analysis is a statistical technique in which data from similar, but not identical, independent studies are pooled in the hope that the assumption of homogeneity and an increase in the number of cases studied might bring into statistical significance observations previously lacking significance because of limited numbers. The difficulty arises from the inevitable differences in experimental design and observations that do in fact exist. The principal problem rests not with the generation of statements of statistical significance, but with deciding what they mean in view of the arguable assumptions of homogeneity. In that respect, it might be said the more meta-analysis in this topic area the better, and this study serves nicely to complement the article reviewed previously (Abstract 2–4). A third meta-analysis[1] was aimed primarily at the role of corticosteroids and tocolytics in the treatment of preterm premature rupture of membranes and did not yield clear conclusions regarding antibiotics. In contrast to the University of Tennessee study (Abstract 2–4), this study excludes those studies in which tocolytics or steroids were used to avoid the implicit assumption of randomness in the distribution of those covariants necessary to the Memphis study. Additionally, these University of Vienna investigators used nonparametric statistics to test for homogeneity, discarding those which failed to meet that test. The concordance of results between the 2 analyses is encouraging. Both studies found antibiotic use associated with a decrease in the incidence of neonatal sepsis and intraventricular hemorrhage. The issue of delay in the interval between rupture of membranes and delivery is stated but the data not shown. Unlike the study by Mercer et al. (Abstract 2–4) these investigators did not have outcome data that enabled them to demonstrate an impact on chorioamnionitis or neonatal pneumonia. In both studies, no impact of antibiotics on neonatal mortality, the incidence of respiratory distress syndrome, or of necrotizing enterocolitis was seen. Even to a skeptic, the sum of these 2 studies demonstrates that antibiotics not only delay the interval from rupture of membranes to the onset of labor, but also have substantive newborn benefits as well.

T.H. Kirschbaum, M.D.

Reference

1. Ohlsson A: Treatments of preterm premature rupture of the membrane: A meta-analysis. *Am J Obstet Gynecol* 160:890, 1989.

Endothelial Cell Proliferation Is Suppressed by Plasma But Not Serum From Women With Preeclampsia
Smárason AK, Sargent IL, Redman CWG (Univ of Oxford, England)
Am J Obstet Gynecol 174:787–793, 1996   2–6

Objective.—Research evidence suggests that a circulating endothelial cell "toxic" factor may be involved in preeclampsia. This placenta-derived factor could contribute to maternal endothelial cell disturbances through suppression of endothelial cell proliferation. The toxic factor most likely arises from the syncytiotrophoblast. Endothelial cell inhibitory activity was sought in the serum and plasma of women with preeclampsia.

Methods.—Serum and plasma studies were done in 20 women with proteinuric preeclampsia and in matched pregnant and nonpregnant controls. Endothelial cell proliferation assays were done to assess endothelial cell inhibitory activity. The placental origin of the inhibitory factor was investigated by assessing recovery of endothelial cell inhibitory activity from syncytiotrophoblast microvesicles that were added to male blood and then prepared as plasma or serum.

Results.—Initial studies showed no inhibition of endothelial cell proliferation by serum samples from women with preeclampsia. However, subsequent studies found that plasma specimens from preeclamptic

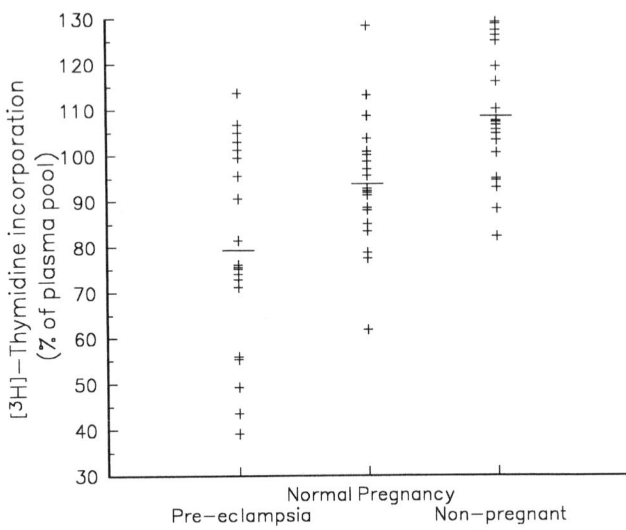

FIGURE 5.—Effect of 20% peripheral vein plasma from women with preeclampsia, matched pregnant controls, and nonpregnant controls on endothelial cell proliferation (tritiated thymidine incorporation). *Long horizontal bars,* mean for each group. (Courtesy of Smárason AK, Sargent IL, Redman CWG: Endothelial cell proliferation is suppressed by plasma but not serum from women with preeclampsia. *Am J Obstet Gynecol* 174:787–793, 1996.)

women produced significantly greater suppression of endothelial cell growth at 20% dilution than did plasma specimens from control women (Fig 5). When syncytiotrophoblast microvesicles were added to blood, their inhibitory activity could be recovered from plasma but not from blood.

Conclusions.—A placenta-derived factor seems to cause maternal endothelial dysfunction in women with preeclampsia. Plasma samples from women with preeclampsia have endothelial cell inhibitory activity, whereas serum samples do not. The next step is to determine whether the endothelial cell inhibitory factor on the syncytiotrophoblast microvillous membrane and in the plasma of preeclamptic women is, in fact, the same and whether the plasma factor does come from the placenta.

▶ Hearkening back to the days when pregnancy induced hypertension was called toxemia of pregnancy, the search for a blood borne substance toxic to maternal endothelial cells continues, and this is the most recent and interesting approach. The early observation of Roberts et al. that serum from preeclamptic women inhibits endothelial cells proliferation has largely been discarded for lack of confirmation.[1] This Oxford group has demonstrated that a preparation of microvillus cell membranes from the placental syncytiotrophoblast, with or without coincident preeclampsia, inhibits but does not block endothelial cell proliferation in cell culture. It seems to disrupt endothelial cell intercommunications in culture without actually producing death of cells. The authors explore the proposition that syncytiotrophoblast fragments are shed more readily in preeclampsia than in normal pregnancy,[2] exerting their effect on endothelium, certainly in pulmonary and perhaps also the systemic vasculature. Implicit is the assumption that this injury is enough to cause vasoconstriction. The hypothesis requires blood transportation of the inhibitory factor, which they find not in serum, but in plasma from women with preeclampsia in larger amounts than in normotensive pregnancy. The experimental observation here is inhibition of tritiated thymidine uptake in endothelial cell cultures in decreasing rank order among preeclamptic women, normal pregnant women, and nonpregnant women. Generous overlap was noted among those 3 groups, and the authors do not claim statistical significance in this observation. They propose the trophoblastic fragments may be enmeshed and inactivated in fibrin, or the inhibitory factor destroyed in serum by the clotting factors activated in the coagulation cascade necessary to convert plasma to serum. The search for a hypertension "toxin" is sure to continue and this is the most recent chapter in that enterprise.

T.H. Kirschbaum, M.D.

References

1. 1990 YEAR BOOK OF OBSTETRICS AND GYNECOLOGY, pp 29–31.
2. Sorget IL, et al: *Ann NY Acad Sci* 731–754, 1994.

Altered Circulating Thrombomodulin Levels and Antithrombin-III Activity as Evidence for Varied Activation of the Coagulation Cascade in Severely Versus Mildly Pre-eclamptic Pregnancies
Hsu C-D, Johnson TRB, Hong S-F, et al (Johns Hopkins Univ, Baltimore, Md; Yale Univ, New Haven, Conn)
J Matern Fetal Invest 5:140–143, 1995   2–7

Introduction.—Recent studies have implicated endothelial cell injury or activation in the pathogenesis of preeclampsia, a disorder characterized by activation of the coagulation cascade. Changes in 2 natural anticoagulant factors, thrombomodulin (TM) (an endothelial cell surface glycoprotein) and antithrombin III (AT-III) (synthesized by the liver and circulated systemically), were studied in relation to the activation of the coagulation cascade in patients with mild and severe preeclampsia.

Methods.—Thirty patients with preeclamptic pregnancies and 30 normotensive healthy pregnant patients were matched in the third trimester for maternal age, gestational age, parity, and race. Twenty women had mild preeclampsia and 10 had severe preeclampsia. Blood samples were drawn from all participating patients and were analyzed for TM with a 2-site enzyme-linked immunosorbent assay and for AT-III activity with a Microlatex particle–mediated immunoassay.

Results.—Compared with their matched controls, the patients with severe, but not mild, preeclampsia had significantly higher levels of circulating TM and lower levels of AT-III activity. In patients with severe, but not mild, preeclampsia, circulating TM levels correlated inversely with AT-III activity and positively with serum creatinine levels.

Conclusions.—Differing changes in AT-III activity and serum TM levels and the inverse correlation between them suggest that women with severe preeclampsia have a different degree of coagulant activation resulting from a different degree of vascular endothelial damage.

▶ This study simultaneously offers confirmation of endothelial injury in severe preeclampsia and provides a theoretical explanation for the disturbance in the relationship between procoagulants and anticoagulants noted in the form of coagulopathy in 20% to 30% of preeclamptics. Thrombomodulin is an endothelial cell surface glycoprotein capable of binding thrombin in a complex that is in turn capable of converting protein C, a vitamin K–dependent product of the liver, together with its cofactor protein S, to an activated form. The activated protein C in turn is capable of inhibiting procoagulant factors V_a and VIII_a. In that way, the TM complex inhibits thrombin production and clotting.

Thrombomodulin's presence in increased amounts in the blood of severe but not mild preeclamptics indicates at once its increased circulatory release by damaged endothelium, the likely progenitor of preeclampsia, and its ability to inhibit the coagulation cascade, which may result in disseminated intravascular clotting. This is important because endothelial injury releases tissue factor (thromboplastin or factor III) from endothelial cells and perivascular fibroblasts that, left unopposed, activates the generation of thrombin and conversion of fibrinogen into endofibrin.

Antithrombin III is a product of the liver that, especially in the presence of heparin, inactivates several activated procoagulant factors (VIIa, IXa, Xa, XIa) and, through prevention of thrombin formation, acts as an anticoagulant. It was this property of heparin that led the late Dr. Duncan Reid to advocate heparin in states of consumptive coagulopathy due to disseminated clotting, a risky proposition since it depended on sufficient amounts of AT-III, a very labile molecule in states of coagulopathy. In both mild and severe preeclampsia, AT-III was reduced in concentration in these preeclamptics, presumably consumed in its combination with free thrombin and further inhibited in its production in the face of impaired renal function. Now that thrombin, AT-III, and TM can all be measured and are available for administration, it's possible that AT-III might be employed to counterbalance the surplus thrombin release in severe preeclampsia, which has the capacity to lead to disseminated intravascular clotting, consumptive coagulopathy, and severe hemorrhage in those patients.

T.H. Kirschbaum, M.D.

A Comparison Between the Haemodynamic Effects of Oral Nifedipine and Intravenous Dihydralazine in Patients With Severe Pre-eclampsia

Visser W, Wallenburg HCS (Erasmus Univ, Rotterdam, The Netherlands)
J Hypertens 13:791–795, 1995

2–8

Purpose.—Pregnant patients with severe preeclampsia usually receive hydralazine or dihydralazine for rapid reduction of blood pressure. How-

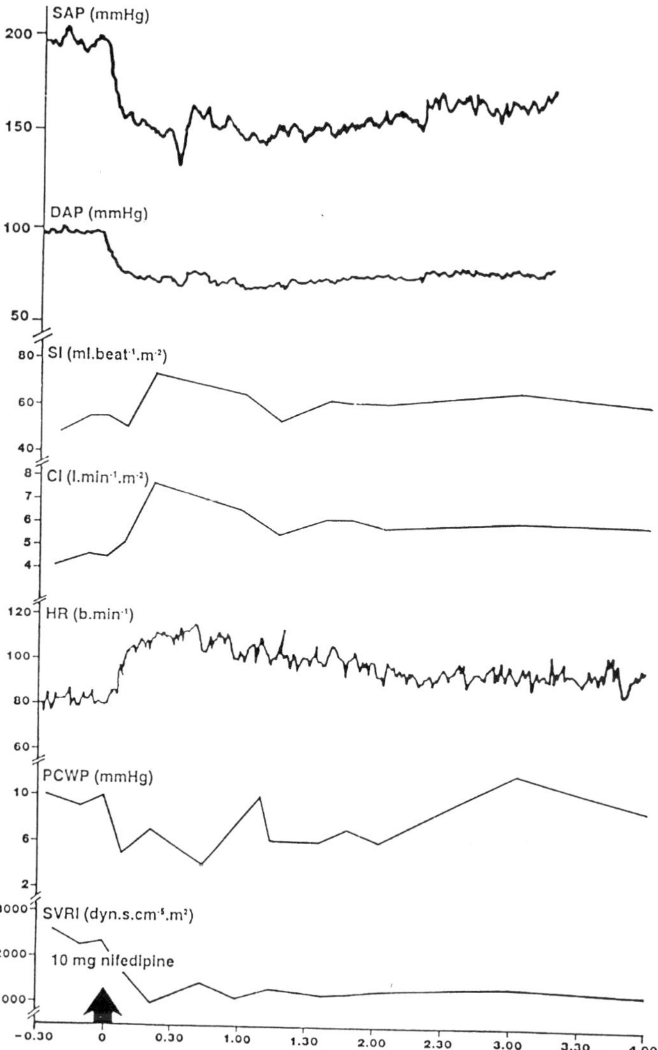

FIGURE 1.—Example of the hemodynamic effects of nifedipine in a preeclamptic patient. At time 0, 10 mg of nifedipine was given. *Abbreviations: SAP,* systolic intra-arterial pressure; *DAP,* diastolic intra-arterial pressure; *SI,* stroke volume index; *CI,* cardiac index; *HR,* heart rate; *PCWP,* pulmonary capillary wedge pressure; *SVRI,* systemic vascular resistance index. (Courtesy of Visser W, Wallenburg HCS: *J Hypertens* 13:791–795, 1995.)

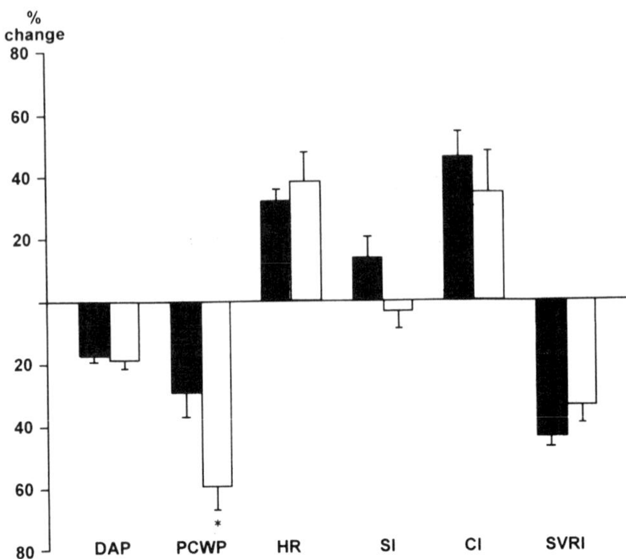

FIGURE 2.—Comparison between the maximum change in hemodynamic values obtained in 10 patients (*filled bars*) with oral nifedipine and 10 patients (*open bars*) with IV dihydralazine. Values are expressed as means ± standard error of the mean. *P < 0.02 vs. nifedipine. *Abbreviations: DAP,* diastolic intra-arterial pressure; *PCWP,* pulmonary capillary wedge pressure; *HR,* heart rate; *SI,* stroke volume index; *CI,* cardiac index; *SVRI,* systemic vascular resistance index. (Courtesy of Visser W, Wallenburg HCS: *J Hypertens* 13:791–795, 1995.)

ever, the onset of action of these drugs is 20–30 minutes after IV administration, the effect on blood pressure is variable, and there is a risk of severe hypotension and hypovolemic shock. The calcium antagonist nifedipine is a potent and rapid-acting vasodilator that has been recommended for use for hypertensive emergencies in pregnant and nonpregnant patients alike. Single-dose oral nifedipine was examined as an alternative to IV hydralazine in pregnant women with severe preeclampsia.

Methods.—Twenty patients with severe preeclampsia in 1 high-risk obstetric unit were prospectively studied. All were at 27–35 weeks' gestation and had normal cardiac filling pressures without fetal distress. After placement of a pulmonary artery thermodilution catheter and a radial artery line, 10 patients chewed a 10-mg capsule of nifedipine and 10 received dihydralazine by IV infusion, 1–3 mg/hr. The patients' arterial pressures, heart rate, cardiac output, and pulmonary capillary blood pressure were measured before and after this treatment. The fetuses underwent continuous cardiotocographic monitoring.

Results.—The characteristics of the 2 groups were similar on admission. Patients receiving nifedipine showed a significant decline in arterial blood pressure starting 4–5 minutes after oral administration. Blood pressures reached their lowest point at 10–15 minutes and then remained stable for 2–4 hours (Fig 1). Nifedipine and dihydralazine yielded comparable reductions in arterial blood pressure and systemic vascular resistance and similar increases in heart rate and cardiac output. Patients receiving dihydralazine had a significantly greater decrease in pulmonary capillary wedge pressure (Fig 2). None of the patients in the nifedipine group showed signs of fetal distress, compared with 5 of those in the dihydralazine group.

Conclusions.—From a hemodynamic viewpoint, nifedipine appears to be a useful drug for the treatment of hypertensive emergencies in pregnant women. It can be given orally, has an almost immediate onset of action, offers potent selective vasodilation, improves maternal circulation, and has no adverse effects on uteroplacental circulation. The use of nifedipine should be studied in preeclamptic patients with volume contraction, particularly those with severely growth-retarded fetuses.

▶ Though the calcium channel blocking agent nifedipine has shown a few inexplicable instances of fetal death associated with acidosis in pregnant animals in experimental studies and there are concerns regarding its use in hypertensive nonpregnant patients, it is a smooth orally active agent with a relatively predictable and significant effect on blood pressure. In this study, it proved at least equally effective as hydralazine in lowering systemic vascular resistance, increasing cardiac output, and reducing cardiac preload. Note that this unit performs volume expansion in severe preeclamptics when pulmonary catheter wedge pressure is less than 8 mm Hg[1-3] to prevent marked decreases in blood pressure with use of antihypertensive agents. This was required in 4 of 10 women with severe preeclampsia receiving nifedipine and was executed in none of the women receiving hydralazine. Note that the increased cardiac index was due solely to increased heart rate with hydralazine, but patients receiving nifedipine also benefited by an increase in stroke volume. Five of 10 women treated with hydralazine showed decreased heart rate variability and late decelerations in fetal heart rate tracings obtained after administration of this agent. This suggests, in a series too small for interpretation of the finding, that some of the hydralazine recipients may well, like 40% of those receiving nifedipine, have benefited by plasma volume expansion for their hypovolemia. Despite the advantages of the use of this drug, there continue to be reservations that obstetricians should weigh carefully before using nifedipine for the care of their hypertensive pregnant patients.

T.H. Kirschbaum, M.D.

References

1. 1991 Year Book of Obstetrics and Gynecology, pp 39–41.
2. 1993 Year Book of Obstetrics and Gynecology, pp 86–90.
3. *Focus & Opinion: Obstetrics and Gynecology,* 1(5):9, 1995.

Effect of Calcium Supplementation on Pregnancy-Induced Hypertension and Preeclampsia: A Meta-Analysis of Randomized Controlled Trials

Bucher HC, Guyatt GH, Cook RJ, et al (McMaster Univ, Hamilton, Ont, Canada; Univ of Waterloo, Kitchener, Ont, Canada)
JAMA 275:1113–1117, 1996   2–9

Background.—A recent meta-analysis concluded that calcium supplementation reduced the proportion of women with new-onset hypertension and preeclampsia in pregnancy. However, that analysis was limited in its assessment of the studies' validity, and in its exploration of the reasons the findings varied. Because new randomized trials of calcium supplementation in pregnancy have been reported since that meta-analysis was published, a new systemic overview was conducted.

Data Sources.—Publications were identified through a MEDLINE and EMBASE search of studies published between 1966 and 1994. The authors of eligible trials were contacted to ensure data accuracy and completeness. Fourteen randomized studies were included in the analysis, with a total of 2,459 women enrolled in these studies. Unpublished trials were also identified with the help of the eligible trial authors.

Data Synthesis.—Differences in blood pressure changes between patients receiving calcium and those in control groups were weighted by the inverse of the variance. The pooled analysis demonstrated a -5.4 mm Hg decrease in systolic blood pressure and a -3.44 mm Hg decline in diastolic pressure. Compared with women given placebo, women given calcium supplementation had a 0.38 odds ratio for the development of preeclampsia.

Conclusions.—Systolic and diastolic blood pressures, as well as preeclampsia, are reduced by calcium supplementation during pregnancy. Calcium supplementation should be considered for pregnant women at risk of preeclampsia. However, more studies are needed to establish the effect of calcium on maternal and fetal morbidity.

▶ This meta-analysis by a group of McMaster University scientists follows the application of that technique to a series of studies of the effect of 1–2 g per day of calcium supplement on nonpregnant individuals. There they found significant reduction in systolic blood pressure in the randomized patients receiving calcium supplementation, an average of -1.27 mm Hg. No significant change in diastolic blood pressure appeared to result and the authors concluded the effects were too small to support recommending calcium supplementation to patients with mild hypertension. Here, they find the results sufficiently compelling to recommend 1.5–2 g of calcium supplement per day in pregnancy in an effort to prevent preeclampsia. The inevitable problems of meta-analysis in aggregating heterogeneous studies, as though there were no differences among them, appear somewhat larger here than in the earlier publication. Strong evidence for data heterogeneity was found for both systolic and diastolic blood pressure and a number of covariants were found, especially in the diastolic blood pressure data.

As before, unpublished data that had not been peer reviewed were included for analysis by the investigators. Most important, observer blinding to test vs. placebo status was not required for entry. This increased the likelihood that observer bias played a role in the conclusions. Two preliminary reports were included, in addition to 3 studies where blood pressure measurements were deemed inadequate but "...reported data about adverse outcomes that we did include" was entered. What this means is unclear. Criteria for the diagnosis of preeclampsia, not a trivial matter, are not described. A pooled estimate of reduced risk of preeclampsia of 0.3 seems large for the relatively small reductions in mean blood pressure identified here. These data have been used to justify a prospective randomized trial of calcium supplement designed to evaluate morbidity outcome variables. Perhaps that will bolster the recommendations made here with what seems to be arguable evidence.

T.H. Kirschbaum, M.D.

HLA-G Deletion Polymorphism and Pre-Eclampsia/Eclampsia
Humphrey KE, Harrison GA, Cooper DW, et al (Macquarie Univ, Sydney, Australia; Univ of New South Wales, Sydney, Australia; Royal Women's Hosp, Carlton, Australia; et al)
Br J Obstet Gynaecol 102:707–710, 1995   2–10

Objective.—The placenta has been implicated in the pathogenesis of preeclampsia/eclampsia because of the presence of abnormal trophoblastic implantation. Placental trophoblastic cells usually block highly polymorphic class I HLA genes that prompt graft rejection, and HLA-G is suspected as the gene for eclampsia. The relationship between HLA-G polymorphism and pedigrees with eclampsia/preeclampsia was studied.

Methods.—The study included 196 individuals, including 58 women, 24 of whom had had severe preeclampsia and 5 of whom had had eclampsia in their first pregnancy. From 10 multicase pedigrees, there were 13 firstborn children, 21 husbands, and 46 relatives of patients who had had eclampsia/preeclampsia. Controls were 25 normal pregnant women, 15 husbands of normal pregnant women, and 47 staff and students. Genotypes for HLA-G were determined.

Results.—No significant differences in HLA-G genotypes were found in the 7 groups.

Conclusion.—No association between the presence of the HLA-G genotype and the occurrence of eclampsia/preeclampsia was found.

▶ At least a major part of the immune tolerance afforded the fetal allograft is the suppression of the usual major histocompatibility antigens, HLA-A, -B, and -C, which, if such paternal antigens were expressed by the fetus and/or its placenta, would likely evoke a rejection reaction by the mother. Instead, a unique antigen class, HLA-G, is expressed by the placenta from among the options in the major histocompatibility complex contained in chromosome 6. Since it was thought to have the same structure among different individuals (monomorphism), its HLA-G expression prevents the discernment of non-self by the gravidas' cellular immune system. However, some HLA-G polymorphisms have been identified, among them a 14–base pair deletion in exon 8 of the HLA-G gene that is untranslated during gene expression since it lies downstream from 2 gene messages (stop codons) that terminate translation before exon 8 is reached. The question explored here is whether this gene deletion allows host immunoreactivity to paternal antigens to take place, resulting in maternal endothelial injury and, thus, preeclampsia. Ten pedigrees, 7 containing the atypical HLA-G gene, were studied, and neither linkage analysis nor gene frequency analysis in parents or fetuses supported the proposition that the HLA-G deletion was a "preeclampsia gene." However, the possibility of an isolated fetal gene defect as causative is not excluded and needs to be explored. That is suggested by a small group of monozygotic twins who were reported to have been discordant for preeclamptic pregnancy.[1] Other mutations in the HLA gene complex need to be explored in the search for a gene locus for preeclampsia. In the future, you will certainly be reading more about this approach to understanding the genetic basis for preeclampsia.

T.H. Kirschbaum, M.D.

Reference

1. Thornton JG, Onwude JL: Pre-eclampsia discordance among identical twins. *BMJ* 303:1241, 1991.

Maternal Serum Thromboxane B$_2$ Reduction Versus Pregnancy Outcome in a Low-Dose Aspirin Trial
Hauth JC, Goldenberg RL, Parker CR Jr, et al (Univ of Alabama, Birmingham)
Am J Obstet Gynecol 173:578–584, 1995   2–11

Background.—Low-dose acetylsalicylate has been reported to reduce the incidence of preeclampsia in selected populations. To determine whether this beneficial effect could be detected in a large unselected sample of pregnant women who ingested low-dose aspirin, a marker of study compliance, maternal serum thromboxane B$_2$ (TxB$_2$), was chosen and assessed.

Methods.—Six hundred six women with singleton gestations were randomly assigned at 24 weeks to take either 60 mg of aspirin or placebo. To determine compliance, maternal serum TxB$_2$ was measured at baseline, at 29 to 31 weeks, at 34 to 36 weeks, and at delivery. After delivery, patients were categorized in a blinded fashion as having either more or less than a longitudinal twofold reduction in TxB$_2$ from the baseline level.

Results.—Of the original 606 participants, 558 had sufficient TxB$_2$ assessments to be used for the study. In the aspirin group, 79% of the

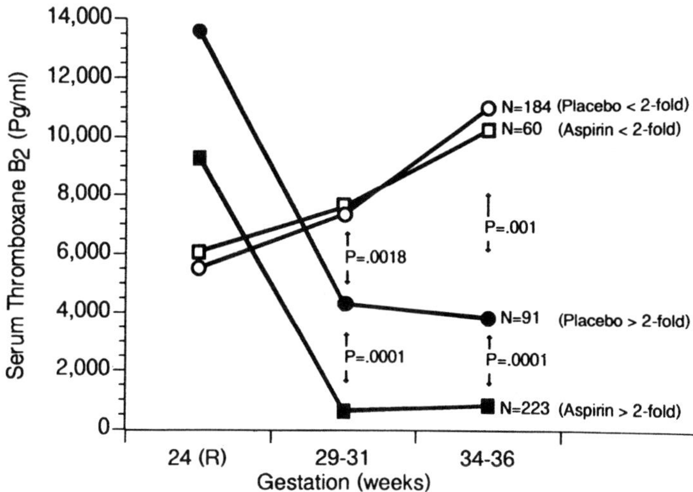

FIGURE 2.—Median maternal serum thromboxane B_2 levels in women assigned to either aspirin or placebo who had less than longitudinal twofold reduction or twofold or greater reduction from randomization (R) values at 24 weeks' gestation. (Courtesy of Hauth JC, Goldenberg RL, Parker CR Jr, et al: *Am J Obstet Gynecol* 173:578–584, 1995.)

women had a twofold or greater reduction in TxB$_2$ levels, whereas in the placebo group, only 33% had a twofold or greater reduction (Fig 2). Women, from either group, who had a twofold or greater reduction in TxB$_2$ levels had infants with higher birth weights and had less preeclampsia and fewer preterm deliveries than did women without the twofold reduction in TxB$_2$ levels (Fig 3).

Conclusions.—Women with a twofold or greater longitudinal reduction in maternal serum TxB$_2$ levels, a marker for compliance in a low-dose

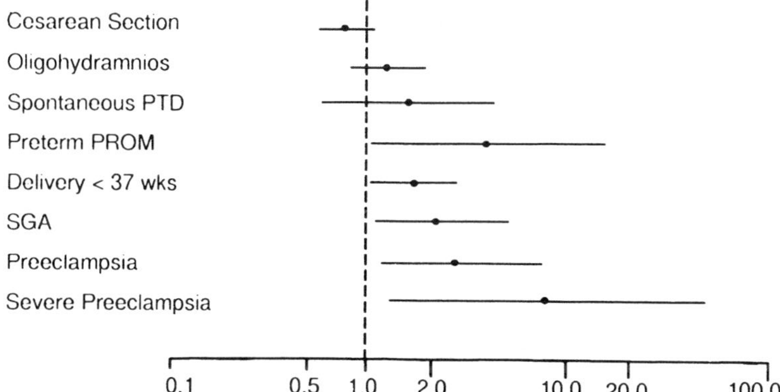

FIGURE 3.—Relative risk of selected pregnancy outcomes associated with less than twofold serum thromboxane B_2 reduction. *Abbreviations: PTD*, preterm delivery; *PROM*, premature rupture of membranes; *SGA*, small for gestational age. (Courtesy of Hauth JC, Goldenberg RL, Parker CR Jr, et al: *Am J Obstet Gynecol* 173:578–584, 1995.)

aspirin study, had significantly less preeclampsia and fewer premature and low-birth-weight infants than did women who did not have this twofold reduction during their pregnancies.

▶ Aspirin acts by irreversibly acetylating and inactivating platelet cyclooxygenase activity, blocking thromboxane production at low concentration and prostacycline production at higher concentrations. Because of some preliminary studies indicating that low-dose aspirin, by reducing TxA_2 production and its metabolite TxB_2 in blood, reduces the arterial vasoconstriction in preeclampsia, a number of trials designed to reduce preeclampsia by using prophylactic low-dose (50–100 mg/day) aspirin have been reviewed in the YEAR BOOK.[1–3] All of them failed to show benefit.

An exception to this generality is the study by Hauth et al., which is subject to analysis controlled for reduced TxB_2, here employing 558 of the original 604 nullipares reported earlier by them. Patients selected for this study had determinations of TxB_2 available through the course of the earlier reported experience. The purpose was to test the presumption that 50 mg of aspirin per day would uniformly reduce TxB_2 in gravidas and to be certain of compliance in using the medication by making that measurement. Controlling the study for previously uncontrolled reduced thromboxane production produced surprising results. Using an admittedly arbitrary level of reduction of greater than 50% of TxB_2 concentration from the pretreatment value, the authors found that one third of women receiving placebo had reduction of TxB_2 to that level, as did 79% of aspirin-treated women. Whether placebo-based reductions represented random variability of thromboxane production, reflected use of a small dose of aspirin for headache or myalgia, or reflected individual metabolic alterations spontaneously protective against the risk of preeclampsia is uncertain. Clearly, spontaneous reduction of TxB in placebo-treated women narrowed the difference between placebo and aspirin and has the effect of concealing the value of aspirin in this regard. In any event, regardless of whether aspirin did or did not induce reduction of TxB_2, this reduction results in a significant decrease in the risk of preeclampsia, consequent growth retardation, preterm birth, and, somewhat unexpectedly, preterm rupture of membranes. This fine piece of work by a very competent clinical investigator should provoke renewed interest in the use of aspirin prophylaxis in women at risk for the development of preeclampsia.

T.H. Kirschbaum, M.D.

References

1. 1993 YEAR BOOK OF OBSTETRICS AND GYNECOLOGY, pp 47–48.
2. 1994 YEAR BOOK OF OBSTETRICS AND GYNECOLOGY, pp 57–58.
3. 1995 YEAR BOOK OF OBSTETRICS AND GYNECOLOGY, pp 58–60, 64–66.

The Angiotensin Sensitivity Test and Low-Dose Aspirin Are Ineffective Methods to Predict and Prevent Hypertensive Disorders in Nulliparous Pregnancy
Kyle PM, Buckley D, Kissane J, et al (John Radcliffe Hosp, Oxford, England; Queen Charlotte's and Chelsea Hosp, London)
Am J Obstet Gynecol 173:865–872, 1995   2–12

Background.—Some women who later have preeclampsia exhibit increased vascular reactivity to angiotensin II. An elevated pressor response is apparent from 26 to 28 weeks' gestation, several weeks or longer before clinical abnormalities develop. Later studies of the angiotensin sensitivity test have failed to replicate the original findings. It has been claimed that aspirin in low dosage can prevent gestational hypertension and preeclampsia.

Objectives and Methods.—The angiotensin sensitivity test was performed at 28 weeks' gestation in 495 healthy nulliparous women. The infusion was begun at 4 ng/kg/min and increased by 2-ng increments every 5 minutes up to 14 ng/kg/min, or until the diastolic pressure increased by 20 mm Hg, when the infusion was stopped. If the effective pressor dose was 10 ng/kg/min or less, the test results were considered positive. Test-positive women were randomly selected to receive 60 mg of aspirin or a placebo tablet each day up to 38 weeks' gestation.

Results.—Eighty women were confirmed as being angiotensin-sensitive, and 44 of them received aspirin. Test-positive women were heavier than the others and slightly younger, but no other differences were noted. The test was only 22% sensitive for preeclampsia and had a positive predictive value of 19%. Its specificity was 85%, and its negative predictive value was 87%. In the randomized trial, all 5 women in whom proteinuric preeclampsia developed had received aspirin.

Conclusions.—The angiotensin sensitivity test has not proved useful in screening for preeclampsia in nulliparous women. Daily low-dose aspirin has not prevented the disorder.

▶ This work appears to represent a subset of patients previously reported in the results of the Collaborative Low-Dose Aspirin Study in Pregnancy (CLASP).[1] That large complex study, combining prophylactic and therapeutic protocols from 5 continents excluding North America, resulted in generally negative results. Here the issue is whether the apparent loss of tolerance to the hypertensive effects of angiotensin II in the early third trimester of pregnancy enables a selection of a subset of women with a strong enough likelihood to develop preeclampsia that they might demonstrate the effectiveness of aspirin treatment in a controlled study. The angiotensive sensitivity test performed miserably with a sensitivity of 22% and false positive rate of 81%. Not surprisingly, women selected in this way failed to show benefit from low-dose aspirin. Before rejecting aspirin's use as a preventive, the reader should review the work of Hauth et al.[2, 3]

T.H. Kirschbaum, M.D.

References

1. 1995 YEAR BOOK OF OBSTETRICS AND GYNECOLOGY, pp 71–74.
2. *Focus & Opinion: Obstetrics and Gynecology* 2(1):26–27, 1996.
3. Hauth JC, Goldenberg RL, Parker CR Jr, et al: Maternal serum thromboxane B2 reduction versus pregnancy outcome in a low-dose aspirin trial. *Am J Obstet Gynecol* 173:578–584, 1995.

Pregnancy in Sickle Cell Disease in the UK: Results of a Multicentre Survey of the Effect of Prophylactic Blood Transfusion on Maternal and Fetal Outcome

Howard RJ, Tuck SM, Pearson TC (Royal Free Hosp, London; St Thomas's Hosp, London)
Br J Obstet Gynaecol 102:947–951, 1995   2–13

Background.—Pregnant women with major sickle cell disease (homozygous S disease, HbSC disease, and sickle cell β-thalassemia) are at increased risk of antenatal and postnatal sickle cell crises, urinary tract infections, pulmonary complications, anemia, proteinuric hypertension, and maternal death. Fetal complications include premature delivery, low birth weight, increased rate of cesarean section, fetal distress in labor, and increased fetal mortality. The use of prophylactic transfusions to improve maternal and fetal sickle cell complications is controversial.

Objective.—The study objective was to assess the outcome of pregnancies in women with sickle cell disease during 1991–1993 and to evaluate the effect of prophylactic blood transfusion programs on maternal and fetal complications and outcomes. Twenty-two hospitals participated in the study.

Methods.—Eighty-one pregnancies in patients with sickle cell disease were compared with 100 pregnancies in women of African descent who did not have hemoglobinopathies. Pregnancies complicated by sickle cell disease were categorized by the type of hemoglobinopathy and by their transfusion programs. The main outcome measures included antenatal and postnatal complications of sickle cell disease, proteinuria hypertension, protein deficiency, emergency delivery by cesarean section, fetal distress, birth weight, and perinatal and maternal mortality. Three transfusion programs were used: prophylactic transfusion from the first or second trimesters; prophylactic transfusion from the third trimester; and no prophylactic transfusions or only occasional transfusions for specific indications. Prophylactic blood transfusion was performed by manual exchange transfusion to increase the level of circulating normal Hb. This was usually accomplished over a period of several weeks, but in some serious cases it was performed in a matter of days.

Results.—Two maternal deaths occurred among the 81 sickle cell pregnancies. Antenatal sickling complications occurred in 46.2% of the pregnancies and were most common in the third trimester. Postnatal sickling complications occurred in 7.7% of the pregnancies. Pregnancies in women with sickle cell disease were significantly more likely than those in the comparative group to be associated with anemia, low birth weight, proteinuria hypertension, and preterm delivery. There was a trend for third-trimester transfusion prophylaxis to decrease sickling complications. This trend was most noticeable in patients with homozygous S disease, and the benefits were most apparent when transfusions were administered after the 28th week of gestation. No evidence indicated an improvement by first- and second-trimester prophylactic transfusion.

Conclusion.—Sickle cell disease is a serious complicating factor in pregnancy and perinatal maternal mortality. Sickle cell disease is associated with increases in preterm delivery, low birth weight, proteinuric hypertension, anemia, and the need for cesarean section as an emergency procedure. Prophylactic transfusion administered after the 28th week of gestation may decrease sickling complications of the third trimester, especially in women with homozygous S disease. No benefits, however, were seen from prophylactic transfusion administered during the first and second trimesters.

▶ This retrospective cohort study of 78 singleton pregnancies in 77 women once again approaches the value of prophylactic transfusion aimed at the prevention of crises and the improvement of perinatal outcome. It is a somewhat bold step in view of the recent prospective randomized study that failed to demonstrate benefit.[1]

The retrospective design complicates analysis because the study population included women with SS, SC, and β-thalassemia Hb, with transfusion begun in the first or second trimester in 30 cases and in the third trimester in 9. The absence of a prospective protocol makes it likely that intrapartum exchange transfusion was sometimes indicated by symptom development and not truly prophylactic. Although exchange transfusion was done to increase the fraction of Hb A in maternal blood, the desired percentage, presumably varying a great deal among the 22 reporting hospitals, is not recorded. The usual associations of SS and SC disease with growth retardation, pregnancy-induced hypertension, and preterm labor are noted, and the outcomes for 3 twin pregnancies were particularly abysmal. Although the number of cases is insufficient to reach statistical significance, there are fewer cases of painful crises among those receiving exchange transfusion in the third trimester than among those who did not. Earlier exchanges in first and second trimester showed no benefit. Lung pathology (embolism, lung infarcts, and pneumonia) was a particularly grave complication.

The diversity of these cases seems to doom a patterned approach to their management. The best results still seem to follow attempts to define what is meant by crisis rigorously and particularly (pyelitis, bone infarction, pneumonia, hemolysis, and so on) and to treat individually the complications that arise in these complicated pregnancies.

T.H. Kirschbaum, M.D.

Reference

1. Koshy M, Burd L, Wallace D, et al: Prophylactic red-cell transfusions in pregnant patients with sickle cell disease. *N Engl J Med* 319:1447–1452, 1988.

Pregnancy in Sickle Cell Disease: Experience of the Cooperative Study of Sickle Cell Disease

Smith JA, Espeland M, Bellevue R, et al (Columbia Univ, New York; Bowman Gray School of Medicine, Winston-Salem, NC; State Univ of New York, Brooklyn; et al)

Obstet Gynecol 87:199–204, 1996   2–14

Background.—Previous reports vary as to the maternal and fetal mortality and complications associated with sickle cell disease in pregnant women. The maternal and fetal outcomes of 445 pregnancies from the Cooperative Study of Sickle Cell Disease were reviewed.

Methods.—Pregnant women from 19 centers were recruited for the prospective study. Information on the patients' steady state and on sickle- and non–sickle-related events was collected by a structured study protocol. Antepartum and intrapartum complications were assessed for pregnancies carried to delivery. The fetal outcomes of gestational age, birth weight, and Apgar score were assessed, along with the effects of genotype on event rates.

Results.—Sixty-four percent of pregnancies progressed to delivery; about 29% ended in elective abortion; 7%, in miscarriage; and 1%, in stillbirth. The rates of non–sickle-related complications in the study group, both antepartum and intrapartum, were similar to those of a group of black women without sickle cell disease. Two of the pregnant women died, 1 as a direct result of her sickle cell disease. Sickle-related maternal morbidity was the same during pregnancy as before. Of pregnancies carried to term, 99% resulted in the birth of a live infant. Mothers with the SS genotype had small for gestational age (SGA) infants in 21% of cases. Genotype had no significant effect on 5-minute Apgar score. The risk factors for having an SGA infant were preeclampsia and acute anemic events.

Conclusions.—Women with all major genotypes of sickle cell disease tolerate pregnancy well. The offspring appear to be healthy, although those whose mothers have the SS genotype are at increased risk of being SGA. Thus, the previous recommendation that women with sickle cell disease should avoid pregnancy or have an abortion seems unwarranted. However, further study is needed to define the possible interactions of risk factors for SGA status and the long-term outcomes of infants at risk.

▶ This large, randomized, cohort study conducted under the auspices of the Sickle Cell Branch of the National Heart, Lung, and Blood Institute is likely to be a standard source for the management of sickle cell pregnancies for years to come. The 297 enrolled women had 445 pregnancies of record, and when the data are diminished by a 28.8% elective abortion rate and normal rates of spontaneous abortion and fetal death, 283 pregnancies remained for analysis.

As usual, complications were more often noted with the sickle cell anemia genotype than with hemoglobin SC disease, and both chronic and acute anemia were more often encountered in the former; no tendency for differing rates of complications among the 3 trimesters of pregnancy was seen. When time-related rates of painful crises were calculated, they were unaltered during pregnancy, and the incidence of acute chest pain and anemia were decreased compared with the nonpregnant state. Growth retardation was noted in gravidas with SS and Sβ-thalassemia, with 21% of neonates having birth weights below the 10th percentile for blacks. The tendency to preterm birth was most marked with maternal SS disease. Preeclampsia and acute anemia during pregnancy were risk factors for intrauterine growth retardation.

Rates of pyelonephritis and abnormal placentation were not increased above normal. In those pregnancies delivered past 28 weeks of gestational age, perinatal survival, exempting only neonatal jaundice, was normal and parameters of early neonatal life were indistinguishable from those of controls. In general, this large, current study should provide support for women with SS disease or its variants who decide, after counseling, to undertake a pregnancy.

T.H. Kirschbaum, M.D.

Prospective Studies of the Association Between Anticardiolipin Antibody and Outcome of Pregnancy

Yasuda M, Takakuwa K, Tokunaga A, et al (Niigata Univ, Japan)
Obstet Gynecol 86:555–559, 1995   2–15

Background.—A role for the immune system has been postulated in a number of adverse pregnancy outcomes including preeclampsia, spontaneous abortion, restricted fetal growth, and fetal death. Several of these events are major complications of systemic lupus erythematosus. Antinuclear antibodies and anticardiolipin antibody are found more often in women having spontaneous abortions, and possibly in those with preeclampsia and restricted fetal growth as well.

Methods.—Titers of anticardiolipin antibody were prospectively related to pregnancy outcomes in 860 pregnant women. Women with a history of recurrent fetal wastage who had received immunosuppressive treatment for positive anticardiolipin antibody were excluded. Titers were estimated by enzyme-linked immunosorbent assay.

Findings.—Anticardiolipin antibody was identified in 7% of women, including 3 of the 10 who had autoimmune disease. One fourth of antibody-positive women aborted spontaneously, compared with 10% of antibody-negative women, a significant difference. The respective rates of preterm delivery were 12% and 4%, also a significant difference. Preeclampsia also occurred significantly more often in antibody-positive women (12% vs. 2%). The relative risk of severe preeclampsia was 22. Restricted fetal growth was observed in 12% of antibody-positive women and 2% of the antibody-negative group. There were 2 fetal deaths in the antibody-positive group and 1 in the antibody-negative group.

Conclusion.—Monitoring of anticardiolipin antibody during pregnancy may help predict the occurrence of spontaneous abortion, preeclampsia, and restricted fetal growth.

▶ This report adds a large prospective study of 860 gravidas and arises from a program of a routine anticardiolipin antibody (aCL) testing at or prior to 9 weeks' gestational age at the Niigata University School of Medicine. Comparison to an earlier similar study of 737 women at Yale University,[1] where a 2.2% incidence of asymptomatic women who were aCL-positive was reported, suggests that the 7% incidence in this study comes from selective referrals for care to this university center. If that's true, the results may not be generalizable.

Of the tested Japanese women, 10 had overt autoimmune disease, but only 3 of these were aCL-positive. Positive aCL antibody status conferred on the 60 women detected an increased likelihood of pregnancy complications, including a twofold increased risk for abortion, a threefold increased risk for preterm delivery, and a sixfold increased risk for preeclampsia and intrauterine growth retardation. However, it should be remembered that 75% of all aCL-positive and 96% of aCL-negative women lacked these complications of pregnancy. Antiphospholipid antibody testing was not performed, but it appears there are technical problems in its detection, with the Yale group finding the activated partial thromboplastin time determination excessively insensitive and the University of Colorado group[2] reporting a 24% antibody-positive rate with many reversions to antibody negativity during pregnancy.

Women who are aCL antibody–positive are clearly a heterogenous group, some of them destined to have a deleterious pregnancy outcome. However, with a sensitivity of 26% and a predictive value of a positive finding of 34%, there seems little support for routine testing of pregnant women from this experience.

T.H. Kirschbaum, M.D.

References

1. Lockwood CJ, Romero R, Feinberg RF, et al: The prevalence and biologic significance of lupus anticoagulant and anticardiolipin antibodies in a general obstetric population. *Am J Obstet Gynecol* 161:369, 1989.
2. 1995 YEAR BOOK OF OBSTETRICS AND GYNECOLOGY, pp 103–104.

Amniotic Fluid Interleukin-6: Correlation With Upper Genital Tract Microbial Colonization and Gestational Age in Women Delivered After Spontaneous Labor Versus Indicated Delivery
Andrews WW, Hauth JC, Goldenberg RL, et al (Univ of Alabama, Birmingham; Wayne State Univ, Detroit; Natl Inst of Child Health and Human Development, Washington, DC)
Am J Obstet Gynecol 173:606–612, 1995   2–16

Background.—Interleukin-6 (IL-6) stimulates prostaglandin release by human amnion and has been reported to be increased in the amniotic fluid

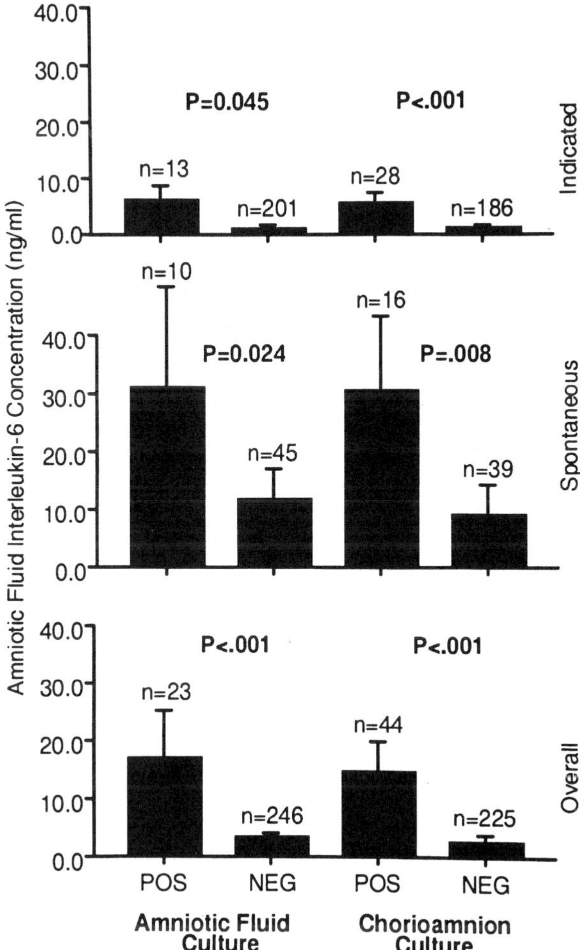

FIGURE 3.—Mean amniotic fluid interleukin-6 concentrations in women with positive (*POS*) or negative (*NEG*) amniotic fluid and chorioamnion cultures. *Abbreviations: overall*, overall study population; *spontaneous*, women with the spontaneous onset of labor; *indicated*, women with indicated deliveries. (Courtesy of Andrews WW, Hauth JC, Goldenberg RL, et al: *Am J Obstet Gynecol* 173:606–612, 1995.)

of women with preterm labor associated with infection. To determine whether IL-6 concentration is elevated in women with spontaneous labor and to determine the relationship between IL-6 levels and microbial infection, amniotic fluid samples from women undergoing cesarean deliveries were cultured and evaluated for IL-6 levels.

Methods.—The chorioamnion and amniotic fluid were cultured for bacteria, fungi, mycoplasmas, *Chlamydia trachomatis,* and *Trichomonas vaginalis* in 269 women with singleton gestations with intact membranes. Amniotic fluid IL-6 levels were assessed. Fifty-five women had spontaneous labor and 214 did not have spontaneous labor. All had cesarean delivery.

Findings.—Amniotic fluid IL-6 levels were significantly higher in women with spontaneous labor than in those without spontaneous labor. Interleukin-6 levels were inversely proportional to gestational age in women with spontaneous labor but not in women without spontaneous labor. Interleukin-6 levels were significantly higher in women with either a positive chorioamnion or positive amniotic fluid culture than in women with negative cultures (Fig 3).

Conclusions.—Elevated amniotic fluid IL-6 levels were associated with spontaneous preterm labor in women with microbial infection of either the chorioamnion or the amniotic fluid. Amniotic fluid IL-6 levels may be a useful marker of microbial infection of the upper genital tract and of infection-mediated preterm labor, especially in women with negative amniotic fluid cultures.

▶ Using material obtained with sterile technique from the placenta and amniotic fluid and with intact fetal membranes at the time of abdominal birth in term and preterm labor, these authors provide an additional firm contribution to an already-clear series of interrelationships concerning preterm birth. The 20% of women in spontaneous labor provides important controls. Although intrapartum cephalosporin was used in 86% of the 269 deliveries, it was administered after transabdominal amniocentesis.

Interleukin-6 is a cytokine produced by leukocytes and macrophages in the presence of inflammation with or without infection. It is elevated in concentration in amniotic fluid in women in spontaneous labor, but not in the absence of labor and not in the presence of failed induction of labor. Amniotic IL-6 concentration was inversely related to the duration of gestation, a finding nicely explained by Hillier's demonstration of the high incidence of latent infection in premature and immature birth.[1] Her finding is confirmed here. This study further strengthens the argument that latent infection is a common cause of preterm labor and delivery by eliminating the chance of inadvertent seeding of the placenta or amniotic fluid from lower reproductive tract flora.

T.H. Kirschbaum, M.D.

Reference

1. 1990 YEAR BOOK OF OBSTETRICS AND GYNECOLOGY, pp 34–36.

Early Fetal Circulation in Pregnancies Complicated by Retroplacental Hematoma
Rizzo G, Capponi A, Soregaroli M, et al (Universitá di Roma; Universitá di Ancona, Roma)
J Clin Ultrasound 23:525–529, 1995   2–17

Background.—The presence of a retroplacental hematoma might affect early development of the fetal circulation. To examine this issue, transvaginal Doppler ultrasonography was performed in cases of retroplacental hematoma, and the results were compared with hematoma volume and pregnancy outcome.

Study Group.—The study group was composed of 38 singleton pregnancies; in each the mother had a known last menstrual period, a live fetus, a retroplacental hematoma, successful Doppler recordings, and a complete perinatal follow-up. The menstrual age was 9 to 14 weeks. The time between bleeding and ultrasonography was 1 to 14 days. Fetal blood flow velocity waveforms were measured in the umbilical artery, descending aorta, middle cerebral artery, and inferior vena cava.

Findings.—There was no significant relationship between any Doppler values and the size of the hematoma or the pregnancy outcome. No significant relationship was found between hematoma size and pregnancy outcome.

Conclusions.—Fetal blood flow velocity waveforms from the umbilical artery, descending aorta, middle cerebral artery, and inferior vena cava are not significantly altered by retroplacental hematomas. The presence of retroplacental hematomas does not appear to have an adverse effect on pregnancy outcome. These results do not support the use of Doppler ultrasonography in early gestation pregnancies complicated by bleeding and retroplacental hematomas.

▶ This ultrasonic study of women threatening to abort offers a couple of puzzling findings. Thirty-eight women with first-trimester bleeding showed evidence of loss of echogenicity between placenta and uterine wall. The method of quantitating the volume of the presumed hematoma was crude, but on average the volume of such a hematoma was roughly a cube the size of 4 cm. What's remarkable is that only 30% of such women aborted and that the remainder went uneventfully to term. If it's true that 20% of women with first-trimester bleeding have ultrasonic evidence of hematomas[1] and only one third abort, this mechanism accounts for only half the incidence of reported clinically defined spontaneous abortion. It seems possible then that false interpretations of first-trimester scans are frequent, and in addition to the inability to discern any changes in fetal circulation velocity, ultrasound now offers us less than we think in terms of prediction of the likelihood of abortion, given a woman threatening to do so.

T.H. Kirschbaum, M.D.

Reference

1. Goldstein SR, Subramanyam BR, Raghavendra BN, et al: Subchorionic bleeding in threatened abortion: Sonographic findings and significance. *AJR* 141:975, 1983.

Maternal, Placental, and Neonatal Associations With Early Germinal Matrix/Intraventricular Hemorrhage in Infants Born Before 32 Weeks' Gestation

Salafia CM, Minior VK, Rosenkrantz TS, et al (Univ of Connecticut, Farmington; Georgetown Univ, Washington, DC; Texas Children's Hosp, Houston)
Am J Perinatol 12:429–436, 1995   2–18

Background.—Histologic placental lesions may be significantly associated with the incidence of early or late germinal matrix/intraventricular hemorrhage (GM/IVH) in premature neonates independent of maternal or neonatal factors. The relationship of clinical antenatal, postnatal, and histologic placental variables to the incidence of early and late GM/IVH in infants born before 32 weeks' gestation was investigated.

Methods.—The records of 406 singleton live-born nonanomalous neonates born before 32 weeks' gestation and their mothers were retrospectively studied. Germinal matrix/intraventricular hemorrhages of grades 1 to 4 diagnosed ultrasonographically fewer than 72 hours after birth were defined as "early," and hemorrhages diagnosed after 72 hours of life were defined as "late."

Findings.—Of the overall group, 10.8% had early GM/IVH, and 4.9% had late GM/IVH. In a stepwise logistic regression analysis, 5 factors were found to be independently related to increased early GM/IVH risk: histologic acute inflammation, gestational age in days, antenatal steroid treatment fewer than 48 hours before birth, volume expansion in the neonate, and magnesium sulfate tocolysis. When the grade of GM/IVH was considered in the stepwise regression analysis, the order of the variables changed, with gestational age and the use of pressor therapy more strongly correlated with higher grade of GM/IVH than amnion inflammation. Factors unrelated to early GM/IVH in univariate and multivariate analyses included mode of delivery, presentation, main indication for delivery, presence/augmentation of labor, mean biophysical profile scores, mean umbilical arterial and venous blood gas values, and surfactant treatment. The neonatal variables correlated with amnion inflammation were volume expansion at delivery and in the first 3 days of life, low mean systolic pressure, low mean oxygen pressure, low initial hematocrit and cord pH, and increased initial white blood cell count and toxic granulations of neutrophils. Gestational age was the only factor significantly associated with late GM/IVH. No maternal or placental factors had significant associations with late GM/IVH.

Conclusions.—The incidence of early but not late GM/IVH is increased in neonates with placentas with acute amnion inflammation who receive volume expansion and who are born to mothers receiving less than 48 hours of exposure to antenatal steroids and selected for magnesium sulfate tocolysis. Amnion inflammation is significantly associated with early GM/IVH as well as early neonatal abnormalities in oxygenation, perfusion, and effective blood volume. Intra-amniotic infection results in advanced preterm labor. Because of the inflammation, tocolysis is ineffective in such cases. Intra-amniotic inflammation may sensitize the fetus to postpartum stresses or initiate early GM/IVH in utero by cytokine effects on cardiovascular instability.

▶ This is one of a flurry of publications arising from the analysis of 406 women delivering at fewer than 32 weeks' gestation at the Farmington Connecticut Health Center over a 5½-year period. In this retrospective cohort study, a very large number of variables was explored among 44 cases of IVH occurring early (fewer than 72 hours of life) and 21 cases occurring late, that is between 4 and 18 days of life. Gestational age and amnionitis were of course highly correlated with each other (colinear) as risk factors, and the special care required in the multivariate regression analysis of colinear variables was apparently not exercised. There are some problems in the certainty of the diagnosis of infection here where only 48% of women with early IVH had amniocentesis with the diagnosis of infection made by uncertain criteria. Further, only 36% of placentas from these infants were culture-positive. In univariate analysis, the mean gestational age for early IVH was 26.5 weeks vs. 28.4 weeks for all others. In comparing the 21 cases with early IVH, 103 of 340 women in the comparative group would have delivered at or prior to 26.5 weeks assuming normal distribution and would have tended to swamp out the effect of gestational age on analysis. When stepwise logistic regression was done beginning with amniotic infection, there was little residual deviation accountable by early gestational age; had gestational age been the initial step, the conclusions would likely have been reversed. When multiple regression was done against the severity of IVH (65% were only Papile class I and II) and against late IVH, gestational age proved to be the only significant correlate of late IVH. The turgid language obscures the obvious. Early neonatal IVH is related to immature birth and the placental infection that most often causes it. Placental morphology and other maternal factors are relatively unimportant. Late IVH most often reflects neonatal ICU attempts to deal with these often infected and fragile neonates.

T.H. Kirschbaum, M.D.

Comparison of a Modified DNA Hybridization Assay With Standard Culture Enrichment for Detecting Group B Streptococci in Obstetric Patients

Kircher SM, Meyer MP, Jordan JA (Univ of Pittsburgh, Pa; Magee-Women's Research Inst, Pittsburgh, Pa)
J Clin Microbiol 34:342–344, 1996   2–19

Purpose.—In the United States, group B streptococcus (GBS) is the major cause of neonatal pneumonia, sepsis, and meningitis and is a common cause of maternal infection as well. Each year, GBS is responsible for up to 15,000 cases of neonatal sepsis. Up to half of neonates with GBS disease developing within the first week of life will die, and up to half the survivors of GBS meningitis will be left with permanent after effects. Because GBS infection is fulminant and because it is usually transmitted vertically, some rapid assay to determine GBS status in laboring women would be valuable. The commercially available ACCUPROBE (AP) kit was tested for this purpose.

Methods.—The AP test, which uses a nucleic acid hybridization GBS 16S ribosomal RNA from pure GBS isolates, was modified for clinical use in detecting GBS in obstetric patients. Mixed cultures were used instead of pure isolates, the culture enrichment time was shortened, and a sample concentration step was added. The comparative study included 402 women in the third trimester of pregnancy, from whom vaginal and rectal swabs were co-cultured and tested for GBS ribosomal RNA.

Results.—Sensitivity fell from 95% with the standard 8-hour enrichment protocol to 73% with the shortened 3-hour enrichment protocol. Specificity was 98% for the 8-hour protocol and 99% for the 3-hour protocol. Although high levels of normal flora in the vaginal-rectal cultures did not interfere with the specificity of the test for GBS, the assay was less accurate with bloody specimens.

Conclusions.—The modified AP test can detect most cases of maternal GBS colonization within 4 hours. This test is of value in identifying the most heavily colonized cases, thus indicating women who are the most likely to transmit GBS to their offspring. The newly modified test could result in important changes in the medical management and antibiotic therapy of pregnancies with maternal GBS colonization.

▶ This probe is a promising candidate to achieve identification of GBS in vaginal and rectal swabs of women in labor sufficiently early to allow effective antibiotic therapy before delivery. The trick is to use a single-stranded DNA nucleotide probe labeled with acridine, complementary to a segment of ribosomal RNA in the streptococcal organism. Although the probe was designed to be applied to pure cultures of GBS, the innovation here is to apply the probe to a mixed culture of all organisms grown together in broth medium, saving the 18 to 24 hours needed for colony selection from mixed cultures and subculture to obtain pure GBS colonies. When 3 hours are used for mixed culture growth and bacterial cells are lysed, the authors take advantage of the resistance to hydrolysis to be conferred on the hybridization product of the probe to the bacterial RNA segment. An acridine fluorescent label is used to detect the presence of hybrid. The 74% sensitivity, 4.5% false positive rates, and 9.6% false negative rate, compared with the results of overnight standard culture, seem a reasonable cost to pay for an answer to the GBS identification in less than 4 hours after obtaining the sample. The probe is commercially available in a kit.

T.H. Kirschbaum, M.D.

Prevention of Premature Birth by Screening and Treatment for Common Genital Tract Infections: Results of a Prospective Controlled Evaluation
McGregor JA, French JI, Parker R, et al (Univ of Colorado, Denver; Denver Dept of Health and Hosps)
Am J Obstet Gynecol 173:157–167, 1995   2–20

Introduction.—Preterm birth, earlier than 37 weeks' gestation, is associated with bacterial vaginosis, common reproductive tract infection, and associated inflammatory responses. The prevalence of common lower genital tract infections and bacterial vaginosis was evaluated, as were the effects of systematic screening and treatment to improve pregnancy outcomes of women with these diseases.

Methods.—A total of 1,260 women were enrolled in a prospective, controlled treatment trial. They were examined at the initiation of prenatal care for lower genital tract microorganisms and bacterial vaginosis during the first 7 months of the program, which was considered the observation phase. Reexaminations were continued at 22–29 weeks and after 32 weeks' gestation. During the second 8 months of the study (the treatment phase), women who were infected were given the recommended Centers for Disease Control and Prevention treatments. For bacterial vaginosis, the treatment was 300 mg of clindamycin orally twice each day for 7 days. Univariate and multivariate methods were used to analyze data according to intent to treat.

Results.—Pregnancy loss at fewer than 22 weeks of gestation was associated with bacterial vaginosis, present in 32.5% of the women at enrollment. The risk of preterm birth and preterm premature rupture of membranes was associated with bacterial vaginosis in the observation phase. Within the observation-phase group, 21.9% of preterm births were attributed to bacterial vaginosis. During the treatment phase of women with bacterial vaginosis, there were fewer preterm births and fewer preterm premature ruptures of membranes. The highest risk of preterm birth was associated with women with bacterial vaginosis and trichomoniasis. Within this group, 28% had preterm birth. In the treatment phase of both conditions, however, preterm births were reduced to 17%. Reduced preterm birth was associated with earlier patient enrollment and oral antibiotic treatment.

Conclusion.—The presence of bacterial vaginosis was associated with increased risks of pregnancy loss at fewer than 22 weeks, with preterm birth, and with preterm premature rupture of membranes.

▶ The relationship between bacterial vaginosis and preterm labor has always proven tenuous, marked as it is with univariate analyses of multivariate problems,[1] multivariate analysis excluding co-infection using only Gram's stain for diagnosis[2] and univariate analysis with confidence levels of risk ratios as low as 1.1, and reporting preterm labor without premature birth weights.[3] More to the point, prophylactic therapy based on vaginal microbiology has failed to provide any evidence of benefit.[4, 5]

Here a very complex experimental design exceeds the power of statistical methods used to analyze it. Data from a 7-month observational study during which some patients were treated for bacterial vaginosis, trichomonas, and yeasts are compared with data from an 8-month treatment protocol where all such women were treated, as were those who were group B strep–positive. There is no significant difference in the overall incidence of preterm delivery in the 2 groups (12.6% vs. 9.5%), and only when idiopathic preterm births are compared (and it's not clear precisely which births are excluded) is improvement in the treatment group claimed by the authors. It proves impossible to do multivariate analysis for co-infection despite its common occurrence since there are too few cases without co-infection to analyze. This is evidence of need for a larger study. Similarly, the impact of therapy during the observational phase, nonwhite status, premature rupture of membranes, and various treatment modalities appear not to have been treated as covariates, though clearly they are. This study purports to contribute more than it can prove and is another insubstantial piece of evidence that treating bacterial vaginosis prevents preterm delivery.

T.H. Kirschbaum, M.D.

References

1. McGregor JA, French JI, Richter R, et al: Antenatal microbiologic and maternal risk factors associated with prematurity. *Am J Obstet Gynecol* 163:1465, 1990.
2. Hay PE, et al: *BMJ* 308:295, 1994.
3. Gravett MG, et al: *JAMA* 256:1899, 1986.
4. 1992 YEAR BOOK OF OBSTETRICS AND GYNECOLOGY, pp 78–79.
5. *Focus & Opinion: Obstetrics and Gynecology* 1(6):416, 1995.

Placenta Previa, Maternal Smoking and Recurrence Risk
Lilja GMC (Univ of Lund, Sweden)
Acta Obstet Gynecol Scand 74:341–345, 1995   2–21

Introduction.—Although the cause of placenta previa is a topic of debate, various types of previous uterine trauma or disturbances of the uterine vasculature may be associated with recurrent placenta previa in later pregnancy. Few studies have examined the risk of recurrence among women with placenta previa. Previous reports have found that maternal smoking during pregnancy is related to placenta previa. Registry data were used to study the recurrence risk of placenta previa and the risk of placenta previa in women who smoked during pregnancy.

Methods.—Both cohort and case-control designs were used to analyze data from the Swedish Medical Birth Registry. This database provided prospectively collected information on previous pregnancies and smoking habits, thus avoiding recall bias. The general epidemiologic characteristics of placenta previa were examined, along with the effects of maternal smoking and the risk of placenta previa for siblings born after an affected proband.

Results.—Of 1,825,998 infants delivered from 1973 to 1990, 5,683 had placenta previa. The incidence of placenta previa during these years was 0.3%, overall and for twins. Maternal age and parity were independent risk factors for placenta previa. The odds ratio for placenta previa associated with previous cesarean section was 1.82. The recurrence rate of placenta previa was 2.4%, 8 times higher than the rate in the general population. Half of the recurrence risk of placenta previa in siblings resulted from cesarean section.

The effects of maternal smoking were analyzed for 1983–1990. The odds ratio for placenta previa among smoking mothers was 1.53. The effects of smoking on the risk of placenta previa increased with increasing parity but not with maternal age. The risk of placenta previa increased with the number of cigarettes smoked per day.

Conclusions.—The risk of recurrent placenta previa for women with a history of this condition is about 7 times higher than the risk of placenta previa in the general population, after stratification for year of birth. About half of this risk is related to cesarean section. As in other studies, maternal smoking is a significant risk factor for placenta previa. The available epidemiologic data suggest a multifactorial origin of placenta previa.

▶ Although there have been several reports of an association between smoking and placenta previa, this one, based on 828,201 births recorded by Sweden's Medical Birth Registry, is the most convincing of the lot. Not only is the quality of the data obtained from 1983 to 1990 very high, but the analyses were thoughtfully done. When covariants of smoking, increased maternal age, parity, year of birth, and cesarean section were controlled, a significantly increased risk of occurrence of placenta previa was found amongst smokers greater than 30 years of age and with parity equal to or greater than 2. The overall increase in risk of occurrence was 53% and the increased risk was 72% for those smoking more than 10 cigarettes a day. That is to say there appeared to be a dose-response relationship. A similarly increased risk was demonstrable in pregnancies before the primary birth of interest and in subsequent pregnancies, though part but not all of this enhanced risk was explicable based on the relationship of the increased risk of cesarean section. Though hypotheses abound to rationalize this relationship, it's honest to say there is no mechanistic explanation for this effect, but smokers should be warned.

T.H. Kirschbaum, M.D.

Did Preterm Deliveries Continue to Decrease in France in the 1980s?
Bréart G, Blondel B, Tuppin P, et al (INSERM, Paris and Toulouse, France)
Paediatr Perinat Epidemiol 9:296–306, 1995   2–22

Introduction.—A program of perinatal care intended to provide more complete training of medical staff and to ensure better prenatal care was instituted in France between 1972 and 1981. Part of the program involved making better equipment available in maternity wards.

Methods.—Three surveys were conducted in 1972, 1981, and 1988–1989 involving representative samples of single live births in 10 regions of the country.

Findings.—The rate of preterm birth decreased from 7.9% in 1972 to 5.8% in 1981 and further to 4% from 1988 to 1989. The rates of infants weighing less than 2,500 g at birth were 5.4% in 1972, 4.3% in 1981, and 4.7% from 1988 to 1989. Preterm infants born in 1988–1989 had a lower average birth weight than did those in the earlier surveys. The reduction in preterm births could not be ascribed to changes in the way gestational age was estimated. The proportion of inductions and cesarean section deliveries before labor increased slightly more for preterm births than for births after 36 weeks' gestation. The average birth weight of preterm infants was lower when labor was not spontaneous, especially for those born in 1988–1989.

Discussion.—The increasing use of ultrasound may have contributed to the apparent reduction in the average birth weight observed in preterm infants in this survey.

▶ From 1971 to 1981, the French Republic, in an effort stimulated by the renowned French pediatrician, Professor Alexander Minkowski, implemented a perinatal program designed to improve perinatal survival by increasing medical staff training and improving obstetrical equipment and prenatal care. Also included was a government-sponsored program of expanded maternity leave from employment for pregnant women. In 1969, a well-known French obstetrician, Dr. Emile Papiernik, introduced his recommendations for prenatal care designed to reduce preterm birth by employing risk assessment, educating high-risk mothers to recognize uterine contractions and, by reducing the efforts of daily life, to diminish them. His suggestions for improving the nature and timing of prenatal care access led to an invitation from the National Institute of Child Health and Development to visit Bethesda, Maryland, where he gained some followers. They, however, were unable to reproduce his success in this country.[1-3] The results of his approach used from 1971 to 1982 in Haguenau, an Alsacian city close to Strasbourg, were published in 1989.[4]

This study reported the results of surveys done in 10 regions across France from 1972, when preterm deliveries were said to occur in 7.9% of birth, and postdate deliveries in 10.2%, until 1989, when the preterm delivery rate was 4% and postdate deliveries occurred in 2.9%. Clearly the problem here is with pregnancy dating, initially done only from chart review of the obstetrician's estimate without benefit of newborn exam and without ultrasound. In 1971, the incidence of uncertain dates was 12.1% in a survey conducted that year. Excluding large-for-gestational-age infants as likely errors in fixing dates of gestation reduced the reported change in preterm delivery incidence from 6.5% to 3.9% over 17 years. The authors think that errors in determining and therefore defining prematurity and small-for-gestational-age pregnancy do not account for this apparent improvement but cannot of course prove it. The authors assume that no other alterations in the environment from 1971 to 1981 accounted for the apparent changes. It's not clear what role, if any, the Haguenau experience plays in all this, but this analysis raises questions about the role of the Papiernik approach, and indeed of the French Perinatal Program, in altering preterm delivery rates in France. What has been described as reduction in preterm birth may instead have been improvement from 1972 to 1988 in the precision of dating pregnancies, progressively removing from recorded preterm births those with underestimates of gestational age and those growth retarded at or past 37 weeks.

T.H. Kirschbaum, M.D.

References

1. 1987 YEAR BOOK OF OBSTETRICS AND GYNECOLOGY, pp 60–62.
2. 1989 YEAR BOOK OF OBSTETRICS AND GYNECOLOGY, pp 136–137.
3. 1991 YEAR BOOK OF OBSTETRICS AND GYNECOLOGY, pp 131–133.
4. Papiernik E, Keith L, Banyar J, et al (eds): Effective prevention of preterm birth: The French experience at Haguenau. White Plains, NY, March of Dimes Birth Defects, Original Article series, 25(1), 1989.

3 Medical Complications of Pregnancy

A Comparison of Magnesium Sulfate With Phenytoin for the Prevention of Eclampsia
Lucas MJ, Leveno KJ, Cunningham FG (Univ of Texas, Dallas)
N Engl J Med 333:201–205, 1995
3–1

Introduction.—In pregnant women with hypertension, magnesium sulfate is widely used to prevent eclamptic seizures. However, few studies have compared the efficacy of magnesium sulfate with that of other drugs, such as the conventional antiepileptic drugs diazepam or phenytoin, which are more commonly used in the United Kingdom. Magnesium sulfate was compared with phenytoin for the prevention of seizures in hypertensive women during labor.

Methods.—Women with hypertension were randomly assigned to receive magnesium sulfate or phenytoin during delivery. The regimen was 10 g of a 50% solution of magnesium sulfate in doses divided in the upper outer quadrant of each buttock. Thereafter, every 4 hours, 5 g of a 50% solution was injected. For severe preeclampsia, a loading dose of 4 mg of IV magnesium sulfate was given as a 20% solution. The phenytoin regimen was 1,000 mg of undiluted phenytoin pumped piggyback with a volumetric pump at a rate of 200 mL/hr over 1 hour; 10 hours later, a maintenance dose of 500 mg of phenytoin was given in a capsule. Anticonvulsant therapy was continued for 24 hours post partum for both regimens.

Results.—Eclamptic convulsions occurred in 10 of 1,089 women assigned to the phenytoin regimen, whereas none of the 1,049 women assigned to magnesium sulfate had eclamptic convulsions. Between the 2 study groups, there were no significant differences in any risk factors for eclampsia. In the 2 groups, maternal and infant outcomes were also similar. In the 10 women with eclampsia despite the phenytoin prophylaxis, a number of peripartum complications were seen, including cesarean section, low-birth-weight infants, partial abruptio placentae, and need for blood transfusions.

Conclusion.—For the prevention of eclampsia in hypertensive pregnant women, magnesium sulfate is superior to phenytoin. The long-practiced use of magnesium sulfate in the prevention of eclampsia is validated by these results. Until now, the effectiveness of phenytoin as prophylaxis against eclampsia has only been studied in small groups.

▶ This is an American counterpart to the report of the Eclampsia Trial Collaborative Group study[1] that was based on the analysis of employment of anticonvulsants in 1,680 eclamptic gravidas in Africa, Asia, and South America. Like the earlier collaborative study, this Dallas experience confirms the superiority of magnesium sulfate in the prevention of initial and recurrent eclamptic seizures and helps confirm the Texas unit's conviction that a serum magnesium concentration greater than 4 mEg/L will, with very rare exception, preclude seizure activity. Although the perinatal mortality rate in the Collaborative Group study was nearly twice that found in this one (27% vs. 13.8%) and there was a maternal mortality of 4.1% in the Third World countries, no significant differences were seen between the results of magnesium sulfate and other agents in either study. Although the prevention of seizures is important in eclampsia and severe preeclampsia, and magnesium sulfate is superior to phenytoin and diazepam in that respect, anticonvulsants are not the sole important factor in the prevention of maternal and perinatal mortality in eclamptics. Clearly, careful management of cardiovascular, renal, and hematologic complications as well as the appropriate timing of delivery remain important determinants of successful management.

T.H. Kirschbaum, M.D.

Reference

1. *Focus & Opinion: Obstetrics and Gynecology* 1(6):418, 1995.

Plasma Cyclic GMP Concentrations and Their Relationship With Changes of Blood Pressure Levels in Pre-eclampsia
Schneider F, Lutun P, Baldauf J-J, et al (Hôpitaux Universitaires de Strasbourg, France)
Acta Obstet Gynecol Scand 75:40–44, 1996   3–2

Background.—Several authors have suggested an imbalance in vascular tone regulation as being involved in the pathogenesis of preeclampsia. If this were so, a loss of efficiency of the L-arginine-nitric oxide pathway could lead to inactivation of guanylyl cyclase in vascular smooth muscle cells and lower plasma cyclic 3'-5' guanosine monophosphate (cGMP) levels. However, previous studies have demonstrated increased plasma levels of cGMP in women with preeclampsia. The purpose of this study was to further examine the role of cGMP in the pathogenesis of pre-eclampsia.

Methods.—The study population consisted of 16 women pregnant with preeclampsia with a mean gestational age of 32.6 weeks; 16 normotensive pregnant controls matched for age, gestational age, body weight, and means of delivery; and 6 nonpregnant controls. Arterial blood pressure was measured before the initiation of antihypertensive drug therapy and once daily thereafter until day 4 after delivery. Blood samples collected concomitantly were measured for plasma cGMP, atrial natriuretic peptide (ANP), creatinine, and uric acid levels. In addition, urinary cGMP levels in aliquots from 24-hour urine collections were measured to calculate the renal clearance of cGMP.

Results.—At baseline, women with preeclampsia had significantly higher plasma cGMP and ANP levels than either the pregnant normoten-sive controls or the nonpregnant controls. After the initiation of antihy-pertensive therapy, plasma cGMP levels decreased concomitantly with decreasing blood pressure. By the time the mean arterial pressure reached the normal level, plasma cGMP levels also had normalized. Baseline plasma ANP levels in women with preeclampsia were increased, confirm-ing increased guanylyl cyclase activity, but renal impairment was ruled out because creatinine clearance was normal in all cases. No statistically significant correlation was found between baseline or subsequent plasma cGMP concentrations and any of the parameters reflecting the severity of the gestational hypertension in these patients.

Conclusions.—Plasma cGMP concentrations are increased, rather than decreased, in women with preeclampsia, indicating enhanced guanylyl cyclase activation by ANP, rather than a lack of production of this enzyme, as previously proposed.

▶ Here is another set of data supporting the contention that although endothelial nitric oxide production may be important in maintaining vasodi-lation in normal pregnancy, its deficit resulting from endothelial cell injury does not have a role in the arterial constriction or vasoconstriction of pre-eclampsia. Nitric oxide acts by stimulating the production of guanylyl cyclase enzyme activity which, in turn, leads to the production of increased amounts of cGMP. This in turn generates a cGMP-specific protein kinase that drives phosphorylation of segments of the cells' apparatus, among them myosin light-chain kinase, which leads to muscle cell relaxation.

In comparing women with preeclampsia with normal pregnant women, 16 women with preeclampsia—including 3 with thrombopenia and hemolysis—were found to have an increased concentration of plasma cGMP, not the decreased concentrations that would be the case had nitric oxide served as the intermediate between endothelial cell injury and vasoconstriction. Al-though it is not possible to prove that nitric oxide is not an intermediate in the pathophysiology of preeclampsia, this study certainly fails to support such a hypothesis.

T.H. Kirschbaum, M.D.

Central and Peripheral Hemodynamics in Severe Preeclampsia

Yang J-M, Yang Y-C, Wang K-G (Mackay Mem Hosp, Taipei, Taiwan, Republic of China)

Acta Obstet Gynecol Scand 75:120–126, 1996   3–3

Introduction.—The key to successful management of pregnancy-induced hypertension is antihypertensive therapy, and different antihypertensive drugs have different effects on uteroplacental perfusion. A new technique, Doppler velocimetry, is a useful tool for measuring blood flow, vascular resistance, and central hemodynamics. It may be of value in monitoring and planning treatment for patients with preeclampsia. Doppler velocimetry was used to examine relationships among central hemodynamics, uteroplacental circulation, and perinatal outcomes in pregnancies complicated by severe preeclampsia.

Methods.—The study included 31 pregnant women with severe preeclampsia. The patients had no history of medical disease and had not received any antihypertensive treatment before hospitalization. Each underwent laboratory studies of blood chemistry and hematogram at admission. In addition, Doppler velocimetry was used to study the maternal hemodynamics and the umbilical and uterine arteries. Antihypertensive treatment with hydralazine, atenolol, and labetolol was given according to the central hemodynamic findings. Information on the patients' general status, the Doppler ultrasound findings, and the perinatal outcomes was analyzed.

Results.—The patients were divided into 3 groups according to their systemic vascular resistance. Fifty-two percent had high vascular resistance (more than 7.5 dynes/sec/cm^{-5}); 16% had normal vascular resistance; and 32% had low vascular resistance (less than 5.0 dynes/sec/cm^{-5}). Patients with high vascular resistance were likely to have reduced left ventricular function and cardiac index. Forty-two percent of patients in the high vascular resistance group had small-for-gestational-age infants, compared with none of those in the low vascular resistance group. The association between high vascular resistance and poor fetal growth seemed to result from underperfusion caused by decreased uteroplacental flow. Maternal hemoconcentration was a common related finding.

Conclusions.—The central hemodynamic findings vary among (and even within) pregnant women with preeclampsia. The uteroplacental circulation is subject to regional vasospasm before the systemic circulation is. For patients with high uterine artery resistance, it may be possible to maintain adequate uteroplacental perfusion through a high cardiac output in low systemic vascular resistance.

▶ Women with severe preeclampsia are not uniform with respect to cardiac output, peripheral vascular resistance (PVR), and plasma volume, the primary determinants of hypertension,[1] and this study attempts to define differences in cardiac output and PVR. The techniques are reasonably effective because the fixed position of the adult aorta, its flat velocity profile, and relatively little systolic diameter change allow fairly accurate estimates of cardiac output using Doppler velocimetry.[2] The failure to control plasma volume remains a problem in this study because plasma volume varies inversely with systemic vascular resistance (SVR) and directly with cardiac output, but the results are still of interest. Initial cardiovascular measurements in the 13 women with severe preeclampsia were made prior to antihypertensive medication, but had magnesium sulfate been given, its tendency to increase plasma volume and cardiac output may have explained the low PVR and high cardiac output seen in 5 of 31 patients and the normal PVR and normal cardiac index in 14 others. In any event, reduced birth weight and emergency cesarean section were confined to those women with normal or high PVR. No significant differences were seen in umbilical artery Doppler values among the 3 groups studied, and expectant management in 16 cases resulted in some deterioration of PVR. Its not clear why atenolol, a beta-adrenergic blocker, was chosen for hypertensive women with low SVR and high cardiac output from which combination one would expect little benefit. Aside from low birth weight and small gestational age among those with high to normal SVR, no differences in newborn outcome were noted.

The work of Easterling et al.[3] in measurements of this sort has always stood apart from that of other workers since they recorded very high values for cardiac output and assumed that these were the cause of hypertension. It is interesting that superimposing values for this study on the Easterling diagrams would lead to predictions of normal blood pressure in contrast to those same measurements by Wallenberg et al.[4] where agreement with this study is good. These data add to the conviction held by many of us that a systematic error in the Seattle data yields false high cardiac output estimates for women with preeclampsia and mistakenly attributes the cause of pregnancy hypertension to those estimates.

T.H. Kirschbaum, M.D.

References

1. 1993 YEAR BOOK OF OBSTETRICS AND GYNECOLOGY, pp 86–90.
2. 1989 YEAR BOOK OF OBSTETRICS AND GYNECOLOGY, pp 64–65.
3. 1988 YEAR BOOK OF OBSTETRICS AND GYNECOLOGY, pp 54–57.
4. 1993 YEAR BOOK OF OBSTETRICS AND GYNECOLOGY, p 86.

Long-Term Outcome of Mothers of Children With Complete Congenital Heart Block

Press J, Uziel Y, Laxer RM, et al (Univ of Toronto)
Am J Med 100:328–332, 1996

3–4

Purpose.—Complete congenital heart block (CHB) occurs as an intra-uterine complication of neonatal lupus erythematosus syndrome, probably caused by transplacental passage of maternal antibodies to SSA/Ro and SSB/La ribonucleoproteins. Some reports have suggested that the mothers of children with CHB are at risk of connective tissue diseases, especially systemic lupus erythematosus (SLE) or Sjögren's syndrome (SS). However, these studies were small or had problems with referral bias. The short- and long-term health outcomes of mothers of babies born with CHB were analyzed.

Methods.—The study included 64 mothers of 64 babies born with CHB. Information for the analysis was obtained from the mothers by questionnaire or telephone interview and/or from the attending physicians. The mothers were classified as having a definite rheumatic disease, as having an undifferentiated autoimmune syndrome (UAS), or as being healthy. Serum samples from 53 mothers were analyzed by enzyme-linked immunosorbent assay (ELISA) for anti-Ro and anti-La antibodies.

Results.—The mothers' mean age at delivery was 28 years, at which time 66% were healthy. Three percent had SLE, 3% had linear scleroderma, 3% had rheumatoid arthritis, 5% had a history of rheumatic fever but were currently well, and 2% had SS. Nineteen percent of the mothers had a UAS at the time of delivery, with symptoms including arthralgias, myalgia, photosensitivity, skin vasculitis, and Raynaud's phenomenon. The mothers' mean age at the time of the study was 38 years. Of the 12 mothers who had UAS at delivery, 3 had progressed to SLE, 2 had SS, and 1 had gone into remission. Of the 42 mothers who had been healthy at delivery, 1 had SLE, 1 had hyperthyroidism, 1 had ankylosing spondylitis, and 3 had a UAS. Mean follow-up was approximately 120 months for the mothers who remained healthy and for those in whom autoimmune diseases developed.

Sixty percent of women tested were positive for anti-Ro and/or anti-La antibodies. At the time of the study, 26% were symptomatic. Serum samples obtained at delivery were positive for anti-Ro and/or anti-La antibodies in 12 of 13 patients.

Conclusions.—Most mothers of children with CHB who are healthy at delivery remain healthy over the long term. Systemic lupus erythematosus may develop in approximately one fourth of mothers who have a UAS at the time of delivery compared with a very small proportion of initially healthy mothers. The rate at which autoimmune disease developed in asymptomatic mothers after the birth of a child with CHB was lower in this study than in previous reports. Mothers who have UAS need close follow-up, however.

▶ This follow-up of 64 women for an average of 10 years after having delivered a child with CHB offers a rare chance to look in detail at their future status. With deliveries occurring from 1964–1993 only 53 gravidas were available for blood sampling. At the time of follow-up exam only 22 women had both Ro and La antibodies, and an additional 10 had only Ro. Only 26% had symptoms of an autoimmune disease despite the presence of 1 or both antibodies in 60% of women tested an average of 10.1 years after delivery. The incidence of healthy women decreased with time but only from 66% at delivery to 56%. The incidence of diagnosable SLE increased from 3% to 11%, and of an undifferentiated autoimmune disorder from 9% to 10%, as some women in this category acquired signs and symptoms of lupus or

Sjögren's syndrome or became normal. What emerges is the wide diversity of autoimmune syndromes associated but relatively infrequently with fetal congenital heart block and the relatively small number of women with SLE at delivery years later. Clearly we tend to ignore that diversity and overemphasize SLE in thinking of the origin of the fetal cardiac affliction. As the authors suggest, we would do better to think of the newborns as showing immune mediated CHB rather than exhibiting a complication of systemic lupus.

T.H. Kirschbaum, M.D.

Pulmonary Hypertension, Cardiac Disease and Pregnancy

Tahir H (Universiti Kebangsaan Malaysia, Kuala Lumpur)
Int J Gynecol Obstet 51:109–113, 1995

3–5

Objective.—Pulmonary hypertension is generally believed to have high morbidity and mortality for mother and fetus alike and is considered to be one of the more severe forms of cardiac disease, indicating the need for prevention or termination of pregnancy. Eisenmenger's syndrome carries a maternal mortality 10 times higher than that of tetralogy of Fallot, even though both are congenital cyanotic heart diseases. The adverse effects of pulmonary hypertension for the mother or fetus or both were studied.

Methods.—Twenty women with co-existing pulmonary hypertension were identified from 268 cases of maternal cardiac disease seen in 1 antenatal clinic during a 3-year period. Their maternal and fetal outcomes were compared with those of a control group of 20 mothers without pulmonary hypertension (Table 1).

Results.—The 2 groups were similar in terms of maternal age, parity, ethnicity, type of cardiac disease, and fetal sex, although the mothers with

TABLE 1.—Types of Heart Disease

	Pulmonary hypertension $n = 20$	Controls $n = 20$
Congenital		
Ventricular septal defect	0	0
Atrial septal defect	4	2
Patent ductus arteriosus	1	1
Eisenmenger's syndrome	3	0
Pulmonary stenosis	0	2
Mitral valve prolapse	0	2
Aortic incompetence	0	1
Rheumatic		
Mitral stenosis	7	5
Mitral incompetence	0	1
Mixed mitral valve disease	4	4
Mixed mitral/aortic valve disease	1	2

(Reprinted from Tahir H: Pulmonary hypertension, cardiac disease and pregnancy. *Int J Gynecol Obstet* 51:109–113, 1995. With kind permission from Elsevier Science Ireland Ltd., Bay 15K, Shannon Industrial Estate, Co. Clare, Ireland.)

TABLE 3.—Maternal Morbidity and Mortality

	Pulmonary hypertension $n = 20$	Controls $n = 20$	P-value
Mode of delivery			
Spontaneous vertex	13	16	NS
Instrumental	4	2	<0.05
Lower segment cesarean section	3	2	NS
Functional class			
1	7	13	NS
2	6	5	NS
3	1	1	NS
4	6	1	<0.05
Congestive cardiac failure	2	0	NS
Maternal mortality	1	0	NS

Abbreviation: NS, not significant.
(Reprinted from Tahir H: Pulmonary hypertension, cardiac disease and pregnancy. *Int J Gynecol Obstet* 51:109–113, 1995. With kind permission from Elsevier Science Ireland Ltd., Bay 15K, Shannon Industrial Estate, Co. Clare, Ireland.)

pulmonary hypertension were more likely to be in New York Heart Association functional class 4 (Table 3). One mother with Eisenmenger's syndrome died. Instrumental deliveries and low birth weight were more likely in the women with pulmonary hypertension than in the controls. However, except for the patient with Eisenmenger's syndrome, no significant differences were found between the 2 groups in maternal morbidity or mortality, premature delivery, or perinatal mortality (Table 4).

Conclusions.—Among pregnant women with cardiac disease, those with co-existing pulmonary hypertension probably have better maternal

TABLE 4.—Fetal Morbidity and Mortality

	Pulmonary hypertension $n = 20$	Controls $n = 20$	P-value
Gestational age (weeks)			
<38	3	3	NS
38–42	17	17	NS
>42	0	0	NS
Mean	38.1	38.0	NS
Birth weight (g)			
<2500	8	3	<0.01
2500–3999	12	17	<0.01
>3999	0	0	NS
Mean	2600	2745	NS
Perinatal mortality			
No.	1	1	NS
Rate (/1000)	50	50	

Abbreviation: NS, not significant.
(Reprinted from Tahir H: Pulmonary hypertension, cardiac disease and pregnancy. *Int J Gynecol Obstet* 51:109–113, 1995. With kind permission from Elsevier Science Ireland Ltd., Bay 15K, Shannon Industrial Estate, Co. Clare, Ireland.)

and fetal outcomes than is generally believed. Eisenmenger's syndrome is the exception. The good results in this study were achieved with a multidisciplinary team including cardiologists, neonatologists, anesthetists, and obstetricians with an interest in the subject.

▶ Pulmonary hypertension often is described as a finding sufficiently grave as to make conception or continued pregnancy contraindicated. That precept rests with observations often made decades ago (see Burch,[1] for example), and more current data using modern diagnostic and therapeutic options are infrequent.

This comparative cohort study of heart disease with and without pulmonary hypertension makes clear some of the problems of data evaluation. Pulmonary hypertension may complicate any of a number of congenital or acquired cardiac lesions, each with implications and hazards of their own. It would be ideal to study women with primary pulmonary hypertension without associated intracardiac lesions, but those are infrequent, and often one is left with the need to compare mixed sets of disparate patients.

Here an effort is made to match controls by New York Heart Association functional class, and the surplus of functional class 4 patients also in frank congestive heart failure among patients with pulmonary hypertension biases the results against the hypertensive group. Perinatal outcomes are generally good, with a surplus of premature births in the hypertensive group. The 1 maternal death reflects the nightmare of acute right heart failure occurring post partum. Increasing pulmonary vascular resistance tends to a high right atrial pressure with shunting from the right to the left atrium of relatively oxygen unsaturated blood. At the same time, as systemic hypoxemia resulting from shunting raises systemic vascular resistance, pulmonary venous return to the left atrium is reduced, as is left ventricular outflow, for which it serves as preload. Transfusion will not improve left ventricular filling and phlebotomy may reduce right atrial pressure a bit, but it may further decrease blood oxygen capacity and oxygen delivery.

Ultimately, patients with pulmonary hypertension must be handled on the basis of their own individual findings. The diagnosis of pulmonary hypertension in this Malaysian series was apparently made by Doppler velocimetry of the regurgitant tricuspid jet occurring during ventricular systole, and should have been confirmed by pulmonary artery catherization. Cardiac output determinations would have been most helpful. About all that can be said for certain from these data is that the uniform injunction against pregnancy in the face of pulmonary hypertension is not warranted.

T.H. Kirschbaum, M.D.

Reference

1. Burch GE: Certain principles in the management of heart disease and pregnancy. *Am Heart J* 100:775, 1980.

Incidence of Pregnancy-Induced Hypertension Among Gestational Diabetics

Schaffir JA, Lockwood CJ, Lapinski R, et al (Mount Sinai School of Medicine, New York)
Am J Perinatol 12:252–254, 1995

3–6

Objective.—Although patients with pregestational diabetes have an increased incidence of hypertensive disorders in pregnancy, it is unclear whether the same applies to patients with gestational diabetes. The incidence and risk of hypertensive disorders among gestational diabetics were investigated in a retrospective case-control study.

Methods.—Gestational diabetes mellitus was diagnosed in 197 prenatal patients between January 1, 1989, and December 31, 1991. The outcome for this group was compared with that of 197 women in the control group.

Results.—No significant difference in preeclampsia or increase in baseline blood pressure was found between groups when those beginning insulin therapy were grouped with those who controlled diabetes by diet alone. Equal numbers of patients with chronic hypertension were found in both groups. The maximum mean arterial blood pressures were significantly higher in the third trimester for the diabetic group than for the control group. The mean arterial blood pressures were also significantly higher in patients with diabetes who were insulin-dependent as compared with those who controlled the disease through diet alone and higher in patients diagnosed with diabetes before 24 weeks as compared with those with diabetes diagnosed after 24 weeks of pregnancy.

Conclusion.—Patients with gestational diabetes do not appear to more frequently have hypertension develop during pregnancy. Although these patients have increases in the mean arterial blood pressure in the third trimester, the relationship to outcome is not clinically relevant and does not merit increased monitoring for preeclampsia.

▶ Given the relationship between insulin resistance, hyperinsulinism, and hypertension that has emerged from studies in the nonpregnant human, this study attacks the question of whether gestational diabetes mellitus (GDM) provides sufficient impetus for that change. The strength of the work rests with careful separation of chronic hypertension from preeclampsia or superimposed preeclampsia and the control of age, race, parity, and nonpregnant weight as covariates. Though preeclampsia as rigorously defined did not show a greater incidence in the 197 GDM patients studied, the underlying relationship between hyperinsulinemia and hypertension was confirmed and supported by finding higher mean arterial pressures among A2 diabetics, i.e., those requiring insulin therapy, than among A1 or diet-controlled gestational diabetics. Further, earlier diagnosis of GDM, a factor that increases the likelihood of maternal exposure to hyperinsulinism, also was related to increased maternal arterial pressure. This study adds to the evidence that the interrelationships of syndrome X[1] apply equally to pregnant and nonpregnant individuals.

T.H. Kirschbaum, M.D.

Reference

1. *J Hypertens* 8:768, 1995 (in press).

Pregnancy Outcomes in the Diabetes Control and Complications Trial
The Diabetes Control and Complications Trial Research Group (Bethesda, Md)
Am J Obstet Gynecol 174:1343–1353, 1996   3–7

Background.—Pregnancy in women with insulin-dependent diabetes mellitus is associated with an increased incidence of spontaneous abortions, stillbirths, and congenital malformations. Fetal outcomes may improve if the mother maintains near-normal glycemia during pregnancy. The effects of closely controlling blood glucose levels on the long-term complications of insulin-dependent diabetes mellitus were examined in the Diabetes Control and Complications Trial. The maternal and fetal outcomes of 180 patients who became pregnant during that trial are reported.

Methods.—The analysis included 270 pregnancies in 180 women with insulin-dependent diabetes mellitus. Women who had been assigned to conventional therapy were switched to intensive therapy when they became pregnant or when they started trying to become pregnant. Intensive therapy sought to achieve normal glycemic control by means of frequent insulin injections or continuous subcutaneous insulin infusion, frequent blood glucose self-monitoring, and dietary adjustments. Once they had delivered, all patients returned to their assigned treatment.

Results.—The 270 pregnancies resulted in 191 live births. At the time of conception, mean glycosylated hemoglobin concentration was significantly different between treatment groups: 7.4% for the intensive therapy group vs. 8.1% for the conventional therapy group. During pregnancy, the mean concentration was 6.6% in both groups (Fig 1). In both groups, the median glycosylated hemoglobin concentration was more for women with abnormal outcomes (Fig 2).

Of the 9 congenital malformations identified, 8 occurred in women from the conventional therapy group. The rate of spontaneous abortions was not significantly different (13% in the intensive therapy group and 10% in the conventional therapy group). Infants of women assigned to intensive therapy were born a mean of 1 week earlier, but there were no differences in birth weight, Apgar scores, neonatal hypoglycemia, respiratory distress, bilirubin levels, hypocalcemia, or state of consciousness. Beginning intensive therapy before vs. after conception made no significant difference in fetal outcome.

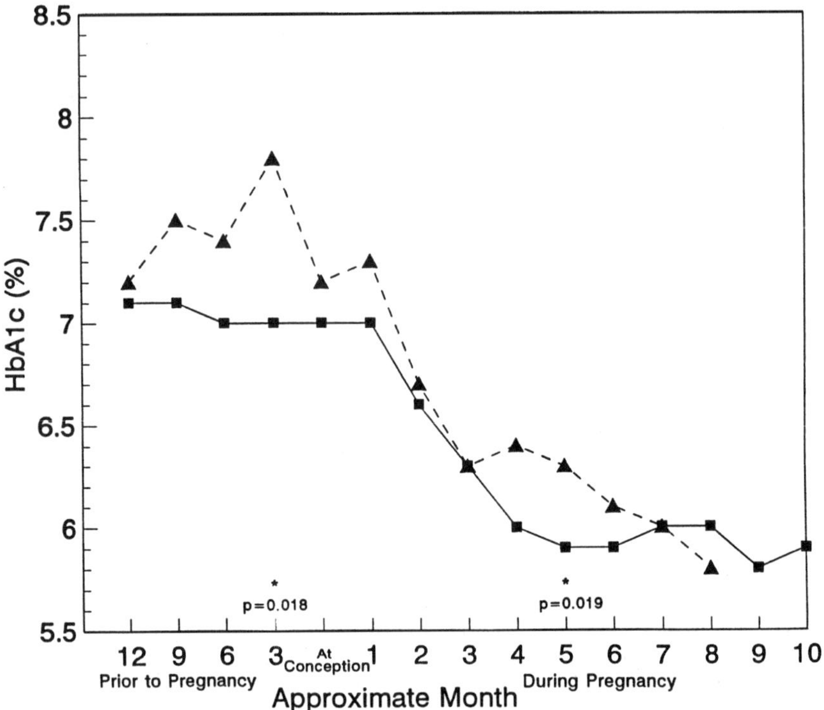

FIGURE 1.—Median hemoglobin A_{1c} (*HbA1c*) for Diabetes Control and Complications Trial pregnancies in intensive treatment group for pregnancies with normal outcomes (n = 88) (*square*) and abnormal outcomes (n = 29) (*triangle*). Abnormal outcomes were defined as ectopic pregnancy, spontaneous abortion for medical reasons, congenital malformation, intrauterine death, and neonatal death. *Asterisk*, $p < 0.02$, Wilcoxon rank-sum test. N-weighted test of stochastic ordering through month 7 during pregnancy: $Z = 2.01$, $p = 0.045$. (Courtesy of The Diabetes Control and Complications Trial Research Group: Pregnancy outcomes in the Diabetes Control and Complications Trial. *Am J Obstet Gynecol* 174:1343–1353, 1996.)

Conclusions.—For pregnant women with insulin-dependent diabetes mellitus, close glycemic control can improve maternal and fetal outcomes. With intensive therapy of the type used in the Diabetes Control and Complications Trial, near normal rates of spontaneous abortions and congenital malformations can be achieved. Having undertaken intensive glycemic control, there seems little benefit from this preconceptional control or outcome of a subsequent pregnancy.

▶ This study, supported by The National Institute of Diabetes Mellitus, Digestion and Kidney Disease of the National Institutes of Health ran from 1983 to 1993 and was aimed at evaluating the merits of strict diabetic control (fasting blood sugar 70–110 mg/dL, 1 hour post cibum serum glucose equal to or less than 140 mg/dL) vs. conventional diabetes management in insulin-dependent diabetes mellitus (IDDM) on the incidence of diabetic complications. The primary result, published in the *New England Journal of Medicine,*[1] showed intensive control associated with a 40% to 76% de-

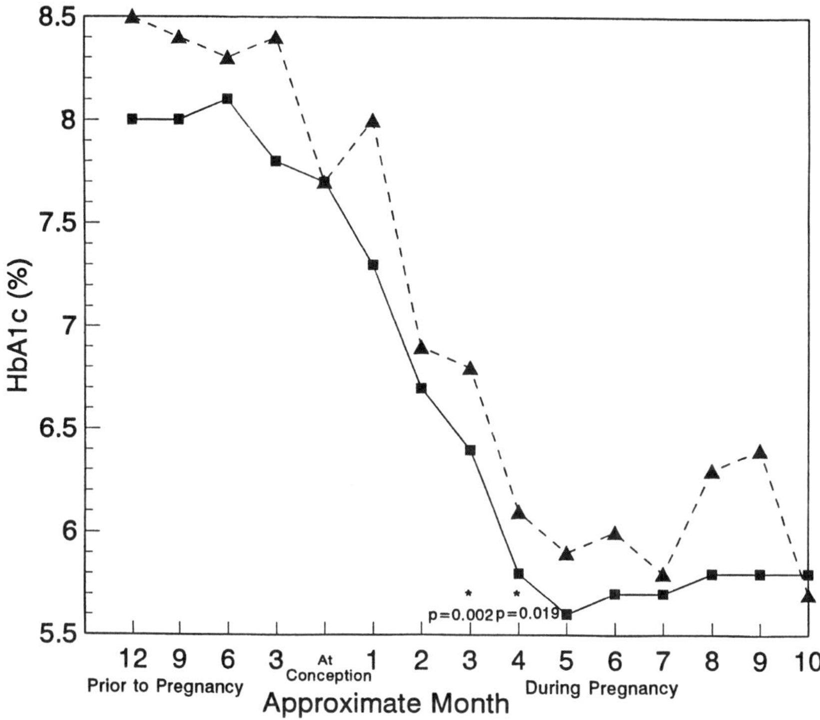

FIGURE 2.—Median hemoglobin A_{1c} (*HbA1c*) values for Diabetes Control and Complications Trial pregnancies in conventional treatment group for pregnancies with normal outcomes (n = 90) (*square*) and abnormal outcomes (n = 37) (*triangle*). Abnormal outcomes were defined as ectopic pregnancy, spontaneous abortion for medical reasons, congenital malformation, intrauterine death, and neonatal death. *Asterisk, p* < 0.02, Wilcoxon rank-sum test. N-weighted test of stochastic ordering through month 7 during pregnancy: Z = 2.41, *p* = 0.016. (Courtesy of The Diabetes Control and Complications Trial Research Group: Pregnancy outcomes in the Diabetes Control and Complications Trial. *Am J Obstet Gynecol* 174:1343–1353, 1996.)

crease in the risk of developing retinopathy, nephropathy, and neuropathy. This report compares pregnancy outcome in those women who, serendipitously or with intent, became pregnant at least 2 years after the randomization and entry into the earlier study. All were urged, if randomized to conventional care, to switch to intensive care, and 26 of 86 women did. Comparisons were made between 135 pregnancies among 92 women in the intensive care group and 135 pregnancies in 99 women in conventional care. There was no difference in the neonatal death rates, and although there were more anomalies among the conventional care group, 37% of these were not attributable to diabetes. The anomaly rate was low and the difference was not significantly different between the 2 groups. Spontaneous abortion rates were 13.3% for intensive and 10.4% for conventional care. No differences were seen among newborn outcome variables, maternal complications of pregnancy, or labor and delivery events. Maternal hypoglycemia was slightly more common among those receiving conventional care but not significantly different from its comparative group. Median hemoglobin A_{1c}

levels were higher on average in those women with abnormal outcomes regardless of care group assigned, and women with conventional care had higher hemoglobin A_{1C} values prior to pregnancy but not past 3 months' gestation. The results are a blow for those who believe in preconceptional care in that there were no differences in outcome in women randomized to conventional care who initiated intensive care preconception vs. those who began it after having conceived. There is reason to urge women with IDDM in pregnancy to strict control regimens, but the benefit rests more in preventing long term diabetic complications than in improving immediate pregnancy outcome.

T.H. Kirschbaum, M.D.

Reference

1. The Diabetes Control and Complication Trial Research Group: The effect of intensive treatment of diabetes on the development and progression of long-term complications in insulin-dependent diabetes mellitus. *N Engl J Med* 329:977, 1993.

Insulin Secretion in Insulin-Resistant Women With a History of Gestational Diabetes

Byrne MM, Sturis J, O'Meara NM, et al (Univ of Chicago)
Metabolism 44:1067–1073, 1995
3–8

Introduction.—Reports are varied regarding the rates of women with a history of gestational diabetes mellitus (GDM) in whom non–insulin-dependent diabetes mellitus later develops. Women with a history of GDM were evaluated for alterations in insulin secretion, action, and clearance.

Methods.—Seven women with a history of GDM and 7 controls matched for weight, age, sex, and race underwent 3-hour glucose, C-peptide, and insulin determinations that were drawn at 30-minute intervals. These insulin secretory responses to oral glucose were also evaluated during a 24-hour period in which 3 mixed meals were served and blood levels were measured at baseline, then at 20-minute intervals throughout. Responses to frequently sampled IV glucose tolerance testing were also determined.

Results.—The fasting plasma glucose concentrations of the oral glucose tolerance test were similar in research subjects and controls. After ingesting glucose, 2 research subjects had normal glucose tolerance and 5 had nondiagnostic oral glucose tolerance tests. Normal oral glucose tolerance tests were determined in all controls. The incremental area under the curve (AUC) for glucose was significantly greater in research subjects from 0 to 180 minutes, as compared with controls. In research subjects, the incremental AUC plasma insulin responses after glucose ingestion were about double those of controls. The incremental AUC plasma C-peptide response was also higher in research subjects, compared with controls.

The mean 24-hour glucose levels were significantly higher in research subjects, compared with controls. This level was also affiliated with higher

24-hour mean levels of insulin and C-peptide and with increased total secretion of insulin. Glucose and insulin responses to frequently sampled IV glucose tolerance testing indicated diminished tissue sensitivity to insulin. Compared with controls, research subjects had decreased impairment in S_1 and lower $AIR_{glucose}$. Research subjects had normal temporal profiles of meal responses, including normal ultradian insulin secretory oscillations, normal insulin clearance, and normal proinsulin-to-insulin molar ratio.

Conclusion.—This cohort of women with a history of GDM was insulin-resistant and demonstrated inappropriately low insulin responses to glucose for the degree of insulin resistance. In women with GDM, an inability of the β-cell to adequately compensate for resistance to the action of insulin may be the causative factor in the subsequent development of non–insulin-dependent diabetes mellitus.

▶ Studies of this sort yield the conclusion that, in the course of development of functional hypoinsulinism, and clinical diabetes mellitus, there is a long, smooth progression of change in insulin regulation, only occasionally marked by diagnosable defects (gestational diabetes, reactive hyperinsulinism, latent hyperglycemia, etc.). In normals, the regulation of insulin secretion to match carbohydrate intake varies widely among individuals, all of them normally glycemic despite individual differences in insulin response. When insulin resistance occurs, as, for example, with ovarian hyperandrogenism or pregnancy, the same mechanisms, clearly not driven by hyperglycemia since such women are usually normoglycemic, increase insulin secretion appropriately. When the capacity to increase insulin secretion wanes, gestational diabetes as transient diabetes becomes discernable. After pregnancy, provided pancreatic β-cell exhaustion has not resulted in fixed chemical diabetes, the prior patterns of response persist, as these investigators show. Impaired insulin sensitivity persists and the level of evoked hyperinsulinism is progressively less than is appropriate for the degree of insulin resistance, indicating the failure of β-cell capacity to respond. Basal resting insulin and plasma glucose concentrations remain normal, but glucose loads result in increases in plasma glucose and insulin above control values, although initially not diagnosably abnormal. In response to meals at 10 AM, 2 PM, and 7 PM, insulin concentration and secretion rates, plasma glucose levels, and C-peptide concentrations behave normally; however, with time, nearly 50% of such women develop non–insulin-dependent diabetes if their insulin resistance is compounded by obesity, and 25% will if they are of normal weight. These findings mark the end result in the inability of pancreatic β-cells to respond to demands present at least initially in the absence of hyperglycemia and with failure of that regulatory mechanism to develop frank hyperglycemia. This analysis highlights our need to understand what, besides hyperglycemia, regulates insulin production and release after a carbohydrate load.

T.H. Kirschbaum, M.D.

Identification of Levels of Maternal HIV-1 RNA Associated With Risk of Perinatal Transmission: Effect of Maternal Zidovudine Treatment on Viral Load

Dickover RE, Garratty EM, Herman SA, et al (Univ of California, Los Angeles; Roche Molecular Systems, Somerville, NJ; Long Beach Mem Med Ctr, Los Angeles)
JAMA 275:599–605, 1996

3–9

Background.—The quantity of HIV in the mother's blood at delivery is an important risk factor in mother-to-infant transmission of HIV. In asymptomatic women with HIV infection, zidovudine can cut the risk of perinatal HIV transmission by two thirds. It is important to find out whether there is some critical threshold or pattern of HIV replication in maternal blood that predicts perinatal transmission to the fetus. Associations between the mother's HIV-1 level during gestation and at delivery, zidovudine treatment of the mother, and risk of perinatal HIV transmission were examined using prospectively collected data.

Methods.—The analysis included 97 infants of 92 HIV-1–seropositive mothers prospectively followed up in a larger study of maternal-fetal HIV-1 transmission. In this nonrandomized study, 42 mothers in 43 pregnancies received zidovudine during pregnancy, labor and delivery, or both. In addition, 11 infants received zidovudine prophylactically for their first 6 weeks of life. Polymerase chain reaction was used to quantitate HIV-1 DNA in peripheral blood mononuclear cells. Logistic regression was used to determine the value of virologic and immunologic markers in predicting HIV-1 transmission. The variables analyzed were viral load, CD4+ cell count, and zidovudine use.

Results.—Twenty-two percent of the infants were infected with HIV-1. Seventy-five percent of the mothers who transmitted HIV-1 to their infants had plasma HIV-1 RNA levels at delivery of greater than 50,000 copies per milliliter, compared with 5% of those who did not transmit HIV-1. When the HIV-1 RNA level was less than 20,000 copies per milliliter, viral transmission never occurred. In a subgroup of 50 mothers followed up through gestation, 7 had increasing HIV-1 replication over time, 29 had a decreasing viral load, and 14 had a stable viral load.

Receiving zidovudine during gestation produced a median eightfold decrease in plasma RNA levels, from 43,043 to 4,238 copies per milliliter at delivery (Fig 1). None of the 22 women receiving this treatment transmitted HIV-1 to their infants. In comparison, 4 of 4 women with high HIV-1 levels who were treated with zidovudine transmitted the virus to their infants. This occurred despite the in vitro sensitivity of the virus to zidovudine.

Conclusions.—The risk of perinatal transmission of HIV-1 depends heavily on the mother's HIV-1 RNA levels. Viral thresholds during late gestation, labor, and delivery are associated with a high and a low risk of transmission. Zidovudine treatment can reduce the mother's HIV-1 RNA level before delivery and thus help to protect against transmission of

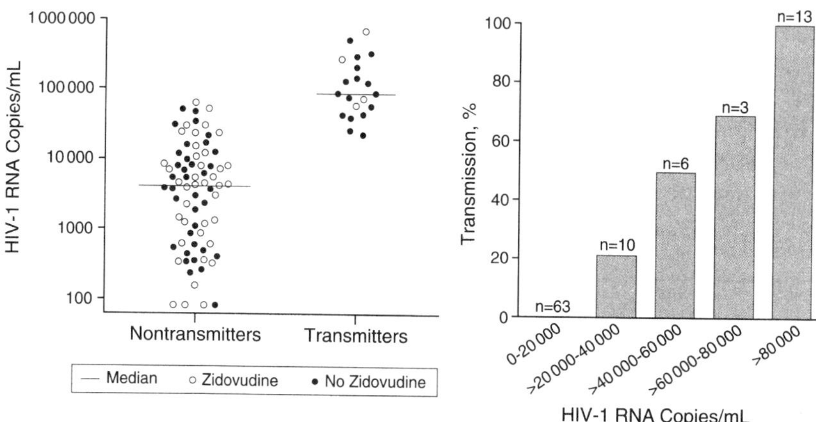

FIGURE 1.—*Left*, maternal plasma HIV-1 RNA levels at delivery in infected nontransmitting and transmitting mothers. Mothers who received zidovudine during gestation or labor and delivery or both are indicated by the *open circles*; mothers who did not receive zidovudine during gestation, labor, or delivery are indicated by the *solid circles*. *Horizontal bars* indicate the median for each of the measured variables. *Right*, Perinatal transmission rate according to HIV-1 RNA levels at delivery. (Courtesy of Dickover RE, Garratty EM, Herman SA, et al: Identification of levels of maternal HIV-1 RNA associated with risk of perinatal transmission: Effect of maternal zidovudine treatment on viral load. *JAMA* 275:599–605, 1996. Copyright 1996, American Medical Association.)

the infection. New preventive approaches are needed for mothers with high or increasing levels of virus or those whose virus does not respond to zidovudine.

▶ As discussed here later (Abstract 10–6), experience with protease inhibitors has caused investigators to look at the dynamics of maternal, fetal, and newborn HIV-1 infection from a new reference point—the density of HIV RNA virions in blood. Here the emphasis is on establishing the risks of maternal-to-fetal transport as a function of maternal viral concentration and correlating the impact of zidovudine (AZT) treatment during pregnancy on both viral concentration and reduction in transmission rates.

The number of HIV-RNA copies per milliliter of plasma sample was estimated using an internal standard of known copy number introduced at the start of polymerase chain reaction. Quantitation of the DNA template for the HIV-1 virus particle (proto-virion) embedded in the host genome through reverse transcriptase action, acting on infecting HIV-RNA, was quantitated through polymerase chain reaction using known quantities of DNA isotopically labeled probes complementary to the viral DNA segments. Then CD4 monocytes were identified by flow cytometry and, assuming each cell contained 1 viral DNA copy, the fraction of total peripheral blood mononuclear cells infected was estimated.

Of the 92 HIV-positive women studied, 45% of them received AZT during pregnancy. Neonates were not treated with AZT. Using plasma HIV-RNA concentration as a discriminator, all 13 women with at least 80,000 viral copies per milliliter had infected infants; none of the 63 women with less than 20,000 HIV-RNA copies per milliliter transmitted their infection to their offspring. An RNA density of 50,000 copies per milliliter proved, by receiver-operating characteristics, an effective predictive level, with 79% sensitivity and 93% specificity, with a 25% false positive rate in predicting the 21.6% overall instance of maternal-to-fetal transmission.

Therapy with AZT reduced the incidence of transmitted infection to 18%. Coincident with maternal AZT were significant decreases in viral plasma RNA copy number, the number of infected CD4 cells, and peripheral blood mononuclear cells. Whether the drug acts by reducing maternal viral load before or during labor or prevents virus from infecting the fetus or infant remains uncertain. Of 20 infected infants, 12 were judged to be infected in utero and 8 intrapartum. Plasma viral RNA was a far better predictor of fetal and infant infection than p24 antigen, CD4 count, or CD 4-proviral quantitation. Not only does this work provide new predictive capacity enabling us to advise HIV-positive women of the risk to infecting their offspring, but it also enables the risk of infectivity to be controlled in studies of prophylactic and therapy of HIV-1 infection in pregnant women.

T.H. Kirschbaum, M.D.

Efficacy of Antenatal Zidovudine in Reducing Perinatal Transmission of Human Immunodeficiency Virus Type 1
Matheson PB, Abrams EJ, Thomas PA, et al (Med and Health Research Assoc of New York City, Inc; Harlem Hosp, New York; New York City Dept of Health; et al)
J Infect Dis 172:353–358, 1995   3–10

Introduction.—The preliminary findings of the AIDS Clinical Trials Group (ACTG) protocol 076 that were released in February, 1994, by the National Institute of Allergy and Infectious Diseases had 3 limitations. First, findings were applicable only to women with moderate or mild absolute CD4+ cell depletion who had not received antenatal retroviral treatment during pregnancy. Second, the relative components of the antepartum, intrapartum, and infant components of treatment with zidovudine could not be determined. Third, long-term in utero side effects of zidovudine exposure were unknown. The effectiveness of antepartum zidovudine was evaluated for its use alone in reducing mother-to-child transmission of HIV-1 among women with various levels of CD4+ depletion.

Methods.—Maternal CD4+ cell counts were obtained prospectively in 432 women with AIDS-defining illness diagnosed before delivery or within 2 weeks post partum. Normal, moderately depressed, and severely depressed CD4+ levels were defined as greater than 499 µL, 200–499 µL, and less than 200 µL, respectively. Infants of mothers who were HIV-1–seropositive were considered HIV-infected if they had 2 different positive blood samples determined by polymerase chain reaction. In mothers who received zidovudine, the dose and timing of treatment with zidovudine were determined by the treating clinician.

TABLE 3.—Transmission Rate of HIV-1 to Infants for 321 HIV-1–Seropositive Women by Zidovudine Use During Pregnancy and CD4+ Lymphocyte Count

CD4+ cell count*	Zidovudine	No zidovudine	OR (95% CI)	Total
<200	3/13 (23)	10/24 (42)	0.42 (0.09–1.9)	13/37 (35)
200–499	3/18 (17)	25/82 (30)	0.46 (0.12–1.7)	28/100 (28)
>499	0/13	27/171 (16)	0.20 (0.01–3.4)†	27/184 (15)
Total	6/44 (14)	62/277 (22)	0.55 (0.22–1.4)	68/321 (21)

Note: Data are number/total (%).
*Closest lymphocyte measurement before or within 2 weeks of delivery (cells per μL.)
†Logit estimation used correction of 0.5.
Abbreviations: OR, odds ratio; CI, confidence interval.
(Courtesy of Matheson PB, Abrams EJ, Thomas PA, et al: Efficacy of Antenatal Zidovudine in Reducing Perinatal Transmission of Human Immunodeficiency Virus Type 1. *J Infect Dis* 172:353–358, 1995: Copyright University of Chicago, publisher.)

Results.—Of 321 women with complete data, the median time of maternal lymphocyte determination was 2 days post partum. The median time from initiation of zidovudine therapy during pregnancy to delivery was 19 weeks. All the mothers who received zidovudine had prenatal care, compared with 82% of those who did not receive zidovudine. Mothers who received zidovudine had significantly lower absolute CD4+ counts, CD4+ percentages, and CD4:CD8 ratios and higher CD8+ cell percentages. They were also more likely to have received a diagnosis of an AIDS-defining illness by 2 weeks post partum. The crude transmission rate for mothers taking zidovudine during pregnancy was 14%, compared with 23% for women not taking zidovudine during pregnancy. The crude transmission rate increased as the CD4+ level decreased: 15% for those with normal counts, 28% for those with moderate CD4+ depletion, and 35% for those with severe CD4+ depletion (Table 3). Mothers with moderately and severely depressed CD4+ depletion were significantly more likely to transmit HIV-1, compared with mothers with normal CD4+ levels. Compared with infants of mothers who did not receive antepartal zidovudine, infants of mothers who received zidovudine during antepartum were significantly more likely to have an elevated mean corpuscular volume within the first 2 weeks of life. Compared with mothers who did not transmit the HIV virus, mothers who transmitted the HIV virus were more likely to have signs of HIV-related illness.

Conclusion.—Combined with the findings of the ACTG protocol 076, these results support the United States Public Health Service guidelines recommending that zidovudine be offered to all pregnant women who are HIV-1–seropositive. It is possible that the maximum effect of zidovudine occurs during the antenatal segment of the ACTG protocol 076 treatment regimen.

▶ Though the Pediatric Aids Clinical Trials Group Protocol 076 Study Group demonstrated the usefulness of zidovudine (AZT) given to HIV-1–positive women with CD4 counts greater than 200 per microliter when administered antepartum and intrapartum coupled with newborn therapy,[1] a number of questions immediately became obvious.[2] This study explores 2 of them. The HIV-positive women with CD counts less than 200 per microliter received therapy, but the numbers of cases were too small to allow direct controlled comparisons. However, when the odds ratio between treated and untreated patients for fetal transmission was adjusted for variant CD4 counts, an odds ratio of 0.36 (confidence interval, 0.14–0.92) emerged against an overall transmission rate of 22% for all 321 patients. This result followed drug therapy given only prior to labor, since neither intrapartum maternal or newborn infant therapy was given to these women and infants treated from 1986 to 1993. It's understandable in this retrospective case-control study that, without therapeutic protocol, only 13 women with CD4 counts greater than 499 per microliter received AZT; the transmission rate in 171 such women not treated with AZT was a surprising 16%. This analysis supports but does not prove that intrapartum AZT for a median duration of 19 weeks' gestation may reduce maternal-to-fetal transmission even with women who have very low CD4 counts.

T.H. Kirschbaum, M.D.

References

1. *Focus & Opinion: Obstetrics and Gynecology* 1(2):103, 1995.
2. 1995 YEAR BOOK OF OBSTETRICS AND GYNECOLOGY, pp 76–77.

Mode of Delivery and Gestational Age Influence Perinatal HIV-1 Transmission

Tovo P-A, and the Italian Register for HIV Infection in Children (Univ of Turin, Italy)

J Acquir Immune Defic Syndr 11:88–94, 1996   3–11

Background.—Mother-infant transmission is a leading cause of HIV infection in children. Mounting lines of evidence indicate that infection occurs late in pregnancy or during labor and delivery in a large percentage of neonates. Cesarean section may offer a means of reducing viral transmission to the fetus and neonates—a possibility that has garnered support in recent investigations. The effects of mode of delivery and other maternal and infant factors on the rate of HIV transmission were prospectively evaluated.

Patients and Methods.—A total of 1,624 neonates born to mothers infected with HIV at or before delivery were prospectively followed from birth. Infants who were older than 18 months of age at the last visit, or who would have been had they not died of an HIV-1–related illness, were included in the perinatal transmission rate analysis. The impact and possible confounding effects of other maternal and infant factors—including pregnancy duration, birth weight, type of feeding, and sex of the infant—on HIV-1 infection also were assessed, as was the risk of infection in first- and second-born infants.

Results.—There were 1,033 infants considered in the analysis. One hundred eighty of the 975 first singleton infants became infected. Eight of 56 second-born infants also acquired infection. Significant and independent associations between higher transmission rates and vaginal vs. cesarean delivery (odds ratio, 1.69), as well as symptomatic vs. asymptomatic mothers (odds ratio, 1.61), were noted in multivariate stepwise analysis. History of maternal drug use, birth weight, breast-feeding (only 37 infants were breast-fed), and infant's sex were not significantly associated with viral transmission. Very premature neonates (32 weeks' gestation or less) had the highest rate of infection, at 30.7%. At week 42, this trend decreased to 11.9%, suggesting a coincident decrease in peripartum transmission.

Conclusions.—Neonates delivered by cesarean section are at less risk of acquiring maternally transmitted HIV-1 infection. Randomized, controlled studies evaluating the protective effect of surgical delivery against HIV-1 transmission are highly recommended.

▶ Here, the data from the Italian Register for HIV Infection in Children are interrogated for evidence of the benefit of cesarean section in reducing the fetal HIV transmission rate reported by others.[1-3] Starting with 1,624 neonates born of 1,480 gravidas who were HIV-positive, most of the conclusions are based on the analysis of 1,033 singleton births with follow-up to at least 18 months of life, sufficient to exclude passive HIV antibody transferred to the infants. Most women were infected through drug use, and the registry did not include women given AZT during pregnancy, as is now recommended.

The infant infection rate was 18.2%, and both maternal symptoms and birth weight of less than 2.5 kg showed significant relationships to increased transmission rates on multivariate analysis. The cesarean section rate of 11.7% was based on data from 274 cesarean sections. Regrettably, multivariate analysis was not done to evaluate the possibility that small fetuses carried by symptomatic HIV-positive mothers might well have had a decreased likelihood of abdominal birth—and to express in this way a confounding relationship to the lower cesarean section transfer rate. However, the conclusion is the same as that expressed in studies previously reviewed here—that abdominal birth is associated with a lower risk of transmission to the neonate.

The role of cesarean section in women receiving AZT desperately needs to be determined. The authors' conclusion that fetal transmission is more common at less than 32 weeks' gestation rests on only 26 infants and needs confirmation as well. There were too few twins or breast-fed infants to comment on those relationships to the likelihood of neonatal infection.

T.H. Kirschbaum, M.D.

References

1. 1993 YEAR BOOK OF OBSTETRICS AND GYNECOLOGY, pp 50–51, 78–79, 221–223.
2. 1994 YEAR BOOK OF OBSTETRICS AND GYNECOLOGY, pp 63–64, 238–239.
3. 1995 YEAR BOOK OF OBSTETRICS AND GYNECOLOGY, pp 76–77.

Vertical Transmission of HIV-1 in Mid-trimester Gestation

Phuapradit W, Chaturachinda K, Taneepanichskul S, et al (Mahidol Univ, Bangkok, Thailand)

Aust N Z J Obstet Gynaecol 35:427–430, 1995   3–12

Introduction.—Reported rates of perinatal transmission of HIV-1 vary widely, from 12% to 65%. Important questions remain about the stage of pregnancy during which the fetus is most vulnerable and the factors that increase the chances of maternal-to-fetal HIV-1 transmission. Viral detection techniques were used to assess in utero transmission of HIV among infected women undergoing elective abortion.

Methods.—The study included 23 HIV-1–seropositive women who elected to have their pregnancies terminated at 18 to 25 weeks' gestation. The abortions were performed by vaginal administration of prostaglandin E1 analogue. Fresh heart blood samples from the fetal bodies were analyzed by polymerase chain reaction of the HIV-1 genome and p24 antigen to assess possible transplacental transfer of HIV-1 infection.

Results.—All but 2 of the women were asymptomatic and had received no antiretroviral therapy. On enzyme-linked immunosorbent assay, all 23 fetal heart blood samples were positive for HIV-1; however, all were negative for polymerase chain reaction and HIV-1 p24 antigen assay. All positive controls gave positive results on these assays.

Conclusions.—In utero transmission of HIV-1 during midtrimester gestation appears to be an infrequent event, if it occurs at all. Most cases of maternal-to-fetal transmission seem to occur during the last weeks of pregnancy or at delivery. Pregnant women with HIV infection should receive zidovudine therapy during the last trimester, during labor, and in the early postnatal period. Midtrimester fetal blood sampling appears to be an inappropriate diagnostic tool for in utero HIV infection.

▶ Although it is clear that fetal infection may occur in utero as early as 11 to 12 weeks of gestational age,[1] most time-linked studies suggest that fetal infection more commonly occurs in the late third trimester, during delivery, or in the neonatal period. This is an important consideration because, if true, it makes fetal diagnosis by cordocentesis in early pregnancy an unreliable measure of ultimate maternal-to-fetal transmission. Then, too, AZT prevention may require that the drug be given to women who are positive for HIV antibody only in the third trimester.

This Bangkok study of 23 midtrimester abortions at 18 to 25 weeks measured HIV-1 antibody, determined HIV p24 surface antigen, and carried out amplification and detection of HIV-1 DNA for fetal diagnosis based on cardiac blood sampling. It is important that sensitivity of the HIV-DNA determination was affirmed using a cell culture line containing a single genome copy of HIV-1 DNA diluted to a concentration of 1 cell per 10 µL. Only 2 of the 23 women had symptoms or chemical evidence of infection or both. In none of the 23 fetuses could p24 antigen or HIV-1 DNA be detected. The authors list 8 earlier studies with consonant results, confirming the relative rarity of early pregnancy maternal-to-fetal transmission of the virus suggested in several previous studies.

T.H. Kirschbaum, M.D.

Reference

1. 1994 YEAR BOOK OF OBSTETRICS AND GYNECOLOGY, pp 136–137.

Human Immunodeficiency Virus Type 1–Infected Cells in Breast Milk: Association With Immunosuppression and Vitamin A Deficiency

Nduati RW, John GC, Richardson BA, et al (Univ of Nairobi, Kenya; Univ of Washington, Seattle; Univ of Manitoba, Winnipeg, Canada)
J Infect Dis 172:1461–1468, 1995   3–13

Introduction.—There is significant risk of mother-to-infant transmission of HIV-1 associated with breast-feeding. However, formula feeding in developing countries carries substantial risk of high infant mortality resulting from infectious disease and malnutrition. Therefore, the World Health Organization currently recommends that women who are HIV-seropositive in areas with high infant mortality breast-feed their infants. To investigate the determinants of HIV transmission through breast milk, the prevalence, concentration, and clinical correlates of virus-infected cells in breast milk were studied among HIV-seropositive mothers.

Methods.—Manually expressed samples of colostrum obtained within 1 week of delivery and of breast milk obtained at 6 to 52 weeks after delivery from 107 HIV-seropositive women were analyzed for the presence of HIV DNA using polymerase chain reaction. Correlations were analyzed between clinical variables and the presence or absence of HIV-1 DNA in breast milk and between clinical variables and virus concentrations in breast milk.

Results.—Of the 212 samples, 123 (58%) had detectable HIV-1 DNA. The prevalence of HIV-1 DNA varied from 71% in the samples obtained at 6 to 9 months to 20% in the samples obtained after 9 months (Fig 1). The prevalence of a high concentration of virus was greatest between 8 and 90 days after delivery and decreased to 0% at 9 months after delivery. Detectable HIV-1-infected cells were significantly correlated with low CD4 cell counts (less than 400 cells/mm^3), high CD8 counts (more than 47%), and low CD4:CD8 ratios (less than 0.5). A significant inverse relationship was found between HIV-1 DNA in colostrum and breast milk and vitamin A levels only among women with less than 400 CD4 cells/mm^3.

Conclusions.—In most breast milk samples, HIV-1 DNA was detected. The prevalence of infected cells remained high from birth until 9 months after delivery, and some samples contained a high concentration of infected cells. Both the prevalence and concentration of breast milk HIV-1 DNA were highly correlated with maternal immunosuppression. Women

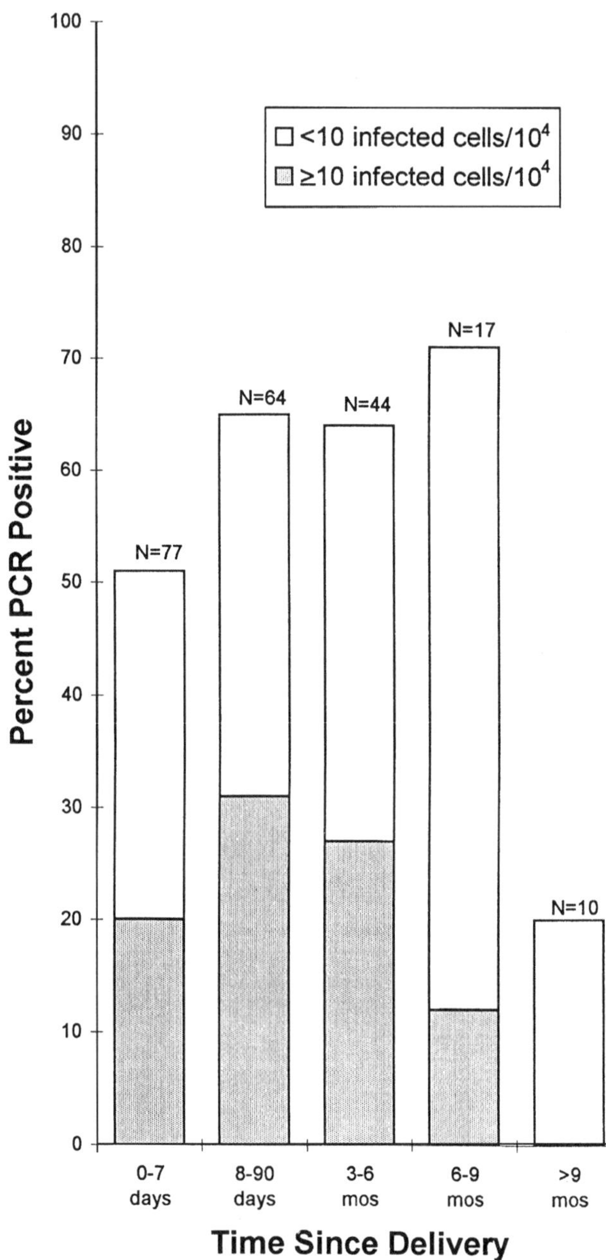

FIGURE 1.—Prevalence and concentration of HIV-1 DNA in breast milk cells. Percentages indicate those with less than 10 or 10 or more infected cells/10,000. *Abbreviation: mos,* months. (Courtesy of Nduati RW, John GC, Richardson BA, et al: Human immunodeficiency virus type 1–infected cells in breast milk: Association with immunosuppression and vitamin A deficiency. *J Infect Dis* 172:1461–1468, 1995. Copyright 1995, The University of Chicago.)

with both advanced HIV disease and prenatal vitamin A deficiency had a particularly high prevalence of infected cells in the colostrum and breast milk, suggesting a possibly higher risk of mother-to-infant HIV transmission in these women.

▶ Although the risk of maternal-to-infant transmission of HIV-1 has been made clear by epidemiologic surveys,[1] this is a first quantitative assay of the incidence of HIV-infected cells and viral DNA in breast milk. It discloses, with respect to infectivity, both high prevalence and long duration into the puerperium. In a population of 107 women from Nairobi who were HIV-positive, none with AIDS, but 39% with symptoms and 16% with CD4 cell counts less than $200/mm^3$, 50% to 70% of 212 breast milk samples showed evidence of HIV DNA after polymerase chain reaction. Nearly 40% of the samples had at least 10 infected cells per 10,000 using serial dilution against HIV-DNA positivity. Only in the interval past 6 months post partum did the number of infected cells, but not viral HIV DNA, begin to decline in concentration.

Nursing after delivery appears to deliver large doses of colostrum-borne virus and infected immune cells to the infant, and breast milk remains a source of pathogens for more than 9 months after delivery. This study re-emphasizes the urgent rationale for the interdiction of nursing by women with HIV, symptomatic or not.

T.H. Kirschbaum, M.D.

Reference

1. 1993 Year Book of Obstetrics and Gynecology, pp 217–219.

Prospective Cohort Study of the Effect of Pregnancy on the Progression of Human Immunodeficiency Virus Infection
Hocke C, and the Groupe D'Epidémiologie Clinique du Sida en Aquitaine (Université de Bordeaux II, France)
Obstet Gynecol 86:886–891, 1995   3–14

Introduction.—Previous studies of the prognostic role of pregnancy in the course of HIV infection have reported contradictory findings. In addition, these studies either did not include a comparison group or had insufficient follow-up to provide statistical power. To further investigate the effects of pregnancy on the progression of HIV infection, the clinical evolution of HIV infection was studied prospectively in cohorts of pregnant and nonpregnant women.

Methods.—Women who were seropositive for HIV and had given birth after the diagnosis of HIV was made were matched with 2 women who were HIV-seropositive who had not conceived after receiving a diagnosis of HIV. The cases and controls were matched for age, CD4 counts, and diagnosis period. The incidences of death, progression to AIDS, and decreasing CD4 counts to less than $200/mm^3$ were compared in the 2 groups.

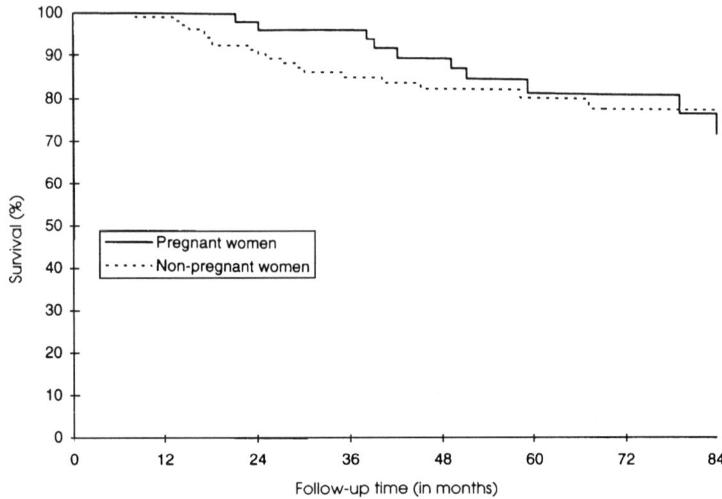

FIGURE 1.—Probability of survival in pregnant and nonpregnant women who were seropositive for HIV. (Courtesy of Hocke C, and the Groupe D'Epidémiologie Clinique du Sida en Aquitaine: *Obstet Gynecol* 86:886–891, 1995. Reprinted with permission from The American College of Obstetricians and Gynecologists.)

Results.—Of the 870 patients in the study population, 90% of the pregnant women and 76% of the nonpregnant women were asymptomatic at diagnosis. The median follow-up after diagnosis of HIV infection was 61 months in the pregnant women and 50 months in the nonpregnant women. No significant differences were found between the 2 groups in the

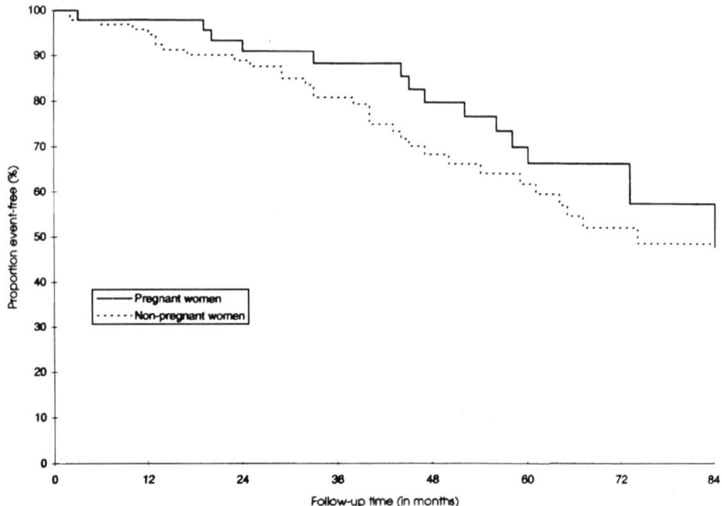

FIGURE 3.—Probability of not reaching a CD4 count less than 200/mm^3 in pregnant and nonpregnant women who were seropositive for HIV. (Courtesy of Hocke C, and the Groupe D'Epidemiologie Clinique du Sida en Aquitane: *Obstet Gynecol* 86:886–891, 1995. Reprinted with permission from The American College of Obstetricians and Gynecologists.)

incidences of death, progression to AIDS, or a drop of the CD4 count to less than 200/mm³. The probability of survival at 5 years was 81.8% in pregnant women and 80.7% in nonpregnant women (Fig 1). The probability of avoiding progression to AIDS at 5 years was 82.6% in the pregnant women and 78.6% in the nonpregnant women. Among the women with a CD4 count greater than 200/mm³ at study entry, the probability of maintaining that status at 5 years was 66.7% in the pregnant women and 62.1% in the nonpregnant women (Fig 3).

Conclusions.—Among women with mild-to-moderate immunosuppression caused by HIV infection, pregnancy did not affect the course of the infection and therefore has no prognostic role.

▶ This study addresses an important question variously answered in the past: does pregnancy adversely affect the course of maternal HIV-1 infection? The authors answer in the negative, but there is 1 concern regarding their data. The prospective study enrolled women who were HIV-positive who had at least 1 delivery after the diagnosis of the infection and matched women who were HIV-positive who were not pregnant in the same time interval, 2 for 1, for age, CD4 count, and time since diagnosis confirmed by Western blot. Although median CD4 counts and years since diagnosis were well matched, clinical stage was not. Ninety percent of those in the pregnant subset of 57 women were asymptomatic, whereas 76% of the nonpregnant group lacked symptoms of AIDS, a statistically significant difference. It is not surprising that pregnancy should more often be undertaken by asymptomatic than symptomatic women who are HIV-positive. With respect to years of survival since diagnosis, AIDS-free survival, and the incidence of CD4 counts less than 200/mm³, no differences were associated with pregnancy, as judged by the Kaplan-Meier test.

Despite concern about matching controls in this cohort study, this is encouraging news to those women who are HIV-positive who become inadvertently pregnant. The high risk of transmitting HIV to newborns should not be forgotten in counseling women who are HIV-positive regarding the imperatives of contraception.

T.H. Kirschbaum, M.D.

The European Collaborative Study: Clinical and Immunological Characteristics of HIV 1-Infected Pregnant Women
Thorne C, Newell M-L, Dunn D, et al (Inst of Child Health, London)
Br J Obstet Gynaecol 102:869–875, 1995   3–15

Background.—An increasing number of European women of childbearing age are being infected with HIV. Heterosexual transmission is becoming the main route of infection for women. The changing clinical and immunologic features and timing of the diagnosis of HIV-infected pregnant women enrolled in the European Collaborative Study were reported.

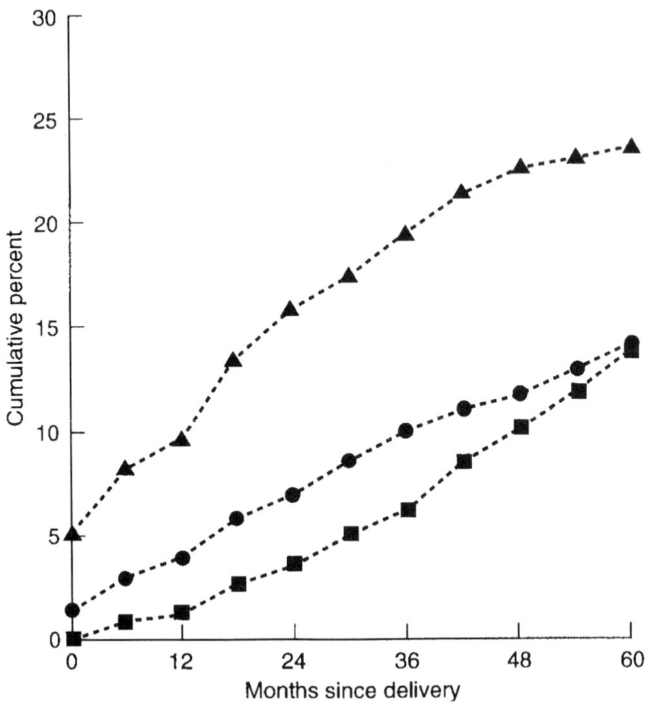

FIGURE 3.—Kaplan-Meier analysis of cumulative percentage of women progressing to Centers for Disease Control stage IV, AIDS, and death, relative to date of delivery. *Triangles*, Centers for Disease Control stage IV: *circles*, AIDS; *squares*, death. (Courtesy of Thorne C, Newell M-L, Dunn D, et al: The European Collaborative Study: Clinical and immunological characteristics of HIV 1-infected pregnant women. *Br J Obstet Gynaecol* 102:869-875, 1995, Blackwell Science Ltd.)

Methods.—Twenty-one centers in 7 European countries participated in the study. Data on 1,690 HIV-infected women and their 1,754 deliveries were analyzed prospectively.

Findings.—From 1984 to 1985, 7% of women with HIV infection were diagnosed before pregnancy, compared with 65% in 1994. The prevalence of breast-feeding, which was associated with the timing of the diagnosis, declined significantly during those years. The mean CD4 count was 510 cells/mm^3. The mean CD4 count declined significantly during the study period. The CD4 count was significantly lower in black women than in white women. Survival analysis indicated that, 5 years after delivery, an estimated 14% of women will have died and 24% will have Centers for Disease Control stage IV disease (Fig 3).

Conclusions.—The timing of HIV diagnosis is critical to reduce mother-to-child transmission through avoidance of breast-feeding. Zidovudine treatment and effective antenatal screening policies have become increasingly important. The rate of progression of disease in the mothers has important implications for their children, both infected and not.

▶ This is the most recent update of the European Collaborative Study of HIV Infection in Pregnancy,[1, 2] which now encompasses 21 centers in 7 countries and includes 1,754 births to 1,690 HIV-positive women. A disproportionate number of these case reports are from Italy and Spain. Unlike earlier reports, this one focuses on the characteristics of the infection in gravid women. Most useful is a by-product of the 89 deaths of mothers reported in cumulative fashion in Fig 3. It shows that, 5 years after delivery, 50% of women will be generally well without progression to AIDS or Centers for Disease Control and Prevention stage 3 disease, 24% will have stage 4 disease, 13% will have AIDS, and 14% will have succumbed. Longitudinal trends show an increasing proportion of HIV-positive women, 65% of them in 1994, will conceive knowing they are HIV-positive. Many of these women are drug users. Breast-feeding has reduced in incidence to approximately 1% in the interval between 1991 and 1994, but it is too early to discern the impact of this step or of prophylactic zidovudine (AZT) use in the 45 women enrolled in that study on infant transmission rates. European screening methods, excluding Sweden where 98% of women were diagnosed before delivery, remain as imperfect as in this country. If the 6 new drugs now available for the treatment of HIV I infection, including the new class of protease inhibitors, and safe sex education do represent the turning of a corner in the treatment of this disease, long-term longitudinal studies of this sort will be the first to demonstrate it.

T.H. Kirschbaum, M.D.

References

1. 1990 YEAR BOOK OF OBSTETRICS AND GYNECOLOGY, pp 196–198.
2. 1993 YEAR BOOK OF OBSTETRICS AND GYNECOLOGY, pp 217–219.

Acyclovir Suppression to Prevent Cesarean Delivery After First-episode Genital Herpes
Scott LL, Sanchez PJ, Jackson GL, et al (Univ of Texas, Dallas)
Obstet Gynecol 87:69–73, 1996   3–16

Background.—It is currently recommended that pregnant women with visible genital herpes lesions or prodromal symptoms at the time of labor have their offspring delivered by cesarean section to prevent possible transmission of the herpes virus (HSV) to the neonate. Gravida patients without visible lesions or prodromal symptoms are allowed to continue in labor because they have a low incidence of neonatal HSV transmission.

Objective.—The study objective was to determine whether suppressive acyclovir therapy given to gravidas at term who had their first episode of genital HSV infection during pregnancy would decrease the need for cesarean section for that indication.

Methods.—In 46 pregnant women who were experiencing their first episode of genital herpes during pregnancy, the diagnosis was confirmed by positive cultures for HSV. The patients were randomly assigned in double-blind fashion to regimens of acyclovir 400 mg or placebo 3 times a day. Twenty-one patients assigned to receive acyclovir and 25 assigned to receive placebo completed the study and yielded assessable results. Study medication was initiated at 36 weeks' gestation and continued until delivery. Vaginal delivery was performed if there was no clinical recurrence of herpes and if no other contraindications were present; otherwise, a cesarean section was performed. Cultures for HSV were obtained from the neonate's conjunctiva, oropharynx, and rectum 24 to 72 hours after delivery. Neonates were also examined for evidence of acyclovir toxicity. The neonate's medical status was reviewed 1 month after delivery.

Results.—None of the 21 patients treated with acyclovir had clinical evidence of recurrent genital herpes at the time of delivery, and all had vaginal deliveries. On the other hand, 9 of the 25 (36%) of those treated with placebo had clinical evidence of recurrent genital herpes at delivery and underwent cesarean section. The difference favoring the acyclovir group was highly statistically significant. No neonate had evidence of herpes infection or acyclovir toxicity either shortly after delivery or 1 month post partum.

Conclusions.—In comparison with treatment with placebo, suppressive acyclovir therapy initiated at 36 weeks' gestation and continued until delivery significantly reduced the need for cesarean section for recurrent genital herpes. None of the neonates in the study manifested evidence of herpes infection, and none of those treated with acyclovir had evidence of acyclovir toxicity.

▶ It is clear that nonpregnant individuals with recurrent genital herpes have decreased frequency of recurrence when they take prophylactic acyclovir. So, it is not surprising that there is suggestion of value in its prophylactic use in pregnancy. The only questions are issues of fetal safety associated with the use of 1.2 g of acyclovir every day for an average of 3.6 weeks during the third trimester. Certainly, the drug appears safe to pregnant women, and the lack of evident fetal effect in the 21 women treated here is encouraging.

It is important that the study was blinded to patients and physicians, but the need for cesarean section in women in labor without lesions but with "prodromal symptoms" of recurrent herpes is arguable. Because no patients without lesions had positive cultures at the time of delivery, some needless cesarean sections were probably done. Although it is impossible to tell how many women without lesions but with prodromal symptoms were in the placebo group, it appears they were disproportionately distributed there and may well have biased the conclusion. At any rate, more data, with patient management based on visible cultured lesions at the time of delivery, would be vital. Note that only 1 of 9 patients with visible lesions at the time of abdominal delivery proved in fact to have a positive culture. The principal value of the study is the evidence of safety to mother and fetus.

T.H. Kirschbaum, M.D.

Outpatient Treatment of Pyelonephritis in Pregnancy: A Randomized Controlled Trial

Millar LK, Wing DA, Paul RH, et al (Univ of Southern California, Los Angeles)
Obstet Gynecol 86:560–564, 1995
3–17

Introduction.—A quarter million cases of acute pyelonephritis occur each year. Nonpregnant patients have been successfully managed as outpatients by combinations of parenteral and oral antibiotics.

Study Design.—Whether pregnant women with acute pyelonephritis can be effectively managed as outpatients was studied in a randomized trial of 120 patients who were seen before 24 weeks' gestation. All participants had clinical findings of upper urinary tract infection and urinalysis findings suggestive of urinary tract infection. Patients were randomly assigned to outpatient treatment or parenteral antibiotic therapy in the hospital. The outpatients received 1 g of ceftriaxone intramuscularly in the emergency department, and at home, they completed a 10-day course of oral cephalexin in a dosage of 500 mg taken 4 times daily. Inpatients received 1 g of IV cefazolin every 8 hours until fever had been absent for 48 hours. After discharge, they took cephalexin orally for 10 days.

Results.—The most prevalent uropathogen by far was *Escherichia coli.* Eleven of 57 outpatients who were followed up (18%) and 20% of 53 inpatients had positive urine cultures. All patients treated as outpatients had a good initial response. Six patients who initially received ceftriaxone were later admitted to the hospital for IV treatment. Six hospitalized patients required a change to gentamicin. Neither sensitivity testing nor bacteremia helped predict treatment failure.

Recommendation.—Women who have acute pyelonephritis develop in the first or second trimester of pregnancy should receive ceftriaxone and cephalexin out of the hospital after an initial period of observation in the hospital. Close follow-up is required to ensure compliance with outpatient antibiotic therapy.

▶ This prospective, randomized, controlled study of outpatient management of pyelonephritis makes the point that it is a safe approach and effective for selected patients, but the authors fail to consider costs and cost equivalents of effort. It's regrettable that different antibiotics were used for inpatients and outpatients, since we are left with uncertainty whether the greater number of prolonged fevers and antibiotic changes in the inpatient group was due to differences in drug effectiveness or failure to obtain adequate outpatient response data. The incidence of bacteremia was 10%, and since patients presenting with septicemia were excluded from study, this means that a sizable number of patients treated as outpatients were potentially septic, as was 1 out of 60 outpatients who developed signs of septicemia during the 4- to 24-hour emergency room observation period. In all, 10% of outpatients required inpatient therapy for a variety of reasons. But outpatient management encumbered increased costs—the extended emergency room observation period and time spent in screening, patient education, and counseling. The costs of at least 3 home health nurse visits and phone monitoring represent certainly necessary but additional expenses for the care of such patients.

The ultimate questions are whether the risks of ambulant care associated with the inability to predict bacteremia and septicemia, the need for reliance on patient and home health care nurses for adequacy of initial drug response, and the recurrent infection often after 48–72 hours of treatment are balanced by cost savings. For me, it's a close call, unsupported here by cost analysis. I suspect, however, that administrators of managed health care systems feel no such reservations.

T.H. Kirschbaum, M.D.

Influence of Pregnancy on the Course of Primary Chronic Glomerulonephritis

Jungers P, Houillier P, Forget D, et al (Necker Hosp, Paris)
Lancet 346:1122–1124, 1995

3–18

Background.—Research on the effects of pregnancy on the course of renal function in women with primary glomerulonephritis has yielded conflicting findings. Some studies indicate a risk of irreversible deterioration in renal function during or after pregnancy, whereas others suggest that pregnancy has no effect in most patients. The incidence of end-stage renal failure (ESRF) in women becoming pregnant was compared with that in women not becoming pregnant after the clinical onset of primary glomerulonephritis.

Methods.—Three hundred sixty patients with various histologic forms for primary glomerulonephritis were enrolled in the study. All had normal renal function, with serum creatinine levels of 0.11 or less, when they were

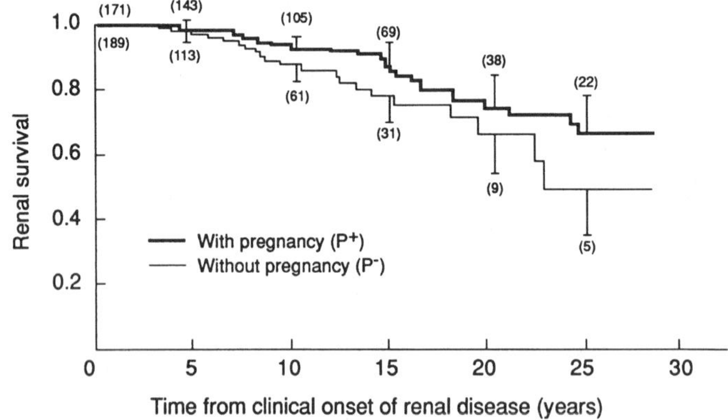

FIGURE 1.—Kaplan-Meier renal survival curves free of end-stage renal failure in groups with and without pregnancy. (Courtesy of Jungers P, Houillier P, Forget D, et al: Influence of pregnancy on the course of primary chronic glomerulonephritis. *Lancet* 346:1122–1124, copyright by The Lancet Ltd., 1995.)

initially seen. One hundred seventy-one women became pregnant after the clinical onset of disease, and 189 did not.

Findings.—Actuarial analyses demonstrated that overall ESRF-free survival did not differ significantly between the women conceiving and not conceiving after diagnosis. In a case-control analysis, pregnancy was not a risk factor for progression to ESRF. However, the type of glomerulonephritis and hypertension were major determinants (Fig 1).

Conclusions.—Pregnancy does not adversely affect the course of renal disease in women with primary glomerulonephritis, at least in those with near-normal renal function at conception. However, it is possible that pregnancy may accelerate progression to ESRF in women who enter pregnancy with impaired renal function. These findings should be included in the counseling of women with renal disease wishing to have children.

▶ This retrospective cohort study of women bearing biopsy-proven diagnoses of chronic glomerulonephritis benefits by the large number of patients cared for on referral in this Parisian Department of Nephrology. The analysis deals only with women of childbearing age with serum creatinine concentration equal to or less than 1.0 mg/dL at the start of the study. The observed dependent variable was the time after disease onset to the development of end-stage renal disease as defined either by the need for dialysis or serum creatinine concentration greater than 4.4 mg/dL. The histologic type of glomerular disease had some prognostic strength, but it was minor compared with the adverse impact of renal vascular hypertension, which often foreshadowed end-stage renal disease. Analyzed in terms of any of these independent variables, there was no measurable impact of pregnancy on the time of occurrence of end-stage renal disease in these women. Note that the same assurance cannot be given to women who exhibit azotemia at the time of conception; for them, the prognosis is much more grave.

T.H. Kirschbaum, M.D.

Effect of Pregnancy on the Long-Term Function of Renal Allografts: An Update

Sturgiss SN, Davison JM (Univ of Newcastle-upon-Tyne, England)
Am J Kidney Dis 26:54–56, 1995   3–19

Background.—In 1992, a case-control study of post-transplant follow-up was done for 36 female renal allograft recipients. During 12 years of follow-up, 18 became pregnant and the other 18 served as the control group. Because no significant differences were found between these 2 groups in renal allograft function, pregnancy did not appear to have a major effect on long-term graft function or survival. Recently, however, authors of a different study found that graft survival favored those who never conceived. Therefore, the follow-up of the participants in the original study was extended another 3 years, and the results of this 15-year follow-up were reported.

Findings.—Data were available for 17 index patients and 17 controls for the additional 3-year period. Over the entire follow-up of 15 years, 1 index patient and 4 controls sustained graft loss. One index patient died with a functioning graft and 3 controls died after graft loss. Plasma creatinine levels increased slightly in both index and control patients within the final 3 years of follow-up, but this difference was not significant. No significant differences were found between the 2 groups in renal allograft function over the 15-year follow-up.

Conclusion.—Pregnancy did not alter renal allograft function over a 15-year follow-up.

▶ It's important in counseling women with renal allografts about the hazards of pregnancy to know whether the viability of their grafts is impaired by pregnancy as compared with prospects for continuing function in women with renal transplants not undergoing the hazards of pregnancy. Earlier publications by this group[1,2] provided reassurance that there was no significant difference in renal functional parameters in 36 women followed for a mean of 12 years post transplant, as compared with matched nonpregnant controls. The average increase in plasma creatinine concentrations and decrease in glomerular filtration were greater in parous than in nonpregnant women; however, the difference lacks statistical significance. This finding and a contrary report subsequently published[3] led these investigators to extend their follow-up to 15 years, and they once more reported no difference attributable to the effects of pregnancy. In the interim, some patients have been lost to follow-up, and there may well have been bias introduced by the tendency for those with marginal renal function to avoid pregnancy. Plasma creatinine concentrations increased by an average of 1% per year in these women. Again, this is strong evidence for the lack of deleterious effect of pregnancy on women with renal allografts.

T.H. Kirschbaum, M.D.

References

1. 1993 YEAR BOOK OF OBSTETRICS AND GYNECOLOGY, pp 114–115.
2. 1994 YEAR BOOK OF OBSTETRICS AND GYNECOLOGY, pp 113–115.
3. Salmela KT, Kyllönen LE, Holmberg C, et al: Impaired renal function after pregnancy in renal transplant recipients. *Transplantation* 56:1372, 1993.

Immunohistological Study in Cases of HELLP Syndrome (Hemolysis, Elevated Liver Enzymes and Low Platelets) and Acute Fatty Liver of Pregnancy

Halim A, Kanayama N, El Maradny E, et al (Hamamatsu Univ, Japan; Natl Yokohama Hosp, Japan; St Marianna Univ, Kawasaki, Japan)

Gynecol Obstet Invest 41:106–112, 1996

3–20

Objective.—The hemolysis, elevated liver enzymes, and low platelet count (HELLP) syndrome and acute fatty liver of pregnancy (AFLP) are 2 serious and fulminant liver diseases of pregnancy that require early diagnosis and termination of pregnancy. The causes of these syndromes are unclear, although recent findings suggest that cytokines play an important role in liver damage related to ischemia and reperfusion. The immunohistochemical cytokine patterns of liver tissue from patients with HELLP syndrome and AFLP were studied.

Methods.—The study included paraffin-embedded hepatic tissue sections from 2 patients (each with HELLP syndrome and AFLP) along with necropsy control tissues from individuals involved in motor vehicle accidents. The cytokine patterns were studied using immunostaining with polyclonal antihuman tumor necrosis factor-α (TNF-α), interleukin (IL)-1β and IL-8, and monoclonal antihuman neutrophil elastase.

Results.—The specimens from patients with HELLP syndrome showed marked neutrophil infiltration, which the specimens from patients with AFLP did not. The HELLP syndrome tissues also showed strong staining with anti–TNF-α and antihuman neutrophil elastase, especially those from a patient with eclamptic HELLP syndrome. In contrast, the AFLP and control tissues showed only weak staining for these cytokines. The HELLP syndrome tissues showed moderate staining for polyclonal anti–IL-1β and IL-8, which was only weak in the AFLP and control specimens. The HELLP cases showed a significant correlation between the number of necrotic hepatocytes and elastase dots in the same randomly selected microscopic fields.

Conclusions.—This immunohistologic analysis suggests that the liver damage occurring in HELLP syndrome is mediated by cytokines and neutrophils. Tumor necrosis factor-α seems to play an important role, either directly or through other cytokines. Cytokine immunostaining is negative in patients with AFLP, suggesting that some other mechanism must be operating.

▶ To at least some of us, HELLP syndrome is a term of little use that describes severe preeclampsia in which intravascular platelet and fibrin deposition fragments erythrocytes and makes them subject to removal from circulation by the reticuloendothelium. Liver injury occurs on the basis of such vaso-occlusive events. The liver pathology is focal and consists of vasoconstriction, small vessel thrombosis, ischemia, and ischemic necrosis, which is periportal at first but then forms a confluent pattern as liver cell necrosis expands. Acute fatty liver of pregnancy seems to arise from a defect in the capacity for mitochondrial beta oxidation of long chain fatty acids which, instead of being chopped into 2 carbon atom fragments, collect and circulate in high concentrations, interfering with liver cell function as their acidity and ester formation cause alterations in mitochondrial structures, glycogen dispersion, and cytoplasmic lipid aggregates.[1-3] Although circulating liver enzymes increase in blood concentration as a result of this dysfunction, irreversible cell death is a late phenomenon that only follows the general systemic effects of free fatty acidosis. This histologic comparison of the liver injury in these 2 disturbances makes that clear. With liver injury in severe preeclampsia there is periportal necrosis and intense leucocytic infiltration together with intense expression of neutrophile elastase and the production of inflammatory cytokines (IL-I β, IL-8, TNF-α). On the other hand, because the insult in acute fatty liver of pregnancy is metabolic, cell dysfunction is denoted by massive elevations in blood fatty acids, SGOT, SGPT, and LDH. Neither liver cell necrosis nor secondary inflammatory changes are seen. Although the morphologic differences have long been known, the lack of inflammatory cytokines described in this study in fatty liver of pregnancy represents a remarkable confirmatory finding. By histology, if too seldom clinically, the distinction between these 2 entities seems very clear.

T.H. Kirschbaum, M.D.

References

1. 1992 YEAR BOOK OF OBSTETRICS AND GYNECOLOGY, pp 69–73.
2. 1994 YEAR BOOK OF OBSTETRICS AND GYNECOLOGY, pp 109–110.
3. 1995 YEAR BOOK OF OBSTETRICS AND GYNECOLOGY, pp 116–117.

Low-dose Aspirin and Prednisone Treatment of Pregnancy Loss Caused by Lupus Anticoagulants
Harger JH, Laifer SA, Bontempo FA, et al (Univ of Pittsburgh, Pa; Central Blood Bank of Pittsburgh, Pa)
J Perinatol 15:463–469, 1995
3–21

Background.—"Lupus anticoagulants" (LAC) often are associated with pregnancy loss that may be repetitive. Therapeutic benefits with low-dose aspirin and corticosteroids have previously been reported.

Objective.—The study objective was to evaluate the safety and efficacy of low-dose aspirin and prednisone in women with a history of pregnancy loss and who had LAC.

Methods.—During the period between 1985 and 1993, 255 patients with 2 or more pregnancy losses were tested for the presence of LAC. Criteria for LAC were an activated partial thromboplastin time (aPTT) that was prolonged beyond the standard established control, and a tissue thromboplastin inhibition index (TTI) that was elevated by at least 1.5 times that of the normal control. The presence of a positive antinuclear antibody test or an elevated concentration of anticardiolipin antibody was not required. Eligible patients were treated with 81 mg of aspirin and 20 or 40 mg of prednisone daily. The prednisone dose was based on the values of the aPTT and TTI. Therapy was initiated as soon as pregnancy was diagnosed. There was no control group. Results were based on a comparison with the outcomes of previous pregnancies.

Results.—Twenty-eight pregnancies were treated in 21 patients. Among the 21 women, there had been a total of 6 previous live births of a total of 69 pregnancies. Of the 63 lost pregnancies, 43 spontaneous abortions had occurred in the first trimester, 17 in the second trimester, and 3 in the third trimester. Therapy was monitored by determinations of aPTT and TTI every 2 weeks and the dose of drugs was adjusted as needed. Among the

28 pregnancies, 4 spontaneous abortions occurred in each of the first 2 trimesters. The 20 other pregnancies resulted in the successful delivery of live neonates.

Conclusions.—Low-dose aspirin and prednisone therapy are safe in the prevention of recurrent pregnancy loss in women who have lupus anticoagulants.

▶ This is a relatively large series of pregnant women bearing abnormal antibodies in pregnancy, and it deserves careful evaluation. There are several design faults, which the authors acknowledge. There are no concurrent controls, and they are badly needed because women with criteria sufficient for admission to this study have been reported to have normal pregnancies without therapy.[1] With only the presence of LAC and a history or previous unexplained pregnancy loss, lacking detailed retrospective record review and placental pathology, it strains credulity to claim that these women had previous pregnancy losses caused by LAC.

Further, in a confusing picture where since 1985 criteria for what has come to be known as the antiphospholipid antibody syndrome have been changing, it is not clear which of several autoimmune processes is being studied here. Only 1 of 21 women had findings sufficient to make the diagnosis of lupus erythematosus. Only 5 had antinuclear antibody, 4 had high titers of anticardiolipid and antibody IgG, and 9 had elevated aPTT. The most consistent finding in this study was prolongation of TTI, and prednisone dose was adjusted longitudinally in part on this finding. However, subsequent to 1985, the relationship of TTI prolongation to antiphospholipid antibody syndrome has become uncertain. Using historical controls, the resulting live birth rate of 72% with 46% preterm births seems favorable, but the implicit question here is whether the data collected in this way suffice to justify the expense and effort in a prospective, randomized trial of this approach. Remember, the authors report far fewer maternal complications associated with the use of prednisone therapy in pregnancy than most. For my part, the absence of controls and the incomplete characterization of patients admitted for study means the experience can be accepted only as the interesting basis for the design of a control-led therapeutic trial, from which convincing evidence of benefit from low-dose aspirin might arise.

T.H. Kirschbaum, M.D.

Reference

1. 1990 Year Book of Obstetrics and Gynecology, pp 89–90.

Therapy and Prevention of Thrombotic Thrombocytopenic Purpura During Pregnancy: A Clinical Study of 16 Pregnancies

Ezra Y, Rose M, Eldor A (Hadassah Univ, Ein-Kerem, Jerusalem)
Am J Hematol 51:1–6, 1996   3–22

Background.—The introduction of plasmapheresis in the treatment of thrombotic thrombocytopenic purpura (TTP) has dramatically reduced the high mortality of this severe multisystem disorder. However, the TTP relapse rate among survivors remains high, ranging from 30% to 60%. Pregnancy appears to be an important precipitating factor in TTP relapse. The management and outcome of TTP in pregnancy between 1985 and 1992 were retrospectively reviewed.

Patients.—During a 7-year period, 17 patients were treated for TTP at 1 institution; 5 had at least 1 episode of TTP during a pregnancy. These 5 women had a total of 16 pregnancies and were treated for a total of 15 TTP episodes; 8 of the pregnancies were complicated by TTP and 8 were not. Episodes of TTP were treated with plasmapheresis, corticosteroids, aspirin, and dipyridamole. Prophylactic therapy included aspirin 100–500 mg/day and dipyridamole 225 mg/day.

Outcome.—No maternal deaths occurred, but 1 woman died of multiple-organ failure during a relapse not associated with a pregnancy. Of the 8 pregnancies not complicated by TTP, 6 ended in the delivery of normal, full-term, healthy infants, 1 ended in intrauterine fetal death, and 1 was electively terminated. Of the 8 pregnancies complicated by TTP, 3 resulted in the normal delivery of a healthy baby. Women who relapsed while receiving prophylactic drug therapy had significantly milder TTP episodes than those who did not comply with the prophylactic drug regimen.

Conclusions.—Women of childbearing age who have survived an episode of TTP should be informed of the high risk of TTP recurrence if they become pregnant. A woman who becomes pregnant should consider terminating the pregnancy, but if she chooses not to, prophylactic therapy with aspirin and dipyridamole should be initiated.

▶ Thrombotic thrombocytopenic purpura is a virulent disease of the hematologic system resulting in thrombopenia, microangiopathic anemia, renal injury, and various signs of neurologic dysfunction. Although it occurs apart from pregnancy, somewhere around 20% of reported cases have occurred in pregnant women. It may occur with subsequent pregnancies, as was the case in 8 such pregnancies in 5 women reported here.

In the late 1980s and early 1990s, plasmapheresis was demonstrated to be of value and has dropped the mortality for TTP with or without pregnancy from 90% into the range of 20% to 30%. Plasmapheresis has also given us a generous clue to the origin of the disease, because the plasma removed is rich in macro aggregates of von Willebrand's factor, an adhesion molecule produced by endothelial cells formerly called factor VIII R:WF. In this terminology, R denotes a ristocetin cofactor.

What appears to take place in TTP is a variant of the hyperacute rejection phenomenon in which as-yet unknown antibody binds to endothelial cells and activates complement. The resulting immune complexes stimulate the production of von Willebrand's factor in mega-multimers, which in turn bind platelets in intravascular aggregates. Red blood cells forced by systolic pressure through these aggregates are fragmented into bizarre forms (schizocytes), which are removed by the reticuloendothelium, resulting in anemia. Fragments of these activated thrombi form and embolize to the brain and the kidneys, producing evidence of injury there. Plasma exchange transfusion removes them from the circulation.

Given a past history, the authors suggest using aspirin and dipyridamole, the latter an agent that reduces the capacity for platelet activation, although recurrences may occur despite this therapy.

Severe preeclampsia may result in microangiopathic anemia and thrombopenia, but in those cases, hypertension is a prominent feature and the hemolytic anemia is less severe than with TTP. A history of previous hemolytic anemia helps make the differential diagnosis in this case. This appears to be a grave complication of the loss of immune privilege for the fetal allograft for which effective therapy, fortunately, is available.

T.H. Kirschbaum, M.D.

4 Fetal Complications of Pregnancy

Intentional Delivery Versus Expectant Management With Preterm Ruptured Membranes at 30–34 Weeks' Gestation
Cox SM, Leveno KJ (Univ of Texas, Dallas)
Obstet Gynecol 86:875–879, 1995   4–1

Introduction.—The management of preterm ruptured fetal membranes is controversial, with many proposed obstetric approaches. The advantages in maternal and neonatal outcomes were compared in pregnancies with ruptured membranes at 30 to 34 weeks' gestation managed with either intentional delivery or expectant management.

Methods.—Over a 3-year period, 129 women with preterm ruptured membranes at 30 to 34 weeks' gestation but without fever, labor, or fetal or maternal complications dictating delivery were randomly assigned to either intentional delivery (61 patients) or expectant management (68 patients). Patients in the intentional delivery group underwent induction of labor if the fetus was in the cephalic presentation; otherwise, they had cesarean delivery. Patients in the expectant management group were not given corticosteroids, tocolytic agents, or prophylactic antimicrobial agents, but maternal vital signs and fetal heart tones were evaluated every 8 hours, and fetal heart rate and uterine activity were monitored for 1 hour daily. Maternal and fetal outcome variables were analyzed in each group.

Results.—In both groups, the mean gestational age at randomization was 31.7 weeks. No significant differences in the mean gestational age were found at delivery: 31.7 weeks in the intentional delivery group and 32 weeks in the expectant management group. Delivery occurred within 24 hours of randomization in all but 2 women in the intentional delivery group but in only 25% of the expectant management group. There was a lower incidence of chorioamnionitis in the intentional delivery group but no difference between the groups in the incidence of puerperal infection. The rate of cesarean delivery was higher in the intentional delivery group. No significant differences in Apgar scores and umbilical artery blood pH levels were found between the 2 groups. One perinatal fetal death occurred in the expectant management group, compared with 3 neonatal deaths in the intentional delivery study group; 3 of the 4 deaths were caused by bacterial sepsis. No differences were noted between the groups in markers of neonatal morbidity.

Conclusions.—No clear advantages were found for either management approach. Although intentional delivery was associated with a shorter maternal hospitalization and a lower maternal and fetal infection rate, it also was associated with a higher rate of cesarean delivery. However, because of the size of the sample, these differences were not statistically significant.

▶ It is a given that premature delivery is likely with preterm premature rupture of membranes. Although antibiotic therapy and expectant management may delay the onset of labor and reduce the incidence of clinical chorioamnionitis and proven newborn sepsis, they do not seem to improve newborn mortality. That is the basis for this legitimate inquiry. To say there was no proof of the value of expectant management at 30 to 34 weeks may well, as the authors indicate, simply reflect a number of cases inadequate to prove efficacy.

Some things are interesting in the authors' data. Twenty-three percent of those treated expectantly delivered before 32 weeks, whereas 29% of those treated by intent for delivery did so. Although modern neonatology is able to afford good prospects for survival at that gestational age range, the results are obtained with considerable cost and some risk of newborn morbidity. In women managed expectantly, cesarean section proved necessary in about 12%, whereas 23% of those in the intent-to-deliver group had abdominal delivery. Although the incidence of infant sepsis was higher in the expectant management group, it was not significantly so, and if the unit had used prophylactic antibiotics, it might well have been lower.

In evaluating treatment of premature preterm rupture of membranes, survival is too crude an independent variable to serve as the basis for judgment. The lack of difference noted reflects population size and a failure to estimate cost and risks in evaluating relative benefits. Regrettably, this study fails to answer this continuing controversy.

T.H. Kirschbaum, M.D.

Intrauterine Growth Restriction in Infants of Less Than Thirty-Two Weeks' Gestation: Associated Placental Pathologic Features
Salafia CM, Minior VK, Pezzullo JC, et al (Univ of Connecticut, Farmington; Texas Children's Hosp, Houston; Univ of Medicine and Dentistry of New Jersey, New Brunswick; et al)
Am J Obstet Gynecol 173:1049–1057, 1995   4–2

Background.—Intrauterine growth restriction (IUGR) is common in preterm neonates. An etiologic association has been hypothesized for suboptimal intrauterine growth and preterm birth, because the placental lesions seen in both premature and neonates with IUGR are similar. The placental lesions were examined in neonates delivered before 32 weeks' gestation to investigate associations between recognized patterns of IUGR and distinct histopathologic features and to examine the independent relationships of preeclampsia and placental lesions to IUGR.

Methods.—All singleton neonates delivered between 22 and 32 weeks' gestation with accurate gestational dating and no maternal history of chronic hypertension, diabetes mellitus, or placenta previa were studied. Preterm delivery was caused primarily by premature rupture of the membranes, preterm labor, preeclampsia, or nonhypertensive abruptio placentae. Birth weight and length were used to classify the infants as appropriate for gestational age (AGA), asymmetric IUGR (birth weight less than the 10th percentile, but length more than the 10th percentile), or symmetric IUGR (both birth weight and length less than the 10th percentile). Other maternal, intrapartum, and neonatal data were extracted from the medical charts. The placentas were examined grossly and histologically. Multiple regression analyses were performed to identify significant predictors of IUGR.

Results.—Of the 420 neonates, 340 (81%) were AGA, 32 (7.6%) had asymmetric IUGR, and 48 (11.4%) had symmetric IUGR. Neonates with symmetric IUGR were more likely to have preeclamptic mothers than were those with asymmetric IUGR or AGA, whereas neonates with asymmetric IUGR were more likely to have mothers with premature labor or premature rupture of membranes than were those with symmetric IUGR. Multiple regression analyses of placental lesions identified independent associations between IUGR and uteroplacental vessel fibrinoid necrosis or atherosis, villous infarct, histologic evidence of abruptio placentae, increased syncytiotrophoblast knotting, and avascular terminal villi. This model predicted 34% of IUGR births. In another multiple regression, adding preeclampsia as a variable, data showed preeclampsia as a strong predictor of fetal growth, predicting 36% of IUGR births. Using data only from patients without preeclampsia, only 7.5% of IUGR births could be predicted by placental lesions.

Conclusions.—Intrauterine growth restriction was significantly associated with more numerous and severe lesions with symmetric IUGR than with asymmetric IUGR. However, the predictive value of the specific histologic lesions diminished relative to preeclampsia.

▶ This is a large study based on selective placental collection for 6 years, relating placental morphology to growth retardation in infants delivered prematurely as a result of preterm labor, preterm rupture of membranes, preeclampsia, or abruptio placentae. Women with diabetes mellitus, chronic hypertension, and placenta previa were excluded. A series of observations of normal maternal decidual structures, umbilical vessels, villus epithelium and stroma, fetal membranes, and fetal normoblasts was compared with 32 cases of asymmetric IUGR (7.6% of all cases) and 48 of symmetric IUGR (11.4%). The authors' reference to the technique of placental examination is not available to me, but 4 blocks of grossly normal placental tissue were examined in blinded fashion. Placental morphometry was not done, raising a serious issue of the representativeness of observations based on only 4 blocks to the entire placental organ. The definition of placental abnormality was developed using "empiric definitions for utero placental [pathology]," based arbitrarily on the presence of 2 or more of a list of 19 findings. No observational support for relationships among those qualitative observations and utero placental insufficiency is offered. In expressing the dependent variable "growth restriction," an index is defined that has no biological referrants but depends solely on the unproven hypothesis that growth restriction is more severe in symmetric than asymmetric growth retardation. Gestational age is excluded from that calculation. Further, birth weight and birth length are converted to percentiles of Z-score distributions without proof that the body measurements are normally distributed. It's not surprising that the growth restriction index suffices to predict only one third of the cases of growth retardation and that, with addition of the diagnosis of preeclampsia, "the significance of placental lesions was either lost or weakened." Only 34% of fetal growth impairment could be explained in terms of placental variables. Though this paper represents a good deal of work, the numbers of unproven and unresearched assumptions deprive it of much meaning. Certainly the findings do not represent "uteroplacental insufficiency."

T.H. Kirschbaum, M.D.

Do Growth-retarded Premature Infants Have Different Rates of Perinatal Morbidity and Mortality Than Appropriately Grown Premature Infants?
Piper JM, Xenakis EM-J, McFarland M, et al (Univ of Texas Health Sciences Ctr, San Antonio)
Obstet Gynecol 87:169–174, 1996
4–3

Introduction.—It is commonly believed that the stress of the intrauterine environment induces accelerated maturation in growth-retarded fetuses, which suggests that, to prevent fetal death, growth-retarded fetuses could benefit from preterm delivery. To sort out the conflicting evidence regarding these assumptions, perinatal morbidity and mortality were compared in growth-retarded and appropriately grown preterm infants at the same gestational age.

Methods.—Data on all pregnancies recorded over a 15-year period were reviewed to identify singleton pregnancies delivered at 24 to 36 weeks' gestation. Of these infants, those with a birth weight at or lower than the 10th percentile were identified as small for gestational age (SGA), and those with birth weights between the 11th and 89th percentiles were identified as appropriate for gestational age (AGA). These 2 groups were compared for perinatal mortality, congenital anomaly, and perinatal morbidity.

Results.—The study population included 1,012 SGA and 3,171 AGA babies born before 37 weeks' gestation. In the SGA pregnancies, 72% of

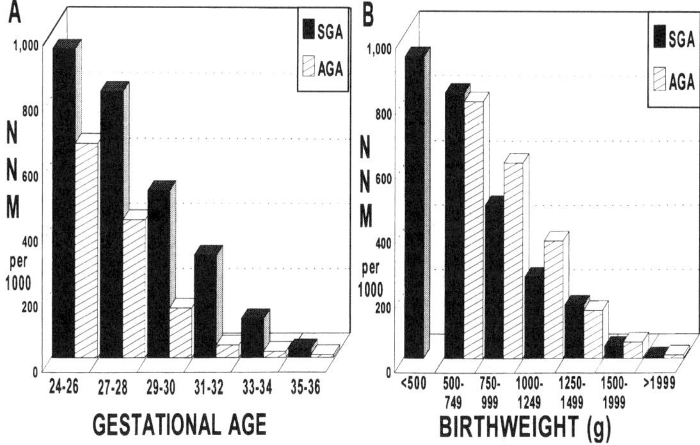

FIGURE 1.—Neonatal mortality (*NNM*) in small for gestational age (*SGA*) and appropriate for gestational age (*AGA*) pregnancies compared by gestational age (**A**) and birth weight (**B**). Neonatal death rates in SGA pregnancies were significantly higher by gestational age ($P < 0.05$) but not by birth weight. (Courtesy of Piper JM, Xenakis EM-J, McFarland M, et al: Do growth-retarded premature infants have different rates of perinatal morbidity and mortality than appropriately grown premature infants? *Obstet Gynecol* 87:169–174, 1996. Reprinted with permission from The American College of Obstetricians and Gynecologists.)

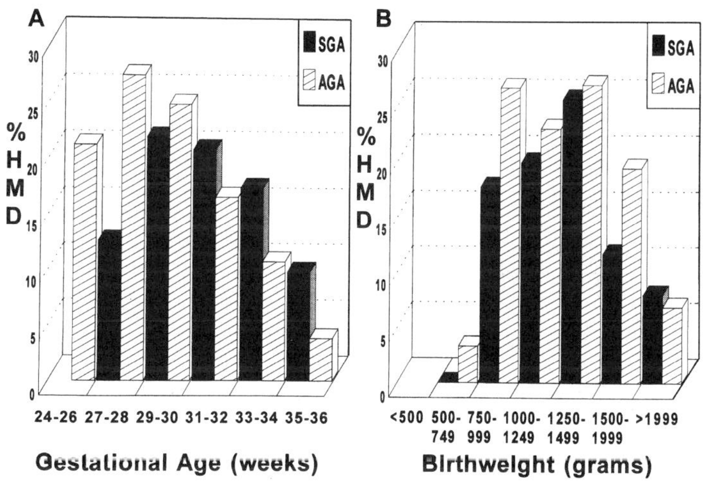

FIGURE 2.—Hyaline membrane disease (*HMD*) rates in small for gestational age (*SGA*) and appropriate for gestational age (*AGA*) infants compared by gestational age (**A**) and birth weight (**B**). Comparison by gestational age revealed an overall significantly higher rate of HMD in the infants who were *SGA* compared with the infants who were *AGA* ($P < 0.05$). In contrast, when compared by birth weight categories, the rate of HMD was lower in the women who had SGA than in those who had AGA pregnancies ($P < 0.05$). (Courtesy of Piper JM, Xenakis EM-J, McFarland M, et al: Do growth-retarded premature infants have different rates of perinatal morbidity and mortality than appropriately grown premature infants? *Obstet Gynecol* 87:169–174, 1996. Reprinted with permission from The American College of Obstetricians and Gynecologists.)

the infants survived and 17% of the fetuses and 11% of the neonates died. In the AGA pregnancies, 83% of the infants survived and 7% of the fetuses and 10% of the neonates died. Compared with the AGA pregnancies, perinatal death rates were significantly higher in the SGA pregnancies at every gestational age, but did not differ significantly in the 2 groups when stratified by birth weight (Fig 1). No significant difference was found in anomaly rates between the 2 groups. Compared with the AGA pregnancies, the SGA pregnancies had more frequent indications for cesarean delivery and fetal heart rate abnormalities, but there were no significant differences between the 2 groups for Apgar score at 5 minutes, birth trauma, and neonatal sepsis. Compared with the AGA infants, the SGA infants had a significantly higher rate of hyaline membrane disease when matched by gestational age, but a significantly lower rate of hyaline membrane disease when matched by birth weight (Fig 2).

Conclusions.—Growth retardation is a significant and independent predictor of perinatal mortality and morbidity. Therefore, elective preterm delivery of SGA fetuses is not justified.

▶ Part of our failure to define treatment algorithms for fetuses and infants with growth retardation that improve their survival is the uncertain disadvantage that growth retardation imposes on a fetus or a neonate. This useful study helps clarify that issue by comparing the impact of impaired birth weight at a given premature gestational age with perinatal mortality and the likelihood of development of hyaline membrane disease. The analysis is based on a 15-year data collection of records of births at less than 37 weeks' gestation, excluding multiple births, patients with diabetes, and "pregnancy with unknown or conflicting dates." It would be good to have more detail about those exclusions for dating because the results of the analysis are likely to be sensitive to that process.

However, the results can be concisely stated. Growth retardation confers the same increased risk of mortality that would apply to a non–growth-retarded premature neonate of the same birth weight. On the other hand, pulmonary maturation as judged by hyaline membrane disease is not compromised by growth retardation but appears to be reflected best by gestational age of the growth-retarded neonate. Because growth retardation and placenta previa and abruption carry with them a sizable risk of fetal death, and because a fetal death cannot also be a neonatal death, logistic regression indicates an adverse effect on neonatal death rates from nonlethal intrauterine events (chorioamnionitis, fetal anomalies). This analysis indicates that hazard to the growth-retarded fetus stems from prematurity risks other than respiratory inadequacy. It is an important concept.

T.H. Kirschbaum, M.D.

Maternal Corticosteroid and Tocolytic Treatment and Morbidity and Mortality in Very Low Birth Weight Infants
Atkinson MW, Goldenberg RL, Gaudier FL, et al (Univ of Alabama, Birmingham)
Am J Obstet Gynecol 173:299–305, 1995   4–4

Background.—Maternal corticosteroid treatment before preterm delivery has been shown to significantly decrease the rates of respiratory distress syndrome (RDS) and neonatal mortality in neonates delivered between 29 and 34 weeks' gestation. The benefits for neonates delivered at 24 to 28 weeks' gestation are uncertain. Although tocolytic agents are widely used, there is little evidence to suggest that they significantly improve neonatal outcomes. Tocolytics are commonly given with the rationale that they will buy time for corticosteroid treatment. The effects of maternal corticosteroid and tocolytic treatment—alone and together—on neonatal morbidity and mortality were investigated in neonates delivered at 24 to 28 weeks' gestation.

Methods.—The analysis included 773 neonates born with birth weights of 500 to 1,000 g from 1979 through 1991. All were live-born between 24 weeks, 0 days and 28 weeks, 6 days. Fifty-six percent of the mothers received neither corticosteroids nor tocolytics, 27% received tocolytics only, 6% received corticosteroids only, and 11% received both corticosteroids and tocolytics. The 2 treatments were investigated for their effects, separately and in combination, on the neonatal outcomes of RDS, intraventricular hemorrhage, persistent ductus, arteriosus, necrotizing enterocolitis, seizures, and death.

Results.—The 4 groups were significantly different in terms of birth weight, gestational age, racial distribution, frequency of multiple gestation, mode of delivery, and obstetric complication rates. Corticosteroids were associated with a significant reduction in mortality when used with or without tocolytics and with a significant reduction in seizures only when used alone. Tocolytic treatment alone was linked to a significant increase in intraventricular hemorrhage. Intraventricular hemorrhage, neonatal death, or both occurred in 71% of neonates in the no-treatment group, 83% of the tocolytic-only group, 48% of the corticosteroid-group, and 56% of the combination-therapy group. Multiple logistic regression analysis showed that combination therapy was associated with a decreased risk of both seizures and mortality. Any tocolytic treatment increased the risk of all grades of intraventricular hemorrhage (odds ratio, 2.23) and of severe intraventricular hemorrhage (odds ratio, 2.10). In contrast, any corticosteroid treatment decreased the risk of intraventricular hemorrhage, with odds ratios of 0.36 for intraventricular hemorrhage and 0.31 for severe intraventricular hemorrhage (Table 5).

Conclusions.—In preterm neonates delivered at 24 to 28 weeks' gestation, maternal corticosteroid therapy is associated with significant benefits in terms of neonatal outcomes, including reductions in intraventricular hemorrhage and neonatal mortality. Tocolytic therapy, when given alone,

TABLE 5.—Adjusted Odds Ratios and 95% Confidence Intervals for Mortality, Respiratory Distress Syndrome (RDS), Intraventricular Hemorrhage, and Seizures Considering Tocolytic and Corticosteroid Use Independently

	Tocolytics	Corticosteroids
Mortality	0.71 (0.47–1.07)	0.49 (0.29–0.82)
RDS, alll cases	0.68 (0.32–1.43)	1.33 (0.64–2.75)
RDS, severe	0.78 (0.45–1.36)	0.63 (0.37–1.09)
Intraventricular hemorrhage, all grades	2.23 (1.40–3.53)	0.36 (0.24–0.55)
Intraventricular hemorrhage, grades III and IV	2.10 (1.26–3.50)	0.31 (0.16–0.60)
Seizures	0.83 (0.45–1.51)	0.37 (0.15–0.92)

Note: Odds ratios are adjusted controlling for gestational age, birth weight, race, sex, mode of delivery, spontaneous vs. indicated delivery, plurality, premature rupture of membranes, preeclampsia, other therapy received, and year of delivery.

(Courtesy of Atkinson MW, Goldenberg RL, Gaudier FL, et al: Maternal corticosteroid and tocolytic treatment and morbidity and mortality in very low birth weight infants. *Am J Obstet Gynecol* 173:299–305, 1995.)

appears to increase the risk of intraventricular hemorrhage. The addition of corticosteroids may lessen the negative effect of tocolytics on intraventricular hemorrhage risk, although this risk is still higher than that associated with corticosteroid treatment alone.

▶ Though several studies have demonstrated the value of corticosteroids in preventing morbidity and mortality in premature and immature births, few if any contain as many infants in the 24–29-week gestational age range as does this study. Further, comparisons to tocolysis alone or in combination with steroids are possible here, and statistical analysis is very well done. Of the 773 women delivering infants less than 1 kg of birth weight between 24 and 28 weeks enrolled in this retrospective case-control study, only 6% received steroids while 38% received tocolytics (magnesium sulfate, β-sympathomimetics, or indomethacin). Women receiving a single 12.5-mg dose of corticosteroids were deemed to have been completely treated, a posture that tends if anything to diminish the apparent value of steroid administration. In general, corticosteroid use alone or with tocolytics reduced infant mortality by 50% and decreased the risk of all grades of intraventricular hemorrhage (IVH) by 65% to 70%. Tocolytics alone were twice as likely to result in IVH, including Papile grades III and IV, and, when combined with steroid use, showed no added benefit. All these reported changes meet a test of statistical significance. This is convincing evidence that tocolysis alone is useless if not dangerous in this gestational age range, and can only be justified if used to afford fetal access to maternal corticosteroids.

T.H. Kirschbaum, M.D.

Prenatal and Perinatal Factors and Cerebral Palsy in Very Low Birth Weight Infants

Grether JK, Nelson KB, Emery ES III, et al (Natl Insts of Neurological Disorders and Stroke, Bethesda, Md; Univ of Vermont, Burlington; Univ of California, San Francisco)
J Pediatr 128:407–414, 1996
4–5

Purpose.—Compared with normal-weight infants, those with birth weights of less than 1,500 g are at a 100-fold increased risk of disabling cerebral palsy. However, most children with very low birth weights (VLBW) will not have CP. The causative variables can be understood only by separating the neonatal factors causing CP from those resulting from earlier physiologic disturbances. Acute infection, which is an important trigger of premature labor, might also be an important risk factor for CP among VLBW infants. This and other risk factors for CP were examined in VLBW infants.

Methods.—The case-control study included 42 VLBW singleton infants with moderate or severe congenital CP. These case subjects represented all VLBW children with congenital CP born in 1 of 4 San Francisco Bay area counties from 1983 to 1985. Their prenatal and perinatal data were collected and compared with those of 75 randomly selected VLBW infants without CP.

Findings.—The odds ratio (OR) for CP among VLBW infants born at level I facilities was 6.3, and that for infants born within 3 hours of the

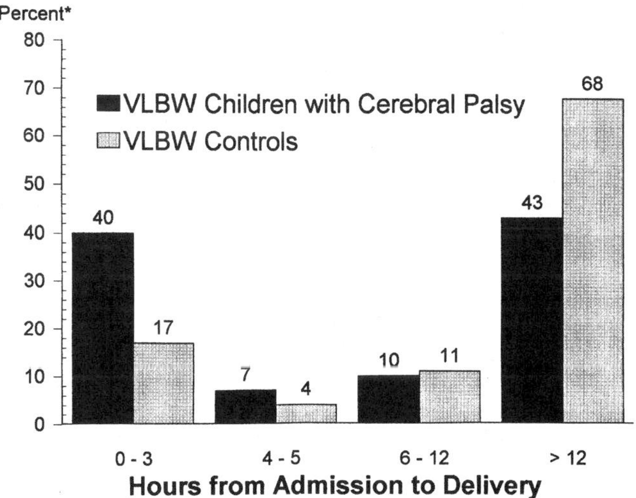

FIGURE.—Hours from initial admission to delivery, percent in very low birth weight (*VLBW*) children with cerebral palsy and in VLBW control subjects (for delivery within 3 hours of admission; OR 3.2, CI 1.4, 7.4). (Courtesy of Grether JK, Nelson KB, Emery ES III, et al: Prenatal and perinatal factors and cerebral palsy in very low birth weight infants. *J Pediatr* 128:407–414, 1996.)

mother's first admission for delivery was 3.2. One fourth of the infants with CP were born within 3 hours after the mother's admission to a level I facility, compared with none of those without CP (Fig). Children delivered more than 4 hours after admission were 4 times more likely to have chorionitis. Fourteen percent of children in the CP group had chorionitis followed by neonatal seizures, including 25% of those with spastic diplegia, compared with none of the children in the non-CP group. Children of pregnancies complicated by preeclampsia were at decreased risk of CP (OR 0.08) as were those whose mothers received magnesium sulfate for the treatment of preeclampsia or preterm labor (OR 0.14). Risk for CP was also increased for infants of women with gravidity greater than 1 (OR 3.9); with a short interval between births (OR 4.1); and with vaginal bleeding on the day of admission (OR 2.9).

Conclusions.—Risk factors for CP among VLBW children were identified in a population-based study. The time spent in the hospital before delivery seems to be an important factor, and one that interacts with other CP-associated risk factors. Also, the infants' neurologic outcomes may be linked to the pathogenic factors predisposing to very premature birth and with the medical events and treatments occurring shortly before birth.

▶ This is another of a series of studies, based on 155,636 births between 1983 and 1985 in northern California, which is useful in comparison with a Collaborative Perinatal Project of 1959–1966 so extensively researched earlier by Dr. Karen Nelson and colleagues.[1] The methodology is to define those single variables with significantly greater likelihood to appear in infants with CP identified in case-control studies than those in control infants (univariate analysis). A next step is to use multivariate analysis to exclude single variables which all express the same and/or another variable (confounding variables). For example, when risk ratios for CP and variable low birth weight infants were sought in the 1959–1966 data, abnormalities of placentation, second trimester bleeding, birth weight less than 2 kilograms in a prior pregnancy, chorionitis, premature rupture of membranes, and major congenital anomalies were all linked univariate predictors. However, all except chorionitis, premature rupture of membranes and major anomalies were excluded on multivariate analysis because they were all linked to the incidence of low birth weight and contain no additional information. This analysis, with additional variables reflecting manner of care, time and place of delivery (level II hospital for entry admission, delivery less than 3 hours after admission), and chorionitis followed by newborn symptoms survived multivariate analysis indicating predictive strength for development of CP. Two other factors—magnesium sulfate for tocolysis or to prevent convulsions and preeclampsia—were significantly negatively associated with CP.[2] Studies of this sort are useful in investigating the etiology of CP and in this study serve to focus attention on events prior to and after labor and delivery. They also show that "our present ability to recognize the important antecedents of CP and to predict the occurrence of the disorder fail to account for the majority of cases and there was an exceeding high rate of false positive identification. We probably do not know what causes most cases of CP."[3] That statement, published 10 years ago, remains true to date.

T.H. Kirschbaum, M.D.

References

1. 1995 YEAR BOOK OF OBSTETRICS AND GYNECOLOGY, pp 135–136.
2. 1996 YEAR BOOK OF OBSTETRICS AND GYNECOLOGY, pp 126–128.
3. 1988 YEAR BOOK OF OBSTETRICS AND GYNECOLOGY, pp 116–118.

Insulin-like Growth Factor-1 Is a Potent Neuronal Rescue Agent After Hypoxic-Ischemic Injury in Fetal Lambs

Johnston BM, Mallard EC, Williams CE, et al (Univ of Auckland, New Zealand)

J Clin Invest 97:300–308, 1996   4–6

Objective.—Recognition of the secondary or delayed phase of neuronal death in infants with acute hypoxic-ischemic or asphyxial brain injury has raised the possibility of using some type of neuronal rescue therapy in the hours after acute injury. The peptide growth factor insulin-like growth factor-1 (IGF-1) may, through unknown mechanisms, play a key role in the rescue of injured neurons of the adult brain. A fetal sheep model of hypoxic-ischemic encephalopathy was used to study the potential effects of IGF-1 as a neuronal rescue agent.

Methods.—In the model, cerebral ischemia was induced in unanesthetized, late-gestation fetal sheep by inflation of carotid artery occluder cuffs. The cuffs were deflated after 30 minutes. Two hours after the onset of cerebral ischemia, the fetus received recombinant human IGF (rhIGF) in a dose of 0.1, 1.0, or 10.0 μg or vehicle only by 1-hour infusion into a lateral cerebral ventricle. The animals were killed for histologic analysis after 5 days.

Results.—Fetuses treated with 0.1 or 1.0 μg of rhIGF-1 had significant reductions in overall neuronal loss, but those receiving the 10.0 μg dose did not. Fetuses receiving the 1.0 μg dose had significantly lower neuronal loss scores in various regions of the brain, including the cortex, hippocampus, and striatum. In comparison, the fetuses receiving the 0.1 μg dose had no improvement in the parietal cortex and thalamus and has less improvement in other areas. The 1-μg dose also was associated with a reduced incidence and delayed onset of seizures and with reduced and delayed secondary cytotoxic edema. The same dose also delayed the secondary peak in systemic blood glucose concentration and delayed and attenuated the secondary peak in blood lactate level (Fig 5).

Conclusions.—Treatment with low-dose rhIGF-1 appears to reduce neuronal death after cerebral hypoxic-ischemic injury in fetal sheep in dose-dependent fashion. If given within 2 hours after the onset of ischemic, rhIGF-1 therapy appears to be effective and nontoxic. With further study,

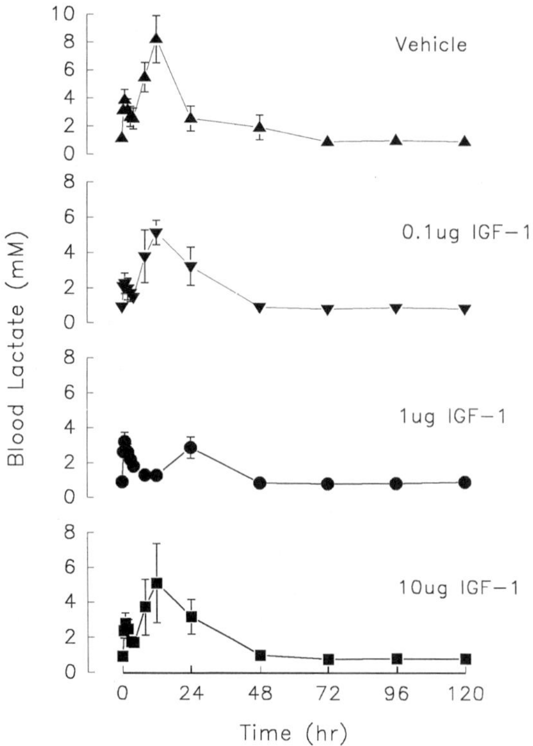

FIGURE 5.—Time course of changes in systemic blood lactate levels after 30 minutes of cerebral hypoxia-ischemia. In vehicle-treated fetuses there was a large secondary peak in blood lactate levels at 12 hours after insult. This was attenuated in the group treated with 0.1 μg recombinant human insulin-like growth factor-1 (rhIGF-1) and delayed and almost abolished in those treated with 1 μg rhIGI-1. (Courtesy of Johnston BM, Mallard EC, Williams CE, et al: Insulin-like growth factor-1 is a potent neuronal rescue agent hypoxic-ischemic injury in fetal lambs. *J Clin Invest* 97:300–308 1996, by copyright permission of The American Society for Clinical Investigation.)

IGF-1 treatment could be considered for use in asphyxiated infants who are identified before the start of the secondary phase of brain injury.

▶ These Auckland investigators have demonstrated, in fetal sheep, that carotid artery occlusion for 30 minutes after vertebral ligation induces 2 phases of changes indicative of nerve cell injury, each phase separated by an interval of 6 to 12 hours.[1] The second, or delayed, interval is associated with the more devastating metabolic and morphologic damage of the two, and this pattern opens the possibility of neuronal prophylaxis against injury using agents administered within that 6-hour interval after the initial insult.

Similar and consonant—though not a complete—observations have been made in the human fetus. The peptide growth factor IGF-1 has metabolic and multiple growth- and repair-stimulating effects thought to be important in modulating fetal growth.[2] Under active investigation in many of its properties by this group, it was inevitable that it be tried for this purpose, and the results are encouraging. One nanogram of rhIGF-1 injected into the fetal lateral ventricles 2 hours after 30-minute carotid occlusion delayed and diminished the rate of seizure activity, which coincided with the delayed increase in cortical impedence. That electrical change measured from the surface of the cerebral cortex denoted cortical intracellular edema largely of glial cells, and IGF-1 appears to impede it. The secondary phase of intracerebral edema was delayed, and both the increase in fetal plasma glucose caused by impaired brain utilization as well as the lactic acidemia after the onset of anaerobic glycolysis were ameliorated by this dose. Finally, morphologic evidence of brain injury was strikingly reduced, especially in the thalamus, amygdala, and dentate gyrus, lateral and slightly cauded to the third ventricle.

Although it is still a hypothesis, the authors believe that IGF-1 acts by impeding apoptosis; that is, gene expression that leads to DNA fragmentation into integral multiple units of 180 base pairs, which results in nuclear pyknosis and the typical "ladder" pattern on gel chromatography. The need for intraventricular administration of this agent will retard its investigation in the human, but these animal experimental results are very important and most promising.

T.H. Kirschbaum, M.D.

References

1. 1992 YEAR BOOK OF OBSTETRICS AND GYNECOLOGY, pp 189–191.
2. 1996 YEAR BOOK OF OBSTETRICS AND GYNECOLOGY, pp 17–19.

Determining the Time Before Birth When Ischemia and Hypoxemia Initiated Cerebral Palsy

Naeye RL, Localio AR (Pennsylvania State Univ, Hershey)
Obstet Gynecol 86:713–719, 1995
4–7

Background.—Cerebral palsy is often attributed to intrapartum ischemia and hypoxemia. Lymphocyte and normoblast counts in neonatal blood may be useful markers to accurately identify when ischemia and hypoxemia damaged fetal brains and caused cerebral palsy.

Methods.—Sixteen neonates were included in the study. The time when antenatal ischemic and hypoxemic brain damage began was known in each case. Blood lymphocyte and normoblastic counts were determined at various intervals after birth and compared with counts from normal newborns, infants with low Apgar scores and no cerebral palsy, and infants with cerebral palsy caused by developmental and other early gestational disorders.

Findings.—Within 2 hours after the onset of brain-damaging ischemia and hypoxemia, lymphocyte counts increased to more than 10,000/mm^3 and normoblast counts to 2,000/mm^3 or more. Lymphocyte counts normalized 24 hours after the damage began. Normoblast counts normalized

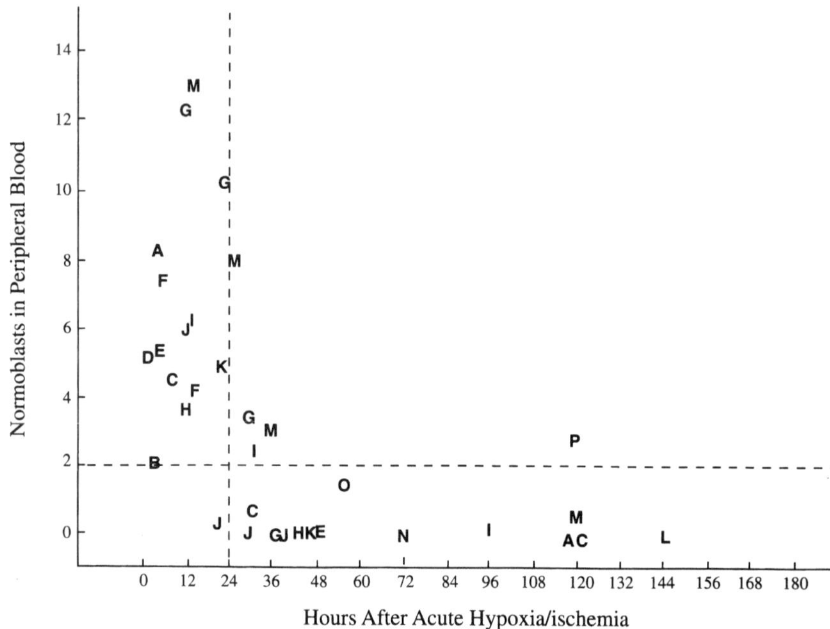

FIGURE 2.—Normoblast counts (× 1,000/mm³) in the blood of neonates after acute antenatal ischemia and hypoxemia. The *letter A-P* represent the 16 patients studied. Eleven of the 16 had more than 1 normoblast count over time. The *dotted horizontal line* at the 2,000/mm³ level reflects the approximate high number of normoblasts per cubic mm for normal control infants. Several overlapping points have been slightly separated to enhance clarity. (Courtesy of Naeye RL, Localio AR: Determining the time before birth when ischemia and hypoxemia initiated cerebral palsy. *Obstet Gynecol* 86:713–719, 1995. Reprinted with permission from The American College of Obstetricians and Gynecologists.)

within 24 to 36 hours. The mean lymphocyte counts in healthy neonates were 4,430 mm³; normoblast counts were 560/mm³ (Fig 2).

Conclusions.—Changes in blood lymphocyte counts were the only reliable indicator of the time of brain injury in this study. Lymphocyte counts increased to more than 10,000/mm³ within 2 hours of the onset of severe ischemia and hypoxemia, normalizing within 24 hours. Lymphocyte counts were especially valuable in identifying the time of injury because the lymphocytosis developed as a single spike that was not sustained beyond 24 hours, even when ischemia and hypoxemia persisted.

▶ As noted here earlier,[1, 2] an increase in cord blood normoblasts offers substantive evidence of recent, usually intrapartum, hypoxemia, which, by stimulating the sympathoadrenal system, causes splenic contraction and autotransfusion of a normoblast-rich population of red cells. Similarly, thrombopenia at birth is consonant with hypoxemia sufficient to cause fetal tissue injury 2 to 3 days prior to birth. Here, the authors cite the report of studies done in a Donner Lab volunteer who spent 5 days at an ambient partial pressure of oxygen of 85 mm Hg in a chamber set to about one-half atmosphere of pressure. Erythropoietin blood concentration was elevated promptly but returned to normal after 3 days, and there was a general elevation of blood-formed elements exempting red cells. The mechanisms by which erythropoietin release and/or production by the kidneys was stimulated are unknown. A control group of 294 cord blood samples among which normoblast data were available in about 30% was compared with a cohort of 16 patients with cerebral palsy. In 70% of these cases, the association with abruptio placentae made it possible to time the onset of occurrence of hypoxemia. Seven cases with cerebral palsy due to CNS anomaly and/or malformation and 35 infants with 1-minute Apgars of 0 to 3 were used as additional controls. Though the control groups were heterogeneous (25% of low-Apgar infants without cerebral palsy had elevated normoblast counts), the authors demonstrate the usefulness of cord blood normoblast determination, fixing a maximum normal value of 2,000 normoblast per cubic millimeter or about 25 per 100 white cells. The predictive strength of lymphocytosis is less certain, its origin somewhat obscure, and transient elevations in low-Apgar infants without cerebral palsy render it less useful. Nonetheless, proving once again the utility of cord blood normoblastemia in establishing recent fetal hypoxemia is a valuable contribution.

T.H. Kirschbaum, M.D.

References

1. 1992 YEAR BOOK OF OBSTETRICS AND GYNECOLOGY, pp 188–189.
2. Lippman HS: *Am J Dis Child* 27:473, 1924.

Delayed Vasodilation and Altered Oxygenation After Cerebral Ischemia in Fetal Sheep
Marks KA, Mallard EC, Roberts I, et al (Hammersmith Hosp, London; Univ of Auckland, New Zealand)
Pediatr Res 39:48–54, 1996

4–8

Background.—In asphyxiated infants and animals, transient hypoxia-ischemia is followed by a delayed impairment in energy metabolism; in sheep, it is followed by a delayed increase in electrical cortical impedance, which reflects loss of cellular ionic homeostasis. The hypothesis that the delayed phase of injury is associated with vasoconstriction and reduced blood and mitochondrial oxygenation was investigated in chronically instrumented, late gestational fetal sheep.

Methods.—Under general anesthesia, 14 singleton fetal sheep were partially externalized, and polyvinyl catheters were inserted into the axillary arteries, amniotic cavity, and brachial vein. Through burr holes, 3 pairs of electrodes were placed on the dura. The fetus was then returned to the uterus. Eight sheep did well postoperatively. Two days after surgery, 30 minutes of ischemia was induced in the 8 sheep by inflation of the bilateral carotid occluders with saline. Four days later, the ewes were killed.

Results.—Cortical impedance increased transiently during ischemia; a delayed increase started an average of 17.5 hours later and peaked at 42.3

hours (Fig 1). The electrocorticogram was depressed both during and after the insult. Two phases of cerebral vasodilation were indicated by increases in the concentration of total cerebral Hb (Fig 2). An early phase started right after early reperfusion and lasted an average of 2.3 hours. A later phase started 12.8 hours after ischemia and lasted 43.1 hours. A prolonged first increase of total cerebral Hb followed by an early and short-lived second postischemic increase was associated with a worse histologic outcome (Fig 3). A delayed increase in mean cerebration oxygen saturation was shown by an elevated concentration of oxyhemoglobin during postischemia day 4. The concentration of oxidized cytochrome aa_3 decreased slightly during the insult, and then, starting 28–30 hours later, fell progressively to reach a minimum at 78–80 hours postischemia.

Conclusions.—In fetal sheep, postischemic delayed cerebral injury is associated with vasodilatation and increased mean cerebral oxygen saturation. However, the progressive fall in the concentration of oxidized

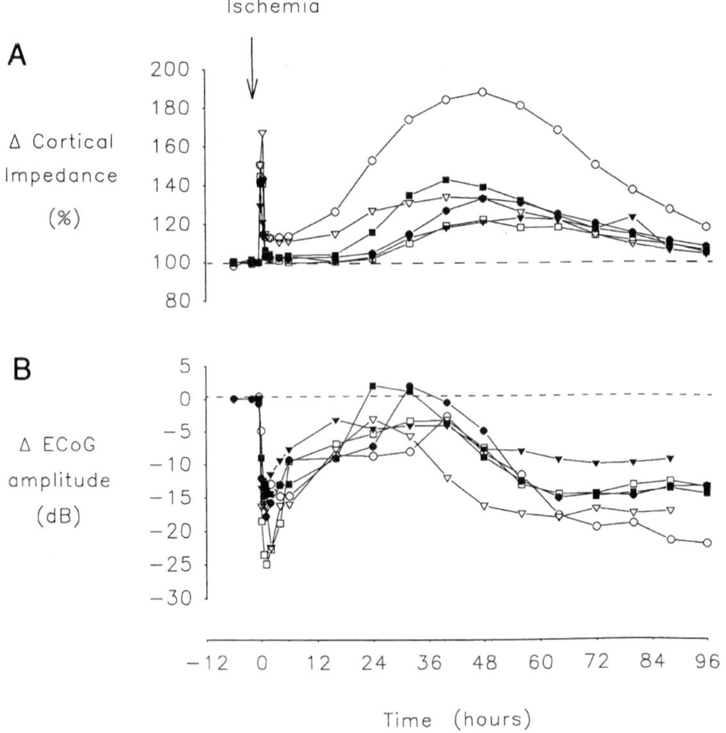

FIGURE 1.—Changes in *A*, cortical impedance, and *B*, electrocortical activity after transient cerebral ischemia. In *A*, the changes in cortical impedance (Δ*CI*) over 96 hours during and after transient cerebral ischemia (*n* = 6) are shown. Symbols represent the mean of averaged data for each fetus as percentage (%) change from pre-insult baseline (100%). There is an increase in CI during the insult, a period of recovery, and a delayed increase commencing several hours later. In *B*, the changes in electrocortical activity (Δ*ECoG*) in decibels (*dB*) from pre-insult zero baseline are shown. The ECoG is depressed during and after cerebral ischemia, recovers toward baseline, and then is finally depressed to an extent that relates to severity of histologic outcome (*P* < 0.01). (Courtesy of Marks KA, Mallard EC, Roberts I, et al: Delayed vasodilation and altered oxygenation after cerebral ischemia in fetal sheep. *Pediatr Res* 39:48–54, 1996.)

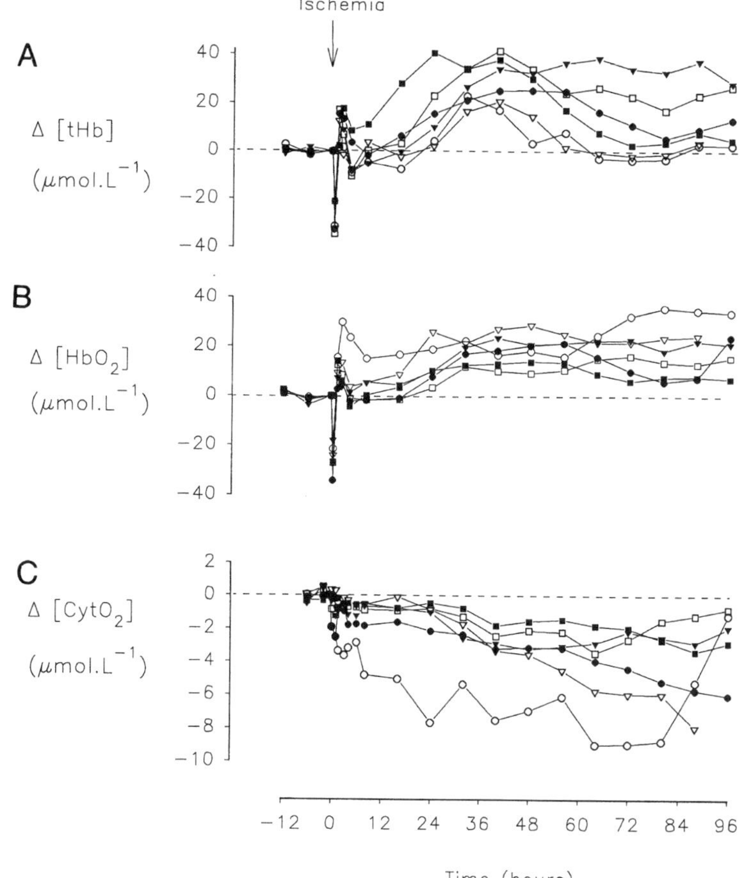

FIGURE 2.—Changes in near infrared spectroscopy variables after transient cerebral ischemia averaged into variable time bias. Changes in *A*, total cerebral Hb (Δ[tHb]), in *B*, oxyhemoglobin ([Hbo$_2$]); and in *C*, oxidized cytochrome oxidase (Δ[Cyto$_2$]) from pre-ischemic normalized baseline ($n = 6$). In each graph, different symbols represent data from each fetus. A fall in [tHb] during ischemia is followed by a first postischemic increase in [tHb], then a return to baseline, and a second postischemic increase in [tHb] commencing several hours later. Then [tHb] returns toward baseline at the end of the study period. In *B*, Δ[Hbo$_2$] demonstrates similar changes although a persistent increase in [Hbo$_2$], when [tHb] returns toward baseline, demonstrates an increase in the mean cerebral oxygen saturation during this time. In *C*, a fall is demonstrated in [Cyto$_2$] during the insult, a period of relative stability and then a progressive fall until 78–80 hours postinsult. *Abbreviations: tHb,* concentration of total cerebral Hb; *Hbo$_2$,* concentration of oxyhemoglobin; *Cyto$_2$,* concentration of oxidized cytochrome *aa$_3$.* (Courtesy of Marks KA, Mallard EC, Roberts I, et al: Delayed vasodilation and altered oxygenation after cerebral ischemia in fetal sheep. *Pediatr Res* 39:48–54, 1996.)

cytochrome *aa$_3$* may indicate decreased mitochondrial oxygenation, cell loss, or alterations in tissue optical characteristics.

▶ Using an intricate experimental model, this group used sheep fetuses with implanted dural electrodes for measuring cerebrocortical electrical

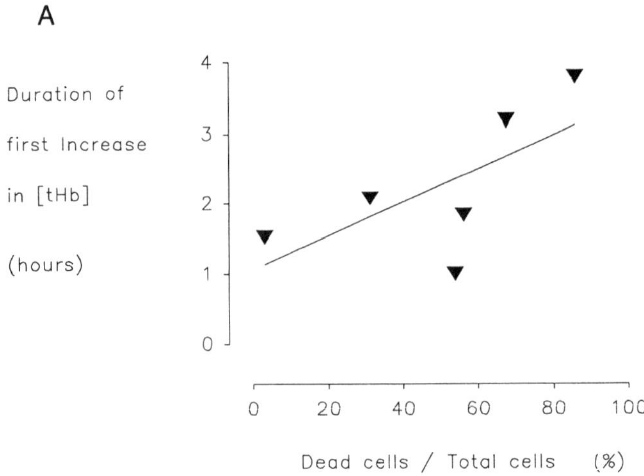

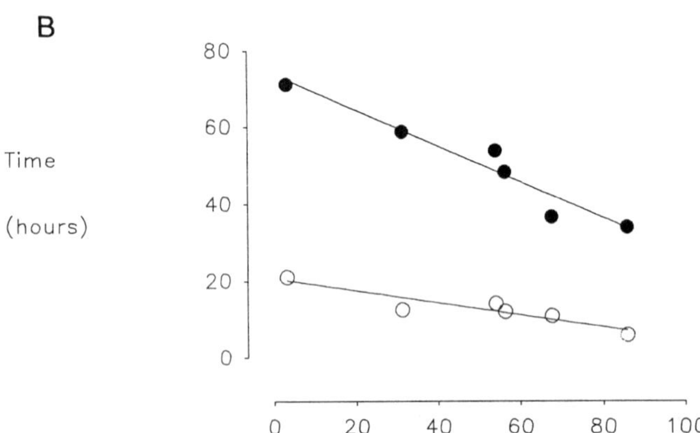

FIGURE 3.—The relation between change in concentration of total cerebral Hb (Δ[tHb]) and histologic outcome after transient cerebral ischemia. In *A* is shown the linear relation between the duration of the first increase in [tHb] ($r = 0.82$; $P < 0.05$) and overall neuronal loss score, and in *B* is shown the relation between time of onset (solid circle) ($r = 0.93$; $p < 0.01$) and duration (open circle) ($r < 0.97$; $P < 0.01$) of the second postischemic increase in [tHb] and overall neuronal loss score. A worse histologic outcome is associated with a prolonged first increase in [tHb] and a second postischemic increase in [tHb] that commences early and is short-lived. (Courtesy of Marks KA, Mallard EC, Roberts I, et al: Delayed vasodilation and altered oxygenation after cerebral ischemia in fetal sheep. *Pediatr Res* 39:48–54, 1996.)

activity and light conduits for doing near infrared spectroscopy on the fetal brain in chronic experimental preparations. An earlier description of their results is seen in the 1992 YEAR BOOK OF OBSTETRICS AND GYNECOLOGY[1] and in 1996 YEAR BOOK OF OBSTETRICS AND GYNEOLOGY.[2] It may be useful to review what can be learned from near infrared spectroscopy as described in the 1996 YEAR BOOK.[3]

Here the focus is on vascular changes in the secondary or delayed phase of cerebral pathophysiology after 30 minutes of bilateral fetal carotid artery occlusion. An immediate transient increase in cortical impedence and electrical activity occurs coincident with the rapid loss of intercellular water and hydration of glial cells. Some resolution of these changes occurs, but they then proceed over the next 24 hours, peaking at a maximum value of 48 hours after the insult by a more prolonged loss of cellular water and reduction of cortical electrical activity and irreversible brain injury. The extent of both changes correlates directly with the degree of brain injury noted on autopsy.

Near infrared spectroscopy discloses the same biphasic pattern with an increase in brain oxyhemoglobin content. This is presumably caused by reduced brain oxygenation, as reflected by the progressive reduction of oxidized cytochrome A3, a marker of mitochondrial oxygenation. The presence of increased brain fetal Hb, both oxidized and reduced, during the delayed phase of brain injury occurs without evident changes in fetal heart rate, blood pressure, or blood gas composition, as shown earlier. For this reason, the authors infer general vasodilatation in injured brain tissue without central cardiovascular alterations. Although use of these chronically implanted sensors imposes some limits on the interpretation of the vascular changes, the authors provide us with the most detailed view yet of the dynamics of ischemic fetal brain injury.

T.H. Kirschbaum, M.D.

References

1. 1992 Year Book of Obstetrics and Gynecology, pp 189–191.
2. 1996 Year Book of Obstetrics and Gynecology, pp 134–137.
3. 1996 Year Book of Obstetrics and Gynecology, pp 169–174.

Patterns of Cerebral Injury and Clinical Presentation in the Vascular Disruptive Syndrome of Monozygotic Twins
Weig SG, Marshall PC, Abroms IF, et al (Univ of Massachusetts, Worcester)
Pediatr Neurol 13:279–285, 1995
4–9

Introduction.—Intrauterine death of a monozygotic twin can have serious effects on the brain and other organs in the survivor. The pathophysiology has not been elucidated, but vascular disruption and infarction of preformed tissue is suspected. Eight neonates with 3 different neurologic presentations were described, and pathogenetic hypotheses were reviewed.

Neurologic Presentation.—Three of the 8 neonates had severe encephalopathy and seizures within their first 24 hours of life. The death of the co-twin occurred less than 48 hours before delivery for 2 of the 3 neonates. An additional 3 neonates had early neurologic complications, with congenital or acquired microcephaly, severe developmental delay, and seizures appearing beyond the neonatal period but before the age of 6 months. In these 3 cases, the co-twin's death occurred several days to many months before delivery. Neurologic anomalies appeared in late infancy in the other 2 neonates, with hemiplegic cerebral palsy occurring in 1 and partial seizures occurring in the other. The death of the co-twin of 1 was discovered unexpectedly at birth and occurred 18 hours before the preterm delivery of the other. Imaging studies of the 8 neonates showed several abnormalities, including multicystic encephalomalacia, bilateral basal ganglia calcification, and large extra-axial fluid collections in 1 neonate with early infancy seizures (Fig 3) and asymmetric periventricular white matter infarction in 1 with late infancy hemiplegic cerebral palsy (Fig 5). With the exception of the groups with late infancy presentations, these neonates had very severe impairments.

Discussion.—Antenatal structural pathology can cause various types of seizure disorders. The time of recognition of brain injury was directly related to the severity of the outcome, with a consistently bleak prognosis for twins with neonatal or early infancy presentations. However, the timing of the death of the co-twin was not clearly related to either the time of presentation or the outcome. Co-twin death that occurred early in pregnancy was associated with neuroimaging evidence of deep white

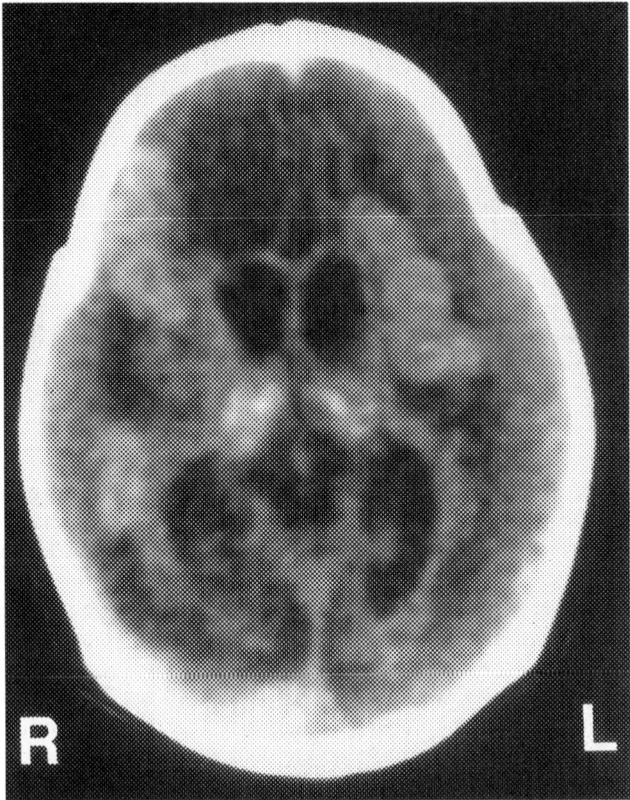

FIGURE 3.—Cranial CT shows severe multicystic encephalomalacia, bilateral basal ganglia calcification, and large extra-axial fluid collections. (Reprinted by permission of the publisher from Weig SG, Marshall PC, Abroms IF, et al: Patterns of cerebral injury and clinical presentation in the vascular disruptive syndrome of monozygotic twins. *Pediatr Neurol* 13:279–285, 1995. Copyright 1995 by Elsevier Science Inc.)

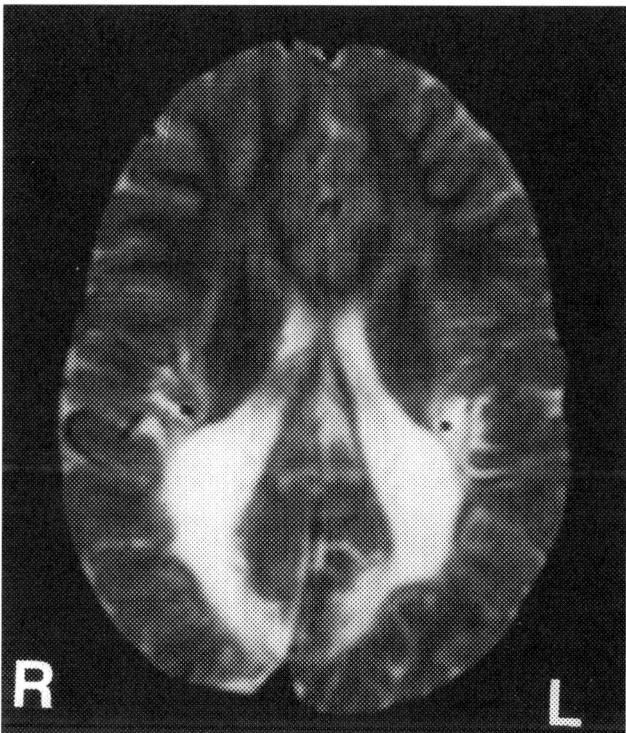

FIGURE 5.—Axial T_2-weighted MRI (TE, 120 ms; TR, 2,500 ms) shows a pattern of asymmetric periventricular white matter infarction. (Reprinted by permission of the publisher from Weig SG, Marshall PC, Abroms IF, et al: Patterns of cerebral injury and clinical presentation in the vascular disruptive syndrome of monozygotic twins. *Pediatr Neurol* 13:279–285, 1995. Copyright 1995 by Elsevier Science Inc.)

matter infarction and ventriculomegaly, whereas co-twin death occurring after 34 weeks' gestation was associated with neuroimaging evidence of multicystic encephalomalacia.

▶ Although no one knows the incidence of brain injury in a monochorionic twin who survives fetal death of his sibling, there is increasing evidence of concern that it might be common. The origin of what most often appears as seizures and devastating brain injury is certainly multifactorial, and this review of 8 such twins illustrates the difficulty in understanding enough about the problem to define rational interventions.

The impact of time between fetal death of 1 twin and brain injury of the second twin is quite variable. The onset of the diagnosis of brain injury in the survivor is often delayed for months to years, during which time the possibilities for other causes of brain damages are abundant. Cocaine and alcohol abuse are important but uncertain cofactors, as is brain injury caused by transient hypoxemia with hypoperfusion, in the neonatal ICU experience of these often prematurely delivered neonates.

The 50% incidence of "vanished twins" means that we may well be underestimating the impact of monochorionicity on fetal injury. Two patterns of neural pathology are beginning to emerge. Early fetal injury, caused by fetal transfusion, disseminated introvascular coagulation, thromboembolus, or cord accident, tends to produce deep white matter necrosis and ventriculomegaly where it occurs earlier than 26 to 28 weeks. After that, multiple cystic encephalomalacia representing multiple vessel disruptions is more common. The authors conclude that, where interuterine fetal death occurs in a monochorionic, diamniotic twin pair, "urgent delivery be considered" at or near term until we understand the incidence and origin of brain injury in the survivor better than at present. It's advice worth considering.

T.H. Kirschbaum, M.D.

Screening for Fetal Trisomies by Maternal Age and Fetal Nuchal Translucency Thickness at 10 to 14 Weeks of Gestation

Pandya PP, Snijders RJM, Johnson SP, et al (King's College Hosp, London)
Br J Obstet Gynaecol 102:957–962, 1995   4–10

Background.—A maternal age of 35 years or older and an increase in fetal nuchal translucency thickness (FNTT) both have been associated with an increase in fetal trisomy 21 and other chromosomal abnormalities.

Objective.—The objective of this study was to screen for trisomy 21 and other chromosomal abnormalities using a combination of maternal age and FNTT as indicators.

Methods.—Fetal nuchal translucency thickness was determined by abdominal or intravaginal sonography performed at 10 to 14 weeks of

TABLE 3.—Relation of Fetal Nuchal Translucency Thickness at 10 to 14 Weeks' Gestation and Karyotype.

		Nuchal translucency		
Karyotype	*n*	≥2·5 mm	>95th centile	>99th centile
Normal	20217	106 (5)	917 (5)	221 (1)
Abnormal	164	127 (77)	127 (77)	100 (61)
Trisomy 21	86	66 (77)	66 (77)	52 (60)
Trisomy 18	40	30 (75)	30 (75)	25 (63)
Trisomy 13	11	9 (82)	9 (82)	8 (73)
Trisomy 20	1	1 (100)	1 (100)	1 (100)
Trisomy 22	1	1 (100)	1 (100)	1 (100)
Turner syndrome	10	10 (100)	10 (100)	9 (90)
47,XXX	1	—	—	—
47,XXY	4	2 (50)	2 (50)	1 (25)
47,XYY	2	2 (100)	2 (100)	—
Triploidy	7	5 (71)	5 (71)	2 (29)
46,XX,4p-	1	1 (100)	1 (100)	1 (100)

Note: Values are shown as *n* (%).
(Courtesy of Pandya PP, Snijders RJM, Johnson SP, et al: Screening for fetal trisomies by maternal age and fetal nuchal translucency thickness at 10 to 14 weeks of gestation. *Br J Obstet Gynaecol* 102:957–962, 1995, Blackwell Science, Ltd.)

gestation. Fetal crown-rump length also was determined by this procedure. In most normal fetuses, the FNTT at this stage of development is less than 2.5 mm (or less than 3 mm when the instruments used are precise only to the millimeter). Fetal nuchal translucency thickness above these values is suggestive of a chromosomal abnormality. Fetal karyotyping was performed during the first trimester in the presence of advanced maternal age (35 years or older), in the presence of increased FNTT, in the presence of a family history of chromosomal abnormality, or at parental request. Appropriate analyses were performed to correlate trisomy 21 and other chromosomal abnormalities with maternal age and FNTT.

Results.—During the study period—from September 1, 1992, to October 28, 1994—a total of 20,804 women were screened. Of these, results were available for analysis in 20,381. First-trimester fetal karyotyping was performed in 2,017 cases. Of these, 729 were done because of increased FNTT; 1,036, for advanced maternal age; 46, for a family history of chromosomal abnormality: and 206, at parental request. A significant relationship was found between abnormal karyotypes and increased FNTT (Table 3). A striking contrast was noted between FNTT in the normal fetus and in those with an abnormal karyotype (Fig 1). In the normal fetus, FNTT increased significantly with crown–rump length. Fetal nuchal translucency thickness was above the 95% centile in 66 of 86 fetuses (77%) with trisomy 21 and in 61 of 78 (78%) of fetuses with other chromosomal defects. On the basis of the combination of FNTT,

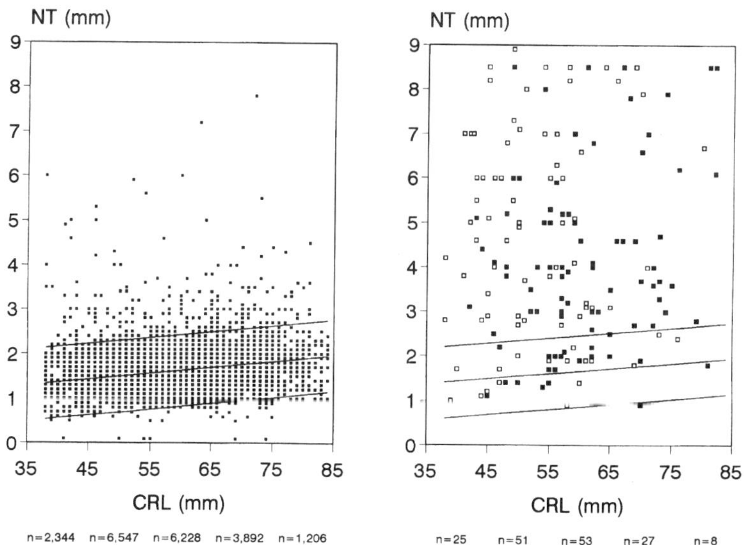

FIGURE 1.—Fetal nuchal translucency in 20,217 chromosomally normal fetuses (**left**), in 86 fetuses with trisomy 21 (**right solid square**), and in 78 fetuses with other chromosomal abnormalities (**right open square**) plotted on the reference range with crown–rump length (median, 5th and 95th centiles). *Abbreviations: NT,* nuchal thickness; *CRL,* crown–rump length. (Courtesy of Pandya PP, Snijders RJM, Johnson SP, et al: Screening for fetal trisomies by maternal age and fetal nuchal translucency thickness at 10 to 14 weeks of gestation. *Br J Obstet Gynaecol* 102:957–962, 1995, Blackwell Science, Ltd.)

crown–rump length and maternal age, the minimal risk was 1/100 for 4.9% of normal pregnancies, in 80% of those with trisomy 21, and in 77% of those with other chromosomal defects.

Conclusions.—During the first trimester, the determination of FNTT in combination with maternal age provides a possibly useful screening technique for the determination of trisomy 21 and other chromosomal defects.

▶ This is a welcome prospective, randomized test of the usefulness of using nuchal translucency on abdominal or vaginal ultrasound at 10 to 14 weeks' gestation to aid in the detection of trisomy 21 and other karyotypic abnormalities. Regrettably, it is hard to evaluate the results. Among those 2,017 women who underwent first-trimester karyotypes, only in 36% of 729 cases was the genetic examination motivated only by ultrasonic nuchal lucency; in 684 women with second-trimester karyotype, only 22% were motivated by the ultrasonic finding because this is a test of efficacy of case findings by ultrasound. It is hard to separate results in those women from others in whom age older than 35 years, family history, anxiety, biochemical testing, and postnatal evidence of dysmorphism and autopsy served as motives for obtaining the karyotype.

Using the sum of all these paths to karyotypic analysis, sensitivity appears to be 77% for trisomy 21 and 78% for other abnormalities, whereas the false positive rate of 0.86% is a reflection of the low prevalence of the abnormal outcome. If one superimposes the frequency distribution plot of nuclear translucencies in normal fetuses with those of 164 abnormal fetuses detected on the basis of any of the several criteria above, the overlap above the 95th percentile boundary seems considerable. What these frequency determinations appear to indicate is a method of some—but modest—sensitivity, which leaves the issue of effective screening for trisomy 21 by this method, as before, uncertain.[1]

T.H. Kirschbaum, M.D.

Reference

1. *Focus & Opinion: Obstetrics and Gynecology,* 1995.

First Trimester Serum Screening for Down's Syndrome
Wald NJ, Kennard A, Hackshaw AK (Univ of London)
Prenat Diagn 15:1227–1240, 1995   4–11

Introduction.—With the quadruple screening approach based on ultrasound determination of gestational age, serum screening for Down's syndrome at 15–22 weeks' gestation can detect 72% of affected pregnancies. Accurate screening before 15 weeks' gestation may be even better. A review of early serum screening for Down's syndrome is reported.

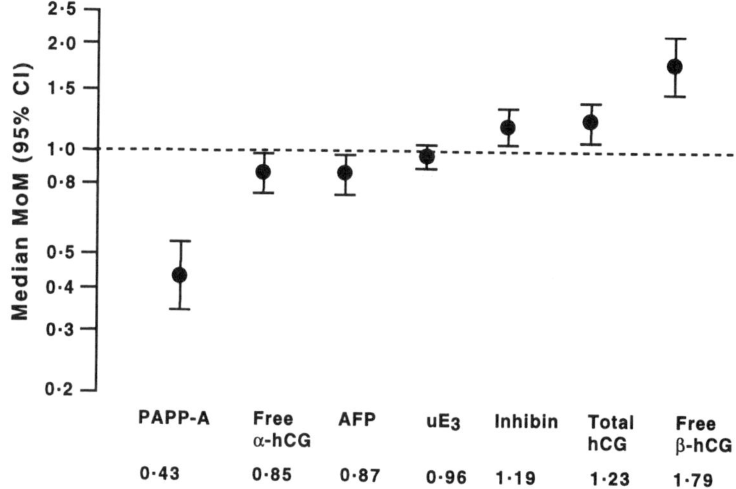

FIGURE 1.—Median serum marker level in 77 Down's syndrome pregnancies at 8–14 weeks of gestation (taken from the FiTSS study, Wald et al., 1996). (Courtesy of Wald NJ, Kennard A, Hackshaw AK: First trimester serum screening for Down's syndrome. *Prenat Diagn* 15:1227–1240, 1995. Reprinted by permission of John Wiley & Sons, Ltd.)

First-Trimester Screening.—The First Trimester Screening Study (FiTSS), the largest study of serum markers for Down's syndrome between 8 and 14 weeks' gestation, analyzed stored serum samples from 77 Down's syndrome pregnancies (Fig 1). The results indicated that the best biochemical markers at this stage were pregnancy-associated plasma protein A (PAPP-

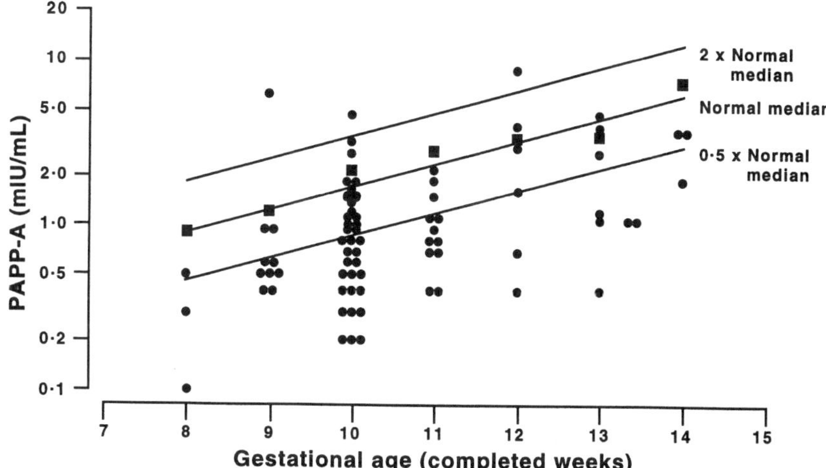

FIGURE 2.—Maternal serum pregnancy associated plasma protein A levels in 77 Down's syndrome pregnancies at 8–14 weeks of gestation (taken from the FiTSS study, Wald et al., 1996). (Courtesy of Wald NJ, Kennard A, Hackshaw AK: First trimester serum screening for Down's syndrome. *Prenat Diagn* 15:1227–1240, 1995. Reprinted by permission of John Wiley & Sons, Ltd.)

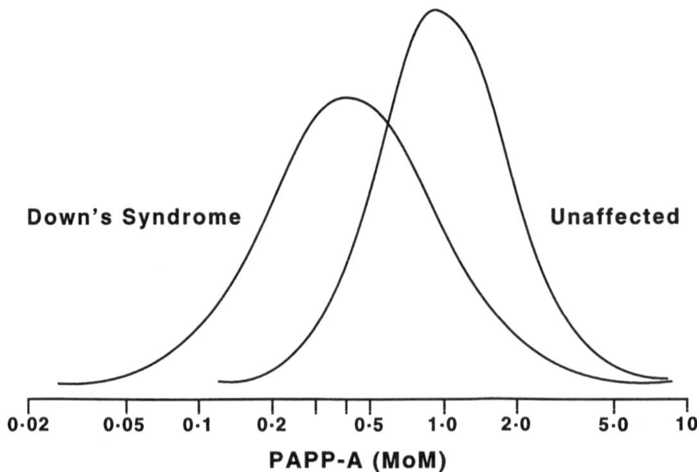

FIGURE 3.—Distribution of serum pregnancy associated plasma protein A levels in 77 Down's syndrome and 383 unaffected pregnancies at 8–14 weeks of gestation (taken from the FiTSS study, Wald et al., 1996). (Courtesy of Wald NJ, Kennard A, Hackshaw AK: First trimester serum screening for Down's syndrome. *Prenat Diagn* 15:1227–1240, 1995. Reprinted by permission of John Wiley & Sons, Ltd.)

A) (Figs 2 and 3) and the free β-subunit of human chorionic gonadotropin (free β-hCG) (Fig 4). The estimated detection rate in the first trimester using PAPP-A and free β-hCG is 62%, with a 5% false positive rate, when used in combination with maternal age. Similar results are noted on a review of the world literature. The 10-week level of dimeric inhibin-A may be of some value, but the other markers studied have less predictive value.

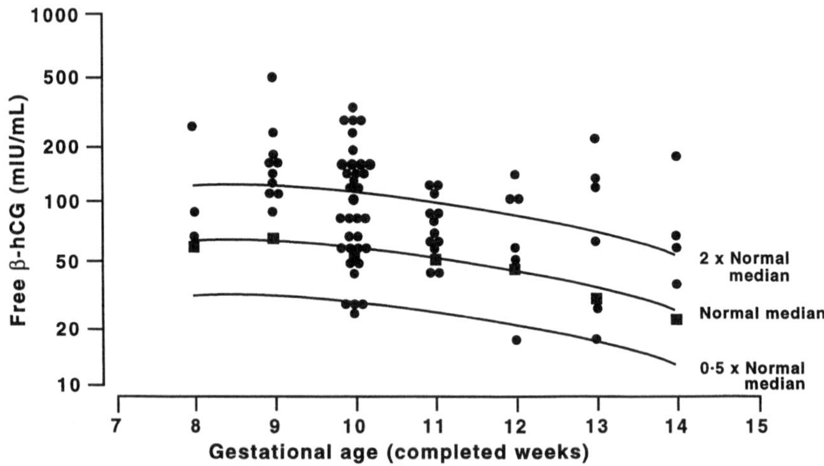

FIGURE 4.—Maternal serum free β-human chorionic gonadotropin levels in 77 Down's syndrome pregnancies at 8–14 weeks of gestation (taken from the FiTSS study, Wald et al., 1996). (Courtesy of Wald NJ, Kennard A, Hackshaw AK: First trimester serum screening for Down's syndrome. *Prenat Diagn* 15:1227–1240, 1995. Reprinted by permission of John Wiley & Sons, Ltd.)

One possibly important new screening marker is nuchal translucency, as measured from a 10-week ultrasound examination. However, the predictive performance of this ultrasound measurement, on its own or combined with biochemical markers, is uncertain.

Conclusions.—Two biochemical measures—PAPP-A and free β-hCG—can be used in early serum screening for Down's syndrome. More information on these techniques, and on nuchal translucency measurement, is needed before they can be recommended for routine use. Once some key issues like these have been addressed, 10-week screening for Down's syndrome will be an advance that improves antenatal care for pregnant women.

▶ Now that the effectiveness of antenatal screening for Down's syndrome between 15 and 22 weeks of gestation is relatively clear,[1] it's a logical extension to look for screening techniques that detect Down's syndrome before 15 weeks. This scholarly consideration of available methodology makes it clear that, because they fail to identify Down's syndrome pregnancies before 15 weeks, maternal serum α-fetoprotein, urinary estriol, and dimeric inhibin assays are of little benefit. The positive conclusions in this study are based on a case-control study of stored serum samples stemming from a collaborative study involving a group of 22 centers in Europe and North America. Seventy-seven Down's syndrome pregnancies, half at 10 weeks' gestation, were compared for predictability with quintuplicate controls matched for gestational age, maternal age, and duration of blood storage. Two serum markers proved useful. Pregnancy associated plasma protein A is a large glycoprotein similar in characteristics to alpha II macroglobulin. It seems to be a placental protease inhibitor of leukocyte elastase and possibly other enzymes. Its potential usefulness stems from its ability to obtund maternal proteolytic action at the placental attachment site. It is decreased in concentration in Down's syndrome just as β-hCG concentrations are slightly increased in the first trimester. Use of these 2 markers gives a 62% detection rate with a 5% false positive rate. The key is the uncertain role of ultrasonic identification of nuchal translucency as a primary predictor. Nicolaides et al. have reported an 86% detection rate with 4.5% false positives using 3 mm of sonolucency as diagnostic of Down's syndrome,[2] but others have failed to confirm these results.[3, 4] The authors suggest we await resolution of these differences in reported value of nuchal ultrasonography because "at present there is uncertainty about its quantitative performance." This paper provides an honest summary of the current status of first-trimester screening for this syndrome.

T.H. Kirschbaum, M.D.

References

1. 1994 YEAR BOOK OF OBSTETRICS AND GYNECOLOGY, pp 157–159.
2. Nicolaides K, Brizot M de L, Patel F, et al: Comparison of chorionic villus sampling and amniocentesis for fetal karyotyping at 10–13 weeks' gestation. *Lancet* 344: 435, 1994.
3. 1993 YEAR BOOK OF OBSTETRICS AND GYNECOLOGY, pp 130–131.
4. Brambot B, et al: *Prenat Diagn* 14:1043, 1994.

Correlation Between Umbilical Arterial Flow and Placental Morphology

Kreczy A, Fusi L, Wigglesworth JS (Univ of Innsbruck, Austria; Hammersmith Hosp, London)
Int J Gynecol Pathol 14:306–309, 1995   4–12

Introduction.—Previous studies have found correlations among abnormal Doppler indices and reduced numbers of arteries in the tertiary stem villi of the placenta. A number of hypotheses explaining this morphologic finding have been proposed. The capillary bed of the placenta was examined in patients with both normal and abnormal Doppler flow studies to correlate these morphologic findings with the Doppler findings and with pregnancy outcome.

Methods.—Nineteen patients with abnormal Doppler flow studies of the umbilical artery blood flow and 11 randomly selected patients matched for gestational age with normal umbilical artery blood flow were studied. At birth, small-for-date (SFD) neonates were identified and the placentas were examined macroscopically, to assess the extent of the visible lesions as a percentage of the placental weight, and histologically, to count the numbers of arteries, vessels, and capillaries per tertiary stem villus in 10 randomly chosen fields.

Results.—There was no relationship between the extent of gross lesions and either Doppler findings or outcome of pregnancy. However, total placental weight correlated significantly with abnormal Doppler findings, to the numbers of arteries and vessels, and to birth weight. The number of capillaries was similar in neonates in the normal and abnormal Doppler groups and were independent of birth weight and gestational age. The numbers of arteries were highly significantly reduced and the number of vessels was less but still significantly reduced in the abnormal Doppler

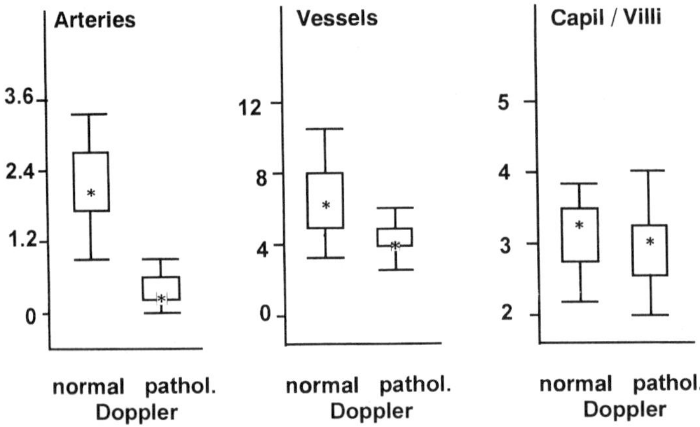

FIGURE 2.—Box charts displaying the distribution of the different counts for arteries, vessels, and capillaries/villi in the group with normal and abnormal Doppler findings, respectively. The *asterisk* indicates the median. The *box* includes 50% of the cases, and the extensions show the total range of the counts. (Courtesy of Kreczy A, Fusi L, Wigglesworth JS: Correlation between umbilical arterial flow and placental morphology. *Int J Gynecol Pathol* 14:306–309, 1995.)

group and also in the placentas of SFD neonates (Fig 2). Abnormal Doppler and SFD status were significantly related.

Conclusions.—The strong correlation of an abnormal pulsatility index and a reduced number of arteries with lower placental weight suggests an early developmental defect. The stable number of villous capillaries may result from a compensatory formation of more capillaries to maintain the fetus's metabolic needs in response to the early developmental arrest of placental angiogenesis. The association with SFD neonates testifies to the limited effectiveness of this adaptive process.

▶ This is a second recently available study of placental morphometry with abnormal umbilical artery Doppler performed by skilled placental pathologists (see Abstract 5–8) in contrast to several earlier reports. Comparing placentas from normals with those from fetuses with pulsativity indices greater than the 95th percentile for gestational age, the authors found no relationship between Doppler signals and the number of stem villi or total villi or in the density of capillary vessels in the 2 groups. They did report a decrease in the number of arterioles and tertiary stem villi without evidence of vessel obliteration in placentas marked by abnormal pulsitivity indices. Comparing with Kaufmann's classification, these are likely immature intermediate villi, present in the second trimester of pregnancy and progressively replaced later by terminal villi that lack arterioles. Regrettably, we know little about gestational ages of the placentas beyond that they were derived from the third trimester (26–40 weeks' gestational age), and the authors disagree regarding the persistence of arteriolar structures in stem villi at this point in pregnancy. Unlike the Kaufmann group, which stained for actin, these investigators found they could not use the Masson trichrome method to differentiate arterioles from capillary structures by the ability of smooth muscle to take up the dye, a possible basis for the differences in their findings. In any event, they fail to agree with the absence of abnormalities in placental resistance elements in such placentas. Clearly there is room for competent pathologists to enter into this disputed area.

T.H. Kirschbaum, M.D.

Flow Cytometry in Diagnosis and Management of Large Fetomaternal Haemorrhage

Johnson PRE, Tait RC, Austin EB, et al (Manchester Blood Centre, England)
J Clin Pathol 48:1005–1008, 1995   4–13

Introduction.—The Kleihauer acid elution test is used to detect and quantify fetomaternal hemorrhage (FMH) and determine the dose of anti-D immunoglobulin to be given. Although the Kleihauer test is sensitive, many sources of error can render it inaccurate, including the inability to differentiate between fetal red blood cells and adult hemoglobin F-

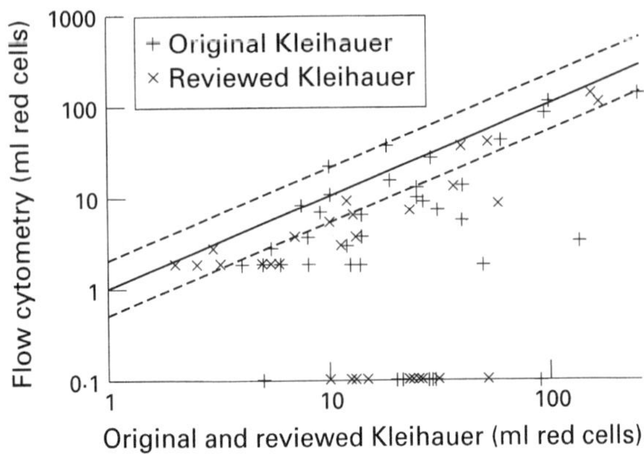

FIGURE 1.—Correlation between results obtained using the original and reviewed Kleihauer tests, and on flow cytometry. The *dotted lines* indicate 50% and 200% of the Kleihauer result. Original Kleihauer test, $r = 0.714$; $r^2 = 0.509$. Reviewed Kleihauer test, $r = 0.915$; $r^2 = 0.837$. (Courtesy of Johnson PRE, Tait RC, Austin EB, et al: Flow cytometry in diagnosis and management of large fetomaternal haemorrhage. *J Clin Pathol* 48:1005–1008, 1995.)

containing cells present in some women. Therefore, the accuracy of indirect immunofluorescence flow cytometry for quantitating FMH was evaluated.

Methods.—Expression of the Rh D antigen was measured by flow cytometry in red blood cells from maternal samples from patients with FMH greater than 4 mL (as detected by Kleihauer testing) after incubation with anti-D serum and fluorescein-labeled anti-human Fab IgG. Mixtures of Rh D-positive cells in Rh D-negative blood and positive and negative controls incubated with AB serum were analyzed. Anti-D immunoglobulin was administered based on the FMH volume as determined by flow cytometry, with further anti-D immunoglobulin administered to patients with positive Kleihauer tests at 48 hours.

Results.—The positive and negative controls demonstrated the excellent differentiation and sensitivity of the flow cytometry technique. Only 26% agreement was found between the results of flow cytometry and of the Kleihauer test originally and 39% agreement between the results of flow cytometry and of corrected Kleihauer tests reviewed centrally with a calibrated microscope (Fig 1). Fifteen patients were given anti-D immunoglobulin doses based on the flow cytometry estimates of FMH volume, which resulted in a 58% reduction in the administration of anti-D immunoglobulin. Six months later, none of these patients required immunization.

Conclusions.—Flow cytometry may provide more accurate quantitation of large FMH, resulting in more rational treatment with anti-D immunoglobulin, particularly in patients with maternal hemoglobin F-containing cells. Further studies of the role of flow cytometry in the detection of FMH are warranted.

▶ All of us have used the maternal Kleihauer assay to estimate the volume of a fetal-to-maternal bleed and found a value that exceeds the total estimated blood volume of the fetus. This study, using Rh-positive cells in the blood of Rh-negative gravidas as a test case, helps us understand why that happens.

For cell sorting, an antibody capable of complexing with fetal but not maternal cells (anti-D here) is needed. This antibody should be labeled with a marker (fluorescein) whose fluorescence can be used to activate the sorter to segregate labeled fetal cells from unlabeled maternal cells and to allow quantitation.

Comparing results with the maternal Kleihauer assay showed that, in 88% of cases, the Kleihauer assay overestimated the volume of the bleed by at least a factor of 2. In 7 cases in which the Kleihauer calculation suggested a fetal-to-maternal hemorrhage of 20–100 mL of fetal blood, none were found by cell sort. In 1 case, a suspected fetal hemorrhage of 254 mL turned out to be 130 mL by flow cytometry.

The implications for the needless overutilization of Rh immune globulin based on the Kleihauer assay are obvious. Flow cytometry is costly and requires careful controls, and the selections of a labeled antibody unique to fetal cells may not be easy. However, we should all realize that there are technical problems that underlie the overestimates derived from maternal Kleihauer cell counts.

T.H. Kirschbaum, M.D.

Maternal and Perinatal Complications in Triplet Compared With Twin Pregnancy

Santema JG, Bourdrez P, Wallenburg HCS (Erasmus Univ, Rotterdam, The Netherlands)
Eur J Obstet Gynecol Reprod Biol 60:143–147, 1995   4–14

Background.—The various methods of assisted reproductive technology in use today are known to be associated with a considerable risk of triplet and higher multiple pregnancies. In an attempt to reduce the maternal and perinatal risks of multifetal pregnancy, parents are being offered the option of reduction of the number of fetuses in the first trimester of pregnancy. To evaluate the risk of continuation of triplet gestation compared with twin or singleton pregnancy, the course and outcome of triplet pregnancies were compared with those of twin pregnancies in a matched-pair analysis.

Methods.—All charts of triplet pregnancies delivered after a gestational age of 20 weeks or more within an 11-year period (January 1981 to December 1991) were retrospectively reviewed. Each triplet pregnancy was matched for maternal parity and age with 2 sets of twins delivered in the same year. The primary end points of the analysis were maternal complications and perinatal outcome.

Results.—Forty triplet pregnancies were delivered during the study and were matched with 80 twin pregnancies. Most of the triplet pregnancies

(82%) were a result of assisted reproduction, compared with 36% of the twin pregnancies. Compared with only 49% of the mothers with twins, 85% of the women with triplets were admitted to the hospital at some time during their pregnancy because of subjective complaints or maternal complications. This difference in antenatal complications was largely a result of the significantly higher incidence of preterm labor in triplets. The incidence of cesarean section was also significantly higher in patients with triplets (62%) than with twins (21%). Compared with twins, triplets had a significantly lower median birth weight (2,030 vs. 1,478 g) and gestational age at delivery (35.5 vs. 32 weeks). Furthermore, the median hospital stay was significantly longer for the triplets, largely because of the lower birth weight.

Conclusions.—Triplets have a lower median birth weight and gestational age at delivery and a longer neonatal stay in the hospital than do twins but no significant differences in major neonatal complications. These data may be helpful in counseling women with a triplet pregnancy who are considering selective reduction to twins. Moreover, because triplet pregnancies are often a result of infertility treatment, these results support the view that methods of assisted reproduction should aim at prevention of multifetal gestation.

▶ As innovations in assisted human reproductive technology have increased the number of multiple pregnancies of high order, counseling parents in regard to current outcomes and the merits of selective fetal reduction has gained new import. This referral center in Rotterdam was able to provide useful information through the collection of 40 triplet pregnancies over an 11-year span, which was sufficient to provide a set of matched comparisons with 80 twin pregnancies over the same time. Triplet pregnancy was associated with a greater risk of preterm labor, longer hospital admissions, increased costs and, inevitably, an increase in low-birth-weight infants. The incidence of fetal death was roughly 3 times higher in triplets than in twins, and this effected a significantly higher perinatal loss rate for triplets (20%) than for twins (8.9%), correcting for birth weight less than 500 g and lethal anomalies. Cesarean sections, 30% of them elective for triplets and 12% for twins, were more common with triplets than with twins.

In brief, the principal impact of triplet pregnancy was expressed in the increased incidence of preterm delivery and not in the incidence of major neonatal complications. Triplet pregnancies encumber parents with increased costs and risk of neonatal loss, and their inadvertent occurrence should certainly be avoided, but as noted earlier here,[1] it's hard to support fetal reduction on any terms other than the personal wishes of the parents. Admittedly, that's an important part of the decision.

T.H. Kirschbaum, M.D.

Reference

1. 1992 YEAR BOOK OF OBSTETRICS AND GYNECOLOGY, pp 167–168.

The Prognostic Factors in the Prenatal Diagnosis of the Echogenic Fetal Lung

Barret J, Chitayat D, Sermer M, et al (Univ of Toronto)
Prenat Diagn 15:849–853, 1995

4–15

Background.—The use of high-resolution ultrasonography for prenatal diagnosis has led to increased detection of echogenic fetal lung (EFL) in the early second trimester. This ultrasonography finding is usually indicative of congenital cystic adenomatoid lung malformation, an intrapulmonary lung sequestration or major airway obstruction. As an aid to parental counseling in these cases, the outcomes of 11 recent cases and a series of cases derived from a literature review were investigated.

Study Group.—Eleven patients referred to the University of Toronto perinatal complex from 1992 to 1993 were studied. Repeated detailed fetal ultrasonography was performed, and associated structural abnormalities, lesion size, lung location laterality, mediastinal shift, and the presence of nonimmune hydrops fetalis (NIHF) were recorded for each case. The English literature was reviewed and patient series containing at least 5 prenatally diagnosed cases of EFL were extracted for purposes of comparison.

Findings.—The gestation age at diagnosis for the 11 cases in the study group was 17 to 32 weeks. Five of the cases were solid and 6 had cystic components. Seven cases had a mediastinal shift, but only 1 case had hydrops associated with it. Three fetuses were aborted. All of the other 8 patients survived without having NIHF develop. In 3 cases, the lung lesions resolved by the third trimester. In 1 case, surgery was required in the immediate postnatal period. In the other 4 cases, the patients are being managed conservatively and have had no complications with a follow-up of 6 weeks to 6 months.

Literature Review.—From an English-language literature review, 60 EFL cases in 3 series were selected. Of these 60 pregnancies, 10 were terminated. Of the other 50 cases, 32% survived past the immediate neonatal period. Among these, 5 had resolution of the lesion in utero and 14 did not require surgery. In only 3 cases that did not have hydrops at diagnosis did it develop during the subsequent pregnancy.

Conclusions.—In the absence of fetal hydrops or other abnormalities, fetuses with a prenatal diagnosis of EFL have a good prognosis. If NIHF is absent at diagnosis, the chance that it will develop subsequently during the pregnancy is low. There is a significant chance that EFL will resolve before delivery. In cases of NIHF, the prognosis is poor.

▶ Though there have been isolated reports of intrapartum spontaneous resolution of cystic adenomatoid malformations (CAMs) of the lung,[1] this is a first successful attempt at amassing enough cases to allow some generalizations to be made in regard to management. In general, ultrasound does not allow one to differentiate congenital lung sequestration from CAM unless the latter is clearly cystic in form. Eleven cases from the University of

Toronto Perinatal Complex were here added to cases available in the literature. Data analysis is complicated by a 30% incidence of therapeutic abortion in those who initially presented. Specific indications for termination included nonimmune hydrops and congenital anomaly, though the latter was not inordinately common. The overall newborn survival after this second-trimester diagnosis was 64% with one fourth of fetuses showing spontaneous resolution of the lesion and the rest some regression. Almost all of the 36% mortality was associated with nonimmune hydrops. Hydrops apparently reflects sufficient pulmonary vascular impairment to result in right heart failure, and its appearance makes all the difference between an excellent prognosis and a hopeless one for want of an effective treatment for the cardiopulmonary complication. It follows that, at present, expectant management is warranted for CAMs and congenital lung sequestration in the absence of hydrops fetalis.

T.H. Kirschbaum, M.D.

Reference

1. 1995 Year Book of Obstetrics and Gynecology, p 150.

Prepregnant Weight in Relation to Risk of Neural Tube Defects
Werler MM, Louik C, Shapiro S, et al (Boston Univ)
JAMA 275:1089–1092, 1996

4–16

Objective.—It has been suggested that obesity may increase the risk of having a pregnancy affected by a neural tube defect (NTD). This is an important public health question because obesity is common and NTDs are among the most frequent and severe congenital malformations. The role of folate intake is also important to determine. The effect of maternal obesity on the risk of NTDs was evaluated in 2 case-control studies: one conducted as part of a birth defect surveillance program and the other as part of a population-based study.

Surveillance Study.—The study included 604 fetuses or infants with an NTD diagnosed within 6 months of delivery, 1,658 control fetuses or infants with other major malformations, and 93 control subjects without major malformations. Women with body weights of 50–59 kg were used as the reference group. The relative risk of NTDs for women weighing 80–89 kg was 1.9 (95% confidence interval [CI] 1.2–2.9). For women weighing 110 kg or more, relative risk was 4.0 (95% CI 1.6–9.9). The risk of NTDs related to body weight applied to women who did and did not receive the recommended amount of 400 µg of folate. For women with body weights of less than 70 kg who took 400 µg of folate or more, risk of NTDs decreased by 40%. For women weighing more than 70 kg, taking the recommended folate amount did not reduce the risk of NTDs.

Population-Based Study.—This study included 538 fetuses and infants with NTDs and 539 control subjects without malformations. The mothers were interviewed within an average of 5 months after their term delivery date. The risk of NTD was approximately doubled for obese women, compared with those with a body mass index of 29 kg/m^2 or less. Odds ratio was 1.9, with a 95% CI of 1.3–2.9. The obesity-associated increase in risk was unrelated to vitamins containing folic acid, diabetes, use of diet pills, dietary folic acid intake, or a previous NTD pregnancy. The odds ratio was unaffected by adjustment for maternal age, education, gravidity, vitamin use, and alcohol use. The link between maternal obesity and NTD was greater for spina bifida and other less common NTDs than for anencephaly.

Conclusions.—Infants born to mothers with heavier prepregnancy body weights are at increased risk of NTDs. The risk of NTDs seems to be doubled for obese women, independent of the effects of folate intake. This modest effect probably makes a significant contribution to the number of NTDs in the population, given that perhaps 10% of women are obese when they become pregnant.

▶ In 2 retrospective case-control studies investigating the role of obesity in the origin of NTDs, the Sloane Epidemiology Unit of Boston University School of Public Health and the California Birth Defects Monitoring Program[1] provide supportive data. The Boston study consisted of 604 cases of NTDs compared with 1,658 infants with birth defects other than NTDs plus 93 normal births and the California study uses 510 cases of NTD compared with about 520 normal births. In both cases, risk ratios based on multivariate analysis together with the 95% CI are provided. By convention, any risk ratio whose CI includes unity (no difference in risk between test and control cases) lacks statistical significance. When viewed in that way, significant data seem patchy and without consistent pattern. In the Boston study only women with prepregnancy weight in the range from 80–89 kg, 100–109 kg, and more than 110 kg, but not 90–99 kg, showed increased risk of having children with NTDs. Above the 89 kg prepregnancy weight range, all comparison involved only 26 cases and 23 controls. In both studies, full folate use was assayed by retrospective questionnaire, usually done approximately 6 months after birth. Full dose obtained this way was unrelated to NTD risk ratios. Only in women with prepregnancy weight less than 70 kg is any folate dose associated with decreased risk of NTDs. Compared to normal and non–NTD anomalous controls, no significant relationships between folic acid use by prepregnancy weight or height are seen, and only in 10 women with body mass index more than 32 kg/m^2, (more than the 29 kg/m^2 level usually used to define obesity) was a significant benefit reported. In the California study, significant reports are similar and rare. Only in the body mass index range less than 29 kg/m^2 but not more was a benefit from folic acid inferred. It's puzzling to me that the Centers for Disease Control and Prevention recommendation for the use of supplemental folate to prevent NTDs was formulated with so little concern for the defects in experimental design in much of the supporting data.[1, 2] It is reminiscent of the claims that folic acid prevented iron deficiency anemia, placental abruption, pregnancy induced hypertension, and a wide range of other fetal anomalies that lie in our past, none of which has stood the test of time.

T.H. Kirschbaum, M.D.

References

1. Shaw GM, Velie EM, Schaffer: Risk of neural tube defect–affected pregnancies among obese women. *JAMA* 275:1093–1096, 1996.
2. 1993 YEAR BOOK OF OBSTETRICS AND GYNECOLOGY, pp 193–194.
3. 1994 YEAR BOOK OF OBSTETRICS AND GYNECOLOGY, pp 137–138, 202–203.

5 Antepartum Fetal Surveillance

The Modified Biophysical Profile: Antepartum Testing in the 1990s
Miller DA, Rabello YA, Paul RH (Univ of Southern California, Los Angeles)
Am J Obstet Gynecol 174:812–817, 1996   5–1

Introduction.—Antepartum testing—the most common forms of which are the contraction stress test, the nonstress test (NST), the fetal biophysical profile, and the modified biophysical profile—is done in an attempt to detect fetal compromise or confirm fetal well-being. The false positive rate can be high, however—up to 90% with some test protocols. The false negative and false positive rates associated with the modified biophysical profile were studied in a large series of high-risk pregnancies.

Methods.—The study included 54,617 modified biophysical profiles done in 15,482 women with high-risk pregnancies from 1990 through 1994. Routine twice-weekly testing started at 34 weeks' gestation. Testing started earlier for some women and later for others, but never before 24 weeks' gestation. The results of the antepartum tests were collected prospectively and tabulated monthly. For the first year of the experience, detailed information on the intrapartum course and the newborn were gathered for all women who were admitted to the hospital and underwent delivery because of an abnormal intrapartum test result.

Results.—Antepartum testing was associated with almost a 7-fold reduction in the rate of fetal death in high-risk pregnancies. The test protocol had a false negative rate of 0.8 per 1,000 women studied. The false positive rate (i.e., the proportion of women who delivered because of an abnormal antepartum test but who showed no evidence of fetal compromise) was 60%. In 1.5% of women undergoing antepartum testing before 37 weeks' gestation, a false positive test result led to preterm delivery.

Conclusions.—As an antepartum test for fetal compromise, the modified biophysical profile has a lower false negative rate than the NST. False negative rates are similar for the modified and complete biophysical profiles and for the contraction stress test. In 1.5% of women, a false positive modified biophysical profile may lead to iatrogenic prematurity. The test is relatively simple and does not require extensive ultrasound experience.

▶ This is an important summary of results of antepartum testing at the Los Angeles County Hospital, consisting of a large number of cases honestly presented from a center with a long history of antepartum monitoring with generally high standards of care. It is a particular strength that, in my opinion, the senior author is the most expert and accomplished interpreter of continuous fetal heart rate monitoring in the world and his expertise is shared among his colleagues. In general, NSTs were done with acoustic stimulation after 10 minutes and abnormals (9.2% of 54,617 tests) submitted for biophysical profile, 98.6% of which were normal. Amniotic fluid indexes are interpreted after Phelan and were normal in 96.7% of 15,431 cases. These data suggest both the large costs involved in this effort and the preponderance of normal findings that evolved. Use of antenatal testing also was quite eclectic, with women with controlled gestational diabetes and those not enrolled until 40 weeks gestational age included. Post datism, which accounted for two thirds of all women tested, accounted for 40% of testing entries and did not begin until the end of the 40th week of gestation. The goal of the program was to prevent fetal death by acting on evidence of fetal compromise before that point. The authors point to a fetal death rate of 1.6 per 1,000 for those 23% of women tested vs. 10.8 per 1,000 for those not tested. However, the untested group includes women who delivered before 25 weeks' gestation to infants with birth weights more than 600 grams, patients admitted with antepartum deaths, patients with lethal anomalies, and those with urgent needs for delivery for whom antipartum surveillance was irrelevant. As constituted, they are not an adequate control group to test the merits of the program. Adjusting the tested cases for anomalies halves the fetal death rate in the control group, but it is not possible to do the same for the 77% of women not monitored antepartum. The reported false positive rate of 60% seems honest and is higher than where reduced amniotic fluid index and late and variable decelerations are predominant antepartum abnormalities. Concepts of true positive and false positive testing results presumes the ability regularly to discern fetal distress antepartum, which, even for this unit, seems a problem. We are left with a large, costly program thoughtfully executed without satisfactory controls to judge its effectiveness. The USC department deserves our thanks for reporting it.

T.H. Kirschbaum, M.D.

Fetal Fibronectin Improves the Accuracy of Diagnosis of Preterm Labor
Iams JD, Casal D, McGregor JA, et al (Ohio State Univ, Columbus; Univ of
Colorado, Denver; Univ of Southern California, Los Angeles; et al)
Am J Obstet Gynecol 173:141–145, 1995   5–2

Introduction.—Early preterm labor has been difficult to diagnose; false
diagnoses are common. The extracellular matrix protein oncofetal fibronectin is normally found in the fetal membranes and decidua, and its
presence in the cervix or vagina after the 20th week is abnormal. The use
of cervicovaginal expression of fetal fibronectin in the diagnosis of preterm
labor was evaluated.

Methods.—One hundred ninety-two women with preterm labor between 24 and 34 weeks' gestation (mean, 30.8 ± 2.9 weeks), cervical
dilatation of less than 3 cm, and intact membranes were evaluated. Using
a monoclonal antibody assay, the presence of fetal fibronectin was determined after cervicovaginal swabs were obtained. The results were compared with uterine contraction frequency and cervical dilatation as indicators of delivery before 37 weeks and interval to delivery.

Results.—The preterm birth rate was 32.3%. In the 45 women with a
positive fibronectin assay, the mean interval from presentation to delivery
was 25.3 days, whereas in the 147 women with a negative fibronectin
assay, the mean interval from presentation to delivery was 52.4 days.
Results of fetal fibronectin expression for delivery at less than 37 weeks
showed there was 44% sensitivity, 86% specificity, 60% positive predictive value, and 76% negative predictive value. In predicting the risk of
delivery within 7 days, the fetal fibronectin assay was especially useful,
with a sensitivity of 93%, a specificity of 82%, a positive predictive value
of 29%, and a negative predictive value of 99%. The fetal fibronectin
assay was notably superior to cervical dilatation of more than 1 cm and
contraction frequency of greater than or equal to 8 per hour.

Conclusion.—In a population of women evaluated for early preterm
labor, cervicovaginal fetal fibronectin predicts delivery within 7 days more
accurately than do contraction frequency or cervical dilatation. The fetal
fibronectin assay may improve the clinician's ability to select patients for
tocolytic drug therapy.

▶ This is a large multicenter trial of the use of the FDC-6 monoclonal
antibody to fetal fibronectin in predicting preterm labor, and the results are
fairly presented. More than half of the patients in preterm labor were
excluded due largely to cervical dilatation and spontaneous premature rupture of membranes. The prevalence of preterm labor in enrollees was 32%.
Taking all 192 cases, the false positive rate of 40% is slightly better but the
false negative rate of 24% slightly worse than reported earlier using this
reagent.[1,2] When the authors use as their goal of predictability the ability to
discriminate delivery within 7 days of the time of the test, they exclude
about half of those delivering prematurely and work with only 14 patients, a
group apparently chosen because only 1 case represented a false negative.

The false positive rate in that group was 71%. Though the authors believe this approach improves the accuracy of diagnosis of preterm labor in comparison to C-reactive protein determination and uterine and cervical exam, the results, for reasons that are fairly clear[3] do not constitute an adequate screening exam for preterm labor.

T.H. Kirschbaum, M.D.

References

1. 1993 YEAR BOOK OF OBSTETRICS AND GYNECOLOGY, pp 36–39.
2. 1994 YEAR BOOK OF OBSTETRICS AND GYNECOLOGY, pp 154–156.
3. *Focus & Opinion: Obstetrics and Gynecology* 1(3):182, 1995.

The Preterm Prediction Study: Fetal Fibronectin Testing and Spontaneous Preterm Birth
Goldenberg RL, Mercer BM, Meis PJ, et al (Natl Inst of Child Health and Human Development, Bethesda, Md; Univ of Alabama, Birmingham)
Obstet Gynecol 87:643–648, 1996   5–3

Background.—Previous studies have suggested that, among women in preterm labor, the finding of cervical or vaginal fetal fibronectin (FFN) identifies a group at increased risk of preterm delivery. One study used fetal fibronectin testing to screen for risk of subsequent preterm labor and delivery in women with high-risk pregnancies. Although FFN was signifi-

TABLE 2.—Predictive Values for Spontaneous Delivery at 34 Weeks or Less for Each of the Fetal Fibronectin Tests

Gestational age at test (wk)	Percent positive	Sensitivity (95% CI)	Specificity	Positive predictive value
24				
Cervical	2.8	0.21 (0.14–0.29)	0.98	0.32
Vaginal	3.5	0.19 (0.13–0.27)	0.97	0.24
Either positive	4.0	0.23 (0.16–0.31)	0.97	0.25
26				
Cervical	3.4	0.20 (0.12–0.30)	0.97	0.22
Vaginal	3.5	0.19 (0.16–0.34)	0.97	0.20
Either positive	4.2	0.22 (0.14–0.32)	0.97	0.20
28				
Cervical	2.6	0.11 (0.05–0.20)	0.98	0.13
Vaginal	3.1	0.17 (0.10–0.28)	0.97	0.18
Either positive	3.9	0.20 (0.11–0.30)	0.97	0.17
30				
Cervical	3.3	0.26 (0.16–0.38)	0.97	0.22
Vaginal	3.4	0.17 (0.09–0.28)	0.97	0.13
Either positive	4.4	0.29 (0.18–0.41)	0.96	0.18

Abbreviation: CI, confidence interval.
(Courtesy of Goldenberg RL, Mercer BM, Meis PJ, et al: The preterm prediction study: Fetal fibronectin testing and spontaneous preterm birth. *Obstet Gynecol* 87:643–648, 1996. Reprinted with permission from the American College of Obstetricians and Gynecologists.)

TABLE 3.—Cervical Fibronectin at 24 Weeks and Subsequent Spontaneous Preterm Birth

	Delivery interval (wks)				
Outcome	24–27	24–29	24–31	24–34	24–36
SPB	19 (0.6%)	28 (1.0%)	50 (1.7%)	127 (4.3%)	303 (10.3%)
Sensitivity of FFN for SPB	0.63	0.54	0.38	0.21	0.10
(95% CI)	(0.38–0.84)	(0.28–0.66)	(0.25–0.53)	(0.14–0.29)	(0.07–0.14)
Relative risk of FFN for SPB	59.2	39.9	21.2	8.9	3.8
(95% CI)	(35.9–97.8)	(25.6–62.1)	(14.3–31.4)	(6.3–12.6)	(2.7–5.3)

Abbreviations: SPB, spontaneous preterm birth; *FFN*, cervical fetal fibronectin; *CI*, confidence interval.

(Courtesy of Goldenberg RL, Mercer BM, Meis PJ, et al: The preterm prediction study. Fetal fibronectin testing and spontaneous preterm birth. *Obstet Gynecol* 87:643–648, 1996. Reprinted with permission from the American College of Obstetricians and Gynecologists.)

cantly related to preterm labor, the test was not sensitive. The ability of FFN as a screening test to predict spontaneous preterm birth in a relatively low-risk population was studied.

Methods.—The study included 2,929 pregnant women at 10 study centers. Beginning at 22–24 weeks' gestation and continuing through 30 weeks, the women underwent biweekly screening for cervical and vaginal FFN. The data were analyzed to determine the link between a positive test at various gestational ages and the risk of spontaneous preterm birth at various intervals after each test.

Results.—At each testing interval, 3% to 4% of FFN tests were positive. There was approximately a 0.7 correlation between cervical and vaginal FFN at each visit, and a 0.17–0.25 correlation between cervical or vaginal FFN at successive visits. A positive FFN test at 22–24 weeks' gestation was 63% sensitive in predicting spontaneous birth at less than 28 weeks' gestation, with a relative risk of 59 for a positive vs. negative test (Table 2). Specificity was in the range of 96% to 98% as the definition of preterm birth was increased from before 28 to before 37 weeks (Table 3). However, positive predictive value increased from 13% to 36% as this definition changed. The definition of preterm birth used and the testing period considered had a significant effect on the relative risk for spontaneous preterm birth after a positive vs. a negative FFN test. However, the relative risk was always significant at more than 4.

Conclusions.—Some spontaneous births occurring before 28 weeks' gestation are predictable by a positive cervical or vaginal FFN test at 22–24 weeks' gestation. The association remains significant, although not quite as strong, as the FFN test is done at later gestational ages. The authors found the predictive strength of FFN testing to be insufficient to warrant screening of asymptomatic pregnant women.

▶ Although the predictability of vaginal-cervical fibronectin has been discussed previously in the YEAR BOOK,[1, 2] this study by the Maternal Fetal Medicine Network of the National Institute of Child Health and Human Development is noteworthy for the nearly 3,000 patients enrolled in a well-designed and evaluated prospective trial. Women with single pregnancies without placenta previa, fetal anomaly, or cerclage were enrolled with ultrasonic confirmation of gestational age prior to the 24th week. They were evaluated for the incidence of spontaneous premature delivery prior to 34 weeks, as a function of FFN test results at 2 week intervals. Two thirds of enrolled gravidas were black. In a group with 10.3% prematurity rate, the incidence of either positive cervical or vaginal test for FFN was 4%. The issue here was not whether there was a correlative relationship between FFN presence in the lower reproductive tract and preterm delivery (because there certainly was), but whether the relationship was strong enough to be useful in screening asymptomatic women. The authors conclude that screening was not warranted for want of effective treatment for those screened, but this begs the issue of the strength of the predictive relationships here. Sensitivity was low for each of the 4 aggregates studied (20% to 29%), and the incidence of false positive tests range between 75% to 82%. In Table 3, extended follow-up to 36 weeks is depicted with overall sensitivity of 10% and greater sensitivity in the 3 weeks after entry, a subset comprised of only 6% of cases of preterm delivery. Because false positive rates are not provided, the predictive value of a positive test cannot be calculated. In a companion paper, the role of simultaneous presence of bacterial vaginosis cannot be shown to increase predictability to acceptable levels with false positive values even when both tests were positive ranging from 95% to 100%.[3] No matter how regrettably, it seems the large number of false positive results robs FFN assays of most of their clinical usefulness.

T.H. Kirschbaum, M.D.

References

1. 1995 YEAR BOOK OF OBSTETRICS AND GYNECOLOGY, pp 66–67, 69–71.
2. 1996 YEAR BOOK OF OBSTETRICS AND GYNECOLOGY, pp 129–130.
3. Goldenberg RL, et al: The preterm prediction study. *Obstet Gynecol* 87:656, 1996.

The Effectiveness of Preterm-Birth Prevention Educational Programs for High-Risk Women: A Meta-Analysis
Hueston WJ, Knox MA, Eilers G, et al (Univ of Wisconsin, Madison; Eau Claire Family Practice Residency, Wis; River Valley Med Ctr, St Croix Falls, Wis; et al)
Obstet Gynecol 86:705–712, 1995   5–4

Purpose.—Education, with or without home uterine activity monitoring, is a major component of strategies to promote early recognition and management of preterm labor. Although these interventions are well accepted by patients, studies of their effectiveness have yielded inconsistent results. Preterm-labor educational programs are inexpensive and low risk, so even a small favorable effect is likely to be cost-beneficial. The effects of preterm-birth education programs on rates of preterm delivery, low birth weight (LBW), and neonatal mortality were evaluated by meta-analysis.

Methods.—A MEDLINE search and supplemental bibliography review identified 31 trials evaluating the effects of preterm-birth prevention programs. However, only 6 of these were randomized, controlled trials of preterm-birth education programs that met the predefined inclusion criteria. Two reviewers assessed the study methods and results independently. The outcomes of interest for meta-analysis were frequency of LBW and preterm birth, neonatal survival, birth weight, gestational age at delivery, and preterm-labor diagnosis rates.

Findings.—All the studies included high-risk pregnancies only. The number of patients ranged from 132 to 2,395, and the study duration ranged from 16 to 54 months. Four studies reported LBW and preterm delivery rates and 3 reported neonatal survival rates. The combined data showed no significant benefits of preterm-birth education in the prevention of neonatal death or the reduction of LBW or preterm delivery rates (Figs 1 and 2). For each of these outcomes, the relative risk was around 1. The interventions did increase the frequency of diagnosis of preterm labor, with a relative risk of 1.71. This was the only significant effect.

Conclusions.—Preterm-birth prevention educational programs can increase the rate of diagnosis of preterm labor for high-risk women. How-

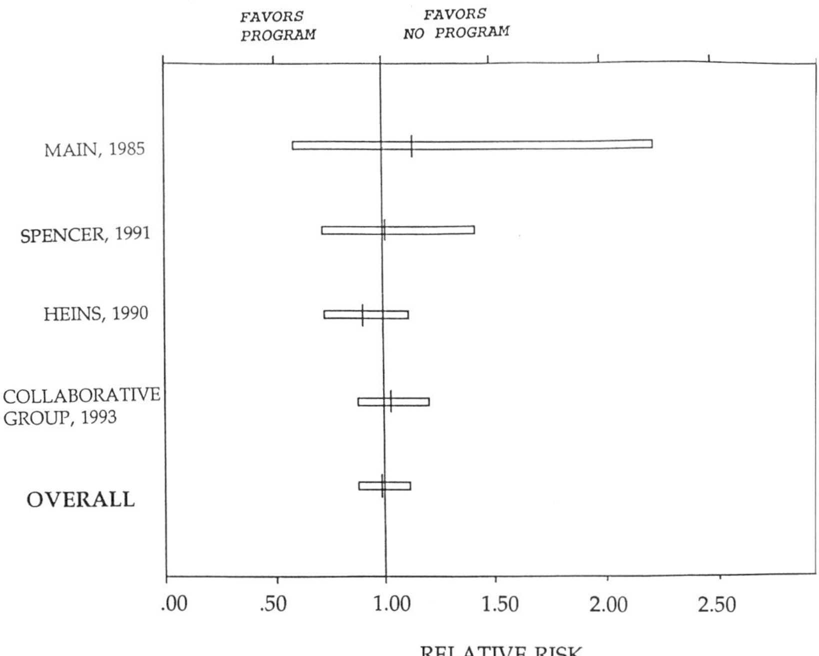

FIGURE 1.—Studies examining preterm delivery rates. Overall relative risk, 1.08; 95% confidence interval, 0.92–1.27 (*P* = 0.34). (Courtesy of Hueston WJ, Knox MA, Eilers G, et al.: The Effectiveness of Preterm-Birth Prevention Educational Programs for High-Risk Women: A Meta-Analysis. *Obstetrics and Gynecology* 86:705–712, 1995. Reprinted with permission from The American College of Obstetricians and Gynecologists.)

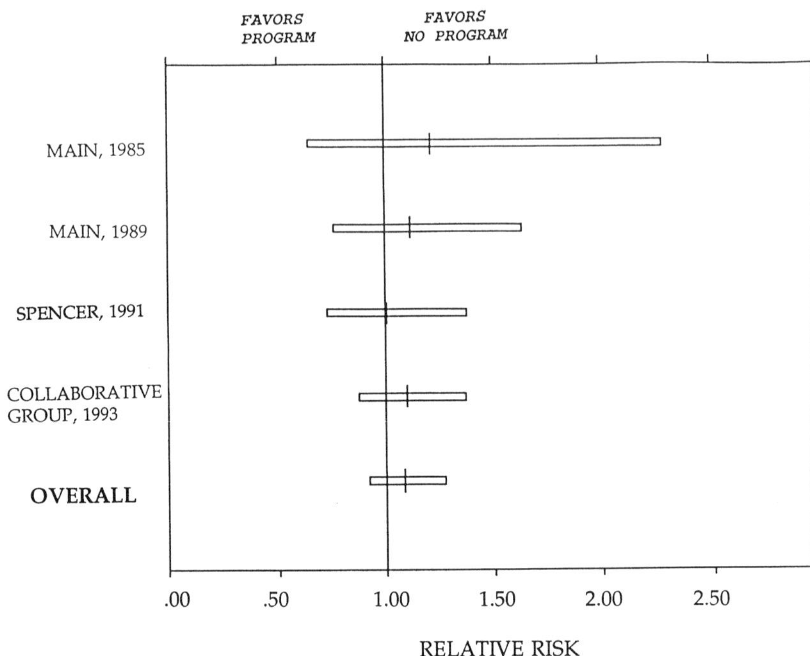

FIGURE 2.—Studies examining low birth weight rates. Overall relative risk, 0.99%; 95% confidence interval, 0.88–1.11 ($P = 0.84$). (Courtesy of Hueston WJ, Knox MA, Eilers G, et al.: The Effectiveness of Preterm-Birth Prevention Educational Programs for High-Risk Women: A Meta-Analysis. *Obstetrics and Gynecology* 86:705-712, 1995. Reprinted with permission from The American College of Obstetricians and Gynecologists.)

ever, they do not appear to reduce the rate of preterm birth. The conflicting results of previous studies are likely explained by methodological and/or population biases.

▶ This meta-analysis of the effectiveness of programs of antenatal education and preterm labor recognition with an eye to improving access to early medical care benefits was performed by a careful evaluation of prior publications and with sound statistical methodology. After dealing with the issue of duplicate publications, which has led to 15 publications from 6 data collections, and excluding uncontrolled studies or those without prenatal outcome measures, they used tests for heterogeneity to prove bias in studies with historical or nonrandom concurrent controls. This latter class of clinical study has always composed the bulk of purported support for this educational approach. Variable outcome measures further restricted the number of suitable studies to 4, 2 of which have been reviewed here earlier.[1,2]

In a group of 2,569 patients with 2,531 controls, no effect on preterm delivery could be shown. Neither was there an effect on the incidence of LBW or gestational age at the time of delivery. Similarly no differences in neonatal survival were seen as a result of a program of preterm labor recognition. The approach, however, results in a nearly twofold increase in the diagnosis of suspected premature labor, unconfirmed subsequently by virtue of the lack of increase in the number of actual preterm deliveries. It seems clear that educational programs after the fashion of Papiernik should, like home uterine activity monitoring, be regarded as failures in the effort to reduce preterm birth.[3–5]

T.H. Kirschbaum, M.D.

References

1. 1991 YEAR BOOK OF OBSTETRICS AND GYNECOLOGY, pp 131–133.
2. 1995 YEAR BOOK OF OBSTETRICS AND GYNECOLOGY, pp 62–64.
3. 1993 YEAR BOOK OF OBSTETRICS AND GYNECOLOGY, pp 152–153, 156–157.
4. 1994 YEAR BOOK OF OBSTETRICS AND GYNECOLOGY, pp 165–166.
5. *Focus & Opinion: Obstetrics and Gynecology* 1(3):163–169, 1995.

A Randomised Controlled Trial of Simple Compared With Complex Antenatal Fetal Monitoring After 42 Weeks of Gestation
Alfirevic Z, Walkinshaw SA (Univ of Liverpool, England; Liverpool Women's Hosp, England)
Br J Obstet Gynaecol 102:638–643, 1995   5–5

Objective.—Although previous studies have suggested that labor should be induced after 41 weeks of gestation to decrease perinatal mortality and rate of cesarean section, there is no general agreement on this approach. There is also no agreement on the proper method of monitoring prolonged pregnancies. Simple monitoring was compared with complex monitoring for pregnancies exceeding 42 weeks in a randomized, controlled study.

Methods.—At 42 weeks of gestation, 145 women were monitored twice weekly until 43 weeks either by cardiotocography and ultrasound to measure maximum vertical pool of amniotic fluid or computerized cardiotocography, amniotic fluid index, fetal breathing movements, fetal tone, and fetal gross body movements.

Results.—Complex monitoring led to significantly more abnormal antenatal results, including abnormal amniotic fluid indices, than did simple monitoring. No significant differences were found between treatment groups with regard to either labor or delivery, although more interventions took place in the complex monitoring group. The amniotic fluid index was 3 times as likely to be termed abnormal with the complex-monitoring method than with the simple-monitoring method.

Conclusion.—The fetal monitoring system used made no difference in pregnancy outcome in prolonged pregnancies, although the complex system gave more abnormal results. Whereas the measurement of amniotic fluid indices can lead to more abnormal reports and obstetric interventions, it is not clear whether either has an effect on neonatal outcome.

▶ This is a third attempt at demonstrating a basis for effective management for postdate pregnancy. Like the other 2 attempts, it fails to define a program of antepartum evaluation that improves outcome.[1, 2] Though the number of cases studied here is fewer than in either the Canadian or National Institute of Child Health and Development network studies referenced, all 145 cases in this study had completed 42 weeks of gestation before enrollment. In contrast, 80% to 90% of women enrolled in prior studies had completed only 41 weeks of gestation and were therefore not quite postdate pregnancies but were included in a policy designed to increase the number of subjects available for analysis. Heart rate analysis was conducted after the manner popularized by G.S. Dawes[3] and compared with the results using the biophysical profile, replacing the NST with the Oxford fetal heart rate analysis method. No benefit was conferred by employing the biophysical profile, but that approach increased the number of abnormal findings, largely reduced evidence of amniotic fluid volume, which in turn resulted in more labor inductions. It's clear we still lack an objective basis for managing postdate pregnancy.

T.H. Kirschbaum, M.D.

References

1. 1993 YEAR BOOK OF OBSTETRICS AND GYNECOLOGY, pp 34–35.
2. 1995 YEAR BOOK OF OBSTETRICS AND GYNECOLOGY, pp 74–76.
3. 1993 YEAR BOOK OF OBSTETRICS AND GYNECOLOGY, pp 144–145, 149–152.

A Multicenter Randomized Controlled Trial of Home Uterine Monitoring: Active Versus Sham Device
Devoe LD, for the Collaborative Home Uterine Monitoring Study (CHUMS) Group (Med College of Georgia, Augusta)
Am J Obstet Gynecol 173:1120–1127, 1995   5–6

Background.—Although initial studies of home uterine activity monitoring suggest that a monitoring device enables earlier detection of preterm labor and lower rates of preterm birth in high-risk patients, critical reviews and meta-analyses have raised important concerns about its use. The contribution of the home uterine activity monitoring device to high-risk care was determined in a new study, which was designed to avoid some of the design flaws of previous research.

Methods.—A total of 1,355 pregnant women were enrolled in the randomized, controlled, double-blind trial. All women were between 24 and 36 weeks' gestation and at high risk for preterm labor or birth. Of the 1,292 women randomized, 1,165 used home uterine activity monitoring devices, and 842 completed the study. All patients had twice-daily nursing contacts and monitoring with the findings revealed or concealed.

Findings.—The active and sham device groups were similar in demographic variables, enrollment and delivery gestational ages, discontinuation rates, risk factors, birth weights, and cervical dilation at enrollment and preterm labor diagnosis (Table 5). The groups were also comparable in cervical dilation changes at the diagnosis of preterm labor, rates of

TABLE 5.—Birth Outcomes for Total Enrollment Group

	Active	Sham
Total deliveries*	551	574
Deliveries		
<37 wk	281 (51.0)	311 (54.2)
≤36 wk	182 (33.0)	225 (39.2)
≤34 wk	74 (13.4)	101 (17.6)
Birth weight (mean)†		
Overall (gm)	2848 ± 747	2732 ± 714
Singletons only (gm)	3040 ± 715	2941 ± 676
Birth weight†		
<2500 gm	204 (31.0)	253 (34.7)
<1500 gm	30 (4.6)	37 (5.3)
Admissions to neonatal intensive care unit†	188 (28.5)	224 (32.0)
Length of hospitalization (days)	13.2 ± 20	17.0 ± 21.1
Neonatal complications†	132 (20.0)	142 (20.3)

Note: Numbers in parentheses are percentages based on the intent-to-treat group.

*These data do not include 23 patients in the active group and 17 patients in the sham group for whom birth and neonatal data were not completely recorded.

†These data reflect 659 individual infants in the active group and 701 individual infants in the sham group.

(Courtesy of Devoe LD, for The Collaborative Home Uterine Monitoring Study [CHUMS] Group: A multicenter randomized controlled trial of home uterine monitoring: Active versus sham device. *Am J Obstet Gynecol* 173:1120–1127, 1995.)

preterm labor and birth, and neonatal intensive care requirements. For all risk factors, the power to detect a difference in cervical dilation of 1 cm or greater at preterm labor diagnosis was 0.99.

Conclusions.—Home uterine activity monitoring data are unassociated with lower rates of preterm birth, greater birth weights or gestational ages at delivery, or fewer complications in infants. This is the largest randomized, controlled U.S. trial of home uterine activity monitoring to date.

▶ Though there have been few conclusive data to support the use of home uterine monitoring in the prevention of preterm labor,[1, 2] it's good to have this large, well-designed, prospective, randomized trial of 1,355 women to prove what should lead to the abandonment of this approach. Patients were entered in the study based on a prior history of preterm labor or preterm delivery, preterm labor in the present pregnancy, or ongoing multiple pregnancy. All women were given the monitoring devices, together with education and instruction in their use, and each transmitted 1 hour of recorded tocodynamometer readings twice daily; half of them went to sham data reception sites. Though there were not enough women with a multiple pregnancy enrolled to meet the requirements of the power calculation for significance, no benefit was seen in those women with active participation in the program compared with sham participants. This is a good source to remember when your patients ask you why you are not using this device.

T.H. Kirschbaum, M.D.

References

1. 1993 Year Book of Obstetrics and Gynecology, pp 152–153, 156–157.
2. 1994 Year Book of Obstetrics and Gynecology, pp 165–166.

Assessment of the Fetal Po₂ Changes by Cerebral and Umbilical Doppler on Lamb Fetuses During Acute Hypoxia

Arbeille P, Maulik D, Fignon A, et al (INSERM, Tours, France; Winthrop Univ, Mineola, NY; CHU Bretonneau, Tours, France; et al)
Ultrasound Med Biol 21:861–870, 1995   5–7

Objective.—In studies performed to date, umbilical and cerebral Doppler indices have been of little value in detecting fetal compromise. In fetuses with evolving hypoxia, redistribution of blood flow occurs to enhance perfusion of the brain and other vital organs, and this response can be detected by comparing the cerebral (CRI) and umbilical (URI) Doppler resistance indices. The cerebroplacental ratio (CPR = CRI/URI) was evaluated as an indicator of fetal hypoxia in an ovine model.

Methods.—Umbilical or maternal aortic flow was reduced by about 70% to produce acute hypoxia in fetal sheep. A Doppler probe was placed on the fetal cervical and abdominal skin over the internal carotid and umbilical arteries, respectively. The maximal and mean Doppler frequencies were measured using a Doptek 3000 spectrum analyzer. Hemodynamic parameters were calculated in real time. Blood gas and blood pressure measurements were made using a catheter inserted into the fetal femoral artery.

Results.—One minute of aortic compression produced a 10% increase in URI, a 10% decrease in umbilical blood flow (UBF), and a 20% decrease in CRI, with no significant change in carotid blood flow (CBF) (Fig 3C). No significant changes occurred in blood pressure, Pco₂, or pH.

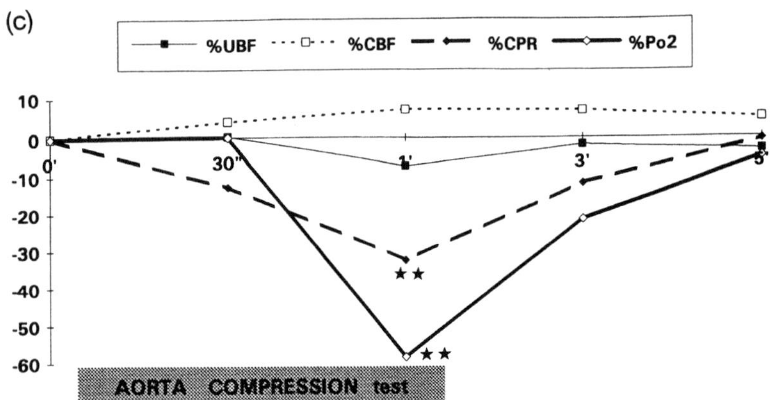

FIGURE 3C.—Aorta compression (*n* = 8). Variations in percentage from the pretest value, of the umbilical mean frequency or umbilical blood flow (*UBF;* NS), carotid mean frequency or carotid blood flow (*CBF;* NS), cerebroplacental ratio (*CPR; P* < 0.001 at 1 minute) and fetal partial pressure of oxygen (*Po₂*) (*P* < 0.001 at 1 minute), during a period of maternal aorta compression. The CPR decreases in proportion with the fetal Po₂ as in the cord compression, but the variations of this parameter are of lower amplitude. In this case, the umbilical flow does not change (**P* < 0.02; ***P* < 0.001). (Reprinted by permission of Elsevier Science, Inc. From Assessment of the Fetal Po₂ Changes by Cerebral and Umbilical Doppler on Lamb Fetuses During Acute Hypoxia, by Arbeille P, Maulik D, Fignon A, et al: *Ultrasound in Medicine and Biology,* 21:861–870. Copyright 1995 by World Federation of Ultrasound in Medicine and Biology.)

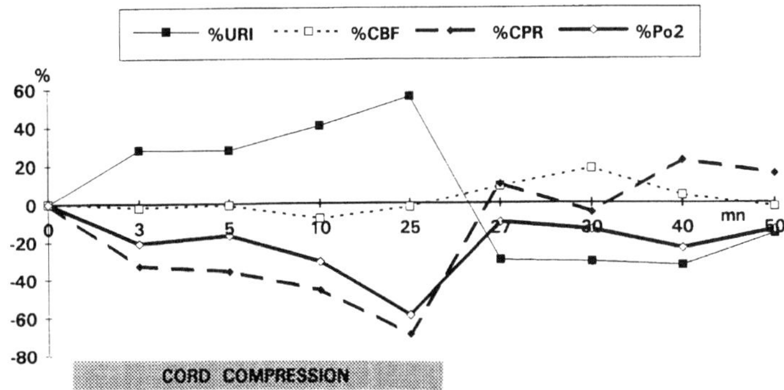

FIGURE 4D.—Cord compression ($n = 8$). Example of fetal hemodynamic response to partial pressure of oxygen (PO_2) changes induced by a progressive and extended cord compression test (25 minutes). Variations of the umbilical vascular resistances (*URI*), carotid mean frequency or carotid blood flow (*CBF*), cerebroplacental ratio (*CPR*), and the fetal PO_2 ($P < 0.001$). Note that the CPR and PO_2 still change in a similar proportion even though the amplitude of hypoxia is higher and the test duration longer, and that the CBF remains stable throughout the test. (Reprinted by permission of Elsevier Science, Inc. From Assessment of the Fetal PO_2 Changes by Cerebral and Umbilical Doppler on Lamb Fetuses During Acute Hypoxia, by Arbeille P, Maulik D, Fignon A, et al: *Ultrasound in Medicine and Biology*, 21:861–870. Copyright 1995 by World Federation of Ultrasound in Medicine and Biology.)

Twelve minutes of cord compression resulted in a 70% to 80% increase in URI, a 60% decrease in UBF, and a 25% decrease in CRI. Again, CBF was not significantly changed, and no significant changes in heart rate, blood pressure, or pH were seen. Of all hemodynamic measures, CPR most closely reflected the acute changes in partial pressure of oxygen (PO_2). The absolute values of CPR and PO_2 correlated well (Fig 4D).

Conclusions.—In fetal sheep, changes in CPR—which reflect the redistribution of blood flow between the placenta and brain—are a significant indicator of the fetal PO_2 changes occurring during hypoxia. The CPR appears to be a promising indicator of the early development of hypoxia, at least acute hypoxia. The results suggest that a 10% to 20% decrease in CPR may correspond to a decrease of comparable amplitude in PO_2. The authors propose that neither CRI nor URI reflect changes associated with fetal hypoxemia associated with decreased maternal aortic or fetal cerebral artery blood flow. They found a correlation between fetal descending aorta PO_2 and CRI/URI.

▶ Many clinicians and investigators continue to equate changes in fetal vessel Doppler velocity indices with rates of blood flow and/or vascular resistance or impedance despite the impressive list of animal experimental experiences summarized here earlier that showed no such relationships exist. Here, in 16 chronic fetal sheep experiments, Doppler transducers were fixed into the skin overlying the umbilical and internal carotid arteries, and inflatable occluders were used to reduce the aortic and umbilical artery mean Doppler velocity to 20% to 30% of normals through maternal aortic and umbilical cord occlusion, respectively. The aortic occlusion experiments resulted in severe fetal hypoxemia, bradycardia, and arrhythmia within 1 minute of onset. The URI increased and CRI decreased but without significant change in fetal blood flow velocity despite increases in fetal blood pressure. Umbilical occlusion was tolerated for 12–25 minutes with a 30% to 50% reduction in fetal blood PO_2, and URI increased sharply while the Doppler velocity signal along the umbilical vessels fell correspondingly. The CRI fell almost as strikingly without change in carotid Doppler velocity readings and with fetal blood pressure essentially unchanged. The authors point to a derived cerebroplacental ratio significantly positively correlated with fetal PO_2 sampled from the fetal descending aorta, but the lack of any regular or significant relationships of umbilical or carotid resistance indices to changes in fetal blood flow rates is once again confirmed and serves as a continuing reservation to the clinical use of these determinations in managing human pregnancies.

T.H. Kirschbaum, M.D.

Elaboration of Stem Villous Vessels in Growth Restricted Pregnancies With Abnormal Umbilical Artery Doppler Waveforms

Macara L, Kingdom JCP, Kohnen G, et al (Univ of Glasgow, Scotland; Technical Univ, Aachen, Germany)
Br J Obstet Gynaecol 102:807–812, 1995

5–8

Background.—There is controversy regarding the relative importance of anatomical and vasomotor mechanisms as a cause of absent end-diastolic velocity in the umbilical artery, which is associated with intrauterine growth restriction (IUGR). The current theories hold that absent end-diastolic velocity is caused either by a selective obliterative process of small stem vessels or by a primary reduction in the vascular development of the villous tree. To establish the validity of 1 of these theories, the vessels within the stem villi were studied immunohistochemically in IUGR and normal pregnancies.

Methods.—Singleton pregnancies of live-born neonates in 3 categories were studied: 8 pregnancies with IUGR, 4 women with preeclampsia and 4 normotensive women, and 8 preterm deliveries matched with the neonates with IUGR for gestational age. Doppler studies were performed in all cases. After delivery, 4 sections of placenta were examined after staining with an anti-α-smooth muscle actin (α-SMA) monoclonal primary antibody to identify stem vessels with lumen diameter ranging from 10 to 160 μm (Fig 1).

Results.—There were no significant differences in the proportion of stem villous vessels or in mean vessel diameter between the IUGR and control placentas. The IUGR placentas did have a significantly reduced volume of peripheral villi, compared with the control group. The stroma of intermediate and terminal villi contained α-SMA-positive cells in 5 IUGR placentas but none of the control placentas.

Conclusions.—Because there was no proportionate shift from low to higher vessel diameters in IUGR placentas, there is no evidence of a selective loss of small arterioles. The reduction in the placental section

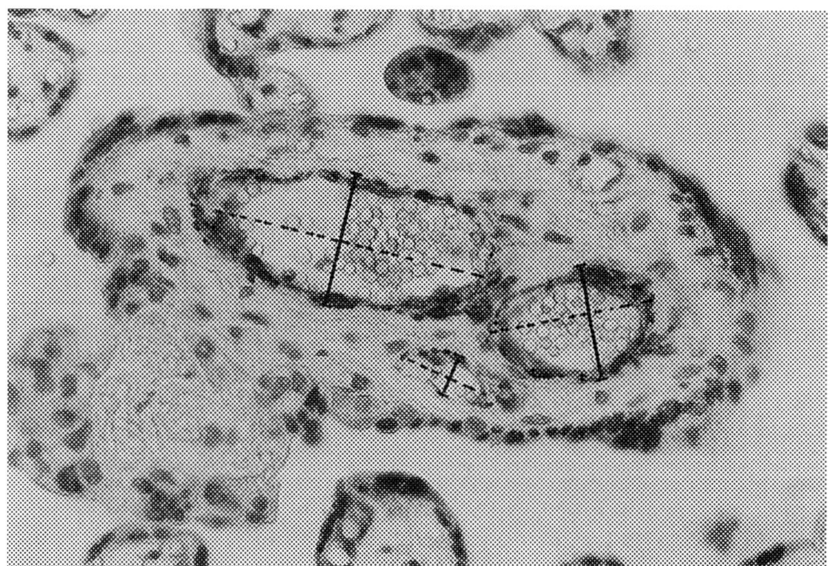

FIGURE 1.—Cross-sectional view of a stem villus containing 3 vessels identified by concentric rings of immunostaining to α-smooth muscle actin. *Hatched line* indicates long axis of vessel profile. *Continuous line* indicates measurement of vessel diameter. Note that the measurement of vessel diameter includes the media. (Courtesy of Macara L, Kingdom JCP, Kohnen G, et al.: Elaboration of Stem Villous Vessels in Growth Restricted Pregnancies With Abnormal Umbilical Artery Doppler Waveforms. *Br J Obstet Gynaecol* 102:807–812, 1995, Blackwell Science Ltd.)

occupied by peripheral villi in IUGR placentas supports the hypovascular theory. In addition, the presence of α-SMA–positive cells within the peripheral villi of some IUGR placentas suggests an ongoing process of vascular remodeling, which may indicate prenatal hypertension.

▶ Among several recent attempts to define a morphologic basis for abnormal umbilical artery Doppler signals and interuterine growth retardation, this one stands out for the quality of its methodology. Also, the pioneering figure in categorizing the development of vascular architecture of the human placenta, Professor Peter Kaufmann from Aachen, is senior author.[1] In brief, stem villi, composing 20% to 25% of the placental tissue, are conduit vessels with muscularized arterioles, and venules that give rise in their first 4 series of divisions to a series of chorionic rami. The next 10 sets of divisions or branchings lead, in mid-pregnancy, to the production of immature intermediate villi. These villi also contain arterioles, venules, and capillaries and are progressively replaced in the third trimester of pregnancy by mature intermediate and terminal villi. These latter structures lack muscularized vessels and contain the terminal capillary structures through which dominant placental exchange with maternal vasculature takes place. Here, staining specific to smooth muscle actin is used to identify vessels whose media contain smooth muscle in stem and immature intermediate villi. Their importance is that only they determine placental vascular resistance and impedance. The comparisons are made of vessel size and diameter between preterm placentas from those with normal Doppler signals and those with absent end-diastolic velocity signals with and without hypertension. Attention is paid to early cord clamping, random selection of villi within grid overlays, prompt fixation, and multiple blocking by an observer blind to clinical details. The placentas from growth-retarded infants were lighter in weight and had significantly less villus tissue than average for gestational age fetal placentas, but no differences in the prevalence of stem and/or mature intermediate villus vessels could be seen. That is, absent end-stage diastolic flow velocity does not appear to stem from changes in those villus vessels that determine umbilical vascular impedance or vascular resistance.

T.H. Kirschbaum, M.D.

Reference

1. Benirschke K, Kaufmann P: *Pathology of the Human Placenta*. New York, Springer-Verlag, 1995.

Umbilical Vein Pulsations and Acid-Base Status at Cordocentesis in Growth-Retarded Fetuses With Absent End-Diastolic Velocity in Umbilical Artery

Rizzo G, Capponi A, Soregaroli M, et al (Univ of Rome; Univ of Ancona, Italy)
Biol Neonate 68:163–168, 1995   5–9

Background.—When pulsations in the umbilical vein are present, growth-retarded fetuses with absent end-diastolic velocity (AEDV) in the umbilical artery appear to have poorer perinatal outcomes. However, no direct data have been collected on the association of umbilical vein pulsations and intrauterine acid-base status. Whether the presence of umbilical vein pulsations is related to a more severe impairment of acid-base status measured at cordocentesis in fetuses with intrauterine growth restriction with AEDV in umbilical artery was studied.

Methods.—Twenty-six fetuses with IUGR free from structural and chromosomal abnormalities were included. All had AEDV in the umbilical artery. In 11 fetuses, or 42.3%, AEDV was associated with pulsations in the umbilical vein. Just after the Doppler recordings were obtained, gas analysis of fetal blood was done.

Findings.—Compared with fetuses without umbilical cord pulsations, those with pulsations had lower pH and partial pressure of oxygen values and higher partial pressure of carbon dioxide (PCO_2) values. All fetuses with pulsations were hypoxemic and hypercapnic. The incidence of acidemia among these fetuses was 90.9%. Although often hypoxemic, 40% of the fetuses with continuous blood flow in the umbilical vein had PCO_2 values in the normal range, and 52.3% had pH values in the normal range (Fig 1).

Conclusions.—Umbilical venous flow analysis enables noninvasive identification of the fetuses with IUGR and AEDV in the umbilical artery with

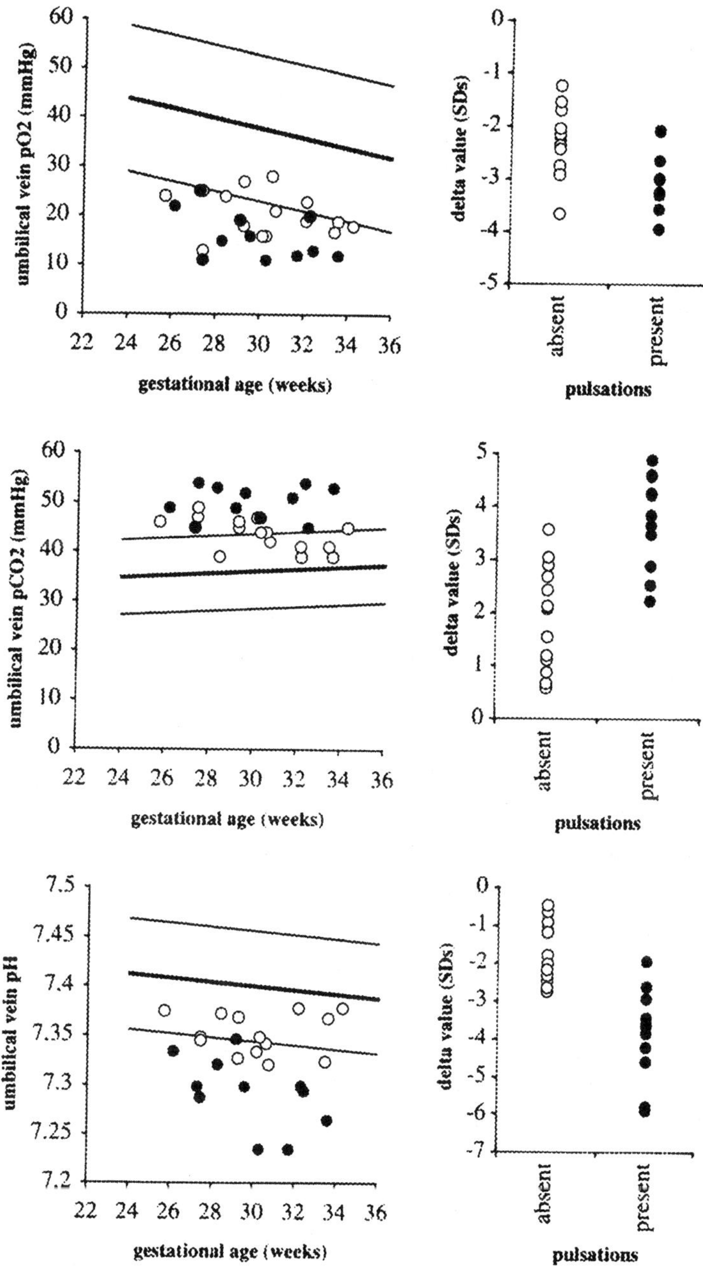

FIGURE 1.—Individual partial pressure of oxygen (Po_2), partial pressure of carbon dioxide (Pco_2), and pH values obtained by cordocentesis in growth-retarded fetuses with (*filled circles*) or without (*open circles*) umbilical vein pulsations plotted on the normal reference limits (mean ± 2 SD) for gestation (**left**) and corresponding delta values (**right**). (Courtesy of Rizzo G, Capponi A, Soregaroli M, et al: Umbilical Vein Pulsations and Acid-Base Status at Cordocentesis in Growth-Retarded Fetuses With Absent End-Diastolic Velocity in Umbilical Artery. *Biol Neonate* 68:163–168, 1995. S. Karger AG, Basel.)

more severely compromised placental oxygenative exchanges. Whether identifying these Doppler changes can be used successfully to optimize the timing of delivery of these fetuses has yet to be established.

▶ Though this paper lacks the information necessary to decide about obstetric management based on fetal Doppler signals, it at least points to the differences between correlation and predictability and between hypoxemia and hypoxia. Cordocentesis data obtained from growth-retarded fetuses yield evidence of hypoxemia that is sufficient to meet tests of statistical significance from normal historical controls. The individual samples do not reveal acidosis, apparently since umbilical vein oxygen content, even at decreased partial pressure of oxygen, still provides sufficient oxygen availability to meet fetal oxygen requirements. That is, the fetuses, though hypoxemic, are not hypoxic. When umbilical vein pulsations are seen, it is assumed that impaired right ventricular output generates a reverse right arterial systolic pressure pulse sufficient to exceed resistance to flow in the ductus venosus producing a retrograde pulse in the umbilical vein. Reed et al. had a similar observation.[1] Fetuses exhibiting this change yield umbilical vein blood with a higher likelihood of acidosis and hypercarbia than those without. However, to act on this finding lacking a prospectively structured control trial requires unproven assumptions about the variability of cardiac output, blood compensation, and fetal cardiac, placental, and maternal uterine artery function. At least in these cases, delivery of those fetuses with AEDV in the umbilical artery but without umbilical vein pulsations would seem hard to justify on the basis of the findings. The authors are correct that the impact of these changes on case management and outcome remains to be determined.

T.H. Kirschbaum, M.D.

Reference

1. 1991 YEAR BOOK OF OBSTETRICS AND GYNECOLOGY, pp 101–102.

The Value of Fetal Arterial, Cardiac and Venous Flows in Predicting pH and Blood Gases Measured in Umbilical Blood at Cordocentesis in Growth Retarded Fetuses
Rizzo G, Capponi A, Arduini D, et al (Universita' di Roma Tor Vergata, Italy; Universita' di Ancona, Italy)
Br J Obstet Gynaecol 102:963–969, 1995   5–10

Background.—There is a paucity of data concerning the possible relationship between acid–base balance in the intrauterine growth-retarded fetus and certain circulatory Doppler-obtained indices, specifically, fetal arterial, cardiac, and venous blood flows.

Objective.—The study objective was to assess the value of Doppler indices obtained from peripheral arterial and venous vessels and cardiac outflow tracts, in the demonstration of acidemia, hypercapnia, and hypoxemia as determined by pH and gas analyses of fetal blood obtained by cordocentesis in growth-retarded fetuses.

Methods.—Forty-eight growth-retarded fetuses were studied. Inclusion criteria were an absence of chromosomal and structural anomalies; an estimated fetal weight of less than the 5th centile; the presence of abnormal waveforms in the umbilical artery; and postnatal confirmation of a birth weight below the 5th centile and the absence of structural anomalies. Doppler recordings were taken from the umbilical artery, descending thoracic aorta, renal artery, middle cerebral artery, cardiac outflow tracts, inferior vena cava, and ductus venosus immediately before cordocentesis. Appropriate analyses were performed to examine the relationship between Doppler indices, blood gas values, and acid–base status.

Results.—An analysis of the various Doppler indices with the measured acid-base parameters indicated that the most significant relationship existed between the percentage of reverse flow in the inferior vena cava and acidemia and hypercapnia. This relationship may be secondary to impaired cardiac function leading to abnormal cardiac and venous flows. Hypoxemia was best predicted by the pulsatility index of the middle cerebral artery. This relationship is consistent with the hypothesis that hypoxemia induces a redistribution of blood flow to vital organs such as the brain and may be monitored by studying the waveforms of the middle cerebral artery.

Conclusions.—The analysis of velocity waveforms from the inferior vena cava and the middle cerebral artery has source relationship to acid–base status in growth-retarded fetuses. This may lead to an accurate antepartum monitoring of such fetuses.

▶ This group of investigators has been very productive in their study of the meaning of fetal Doppler measurements; their interpretation of their data is regularly thoughtful and fair. Here the goal is to compare a series of fetal Doppler measurements with blood gas determinations on umbilical vein blood obtained by cordocentesis in 48 growth-retarded fetuses at or below the 5th percentile at subsequent birth. Longitudinal patterns are inferred from cross-section data but, in terms of available investigational tools, that is an unavoidable problem.

As before,[1,2] unbilical artery pulsatility indices are high, and the middle cerebral artery is low in the pulsatility index in growth retardation compared with those of normal fetuses at the same gestational age. What is most interesting is that umbilical artery pulsitivity index values have no significant relationship to umbilical vein blood gas determinations. Of all the Doppler signals obtained, reverse flow velocity in the inferior vena cava during arterial systole is, as K.L. Reed indicated 5 years ago, the most reliable.[3] The authors are correct in pointing out that nothing in the Doppler measurements assures that clinical management based on the inference of fetal acidosis, true or not, will be useful in clinical management. To reach that level of assurity, an independent randomized trial of this approach is needed.

T.H. Kirschbaum, M.D.

References

1. 1993 YEAR BOOK OF OBSTETRICS AND GYNECOLOGY, pp 155–156.
2. *Focus & Opinion: Obstetrics and Gynecology*, 1995.
3. 1991 YEAR BOOK OF OBSTETRICS AND GYNECOLOGY, pp 101–102.

Uncertain Value of Electronic Fetal Monitoring in Predicting Cerebral Palsy

Nelson KB, Dambrosia JM, Ting TY, et al (Natl Inst of Neurological Disorders and Stroke, Bethesda, Md; Howard Hughes Med Inst, Bethesda, Md; Univ of Pennsylvania, Philadelphia; et al)
N Engl J Med 334:613–618, 1996   5–11

Introduction.—Electronic fetal monitoring was introduced in an attempt to prevent birth injuries caused by hypoxia or asphyxia and thus reduce the frequency of cerebral palsy and mental retardation. The widespread use of fetal monitoring has probably contributed to the increasing rate of cesarean section; however, there has been no accompanying decrease in the incidence of cerebral palsy. There are few reliable data on whether specific fetal heart rate patterns detected by electronic monitoring are useful in predicting long-term neurologic outcomes. The value of fetal monitoring in predicting the diagnosis of cerebral palsy was evaluated in a population-based study.

Methods.—The research subjects were from a population of nearly 156,000 children born in 4 California counties during a 2-year period.

TABLE 4.—Crude and Adjusted Odds Ratios for Cerebral Palsy According to Literature-Identified Risk Factors and Specific Heart-Rate Patterns on Electronic Fetal Monitoring in Singleton Children with Birth Weight of 2,500 g or More*

FACTOR†	UNIVARIATE ANALYSIS			MULTIVARIATE LOGISTIC ANALYSIS		
	CHILDREN WITH CEREBRAL PALSY (N = 78)	CONTROLS (N = 300)	CRUDE ODDS RATIO (95% CI)	ESTIMATES	P VALUE	ADJUSTED ODDS RATIO (95% CI)
	no. (%)					
Bleeding during pregnancy	13 (16.7)	21 (7.0)	2.7 (1.3–5.6)	1.05	0.01	2.9 (1.3–6.4)
Breech presentation	8 (10.3)	10 (3.3)	3.3 (1.3–8.7)	1.06	0.05	2.9 (1.0–8.1)
Gestational age <37 wk	8 (10.3)	12 (4.0)	2.7 (1.1–7.0)	1.01	0.05	2.7 (1.0–7.6)
Meconium	26 (33.3)	52 (17.3)	1.9 (1.3–2.9)	0.45	0.05	1.6 (1.0–2.5)
Maternal infection	14 (18.0)	13 (4.3)	4.8 (2.2–10.8)	1.21	0.01	3.3 (1.4–8.1)
MLD/DV	21 (26.9)	28 (9.3)	3.6 (1.9–6.7)	1.01	0.01	2.7 (1.4–5.4)

*Odds ratios are calculated as the risk of cerebral palsy among children with the risk factor as compared with those without it. Estimates are the coefficients of the fitted logistic regression, and *P* values are for the comparison between case children controls.
†Each factor was analyzed as either absent or present, except meconium, which was coded as absent, light, or heavy.
Abbreviations: CI, confidence interval; *MLD/DV*, multiple late decelerations.
(Courtesy of Nelson KB, Dambrosia JM, Ting TY, et al: Uncertain value of electronic fetal monitoring in predicting cerebral palsy. *N Engl J Med* 334:613–618, Copyright 1996 Massachusetts Medical Society. Reprinted by permission of The New England Journal of Medicine.)

TABLE 5.—Measures of the Association between Multiple Late Decelerations, Decreased Variability in Heart Rate, or Both on Electronic Fetal Monitoring with Cerebral Palsy in Singleton Children with Birth Weights of 2,500 g or More, According to Risk Group*

RISK GROUP	% OF POPULATION	PREVALENCE OF CEREBRAL PALSY (PER 10,000)	SENSITIVITY (%)	SPECIFICITY (%)	POSITIVE PREDICTIVE VALUE (%)
Low	69	3.6	13.8	91.3	0.05
High	31	13.8	34.7	89.1	0.25
Total	100	6.8	26.9	90.7	0.14

*The risk groupings were based on the presence or absence of 5 factors identified in the literature as associated with an increased risk of cerebral palsy: bleeding during pregnancy, breech presentation, gestational age of less than 37 weeks at delivery, maternal infection, and the presence of meconium in the amniotic fluid. Low risk was defined as the absence of the 5 risk factors and high risk as the presence of 1 or more of them. Sensitivity and specificity were calculated within the case-control study, whereas the percentage of the population in each risk group, prevalence of cerebral palsy, and positive predictive value were obtained by projection onto the entire population of children born during the 3-year study period in 4 counties.

(Courtesy of Nelson KB, Dambrosia JM, Ting TY, et al: Uncertain Value of Electronic Fetal Monitoring in Predicting Cerebral Palsy. *N Engl J Med* 334:613–618, Copyright 1996, Massachusetts Medical Society. Reprinted by permission of The New England Journal of Medicine.)

Ninety-five children with moderate to severe cerebral palsy who lived to 3 years old and had birth weights of no less than 2,500 g were identified. They were compared with 378 randomly selected control subjects; 78 of the children with cerebral palsy and 300 of the control children had intrapartum fetal monitoring. The results of fetal monitoring were analyzed in terms of the interpretations made at the time by the attending physicians. Known risk factors for cerebral palsy (including vaginal bleeding during pregnancy, breech presentation, meconium in the amniotic fluid, gestational age less than 37 weeks, and maternal infection) were evaluated for univariate association with cerebral palsy and with electronic fetal monitoring abnormalities.

Results.—Certain fetal monitoring characteristics were associated with an increased risk of cerebral palsy. These were multiple late decelerations in the heart rate (i.e., heart rate slowing well after the start of uterine contractions), odds ratio (OR) 3.9; and decreased beat-to-beat variability, OR 2.7. Cerebral palsy was unrelated to the highest or lowest recorded fetal heart rate. After adjustment for other risk factors, fetal monitoring abnormalities were still associated with an increased risk of cerebral palsy, OR 2.7. The previously identified risk factors were significantly associated with cerebral palsy (Table 4).

However, the fetal monitoring abnormalities identified were not present in all children with cerebral palsy and were present in many children without cerebral palsy. Although 21 children with cerebral palsy had multiple late decelerations or decreased heart rate variability, they accounted for only 0.19% of all infants in the study population with these findings. The associated false negative rate was therefore 99.8% (Table 5).

Conclusions.—Although certain fetal heart rate abnormalities are associated with an increased risk of cerebral palsy, the majority of infants with these findings will not be cerebral palsy patients. If these abnormalities were used as indications for cesarean section, many such deliveries would be performed with no benefit but with significant risk to the mother. The emphasis on the rare outcome of cerebral palsy may be distracting attention from other important factors that could lead to injury or maldevelopment of the infant brain.

▶ This cohort study of infants with cerebral palsy noted by age 3 (born in 1 of 4 counties in the San Francisco Bay area in 1983–1985) has been discussed here earlier.[1] It's particularly valuable because the births occurred during a time when electronic fetal heart rate monitoring was in general use; 90.7% of those infants with cerebral palsy and 86.1% of 300 randomly selected control subjects were monitored. Data were obtained from California birth certificates and a review of hospital records by the staff of the California Birth Defects Monitoring Program. Seventy-eight infants with cerebral palsy were electronically monitored. As before in the collaborative Perinatal Project study 30 years earlier, there was no relationship of cerebral palsy to labor, the absence of electronic fetal monitoring, patient parity, or route of delivery. Fetal heart rate tracings were not externally reviewed in this study, but evaluations recorded at the time of labor were used to assess the monitoring. Maximum and minimum heart rates showed no relationship to the incidence of cerebral palsy, but multiple late decelerations and/or reduced beat to beat variability carried an increased risk for cerebral palsy (relative risk 3.6; confidence interval, 1.9–6.7) in univariate analysis. As in the collaborative study, pregnancy bleeding, breech presentation (not breech birth), prematurity, meconium-stained amniotic fluid, and maternal infection were additional, independently operating univariate risk factors. But these are retrospective appraisals of damage to children, and when the randomly selected incidence figures are extrapolated to the entire population of 155,636 births during those 4 years, it's possible to estimate the predictiveness of abnormal fetal heart rate tracings. The failure of electronic fetal monitoring during labor to predict cerebral palsy emerges in the form of large false positive rates. For all births, the false positive rate for prediction of cerebral palsy from beat-to-beat variability and/or recurrent late decelerations is 99.86%, and for the patients with risk factors, 99.75%. Often, false positive findings lead to cesarean section, which does not clearly reduce the risk of cerebral palsy in turn.[2] If cesarean section were effective in preventing cerebral palsy, the authors estimate 2,324 needless interventions for each cesarean section in a child destined for cerebral palsy. The authors conclude that a focus on electronic fetal heart rate monitoring reflecting birth asphyxsia "may have diverted clinical and research attention from an exploration of factors other than birth exphyxsia that can contribute to maldevelopment or injury of the infant's brain".

T.H. Kirschbaum, M.D.

References

1. 1995 YEAR BOOK OF OBSTETRICS AND GYNECOLOGY, pp 135–138.
2. 1995 YEAR BOOK OF OBSTETRICS AND GYNECOLOGY, pp 135–138.

Predictors of Neonatal Encephalopathy in Full Term Infants
Adamson SJ, Alessandri LM, Badawi N, et al (Inst for Child Health Research, West Perth, Australia; Princess Margaret Hosp for Children, Subiacco, Australia)
BMJ 311:598–602, 1995   5–12

Background.—Most neonatal encephalopathy has been assumed to be caused by intrapartum asphyxia, indicating a high level of obstetric intervention in labor. However, this assumption is now being questioned. There have been few studies of unselected populations examining the contribution of other causes to neonatal encephalopathy. The contribution of factors in family and maternal history, pregnancy, and birth to encephalopathic features in full-term neonates was investigated.

Methods.—Eighty-nine full-term singleton neonates born during 8 months in 1992 who met 1 or more criteria for encephalopathy in the first week of life were included. The criteria were seizures, abnormal conscious state, persistent hypertonia or hypotonia, and feeding or respiratory difficulties of central origin. Infants in a control group were matched by sex, hospital of delivery, time of day and day of the week of birth, and maternal health insurance status.

Findings.—Moderate or severe encephalopathy in the first week of life occurred in an estimated 3.75 per 1,000 full-term live-born neonates. Evidence suggesting important intrapartum hypoxia was noted in 13 infants with encephalopathy and in none without it. The neurologic condition at birth was attributed to events during the intrapartum period in only 5 of these encephalopathic infants. In a univariate conditional logistic regression analysis, the case and control groups differed significantly in maternal vaginal bleeding during pregnancy, maternal thyroxine therapy, congenital abnormalities, labor induction, interval between membrane rupture and delivery, maternal pyrexia in labor, labor augmentation, abnormal intrapartum cardiotocograms, and meconium in labor. Between-group differences in family history of convulsions approached significance.

Conclusions.—Intrapartum hypoxia did not appear to be the cause of neonatal encephalopathy in most affected infants. There may be many causes of this condition originating in the antepartum period.

▶ Most studies of birth trauma use cerebral palsy as an end point for cohort selection, since motor dysfunction in the early neonatal period is usually an unequivocal observation. Here, the dependent variable is more subtle—neonatal difficulties in regulation of consciousness, respiration, unusual response to external stimuli, inability to carry out sucking, and appearance of seizures without evident motor dysfunction observed in the interval from 24 to 48 hours after birth. Called neonatal encephalopathy, its incidence in this cohort of 89 singleton infants born at term without growth retardation was 0.4%, twice the incidence of cerebral palsy. The neonatal mortality for the group was 8%.

The authors' approach has been described here before.[1] Retrospective chart review divided incidents among 5 epochs in time—preconceptional, antepartum, intrapartum, newborn, and neonatal. Birth asphyxia was defined by an abnormal fetal heart rate tracing that a panel of reviewers agreed upon as indicative, or the passage of fresh meconium together with an impaired Apgar score. In fact, cord blood pH and signs of renal hypoxic ischemic injury were also considered. Since only half such infants had cord blood analysis, these diagnostic criteria are arguable in their impact. However, only 13 cases (15% of the total) qualified for the diagnosis of intrapartum hypoxia, and 8 of these (9%) had intrapartum obstetric factors that may have affected the newborn status (postdatism, maternal hypotension, vasa previa, etc.). The incidence of anomalies was 17%.

Just as they did with their study of cerebral palsy, this Western Australia group concluded that hypoxic birth injury was an uncommon cause of this form of newborn cerebral dysfunction. Their conclusion fortifies the now impressive number of investigators who have reached the same conclusion.[2-4]

T.H. Kirschbaum, M.D.

References

1. 1995 YEAR BOOK OF OBSTETRICS AND GYNECOLOGY, pp 131–134.
2. 1988 YEAR BOOK OF OBSTETRICS AND GYNECOLOGY, pp 116–118.
3. 1991 YEAR BOOK OF OBSTETRICS AND GYNECOLOGY, pp 176–177.
4. 1995 YEAR BOOK OF OBSTETRICS AND GYNECOLOGY, pp 135–136, 180–181.

Prenatal Screening for Down's Syndrome Using Inhibin-A as a Serum Marker

Wald NJ, Densem JW, George L, et al (St Bartholomew's Hosp, London; Univ of Reading, England)
Prenat Diagn 16:143–153, 1996
5–13

Purpose.—The 4-marker method of prenatal serum screening for Down's syndrome provides good results, with an estimated detection rate of 65% and a 5% false positive rate. Another potentially useful marker is inhibin-A (the $\alpha\beta_A$ dimeric form), which requires a much smaller volume of serum. Inhibin-A, alone and combined with other serum markers, was investigated as a screening marker for Down's syndrome.

Methods.—The study included stored serum samples obtained at 15–22 weeks' gestation from 77 singleton pregnancies (Fig 1) with Down's syndrome and 385 unaffected pregnancies. The 2 groups were matched for maternal age, gestational age, and length of serum storage. Supplementary data were obtained from 970 white women with unaffected pregnancies. Markers measured were the $\alpha\beta_A$ dimer of inhibin-A; human chorionic gonadotropin (hCG), total and the subunits free α- and β-hCG; α-fetoprotein (AFP); and unconjugated estriol (uE_3).

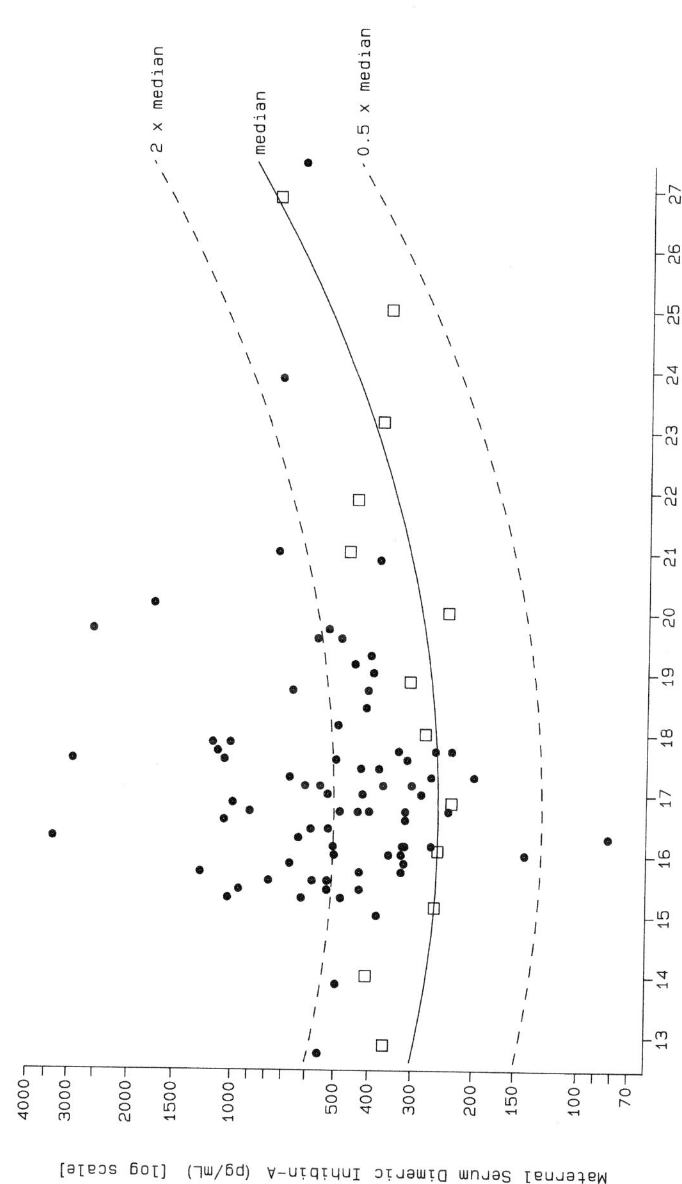

FIGURE 1.—Inhibin-A concentration in maternal serum at 13–27 weeks' gestation in 77 pregnancies with Down's syndrome and regressed median for unaffected singleton pregnancies in relation to gestationa. age. The *squares* are the observed medians for unaffected pregnancies at each completed week of gestation. The *solid circles* are the values for each of the affected pregnancies. The *dashed lines* show twice and half the regressed median value. (Courtesy of Wald NJ, Densem JW, George L, et al: Prenatal screening for Down's syndrome using inhibin-A as a serum marker. *Prenat Diagn* 16:143-153, Copyright 1996. Reprinted by permission of John Wiley & Sons, Ltd.)

Results.—The Down's syndrome pregnancies had increased serum inhibin-A concentrations, with a median of 1.79 multiples of the median. Using AFP, uE_3, total hCG, and inhibin-A (together with maternal age) correctly identified 70% of pregnancies affected with Down's syndrome, with a 5% false positive rate. This compared favorably to a 59% detection rate with the conventional triple test, (i.e., AFP, uE_3, and total hCG plus maternal age). Using an ultrasound-based estimation of maternal age would improve the detection rate of the 4-marker test to 77%, compared with 67% with the triple test, or 79% if the marker values were adjusted for maternal weight. Using the 4-marker test with a detection rate of 70% and an ultrasound estimate of gestational age was associated with a false positive rate of only 6%, compared with 3% with the triple test. The use of free β-hCG vs, total hCG made little difference in the results.

Conclusions.—The 4-marker screening test for Down's syndrome—including inhibin A, AFP, uE_3, and total hCG—seems the most effective test for routine clinical use. The use of inhibin-A rather than free α-hCG would reduce the number of fetal losses to amniocentesis per case detected. This test would be cost-effective if the extra cost incurred were less than approximately £3 per patient.

▶ This carefully done work reveals the advantage of assaying serum dimeric inhibin and the continuing effort of obtaining effective antenatal screening in Down's syndrome pregnancies, especially in women younger than 35 years of age who, despite the low rate of occurrence, account for approximately 80% of such infants at the time of delivery.[1-3] As discussed earlier, inhibin-A is a dimeric glycoprotein containing an α and a dimorphic β fragment, the latter differentiating it from inhibin-B. A product of grandulosan and Sertoli cells as well as the corpus luteum, it plays a role in the regulation of the ovarian cycle. Its placental production results in a concentration in maternal serum bimodal with time, with a peak at approximately 10 weeks' gestation, a slight decrease followed by a steady state of concentration from 15–20 weeks, and then a progressive increase to a maximum at term. Its function in pregnancy is unknown, but 2 sets of investigators have found it increased in Down's syndrome pregnancies.[4, 5] An enzyme immunoassay specific for both parts of the dimer was used and comparisons were made between inhibin-A assays on stored serum and data on measurements of maternal serum α-fetoprotein (MSAFP), urinary estriol, and various hCG components previously reported.[6] The process of establishing fiducial limits is now familiar. Median values and confidence ranges as a function of gestational age are established; tests for normal frequency distribution are made; and estimates of sensitivity, specificity, and false positive rates established for various risk cutoff values, usually 1–195, are needed. Most reports of a 4-marker test using MSAFP, estriol, free hCG, and maternal age correctly predict 65% of cases with 5% false positive rates. Using serum inhibin assays corrected for maternal weight (with which it varies inversely) and using ultrasonic dating of pregnancy, detection increases to 79% with 5% false positives. These are the best results reported by established investigators to date.

T.H. Kirschbaum, M.D.

References

1. 1992 YEAR BOOK OF OBSTETRICS AND GYNECOLOGY, pp 106–107.
2. 1995 YEAR BOOK OF OBSTETRICS AND GYNECOLOGY, pp 157–159.
3. 1994 YEAR BOOK OF OBSTETRICS AND GYNECOLOGY, pp 158–159.
4. Cuckle HS, Holding S, Jones R, et al: Maternal serum inhibin levels in second-trimester Down's syndrome pregnancies. *Prenat Diagn* 14:387, 1994.
5. Wallace EM, et al: *Endocrinology* 144:134, 1995.
6. 1993 YEAR BOOK OF OBSTRETICS AND GYNECOLOGY, pp 138–140.

Measurement of Circulating Inhibin Forms During the Establishment of Pregnancy

Illingworth PJ, Groome NP, Duncan WC, et al (Univ of Edinburgh, Scotland; Oxford Brookes Univ, Oxford, England)
J Clin Endocrinol Metab 81:1471–1475, 1996   5–14

Background.—The circulation concentration of inhibin immunoactivity is markedly increased in pregnancy. The forms of inhibin released into circulation in very early pregnancy, after stimulation of the corpus luteum by exogenous human chorionic gonadotropin (hCG), and in abnormal pregnancy were studied using new inhibin enzyme-linked immunosorbant assays (ELISAs).

Methods and Findings.—Samples were obtained from volunteers and assayed by ELISAs for inhibins A and B and inhibin pro-αC-related immunoreactivity (pro-αC-RI). Inhibin A levels increased steadily during the conception luteal phase to an initial peak 12 days after ovulation. These concentrations then rose rapidly to another peak 43 days after ovulation. A much greater peak of pro-αC-RI concentrations was noted on day 15 after ovulation, declining thereafter. Inhibin B levels were low after ovulation. Subsequently, they were barely detectable in pregnancy. A significant increase in inhibin A and pro-αC-RI resulted from hCG therapy. However, this treatment did not affect inhibin B concentrations. Levels of pro-αC-RI were better indicators of continuing pregnancy viability than either hCG or inhibin A.

Conclusion.—Inhibin A is the principal bioactive form in the circulation in early pregnancy. Inhibin B, by contrast, occurs at very low concentrations. These findings further support the notion that these 2 hormones are distinct in their source and mode of secretion.

▶ The addition of an assay for maternal diameric inhibin A appears to improve prenatal screening for Down's syndrome[1] (see Abstract 5–13). Although it has never been clear why inhibin blood concentrations are elevated with Down's syndrome–afflicted pregnancy anymore than the elevation of hCG or reduction in urinary estriol in this syndrome, this fine study not only charts the course of inhibin A concentration in early pregnancy with very sensitive methodology, it also suggests the basis for increased inhibin concentration during that time. Note the bimodal concentration function for inhibin with 1 maximum at 12 days post ovulation and the second at roughly 8 weeks' gestational age after menses. Maternal hCG administration to a nonpregnant woman causes peripheral inhibin concentration to increase. It seems a likely sequence that the increase in maternal hCG causes increased inhibin production as a result, at least in early pregnancy. It may well be that the enhanced predictability of Down's syndrome using inhibin simply reflects the sensitivity of its response to hCG.

T.H. Kirschbaum, M.D.

Reference

1. 1992 YEAR BOOK OF OBSTETRICS AND GYNECOLOGY, pp 5–6.

6 Fetal Therapy

The Incidence and Spectrum of Neurological Injury After Open Fetal Surgery

Bealer JF, Raisanen J, Skarsgard ED, et al (Univ of California, San Francisco)
J Pediatr Surg 30:1150–1154, 1995   6–1

Background.—Central nervous system injury is an important clinical problem in premature newborns. When under physiologic stress, these infants are highly vulnerable to anoxic and hemorrhagic brain injury. With the development of in utero surgery, there is a new population of premature infants at risk of CNS injury. The incidence and spectrum of CNS injury were retrospectively assessed in fetuses undergoing in utero surgery.

Patients and Findings.—A total of 33 fetuses who underwent in utero surgery at 1 medical center were reviewed. Imaging studies and/or postmortem examination revealed significant CNS abnormalities in 7 patients, all of whom had congenital diaphragmatic hernia. The major CNS abnormalities were periventricular leukomalacia in 3 patients, intraventricular hemorrhage (IVH) with hydrocephalus in 2 patients, IVH without hydrocephalus in 1 patient, and periventricular hemorrhage in 1 patient. Four of the patients had significant episodes of fetal bradycardia or neonatal hypertension, suggesting that asphyxia may have played a role in their neurologic injuries. The other 3 cases of CNS injury occurred with no evidence of fetal distress. These may have been related to tocolytic drugs given to the mother in 2 patients and maternal hypoxia in 1.

Conclusions.—A 21% incidence of CNS injuries was demonstrated in these fetal surgical patients. Preterm newborns and postoperative fetuses appear to be at similar risk of CNS injuries resulting from cerebral circulatory disturbances. Parents must understand the risks of neurologic injury. The presence of CNS injury must be assessed in all fetal surgical patients, before and after birth.

▶ This study makes clear the potential hazard that exists even when reparative fetal surgery is successfully conducted. In this group of 33 pregnancies, there were 16 perinatal deaths and 17 surviving infants. Among the 7 cases with significant evidence of CNS injury, comprising 21% of all cases, there was 1 fetal and 3 early neonatal deaths. Among the remaining 12 perinatal deaths, CNS autopsy findings failed to disclose injury, and other survivors were clinically normal with normal brain scans.

171

Open repair for congenital diaphragmatic hernia was most commonly associated with CNS injury, but 2 cases treated with intratracheal occlusion also suffered brain injury.[1] Not surprisingly, periventricular leukomalacia and IVH were most commonly noted and likely represented transients in brain perfusion during extensive surgery on these fragile infants. These findings add to the likelihood that fetal surgery will not rank as an important member in the roster of invasive fetal therapeutic modalities in the near future.

T.H. Kirschbaum, M.D.

Reference

1. 1995 Year Book of Obstetrics and Gynecology, pp 176–178.

Successful In Utero Therapy of Fetal Heart Block
Copel JA, Buyon JP, Kleinman KS (Yale Univ, New Haven, Conn; New York Univ)
Am J Obstet Gynecol 173:1384–1390, 1995   6–2

Background.—Maternal autoantibodies to Ro and La proteins have been associated with congenital complete heart block. These autoantibodies injure the fetal cardiac conduction system. The outcomes of dexamethasone treatment given to the mothers of 5 fetuses with heart block caused by maternal antibodies were reported.

Methods.—Five fetuses with heart block diagnosed at 20 to 23 weeks and their mothers were included in the trial. All mothers were treated with oral dexamethasone, 4 mg daily, for the remainder of the pregnancy. Results of anti-Ro and/or anti-La testing were positive in all patients.

Findings.—Heart block was complete in 4 fetuses and second-degree in the fifth. The degree of the block was decreased with treatment in 1 fetus with complete block and in the 1 with second-degree block. Hydrops, present in 3 fetuses with complete block, resolved after dexamethasone therapy. Maternal antibody levels were unaffected. Antibody levels were similar in maternal and cord samples at delivery.

Conclusions.—Transplacental glucocorticoid treatment can effectively improve cardiac conduction in fetuses with complete heart block. Because myocarditis may be concurrent, in utero treatment may also improve cardiac contractility, resulting in the rapid resolution of hydrops observed in the current patients. Clinicians should consider therapy with steroids that cross the placenta for newly diagnosed cases of complete heart block with positive antibody screens. A prospective, randomized, multicenter, controlled trial is now needed to test this treatment approach.

▶ Though 5 cases are not enough for firm establishment of this mode of therapy for congenital fetal heart block, this scholarly report from a unit renowned for its success in the diagnosis and treatment of fetal arrhythmias deserves particular attention. Most such cases are associated with maternal antibodies to the ribonucleoproteins SS-A (Ro) and SS-B (La). Maternal-to-fetal transmission of these immunoglobulins either becomes large enough to exert an effect or fetal immunoreactivity matures enough to produce an effect, or both, only after 18 weeks of gestational age. Past that point, the antibodies form a complex with the corresponding antigens on their surface membranes of fetal myocardial cells and induce inflammatory changes. The subsequent scarring, which interferes with atrioventricular conduction, produces various degrees of heart block. The ventricles are then deprived of the atrial systolic phase of diastolic filling, and, especially with idioventricular rates less than 55 beats per minute, the inability to increase ventricular stroke volume sufficient to maintain cardiac output may produce cardiac failure with pericardial and pleural transudation, hydrops, and fetal death. The authors point to their early use of dexamethasone after confirmation of maternal anti-Ro and anti-La antibody as a way of reducing fetal myocardial inflammatory changes and preventing extensive irremediable scarring. They find dexamethasone superior to prednisone since the latter undergoes considerable placental catabolism. β-Adrenergic agents are useful in maintaining a ventricular rate above 55 beats per minute. Where these agents don't suffice to reverse or prevent fetal cardiac failure, the authors opt for delivery. Their results are impressive and this seems advice well worth considering.

T.H. Kirschbaum, M.D.

In Utero Diagnosis and Treatment of Fetal Goitrous Hypothyroidism, Caused by Maternal Use of Propylthiouracil

van Loon AJ, Derksen JThM, Bos AF, et al (Univ Hosp Groningen, The Netherlands)
Prenat Diagn 15:599–604, 1995

6–3

Objective.—Treating Graves' disease during pregnancy with thionamide drugs can cause fetal goiter or hypothyroidism. Because of birth difficulties or neonatal problems, in utero evaluation of fetal thyroid function is desirable but, until now, has been impossible. Successful results were achieved in 1 case of in utero diagnosis and treatment of fetal goitrous hypothyroidism using ultrasound and cordocentesis.

Case Report.—Woman, 35, at 10 weeks of gestation, received a diagnosis of Graves' disease and was treated with 15 mg of carbimazole per day. At 19 weeks of gestation, the woman's medication was changed to 300 mg of propylthiouracil (PTU) per day and increased 2 weeks later to 600 mg/day. At 31 weeks of gestation, an ultrasound examination showed fetal goiter. At 33 weeks, the size of the goiter had increased (Fig 2). The fetus received a diagnosis of hypothyroidism and was treated with an intra-amniotic injection of 250 µg of thyroxine, tested 1 week later to evaluate therapy, and then given 250 µg of thyroxine weekly until 38 weeks. Labor was induced at 39½ weeks, and a male infant weighing 3,090 g was

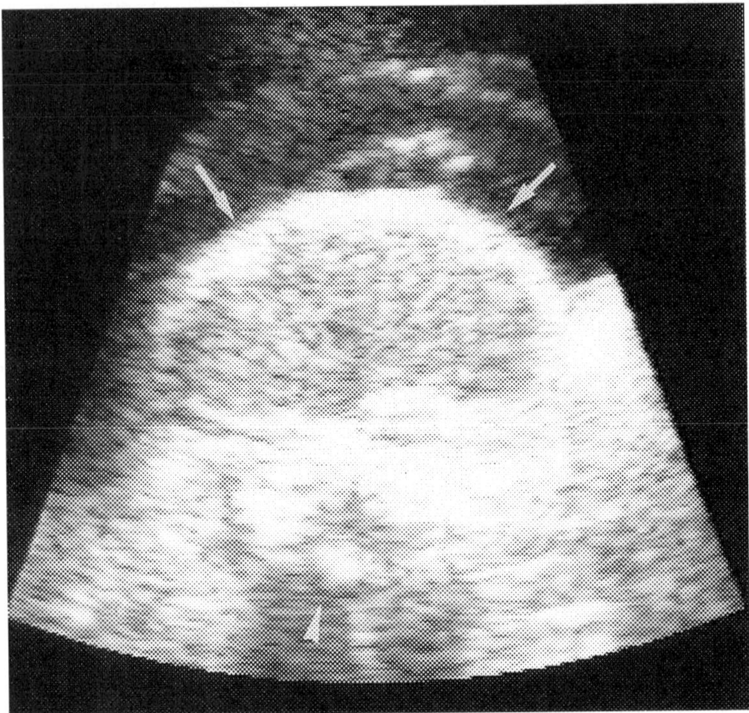

FIGURE 2.—Ultrasonographic image of the fetal neck at 33 weeks' gestation. Transverse section with the spine posterior (*arrowhead*) and the goiter anterior (*arrows*). The umbilical cord is in front of the goiter. (Courtesy of van Loon AJ, Derksen JthM, Bos AF, et al.: *In Utero* Diagnosis and Treatment of Fetal Goitrous Hypothyroidism, Caused by Maternal Use of Propylthiouracil. *Prenat Diagn* 15:559-604, copyright 1995. Reprinted by permission of John Wiley & Sons, Ltd.)

born. He was given 12 μg of thyroxine per kg/day for 3 days and decreasing doses of PTU for 14 weeks to treat hypothyroidism. At 3 and 12 months, his neurologic development was normal.

Conclusion.—Administration of 250 μg of thyroxine weekly was sufficient to treat fetal hypothyroidism induced by PTU treatment of the mother's Graves' disease.

▶ Fetal goiter is infrequently recognized. Though management here was similar to that of a case report reviewed in a previous YEAR BOOK,[1] the neonatal findings in this case were particularly interesting. Treatment for evidently severe maternal Graves' disease was begun at 10 weeks' gestational age and PTU was begun at 19 weeks, ultimately requiring 600 mg/day together with propranolol to control tachycardia. The patient was clinically euthyroid at 26 weeks, but the PTU dosage, which probably could well have been reduced at that point, was continued at 600 mg/day until 34 weeks of gestational age. Following the injunction voiced by Davidson et al.,[1] fetal ultrasound done at 33 weeks showed fetal goiter, polyhydramnios, and an absent stomach bubble, possibly a reflection of reduced fetal swallowing. Percutaneous umbilical blood sampling was done at about 34 weeks to differentiate between hyperthyroid fetal goiter due to placental transfer of the thyroid-stimulating immunoglobulin of Graves' disease and hypothyroid goiter secondary to PTU transfer to the fetus. Treatment with amniotic fluid thyroxine was begun and 1 more percutaneous umbilical blood sampling was done a week later to help evaluate dosage. Thyroxine was continued after birth at 39 weeks because of low newborn T4 developing on day 2 of life, but this was followed by 3 days of hyperthyroidism, apparently the effect of passively transferred maternal Graves' antibody. The infant was thereafter normal.

This case underlines the need to examine the fetal thyroid during the third trimester while treating maternal Graves' disease and helps establish amniotic fluid thyroxine as the treatment of choice for fetal hypothyroidism.

T.H. Kirschbaum, M.D.

Reference

1. 1992 Year Book of Obstetrics and Gynecology, pp 195–196.

Gene Therapy for Cystic Fibrosis: Challenges and Future Directions

Wilson JM (Univ of Pennsylvania, Philadelphia)
J Clin Invest 96:2547–2554, 1995
6–4

Introduction.—Since the gene responsible for cystic fibrosis (CF) was discovered in 1989, approaches to gene therapy for CF have been investigated. The important scientific discoveries and issues examined during the development of in vivo gene therapy for CF using adenoviral vectors were reviewed.

Cystic Fibrosis Pathophysiology.—Although CF affects many organs, its pulmonary manifestations are the most life-limiting and have therefore been the major focus of gene therapy approaches. A protein named the CF transmembrane conductance regulator (CFTR) has been shown to be a primary regulator of membrane ion transport processes. In vitro experiments have demonstrated that a high level of recombinant CFTR expression in only a few cells can initiate a cascade culminating in functional normalization in all cells, suggesting that incomplete gene transfer can be effective in in vivo gene therapy.

The Adenoviral Vector.—Human adenoviruses, because of their natural tropism to the respiratory tract, have been chosen as a vehicle for pulmonary gene transfer. Intratracheal instillation of modified adenovirus complexed to CFTR have not resulted in high levels of gene transfer in the lung.

Immunologic Barriers.—The efficacy of recombinant adenoviruses has been consistently compromised by inflammation and the subsequent loss of transgene expression caused by both cellular and humoral immune responses to adenovirus. Interference with the activation of the CD4 T cells represents another approach.

Conclusions.—Investigations of in vivo gene delivery for gene therapy of CF will have clinical significance for the development of in vivo gene therapy for other diseases. To design rational strategies, more research is required to elucidate host-vector interactions, methods of escaping immune surveillance and modulating immune responses, the basic pathophysiology of CF, and surrogate end points for evaluating clinical efficacy.

▶ In 1989, CFTR gene was identified, and homozygous, deleterious mutations in the gene were identified as a cause of CF. Shortly thereafter, trials in rodents attempting pulmonary CFTR gene insertion into cells lacking the normal gene (transduction), using an adenovirus as vector and taking advantage of its affinity for respiratory epithelium and its ability to infect nondividing cells—provided some optimism. Among the possibilities then viewed were gene therapy in fetuses or infants destined to have CF. Since then, 6 phase I human trials have been conducted, and some problems impeding success have appeared.

Although nasal and tracheal instillation of the adenovirus-CFTR gene complex allows transduction to incur, it is clear from the normal distribution of messenger RNA for the CFTR gene that optimal gene locus is in the submucous glands beneath the respiratory epithelium of the proximal conducting airway, not in surface epithelium or lung parenchyma. It seems apparent that transduction of the exogenous CFTR gene in this way does not occur optimally in the sense of localizing preferentially in submucous glands. The results in vitro and with in vivo graft tissue suggest that as little as 5% of transduction repairs the gene defect, but results are far less productive as natural and adaptive immunity produces cytotoxicity to the adenovirus vector or to the new transgene protein product. The adenovirus is altered genetically to reduce infectivity by deletion of its E1 locus, a gene producing a protein essential for viral cell replication. However, it appears that 1 or more similar gene products are capable of repairing the E1 defect, resulting in a virulent modification and acute respiratory adenovirus infection. But this is progress in understanding what must be done for effective gene therapy. The ultimate prospect for treatment of this common genetic disorder remains very bright.

T.H. Kirschbaum, M.D.

Reversible Tracheal Obstruction in the Fetal Sheep: Effects on Tracheal Fluid Pressure and Lung Growth
Hashim E, Laberge J-M, Chen M-F, et al (Montreal Children's Hosp; McGill Univ, Montreal Quebec)
J Pediatr Surg 30:1172–1177, 1995
6–5

Background.—Infants with congenital diaphragmatic hernia (CDH) have high morbidity and mortality, despite diagnostic and treatment advances. Previous studies have shown that fetal tracheal atresia or ligation is associated with augmented lung growth. An animal model of reversible fetal tracheal obstruction was developed to evaluate the effect of tracheal obstruction on tracheal pressure and lung growth in normal fetuses.

Methods.—Nine pregnant ewes underwent surgery at 108–118 days' gestation to place a Swan-Ganz catheter into the fetal trachea. In 4 fetuses used experimentally, the catheter balloon was inflated. The 5 control fetuses had either uninflated balloons or no catheter placement. Fetal viability was monitored weekly with ultrasonography for 3–4 weeks. The ewes were sacrificed at 137–139 days' gestation, and the trachea, lungs, heart, and liver were removed from the fetus and weighed. Lung volumes were measured. The right middle lobe and left lingula were analyzed for DNA and protein content. Lung tissue sections were examined histochemically and morphometrically.

Results.—The lungs in the fetuses used experimentally were much larger and had volumes 2–3 times greater than those in the control fetuses. Fetal liver and heart weights were similar in the 2 groups. There were no differences between those with uninflated balloon catheters and those without catheters in the control group. Lung architecture was similar in the 2 groups, except that the experimental lungs had more alveoli, thinner septations, and greater airspace fractions. The animals used experimentally had more alveoli because their lungs were larger; the alveolar numerical density was the same in animals used experimentally and as controls, thus preserving the ratio between parenchyma and airspace volume. Experimental and control lungs had similar tissue DNA and protein levels per gram of lung tissue, as well as similar ratios of DNA to protein, indicating that the ratio of cells to extracellular matrix was unchanged.

Conclusions.—Preventing fluid egress in developing fetal lungs enhances lung growth. This tracheal occlusion technique could be modified to be performed with minimally invasive laparoscopic techniques, thereby reducing the risk of uterine instability and preterm labor.

▶ This experimental study in fetal sheep, using chronic fetal tracheal obstruction employing the balloon of the Swan-Ganz catheter and suitably controlled with catheterized uninflated subjects, adds the results of pulmonary microscopic morphometry to what has been noted less rigorously by other investigators.[1] When the fetal trachea is obstructed, it develops an intrathoracic pressure head of 4 mm Hg proximal to the obstruction; in the fetus operated on at 0.75–0.83 of term gestational age, hyperplasia of lung tissue by 2–3 times as measured by wet lung weight follows. The ratio of alveolar to total lung volume is unchanged; that is, the lung tissue is proportionately normal, but alveolar circumference per unit birth weight is doubled and alveolar surface area per unit birth weight increased 2.5-fold. This is true because alveolar surface area is a third-order function of the 1.5-fold increase in alveolar radius. Since DNA-protein ratios are preserved, what has transpired in these experiments is pulmonary hyperplasia, not simply hypertrophy. This study adds strong experimental support for the PLUG (*P*lug the *L*ung *U*ntil it *G*rows) procedure for fetal treatment of congenital diaphragmatic hernia[1] and raises the possibility of treatment of congenital pulmonary atresia in the human fetus.

T.H. Kirschbaum, M.D.

Reference

1. 1995 YEAR BOOK OF OBSTETRICS AND GYNECOLOGY, pp 176–178.

Lung Hypoplasia Can Be Reversed by Short-term Obstruction of the Trachea in Fetal Sheep
Nardo L, Hooper SB, Harding R (Monash Univ, Clayton, Australia)
Pediatr Res 38:690–696, 1995   6–6

Background.—Inadequate fetal lung growth is a common cause of morbidity and mortality in newborns. The volume of liquid retained within the future airways of the fetus is critical for normal lung growth and development. Using fetal sheep, whether short-term obstruction of the fetal trachea, resulting in increased expansion of the lungs, might reverse an existing lung growth deficit in utero was investigated.

Methods.—Seventeen pregnant ewes were operated on at 100 days of gestation. Two catheters were implanted 2–4 cm into the trachea and joined to form an exteriorized tracheal loop. Five days after surgery the animals were divided into 4 experimental groups. In 5 controls, fetal lung liquid was allowed to flow normally through the tracheal loop. The intervention groups had either continuous lung liquid drainage to induce lung hypoplasia (drain group), lung liquid drainage followed by restoration of tracheal flow (drain and reconnect group), or lung liquid drainage followed by tracheal occlusion to accelerate lung growth (drain and obstruct group). Measurements of lung liquid volumes and secretion rates were obtained on days 125, 130, and 134 of gestation; postmortem data were collected on day 135 after killing the ewe and fetus.

Results.—The 4 groups of fetuses were compared for tissue weights and DNA and protein contents. Fetuses in the drain group had significantly reduced wet lung weights and total lung DNA contents compared with controls. In the drain and reconnect group, reestablishment of tracheal flow for 6 days increased fetal lung wet weights relative to the drain group, but not total DNA contents. Lung liquid volumes, wet lung weights, and total protein contents after 6 days of tracheal obstruction were similar in the drain and obstruct group to values in the control group, whereas lung DNA contents were less than control but greater than values of the drain group.

Conclusion.—Twenty-nine days of lung liquid drainage in fetal sheep greatly reduced lung growth, resulting in severe pulmonary hypoplasia. Tracheal obstruction restored normal volumes of lung liquid and reversed the lung growth deficit. Solely restoring tracheal continuity, as in the drain and reconnect group, is analogous to correcting the condition causing the lung hypoplasia and did not increase fetal lung growth.

▶ This study including chronic tracheal catherization in fetal lambs adds further important background information to the prospects of treating pulmonary hypoplasia and/or atresia in human fetuses exposed to long-term oligohydramnios or congenital diaphragmatic hernia. It also brings back fond personal memories garnered at UCLA of Dr. Forrest Adams demonstrating the vast quantities of lung fluid obtainable from fetal tracheal catherization with mild negative pressure, a process recently demonstrated to produce fetal lung hypoplasia.[1] Work previously reviewed here has demonstrated the capacity to reverse pulmonary hypoplasia with fetal tracheal obstruction[2] and showed histologic evidence of lung hyperplasia under those circumstances (Abstract 6–5). Here the question is, how long does it take tracheal occlusion to repair the lung injury caused by withdrawal of fetal lung fluid at 105 to 120 days' gestation at (0.72 to 0.88 term gestation)? Suitable controls for normals at 105 and 134 days of gestational age as well as those for reconnection without plugging of the exteriorized endotracheal catheter loop are offered. The data demonstrate restoration to control values of lung fluid volume, wet and dry weight, and lung DNA and protein content within only 6 days of tracheal occlusion. This remarkably rapid change can only bode well for the prospects for human fetal therapy in the future.

T.H. Kirschbaum, M.D.

References

1. Messinger AC, Harding R, Adamson TM, et al: Role of lung fluid volume in growth and maturation of the fetal sheep lung. *J Clin Invest* 86:1270, 1990.
2. 1995 YEAR BOOK OF OBSTETRICS AND GYNECOLOGY, pp 176–178.

7 Labor, Operative Obstetrics, and Anesthesia

The Relationship Between Physicians' Qualifications and Experience and the Adequacy of Prenatal Care and Low Birthweight
Haas JS, Orav EJ, Goldman L (Harvard Med School, Boston; Univ of California, San Francisco)
Am J Public Health 85:1087–1091, 1995   7–1

Objective.—The relationship between physicians' qualifications and experience and the completion of the recommended number of prenatal visits and the delivery of low-birth-weight infants was evaluated.

TABLE 2.—Relationship Between Physicians' Qualifications and Experience and the Recommended Number of Prenatal Visits and Low Birth Weight

	Adjusted* Odds Ratio (95% Confidence Interval)	
	Recommended No. of Prenatal Visits	Low Birthweight
Board certification		
No	0.67 (0.54, 0.85)	1.20 (1.00, 1.42)
Yes	1.0 ...	1.0 ...
Duration of Practice†		
Short	0.92 (0.65, 1.30)	1.66 (1.32, 2.09)
Medium	1.15 (0.93, 1.44)	1.14 (1.01, 1.29)
Long	1.0 ...	1.0 ...
Volume of practice‡		
Low	1.31 (0.92, 1.86)	1.54 (1.10, 2.16)
Medium	1.00 (0.80, 1.25)	1.19 (0.98, 1.44)
High	1.0 ...	1.0 ...

*Adjusted for maternal age, parity, race, multiple gestation, level of education, marital status, payer, cigarette and alcohol use, site of care, and physicians' qualifications (board certification) and experience (volume of practice and duration of practice).

†Duration of practice: long (licensed before 1979); medium (licensed 1979–1988), short (licensed after 1988).

‡Volume of practice: low (124 deliveries per year); medium (25–118 deliveries per year); high (119–523 deliveries per year).

(Courtesy of Haas JS, Orav EJ, Goldman L: The Relationship Between Physicians' Qualifications and Experience and the Adequacy of Prenatal Care and Low Birthweight. *Am J Public Health* 85:1087–1091, 1995, copyright American Public Health Association.)

Study Design.—All 80,537 deliveries performed by a permanently licensed physician in Massachusetts in 1990 were evaluated. Board certification, volume of deliveries, and duration of practice data were obtained for each physician.

Findings.—Women who received prenatal care from a physician who was not board-certified were less likely to have the recommended number of prenatal visits and were more likely to have a low-birth-weight infant than were those who received care from a board-certified physician (Table 2). Physicians with a smaller delivery volume or shorter duration of practice were also more likely to deliver low-birth-weight infants.

Conclusions.—Both physician qualifications and experience are associated with the quality of prenatal care and with birth outcome. Further research should focus on whether these differences result from differences in patients' self-referrals or from physicians' judgement and efficiency in the delivery of prenatal care.

▶ It's never been easy to prove in objective fashion the benefits of prenatal care, but this large case-control study conducted in 1990 of more than 80,000 Massachusetts births provides some support for that mode of care. The authors employ low birth weight as an outcome measurement because it's more common than either perinatal morbidity or mortality. Of 924 physicians supervising delivery, 49% or 451 were board-certified in obstetrics and gynecology and 6.7% were board-certified in family medicine; 27.3% of deliveries were conducted by those not specialty certified. Patients with prior low-birth-weight pregnancies might be expected preferentially to seek physicians with board certification and/or large-volume practices providing greater-than-average experience. Despite that likelihood, which tends to bias results in the opposite direction, the risks of low-birth-weight delivery (less than 2.5 kg birth weight) were greater among noncertified birth attendant physicians than in those certified and among those with low-volume practices and short duration of practice in Massachusetts than among their opposite counterparts. Though it's not easy to be certain what accounts for the differences, it looks as though these specialty training physicians were doing something right.

T.H. Kirschbaum, M.D.

Perinatal Outcome in Relation to Second-Stage Duration
Menticoglou SM, Manning F, Harman C, et al (Univ of Manitoba, Winnipeg, Canada)
Am J Obstet Gynecol 173:906–912, 1995   7–2

Introduction.—It is generally believed that fetuses are at particular risk of hypoxia during the second stage of labor. This belief is often used as the justification for time limits on the second stage of labor and for high rates of operative vaginal delivery. Obstetricians run some risk of fetal hypoxia if they wait too long during the second stage of labor, and of fetal trauma

TABLE 1.—Perinatal Outcome and Duration of Second Stage

Length of second stage (min)	No. of deliveries	Cumulative percentage of total deliveries	5 min Apgar score <7 (%)	Admission to NICU of nonanomalous babies (%)	Seizures in nonanomalous babies	Deaths of normal fetuses
0–30	1071	17.7	12 (1.1)	8 (0.7)	1	0
31–60	1551	43.4	21 (1.4)	18 (1.2)	2	0
61–90	1052	60.8	11 (1.0)	9 (0.9)	1	0
91–120	753	73.3	10 (1.3)	9 (1.2)	0	0
121–150	517	81.8	11 (2.1)	7 (1.4)	1	0
151–180	410	88.6	9 (2.1)	7 (1.7)	0	0
181–240	379	94.9	7 (1.8)	6 (1.6)	0	0
241–300	147	97.3	0 (0.0)	0 (0.0)	0	0
301–360	79	98.6	5 (6.3)	2 (2.5)	0	0
361+	82	100	2 (2.4)	0 (0.0)	0	0
TOTAL	6041	100	88 (1.5)	66 (1.1)	5	0

Abbreviation: NICV, neonatal ICU.

(Courtesy of Menticoglou SM, Manning F, Harman C, et al: Perinatal outcome in relation to second-stage duration. *Am J Obstet Gynecol* 173:906–912, 1995.)

if they opt for operative vaginal delivery. Risk of fetal mortality and morbidity was analyzed in terms of the length of the second stage of labor.

Methods.—Data on 6,041 nulliparous women reaching the second stage of labor with a live, singleton, cephalic fetus who weighed at least 2,500 g at birth were retrospectively analyzed. The infants were delivered at 1 university teaching hospital within a 5-year period. The perinatal outcomes were determined and related to the duration of the second stage of labor. The second stage was considered to begin when vaginal examination revealed full cervical dilatation.

Results.—There were no deaths during the second stage of labor, and no normally formed infant who survived into the second stage died of any cause. The duration of the second stage was more than 3 hours in 11% of deliveries and more than 5 hours in about 3%. The length of the second stage was not significantly related to measures of neonatal morbidity, including low 5-minute Apgar scores, neonatal seizures, and admission to the neonatal ICU (NICU) (Table 1). Only 1% of infants in whom the second stage lasted 5 hours or longer eventually required admission to the NICU. The longer the second stage lasted, the more it was likely that operative vaginal or cesarean delivery would be performed.

Conclusions.—The length of the second stage of labor per se is unrelated to fetal mortality and morbidity, including asphyxia. Operative intervention is not indicated simply because the second stage of labor has passed some arbitrary time limit. Conservative management of the second stage will result in spontaneous birth for many infants who otherwise would have undergone operative delivery and also in safer instrumental delivery from a lower station in the pelvis for others.

▶ This experience is important in advising those young obstetricians who feel that the second stage of labor should never exceed 120 minutes. Motivated by a midforceps rotation, which produced a cervical cord injury during the second stage of labor 8 years previously, this University of Manitoba unit adopted a tolerant management approach to the second stage of labor. What they demonstrated in term-size infants presenting by the vertex was that after 120 minutes, the incidence of 5-minute Apgar scores less than 7 increased from about 1% to 2% but without impact on perinatal death, neonatal symptoms, or need for NICU admission. It is not the first time this has been observed. If there are no compelling signs of trouble and some progress continues in descent and rotation and/or in descent of the presenting part, it doesn't appear to matter how long the second stage lasts. When progress stops, intervention is indicated. It's a precept from one of my teachers that has stood me in good stead for a long time.

T.H. Kirschbaum, M.D.

A Clinical Trial of Active Management of Labor

Frigoletto FD Jr, Lieberman E, Lang JM, et al (Harvard Med School, Boston; Boston Univ)
N Engl J Med 333:745–750, 1995   7–3

Background.—Active management of labor was developed to reduce the duration of labor. The approach includes strict criteria for diagnosing labor, early rupture of the amniotic membranes, prompt use of high-dose oxytocin in patients with inefficient uterine action, and constant nursing attendance during labor. The efficacy of this protocol for reducing the cesarean section rate in nulliparous women was evaluated in a randomized trial.

Methods.—Nulliparous women without increased risk of preterm or cesarean delivery were randomly assigned to either the active-management group (1,017 patients) or the usual-care group (917 patients) before 30 weeks' gestation. The women in the active-management group received 1-on-1 nursing care throughout labor. Labor was diagnosed when the following criteria were met: painful contractions plus at least 80% effacement, bloody show, or spontaneous rupture of the membranes. Labor was managed with amniotomy within 1 hour of the diagnosis of labor, cervical examinations every 2 hours, and high-dose oxytocin administration if cervical dilation took longer than 1 cm/hr during the first stage of labor and if it took longer than 1 hour for the head of the fetus to reach the pelvic floor after full dilation. Efficacy was evaluated by comparing cesarean delivery rates in the 2 groups; safety was evaluated by comparing the 2 groups for labor and postpartum complications and the outcomes of the infants.

Results.—By intention to treat, the rate of cesarean section was 19.5% in the active-management group and 19.4% in the usual-care group. Among the women actually treated according to their assigned protocol, the rates of cesarean section were 10.9% in the active-management group and 11.5% in the usual-care group, a nonsignificant difference. Failure to progress was the indication for cesarean section in 7% of the active-management group and 8% of the usual-care group. Labor had a median duration of 6.2 hours in the active-management group and 8.9 hours in the usual-care group. There was a lower incidence of fever in the active-management group than in the usual-care group; there were no other significant differences in maternal complications or infants' outcomes.

Conclusion.—The active-management protocol was not effective in reducing the rate of cesarean sections but did result in shorter labor and a reduced incidence of maternal fever.

▶ In 1980, Professors O'Driscoll and Meagher published their description of the active management of labor including data from Dublin's National Maternity Hospital from 1963 to 1976. They disclosed a cesarean section rate of 4%, a forceps delivery rate of 10%, and a perinatal death rate for 1976, corrected for malformations, of 12 per 1,000 live births. Trials of the employment of this approach elsewhere have led to generally successful results,[1,2] but this study is the largest, best-executed randomized control trial to date.

An initial problem is the failure of the Dublin group to define labor onset by cervical dilatation. They accept uterine contractions, partial cervical effacement, and "show" as sufficient for the diagnosis, introducing the 10% false diagnosis of labor by their own account.

A complication in the Boston study is the need to deviate from planned management in either active- or usual-management subsets in 33% to 35% of cases, largely because of the de novo clinical indications for the induction of labor, a criterion for exclusion from this study. It's necessary to include all such cases in their initially assigned subgroups on statistical grounds from which process emerge cesarean section rates of 19.5% for active and 19.4% for usual management. However, the requirement for reporting data in terms of initial intention of therapy was not meant to deal with such large unanticipated ineligibility, and the authors report cesarean section rates of 10.9% and 11.5%, respectively, for those 1,263 gravidas for whom ineligibility did not appear after enrollment. Those with active management had more frequent vaginal exams and artificial rupture of membranes, received more oxytocin earlier, and had mean labor durations of 6.2 vs. 8.9 hours without evidence of additional newborn compromise.

An unavoidable problem is that the decision to do cesarean section, given a single term pregnancy and spontaneous labor, cannot be standardized and controlled internally among patients recruited from 17 prenatal sites, all cared for by their own physicians in the usual-care subset. Neither can comparisons be made to the Dublin group with whom there surely are contrasts in the threshold for cesarean section, very striking during the second stage of labor, as the authors here note. Active management offers some benefits to primigravidas in labor, but in the hands of Boston-area nurse-midwives and obstetricians, a significant reduction in cesarean section incidence was not one of them.

T.H. Kirschbaum, M.D.

References

1. 1989 YEAR BOOK OF OBSTETRICS AND GYNECOLOGY, pp 139–140.
2. 1993 YEAR BOOK OF OBSTETRICS AND GYNECOLOGY, pp 170–172.

Randomized Trial of Epidural Versus Intravenous Analgesia During Labor

Ramin SM, Gambling DR, Lucas MJ, et al (Univ of Texas, Dallas)
Obstet Gynecol 86:783–789, 1995   7–4

Background.—Concerns have been raised about the adverse effects of epidural analgesia during labor. Epidural analgesia was compared with parenteral meperidine in a randomized study of the effects of epidural analgesia on labor.

Methods.—By random assignment, 1,330 women with uncomplicated term pregnancies in spontaneous labor were offered epidural bupivacaine-fentanyl or IV meperidine analgesia during labor. Four hundred thirty-two of the 664 women randomized received epidural analgesia, and 437 of the 666 randomized received meperidine.

Findings.—Epidural analgesia was significantly correlated with prolongation of labor, an increased rate of oxytocin administration, chorioamnionitis, low forceps use, and cesarean delivery. Because a large proportion of women randomized declined analgesia, a multifactorial regression analysis was done on the entire cohort. A twofold relative risk of cesarean delivery continued to be associated with epidural treatment. The effect of epidural analgesia on cesarean delivery was significant for both nulliparous (risk ratio, 2.55) and parous women (risk ratio, 3.81). Pain relief was significantly better with epidural analgesia than with parenteral meperidine (Tables 2 and 3).

Conclusions.—Although epidural analgesia provides superior pain relief, its administration produces significant undesirable effects on labor outcomes. The increased risk of operative delivery may be avoided in

TABLE 2.—Duration of Labor and Complications in Relation to Type of Analgesia

Labor complications	Epidural (N = 432)	Meperidine (N = 437)	P
Interval from admission to delivery			
Mean ± SD (h)	7.2 ± 3.9	5.7 ± 3.3	.001
≥10 h	89 (21%)	39 (9%)	<.001
2-h or longer second stage	31 (7%)	11 (3%)	.001
Oxytocin augmentation	139 (32%)	102 (23%)	.004
Chorioamnionitis*	98 (23%)	21 (5%)	<.001

Note: Data are presented as mean ± standard deviation (SD) or *n* (%).
*Chorioamnionitis: fever of 38°C or higher in labor.
(Courtesy of Ramin SM, Gambling DR, Lucas MJ, et al: Randomized Trial of Epidural Versus Intravenous Analgesia During Labor. *Obstetrics and Gynecology*, 86:783–789, 1995. Reprinted with permission from The American College of Obstetricians and Gynecologists.)

TABLE 3.—Route of Delivery and Complications in Relation to Type of Labor Analgesia

Delivery complications	Epidural (N = 432)	Meperidine (N = 437)	P
Vaginal delivery			
Spontaneous	352 (81%)	407 (93%)	<.001
Outlet forceps*	8 (2%)	8 (2%)	NS
Low forceps†	33 (8%)	5 (1%)	<.001
Shoulder dystocia	2	2	NS
Cesarean delivery	39 (9%)	17 (4%)	.002
Dystocia	21 (5%)	7 (1.6%)	.007
Fetal distress	18 (4%)	10 (2.3%)	NS

Note: Data are presented as *n* (%).

*Outlet forceps: fetal head at the perineum. (American College of Obstetricians and Gynecologists. Obstetric forceps. ACOG committee opinion no. 71, Washington, DC, American College of Obstetricians and Gynecologists, 1989.)

†Low forceps: +2cm to +4cm below the ischial spines.

(Courtesy of Ramin SM, Gambling DR, Lucas MJ, et al.: Randomized Trial of Epidural Versus Intravenous Analgesia During Labor. *Obstetrics and Gynecology*, 86:783–789, 1995. Reprinted with permission from The American College of Obstetricians and Gynecologists.)

women who can tolerate labor pain well or whose discomfort is adequately relieved by treatment with less risky agents. Women should be informed of the risks and benefits associated with epidural analgesia.

▶ It's a rarity to achieve a well-conducted randomized prospective study of intrapartum anesthesia/analgesia of this size, and it makes very clear the costs of effective anesthesia that mothers, but fortunately not their infants, pay. Only women with normal spontaneous term labors with cervix equal to or greater than 5 cm dilation on admission were admitted for study, so the results cannot be applied to gravidas with complicated pregnancies or labors. In 6 months' time, 1,330 women were entered and randomized; protocol failures or altered patient selection occurred in about 35% of both epidural and meperidine subsets, leaving 869 women for final comparison. Meperidine was given in 50-mg doses with promethazine, to a maximum of 200 mg for 4 hours. Bupivacaine/fentanyl epidural supplied superior pain relief, but hypotension was noted in 22% despite fluid preloading of at least 0.5 L of Ringer's lactate. Ephedrine was required in 9 cases. Epidural analgesia resulted in prolongation of labor, an increased incidence of second stage greater than 2 hours, the need for oxytocin augmentation, and presumptive chorioamnionitis in its recipients. The cesarean section rate was doubled after compensating for confounding variables, and the crude odds ratio for forceps delivery was 3.91 among women receiving epidural anesthesia. No difference in newborn outcome was seen. Work of this sort will certainly not reduce the popularity of epidural pain relief, but it enables us to be clear regarding the cost-benefit ratios to which our patients are exposed.

T.H. Kirschbaum, M.D.

Head Entrapment and Neonatal Outcome by Mode of Delivery in Breech Deliveries From Twenty-Four to Twenty-Seven Weeks of Gestation

Robertson PA, Foran CM, Croughan-Minihane MS, et al (Univ of California, San Francisco)
Am J Obstet Gynecol 173:1171–1176, 1995   7–5

Introduction.—Obstetricians often advocate routine cesarean section for the delivery of breech neonates in the very preterm gestational age group because of a perceived increased risk of head entrapment in this group. However, there are few data on the incidence of head entrapment for neonates with a gestational age of 24 to 27 weeks. Therefore, the incidence and outcome of head entrapment in breech neonates at a gestational age of 24 to 27 weeks were analyzed retrospectively.

Methods.—The charts of all 132 viable singleton breech deliveries between the gestational ages of 24 and 27 weeks from 1976 to 1993 were reviewed. Associations between the mode of delivery and head entrapment and among head entrapment, mode of delivery, and adverse neonatal outcome were analyzed.

Results.—Of the 132 breech deliveries, 67.4% were by cesarean section and 32.6% were by the vaginal route. The incidence of head entrapment was 5.6% at cesarean section and 9.3% at vaginal delivery and was not associated with gestational age or type of breech. The only statistically significant risk factor for head entrapment with either mode of delivery was birth weight between 1,000 and 1,249 g. There were no significant differences between neonates with and without head entrapment in the occurrence of fetal distress or other outcome variables.

Conclusions.—The occurrence of head entrapment was not associated with either vaginal or cesarean delivery and did not adversely affect neonatal outcome. Therefore, routine cesarean delivery of breech neonates at less than 29 weeks' gestation is not justified by these data.

▶ The relative merits of vaginal vs. abdominal delivery of very low birth weight infants is a subject of at least weekly discussion in my experience, and this cohort study based on the University of California at San Francisco Data Collection dating back to 1973 provides some useful information to the argument. Head entrapment with vaginal birth is defined as greater than 90 seconds of time lapse between delivery of the body and the head or the need for additional or unusual maneuvers to effect head delivery. With cesarean section, more than 4 minutes from hysterotomy to delivery suffices to make the diagnosis. Though vaginal entrapment appeared to be more common at 27 than at 24–25 weeks of gestational age, there was no difference in the incidence of head entrapment comparing abdominal vs. vaginal birth in this gestational age range. The type of breech presentation appeared to make no difference. Once again, clinical research fails to support the use of cesarean section based solely on the breech presentation in this gestational age range.

T.H. Kirschbaum, M.D.

Breech at Term: Mode of Delivery? A Register-Based Study
Krebs L, Langhoff-Roos J, Weber T (Univ of Copenhagen)
Acta Obstet Gynecol Scand 74:702–706, 1995   7–6

Background.—The best mode of delivery of term fetuses in the breech position is still debated. Neonatal mortality and morbidity in nonmalformed singleton term neonates delivered in breech presentation were reported, and possible correlations between outcome and mode of delivery, parity, and birth weight were investigated.

Methods.—Data were obtained from a Danish cohort of 15,718 normal, singleton term neonates initially seen in the breech position and delivered between 1982 and 1990. All were alive at the onset of labor.

Findings.—Deliveries were vaginal for 3,247 neonates, or 20.7%; elective cesarean in 7,106, or 45.3%; and emergency cesarean in 5,356, or 34.1%. Compared with those delivered by elective cesarean section, those delivered vaginally and by emergency cesarean section had significantly greater rates of mortality, including intrapartum and early neonatal death, and morbidity, as evidenced by low Apgar scores. Parity was unassociated with outcome among vaginal deliveries (Fig 2). However, neonates with birth weights of more than 4,000 g had significantly greater rates of low Apgar scores.

Conclusions.—Vaginal delivery of nonmalformed, term neonates in breech presentation appears to be associated with increased mortality and morbidity. These findings need to be validated and more information must be obtained from the medical records before it is clear whether selection of

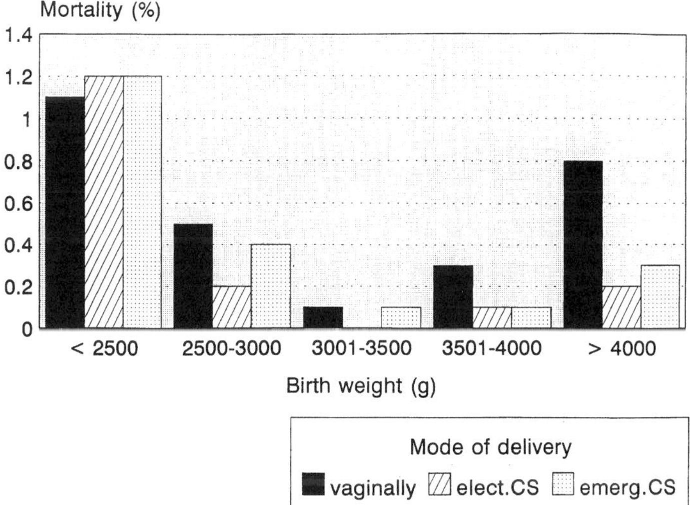

FIGURE 2.—Rates of mortality (intrapartum and early neonatal) in relation to birth weight and mode of delivery. (Courtesy of Krebs L, Langhoff-Roos J, Weber T: Breech at Term: Mode of Delivery? A Register-Based Study. *Acta Obstet Gynecol Scand,* 74:702-706, 1995 Munksgaard International Publishers Ltd., Copenhagen, Denmark.)

parturients, structure of perinatal care, or professional skills need to be improved or whether all singleton term neonates in breech presentation should undergo cesarean delivery.

▶ Though cesarean section has become the dominant approach to delivery of the term fetus presenting by the breech, the lack of conclusive support for that position continues to make it a topic for debate both in Europe[1] and the United States.[2] This large retrospective cohort study of term infants excluding fetal deaths and lethal anomalies tends, to the unwary, to support abdominal as preferred to vaginal birth. As with all retrospective studies, the inability to control confounding variables is the problem that can only be overcome with random assignment of large numbers of cases prospectively. Here, elective cesarean section yields better results than vaginal birth with respect to intrapartum and early neonatal death and reduced Apgar score. When, however, one compares all cesarean sections with all vaginal births, the difference in mortality figures disappears. This highlights the possibility that the incidence of undiagnosed breeches with unintended vaginal birth or vaginal delivery by virtue of insufficient time to get to the operating room may be part of the conclusion. So too might differences in incidences of incomplete breech presentation, frank breeches and nonlethal fetal CNS maldevelopment/anomaly, which tends to predispose to breech presentation. Though they represent only about 0.8% of all deliveries, vaginal delivery of fetuses greater than 4 kg at birth was seen to account for 15% of both mortalities and reduced Apgar scores. It's important to note that no adverse outcome was associated with vaginal deliveries of 838 fetuses less than 2.5 kg by virtue of their vaginal and in comparison to abdominal birth. The authors conclude that a prospective randomized study of nearly 1 million term births would be needed to meet reasonable requirements of power analysis to demonstrate statistical significance in this choice. This debate will continue until we reach that point, and decisions for delivery of such fetuses will continue to be unsupported by anything other than individual opinions and market forces.

T.H. Kirschbaum, M.D.

References

1. Thorpe Beeston JG, Banfield PJ, Saunders NJStG: Outcome of breech delivery at term. *BMJ* 305:746, 1992.
2. Peller D, Van Dorsten JP: *Am J Obstet Gynecol* 173:393, 1995.

Induction of Labor Compared With Expectant Management for Prelabor Rupture of the Membranes at Term
Hannah ME, for the TERMPROM Study Group (Univ of Toronto; Women's College Hosp, Toronto; McMaster Univ, Hamilton, Ontario, Canada)
N Engl J Med 334:1005–1010, 1996   7–7

Introduction.—The fetal membranes rupture before the start of labor in approximately 8% of term pregnancies, and almost all of these women will go into labor within 72 hours. However, as the time between membrane rupture and delivery increases, fetal and maternal infection may become more likely. The effects of labor induction—and of various methods of induction—on infection risk after spontaneous rupture of the membranes at term were examined.

Methods.—The study included 5,041 women with term pregnancies whose membranes ruptured before term. They were randomly assigned to 1 of 3 groups. Two groups underwent induction of labor with IV oxytocin of vaginal prostaglandin E$_2$ gel. The third group was managed expectantly for up to 4 days; induction with oxytocin or prostaglandin E$_2$ was done in case of complications. The 3 groups were compared for neonatal infection, cesarean section rate, and patient evaluations of their treatment.

Results.—Neonatal infection rates ranged from 2% to 3% in all groups and cesarean section rates from approximately 10% to 11%. Four percent of women undergoing induction with oxytocin had clinical chorioamnionitis, compared with almost 9% of those managed expectantly. Rates of postpartum fever were 2% and 4%, respectively. The patients who underwent induction of labor were less likely to say they liked nothing about their treatment than those managed expectantly.

Conclusions.—Induction of labor and expectant management yield comparable rates of neonatal infection and cesarean section in women who experience prelabor rupture of the membranes in a term pregnancy. This is true whether induction is done with oxytocin or prostaglandin E$_2$. Maternal infection is less likely with oxytocin induction than with expectant management. Patient satisfaction ratings are higher with induction of labor than with expectant management.

▶ This is a large, well-designed, prospective randomly controlled study that gains much of its strength from its apparently rigorous execution. For example, bacteriologic information was obtained in 80% of the 5,041 patients studied. For this reason, these data provide a clearer view of the incidence of latent or asymptomatic maternal infection in premature membrane rupture (PROM) than most. In essence, the study fails to show significant difference in outcome between planned inductions or inductions indicated in the 20% of women who failed to enter spontaneous labor after 4 days, regardless of whether oxytocin or PGE$_2$ gel was used. Generally, infection rates were low, 4% to 6% for planned inductions and 8% in women treated expectantly, and 2.6% neonatal infection with neonatal mortality less than 1%. These data suggest that women from lower socioeconomic strata were not frequently enrolled by virtue of their higher anticipated perinatal infection rates. This is also suggested by the 60% incidence of primigravidity at mean age 28 and only a 10% incidence of Group B streptococcus (GBS) positive cultures on antenatal screening. Design of the protocol is based on the premise that women at term with rupture of membranes should be treated by either prompt induction or by 96 hours delay to maximize the chance of spontaneous labor anticipated in 95% of such women after that time. That the policy does not increase the risk of maternal and/or neonatal infection depends on the underlying risk of infection, small in these women, but larger in metropolitan indigent care facilities. All the perinatal mortality occurred in the expectant management group but in only 1 case of neonatal GBS sepsis without clinical chorioamnionitis was the outcome possibly avertable. Regardless of indication, oxytocin results were better than those with PGE_2 gel in terms of shorter interval until labor, time in labor, less time in the neonatal ICU, but not different in terms of a long list of other outcome measures. With an incidence of unripened cervix of 30% on palpation, one would expect that PGE_2 would prove more advantageous than it did here, but it continues to be difficult to prove objectively that it is uniformly true. These results should not be projected to include women at high risk of infection or those with unripe cervix.

T.H. Kirschbaum, M.D.

The Role of Emergency Obstetric Care in Preventing Maternal Deaths: An Historical Perspective on European Figures Since 1751
Papiernik E (Université René Descartes, Paris)
Int J Gynaecol Obstet 50:73S–77S, 1995   7–8

Background.—Maternal mortality has greatly decreased in industrialized countries, possibly because of the general advances in medical care or because of specific technical interventions. The time relationships between the introduction of obstetric techniques and the organization of obstetric care in Europe and the decline in maternal mortality between 1751 and 1980 were reviewed.

Methods and Findings.—Published data were used to determine trends in maternal deaths for 250 years. Between 1751 and 1920, the decline in maternal death rates in European countries was slow. In Sweden, the ratio of maternal deaths per 100,000 live births declined from 1,100 to 100 during this period (Fig 1). The annual reductions of deaths during those 170 years was 0.5%. Between 1920 and 1980, maternal deaths declined by 90%, from 100 to less than 10 maternal deaths per 100,000 births in Sweden. The decrease was even sharper in other industrialized countries. Declines by specific cause of death differed, being greater for hemorrhage and infection and much slower for complications of hypertension. The rate of maternal deaths associated with infection dropped quickly in the 1930s, before antibiotics became available.

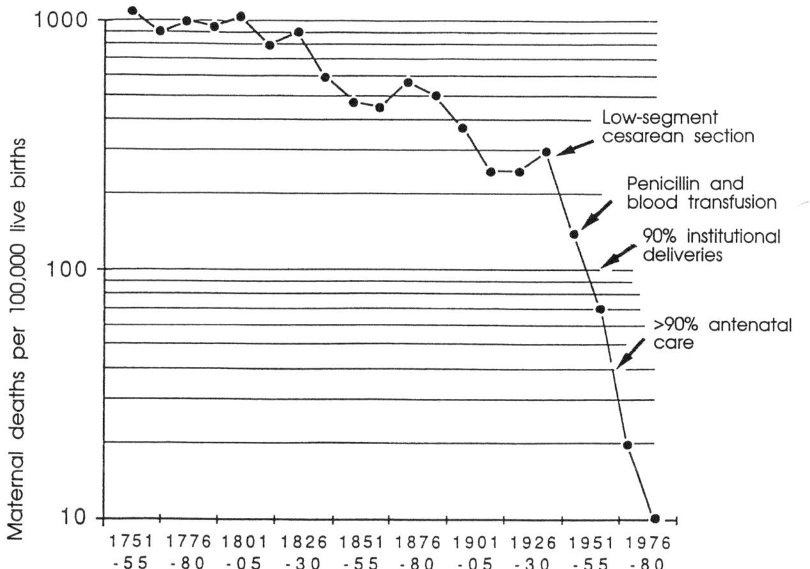

FIGURE 1.—Maternal deaths in Sweden, 1750–1980. (Reprinted from Papiernik E: The Role of Emergency Obstetric Care in Preventing Maternal Deaths: An Historical Perspective on European Figures Since 1751. *Int J Gynecol Obstet*, 50:73S–77S, 1995, with kind permission from Elsevier Science Ireland Ltd., Bay 15K, Shannon Industrial Estate, Co. Clare, Ireland.)

Conclusions.—These historical data as well as data from geographic series suggest that the greatest declines in maternal death rates occurred when essential obstetric functions were introduced. The introduction of low-segment cesarean section at the beginning of the 20th century coincided with the most pronounced decline in maternal mortality. The movement of birth sites from homes to specialized units was also a factor.

▶ In looking for a basis for an historical review of the relationships between obstetric advances and declining maternal mortality, this distinguished French obstetrician has turned to Swedish data submitted to the World Health Organization for the interval of 1750–1980. Representative of Western industrialized nations, the Swedish maternal mortality rates seem roughly comparable to American-derived data, but have a laudably longer reach back into the 18th century. Though forceps were available during America's colonial period and in 18th century Europe, their use did not become common until the 1880s. The value of asepsis was still being debated in the late 1880s in this country, and it became generally accepted around 1900. Together, these contributions likely were part of the slow decline in maternal mortality, compared with what was to follow during the 1900s. In 1926, the Scottish obstetrician J.M. Munro Kerr introduced the transverse lower-segment cesarean section, rendering abdominal birth safer and easier. Though there's danger of the post-hoc fallacy here, the popularity of the Kerr incision marked the start of a rapid decline in maternal mortality. Availability of effective antimicrobials and safe blood transfusion, both by-products of World War II, added to the decline as did effective oral contraception, thanks to the efforts of Pincus, Rock, and Garcia in the late 1950s. The author cites the work of Schwartz[1] to the point that hospitalization for birth is associated with further reduction using Latin American data, but confounding relationships here abound. He does us a service, however in highlighting effectively the major contributions that have brought us to where we are in safeguarding maternal life in the course of delivery.

T.H. Kirschbaum, M.D.

Reference

1. Schwartz R: Mortalidad maternal y cobertura institucional para el parto en 22 paises de la Région de las Americas 1973–1984, Maternal mortality and institutional coverage for delivery in 22 countries in the Region of the Americas 1973–1984, WHO. CLAP-OPS-OMS, 1985.

8 Genetics and Teratology

Identification of Human Parvovirus B19 Infection in Idiopathic Nonimmune Hydrops Fetalis
Jordan JA (Univ of Pittsburgh, Pa)
Am J Obstet Gynecol 174:37–42, 1996   8–1

Purpose.—Parvovirus B19 infection can have serious complications in individuals with pre-existing anemia, patients with immunodeficiency, and pregnant women and their fetuses. Nonimmune hydrops fetalis is now the most common cause of hydrops fetalis. There are many different causes of nonimmune hydrops fetalis, which are often pathologically indistinguishable. No cause is identified in about 44% of cases. To identify cases with parvovirus B19 infection, a number of cases of nonimmune hydrops fetalis were studied.

Methods.—Placental and fetal tissues from 57 cases of nonimmune hydrops fetalis were analyzed by a sensitive polymerase chain reaction (PCR) assay for B19 DNA. Of the 57 cases studied, 34 were regarded as idiopathic and 23 had known noninfectious-based causes.

Findings.—In 18% of cases of idiopathic nonimmune hydrops fetalis, B19 DNA was found. None of the known, noninfectious-based cases had B19 DNA. In all 6 cases identified by PCR, the presence of virus was confirmed by the finding of B19-specific DNA on in situ hybridization or immunocytochemistry. However, histologic examination failed to identify the characteristic viral-like inclusion bodies in 4 of the 6 cases.

Conclusions.—In about one fifth of idiopathic cases of nonimmune hydrops fetalis, B19 DNA is detected. The PCR assay provides a powerful molecular-based tool for the diagnosis of B19-associated nonimmune hydrops fetalis. The PCR is recommended for use in screening for potential B19 infection in maternal-fetal cases, as well as in patients with pre-existing anemia or congenital or acquired immunodeficiencies.

▶ The ability to make the diagnosis of parvovirus B19 using a labeled oligonucleotide probe is not a new contribution to the diagnosis of this increasingly important infection. What is unique here is the use of archival collections of fixed, paraffin-mounted tissue sections of placental and fetal tissues in cases of nonimmune hydrops managed up to 10 years ago.

The technical details are the most important elements of this account of 57 such cases. Particular care, including physical separation of laboratory sites for sample preparation, PCR, and DNA detection, was used to reduce the risk of cross contamination. A unique set of primers, only available as recently as 1995, was used for PCR, and each run incorporated several negative controls. Parallel amplification of the β-globulin gene on chromosome 15 was conducted as a positive control of the amplification process. All samples positive for parvovirus B19 had the diagnosis confirmed by in situ hybridization and immunocytochemistry on the sample slides. For these reasons, the author's estimate that 18% of all cases of nonimmune hydrops contained fetal and placental parvovirus B19 DNA seems reliable.

T.H. Kirschbaum, M.D.

Aromatase Deficiency in Male and Female Siblings Caused by a Novel Mutation and the Physiological Role of Estrogens
Morishima A, Grumbach MM, Simpson ER, et al (Columbia Univ, New York; Univ of Texas, Dallas; Univ of California, San Francisco)
J Clin Endocrinol Metab 80:3689–3698, 1995   8–2

Background.—In many tissues, the conversion of androgens to estrogens is catalyzed by the aromatase enzyme complex. Aromatase cytochrome P450 enzyme is produced by the CYP19 gene. A novel mutation of the CYP19 gene was found in a sister and a brother. Their mother had progressive virilization, which resolved post partum, during both her pregnancies.

Case 1.—Woman, 28, had female (XX) pseudohermaphrodism at birth. As an infant, she had a clitorectomy and repair of her external genitalia. During adolescence, she had progressive signs of virilization and tall stature (her adult height was 177.6 cm, +2.5 standard deviation), but no breast development. Laboratory evaluation revealed hypergonadotropic hypogonadism; ultrasonography showed polycystic ovaries and a prepubertal uterus. The patient's plasma estradiol level was low, but her plasma testosterone, androstenedione, and 17-hydroxyprogesterone levels were elevated. Hormone replacement therapy resulted in breast development, menses, resolution of the ovarian cysts, and suppression of the elevated gonadotropins.

Case 2.—Man, 24, her XY sibling, was 204 cm tall (+3.7 standard deviation), weighed 135 kg (+2.1 standard deviation), was sexually fully mature, and had eunuchoid skeletal proportions and macro-orchidism. His plasma levels of estradiol and estrone were less than 7 pg/mL; his plasma levels of testosterone, androstenedione, 5α-dihydrotestosterone, gonadotropins, and insulin were elevated. His serum total cholesterol, low-density lipoprotein cholesterol, and triglyceride levels were elevated. His bone age was 14 years, and bone densitometric studies suggested osteoporosis.

Findings.—Both siblings had a homozygous single base change at base pair 1123 (C→T) in exon IX of the CYP19 gene. The mutation had 0.2% of the aromatase activity of the wild-type enzyme. In this consanguineous pedigree, the parents are obligate heterozygotes.

Conclusions.—Even with high levels of testosterone, estrogens are important in the sex-steroid gonadotropin feedback mechanism in the male. In both men and women, estrogens are necessary for normal skeletal maturation, the accretion and maintenance of bone mass and density, and control of the bone turnover rate. In the adult male, deficient estrogens may be associated with hyperinsulinemia and abnormal plasma lipids. Placental aromatase protects the female fetus from masculinization and the mother from virilization, estrogen synthesis in the blastocyst, fetus, and placenta is not essential for normal embryonic and fetal development.

▶ Cytochrome P450 aromatase is a ubiquitous enzyme that serves various specific organ functions through the control of local promoter genes that are specific to each organ. In this case, the mutational conversion of cytosine to thymine (transversion) in the DNA of the CYP19 gene located in the long arm of chromosome 15 of both parents resulted in 2 individuals homozygous for the gene defect. With abnormal P450 aromatase proteins present, the conversion of Δ^4 androstenedione and testosterone to estrogens was blocked. Study of those now-adult siblings tells us a great deal about the importance and lack of importance of estrogen in reproduction. Their mother, deprived of the increased placental aromatase activity that converts the excess maternal and fetal adrenal dehydroepiandrosterone sulfate to estrogens, became virilized in midpregnancy but reverted to normal 6 months thereafter.

The female child showed the labioscrotal vulvar fusion and clitoral hypertrophy characteristic of excessive exposure to antigens before 12 weeks of gestational age. But otherwise, normal embryonic growth, sexual differentiation and development proceeded without the production of endogenous estrogen in that young woman. With puberty, when ovarian aromatase becomes important to increased estrogen production, her severe estrogen deficiency led to hypergonadotropism and cystic ovarian changes with androgen-full follicles similar to those in polycystic ovarian disease. Note that the high androgen content was insufficient to inhibit the pituitary gonadotropins for which functions estrogen is much more efficient.

In the male sibling, delayed epiphyseal fusion with osteoporosis points to the role of estrogen, not androgens, in limiting epiphyseal growth and in the control of bone remodeling. At age 24 years, the male shows evidence of insulin resistance, a finding spared his sister by virtue of her estrogen replacement therapy.

Both siblings have heterosexual orientation. This beautiful example of modern genetic investigation nicely shows the extent to which estrogen is not vitally necessary in reproduction and sexual differentiation in the human fetus to the extent that it is in other species.

T.H. Kirschbaum, M.D.

Prenatal Diagnosis of Mitochondrial Fatty Acid Oxidation Defects
Nada MA, Vianey-Saban C, Roe CR, et al (Baylor Univ, Dallas; Hopital Debrousse, Lyon, France; Indiana Univ, Indianapolis; et al)
Prenat Diagn 16:117–124, 1996   8–3

Objective.—Although prenatal diagnosis of inherited biochemical disorders has improved substantially during the past 20 years, many fatty acid oxidation disorders still cannot be diagnosed before birth. For families at risk of disorders of mitochondrial fatty acid oxidation, it is especially difficult to make the diagnosis prenatally if the precise enzymatic defect is unknown. A new approach using skin fibroblasts has had promising results in diagnosing of various fatty acid oxidation defects. The use of this technique for prenatal diagnosis of 2 patients with mitochondrial fatty acid oxidation defects is reported.

Patients.—The study included 2 families who had children with diagnosed or probable fatty acid oxidation defects. Amniocytes were obtained and incubated with stable isotopically labeled palmitate, in the presence of L-carnitine. The acylcarnitine intermediates produced by this technique were analyzed by tandem mass spectrometry. In the family at risk for medium-chain acyl-CoA dehydrogenase (MCAD) deficiency, amniocyte culture yielded an acylcarnitine profile characteristic of MCAD deficiency, with increased concentrations of octanoylcarnitine and decanoylcarnitine. The fetus was later proven to be homozygous for the MCAD A985G mutation on DNA analysis, and MCAD deficiency was confirmed by acylcarnitine and DNA analysis of blood obtained after birth.

The second case was in a family at risk for an unknown fat oxidation defect. In this case, amniocytes produced increased concentrations of long-chain acylcarnitines consistent with a deficiency of very-long-chain acyl-CoA dehydrogenase (VLCAD). This deficiency in amniocytes was confirmed by measurements of enzyme activity. The VLCAD deficiency was also confirmed by examination of the acylcarnitine profiles of postpartum blood and by measurement of enzyme activities in fibroblasts.

Conclusions.—The prenatal diagnosis of mitochondrial fatty acid oxidation defects (specifically, VLCAD and MCAD deficiency) using in vitro probes of fatty acid oxidation in fibroblasts is a new technique that may be useful in identifying mitochondrial fatty acid oxidation defects even in at-risk families in whom no specific defect has been identified.

▶ It's becoming reasonably clear that acute fatty liver of pregnancy reflects the presence of a mutational event in mitochondrial DNA in a heterozygous state that, because of the metabolic load of pregnancy, becomes physiologically important.[1, 2] When present in homozygous form in the infant of a female carrier, usually early onset liver injury and neonatal death result.[3] In either case, the mechanisms are the same and stem from a failure of acyl-CoA dehydrogenase activity that cuts long chain fatty acids into multiples of 2 carbon lengths (β oxidation) that, reacting with coenzyme A, yield acyl-CoA and ultimately ATP through the Krebs cycle. Adenosine triphosphate serves as an important resource for energy acquisition, storage, transfer and release to energize cell functions. The gene for the short chain dehydrogenase is coded on chromosome 12 and in mitochondrial DNA for long and middle-length chain β oxidation. Carnitine, a 7-carbon atom amino acid formed in liver and muscle, is needed for the transport of fatty acids through mitochondrial membranes into the matrix where β oxidation occurs. With defective oxidation, concentrations of free fatty acids complexed or not to carnitine increase to concentrations toxic to liver, kidneys, and myocardium. As lipid metabolism grinds to a halt as a result of failed β oxidation, stored carbohydrate is depleted in ATP generation, leading ultimately to hypoglycemia, severe metabolic acidosis, uremia, and death. Although a mitochondrial gene defect has been identified in the MCAD A985G mutation, it is not useful in direct gene analysis because, like the cystic fibrosis gene, its mutation exists in only 80% of cases of oxidation defects. The authors report a method using cultured fetal amniocytes or maternal or newborn fibroblasts cultured with palmitic acid triply labeled with deuterium and assayed by mass spectroscopy. The purpose is to demonstrate the β oxidation defect by demonstrating the lack of short-chain fatty acids complexed to carnitine in cell culture. The result is independent of the locus of the gene defect or whether it occurs in long- or medium-chain dehydrogenase. This enables the diagnosis to be made in the mother, the fetus as in case 2, or the newborn in time for dietary treatment and for L-carnitine to be used. As techniques of this sort grow in numbers and use, more cases of defective fatty acid metabolism are certain to be reported.

T.H. Kirschbaum, M.D.

References

1. 1992 YEAR BOOK OF OBSTETRICS AND GYNECOLOGY, pp 69–70.
2. 1994 YEAR BOOK OF OBSTETRICS AND GYNECOLOGY, pp 116–117.
3. 1994 YEAR BOOK OF OBSTETRICS AND GYNECOLOGY, pp 211–213.

Fetal RhD Genotyping in Fetal Cells Flow Sorted From Maternal Blood
Geifman-Holtzman O, Bernstein IM, Berry SM, et al (Med Ctr Hosp of Vermont, Burlington; Hutzel Hosp, Detroit; Massachusetts Gen Hosp, Boston)
Am J Obstet Gynecol 174:818–822, 1996   8–4

Background.—Even with the availability of prophylactic Rh immunoglobulin, RhD hemolytic disease of the newborn still occurs in 10.6 of

10,000 live births. Determining fetal RhD status from fetal cells circulating in the maternal blood would avoid multiple invasive procedures and exposure to Rh immune globulins. The accuracy of noninvasive fetal RhD typing in cells obtained by fluorescence-activated cell sorting from the maternal blood was evaluated.

Methods.—The study included fetal cells from 18 Rh-negative pregnant women referred for amniocentesis or cordocentesis. There was 1 twin pregnancy. Fetal cells were isolated from the maternal blood by fluorescence-activated cell sorting. The sorted cells then underwent polymerase chain reaction amplification of a 261 based pair fragment of the RhD gene. Fetal cells showing a positive RhD-amplification product were considered to predict an RhD-positive genotype in the fetus.

Results.—The noninvasive procedure correctly predicted the fetal genotype in 16 of 19 cases: 10 Rh-positive and 6 Rh-negative fetuses. The other 3 fetuses were RhD positive, but no amplification product was detected. The relationship between the amplification product and the RhD-positive genotype was significant.

Conclusions.—Fetal RhD genotyping can be done noninvasively using fetal cells obtained from the maternal blood by fluorescence-activated cell sorting. If no amplification product appears, the presence of fetal material in the specimen must be confirmed. The noninvasive test already has a positive predictive value of 100% and a negative predictive value of 67%, and accuracy should improve with further advances in fetal cell purity and yield.

▶ Identification of the relatively complex Rh gene on chromosome I has enabled application of recombinant DNA techniques to preimplantation embryonic cells,[1] and, in this case, to fetal cells isolated from maternal blood during pregnancy. Specifically, a fluorescein tag is attached to fetal nucleated red blood cells found in maternal blood using a monoclonal antibody specific to fetal cell nuclei. A fluorescent activated cell sorter is used to collect an enriched sample of fetal red blood cells to avoid problems of dilution and maternal cell contamination when DNA is extracted from a mixture of maternal and fetal cells. Polymerase chain reaction is then carried out on DNA extracted from the sorted cells using primers that yield a 261 based pair segment of the D portion of the Rh gene. Using 19 pregnancies in Rh-negative women, sensitivity of detection was 77% and specificity 100%, with no false positives but 33% false negatives. Although this is rapid progress for this approach to noninvasive fetal Rh typing, the high false negative rate precludes clinical use at present. If the rapid rate of progress continues, it should not be long before a clinically useful determination of this sort becomes available to us.

T.H. Kirschbaum, M.D.

Reference

1. 1996 YEAR BOOK OF OBSTETRICS AND GYNECOLOGY, pp 220–221.

The Time of Appearance and Disappearance of Fetal DNA From the Maternal Circulation

Thomas MR, Tutschek B, Frost A, et al (Imperial College London; Univ College London; London Gynaecology and Fertility Centre)
Prenat Diagn 15:641–646, 1995

8–5

Background.—Fetal cell retrieval from the maternal circulation enables noninvasive prenatal cytogenetic or DNA diagnosis. Before such screening can become routine, it must be determined whether sufficient fetal cells are present for analysis and whether the time of cell appearance varies significantly. Whether cells from previous pregnancies persist in the blood must also be determined, along with how soon after pregnancy the cells are cleared from the blood.

Methods.—Thirty women who had become pregnant in an in vitro fertilization program, in whom the exact time of conception was known, were enrolled in a study of the time of appearance and disappearance of fetal DNA from the maternal circulation. Peripheral blood was obtained from the women, and a single-copy Y chromosome DNA sequence was amplified using the polymerase chain reaction. The time of conception was confirmed by serial ultrasound scans.

Findings.—In all women carrying male fetuses, Y chromosome–specific DNA was identified. The earliest detection was at 4 weeks and 5 days. The latest detection was at 7 weeks and 1 day. Eight weeks after delivery, Y chromosome–specific sequences were no longer found in any of the mothers of male infants. None of the women pregnant only with female infants showed Y chromosome sequences.

Conclusions.—Fetal DNA appears in the maternal circulation early in the first trimester and can be detected in all pregnancies tested by 7 weeks. Fetal DNA continues to be detectable throughout pregnancy and is cleared from the maternal circulation 2 months after parturition. If fetal cells can be isolated from maternal contamination and without problems of contamination from previous pregnancies, early noninvasive prenatal diagnosis for aneuploidies and inherited disorders in all pregnancies will be possible.

▶ The ability to isolate fetal cells from circulating maternal blood allows fetal genetic analysis to be done without invading placental membranes or the fetal vasculature.[1, 2] This report deals not with well-established feasibility, but with timing of the first appearance of fetal DNA in maternal blood. As often reported, the identification of fetal cells involves fetuses known to be male with amplification of fetal DNA obtained by maternal venepuncture searching for a known single copy of a DNA sequence known to be derived from the Y chromosome. Using infertility patients in whom conception and implantation times are well known allows the needed precision in pregnancy dating to establish early appearance of fetal DNA. Astonishingly, fetal DNA was detected as early as 33 days after a last menstrual period and was routinely detectable in this group of 18 women by 50 days. This means that as soon as development of the heart has proceeded to the onset of fluid circulation, fetal cells, whether blood cells or trophoblastic, can be detected in the maternal circulation. This finding expands considerably the range of utilization of fetal cells captured in this way. It also anticipates the report that fetal cells may be detected in nonpregnant women years after a pregnancy has been completed. Apparently they represent fetal-to-maternal cell transfer and transplantation in miniature, with long-term growth and survival of clones of fetal cells acquired during pregnancy years earlier.

T.H. Kirschbaum, M.D.

References

1. 1990 Year Book of Obstetrics and Gynecology, pp 178–180.
2. 1993 Year Book of Obstetrics and Gynecology, pp 199–201.

Male Fetal Progenitor Cells Persist in Maternal Blood for as Long as 27 Years Postpartum

Bianchi DW, Zickwolf GK, Weil GJ, et al (Harvard Med School, Boston; Tufts Univ, Boston)
Proc Natl Acad Sci U S A 93:705–708, 1996

8–6

Objective.—It has long been known that fetal cells are present in maternal blood, and this finding has been confirmed using modern molecular genetic techniques. The presence of fetal cells in the maternal blood has important implications not only for diagnosis but also for our understanding of reproductive immunobiology. Persistent fetal cells are found in the maternal circulatory system many years after delivery.

Methods.—The study included 32 pregnant women and 8 nonpregnant women. These women had given birth to boys 6 months to 27 years previously. Antibodies to various cluster differentiation (CD) antigens were used to sort mononuclear cells by flow cytometry. The finding of Y chromosome sequences in PCR-amplified DNA was interpreted as predicting a male fetus or providing evidence of persistent cells from a previous male fetus.

Results.—Male DNA was detected in 13 of 19 pregnant women who were carrying male fetuses and in 4 of 13 women who were carrying female fetuses. All of the women with female fetuses had had previous pregnancies with male fetuses or pregnancies that had ended in abortion. Six of the 8 nonpregnant women who had previously given birth to male infants had male DNA in their CD34+CD38+ cells, including 1 women whose last son was born 27 years previously.

Conclusions.—Women may continue to have circulating fetal CD34+ or CD34+CD38+ cells for many years after pregnancy. The findings present the possibility that pregnancy may result in a long-term, low-grade chimeric state in child-bearing women. This "microchimerism" may play an important role in the mother's immune tolerance of the fetus.

▶ In work done more than 20 years ago,[1] quinacrine fluorescence of the distal two thirds of the long arm of the Y (male) sex chromosome was reported in nuclei from the blood of parous women for up to 1 year after delivery of a male infant. This report is part of a collaborative National Institutes of Health project aimed at collecting fetal cells from the blood of pregnant women to allow noninvasive fetal diagnosis and to obtain fetal hematopoietic stem cells for transplantation therapy. Such cells, expressing the appropriate clonal designator (CD34+) for transplantation, are useful in treatment of hemoglobinopathies and genetic immune deficient states. In this study, the identification of the Y chromosome used PCR using primers specific to a DNA sequence on the Y chromosome (Y49a) on cells sorted from maternal blood using fluorescent antibody to CD34+ and CD38+. This latter designator is characteristic of differentiated lymphoid cells. Gel electrophoresis (Southern blot) was then done. The work is conspicuous for carefully designed controls for male contamination, nonspecific fluorescence, PCR false positive amplification, and observer bias. Using these techniques, male DNA was found in 4 of 13 women pregnant with female children, 2 with previous male infants and 2 others whose pregnancies ended in abortion and the sex of the fetuses was not known. In 8 nonpregnant parous women, male DNA was found in 6, proving the presence of chimerism, or the presence of cells from more than 1 zygote surviving in the same individual. Almost certainly these represent quantitatively small microtransplants of fetal cells transferred to mothers from male fetuses during a prior pregnancy.

The "grandmother theory" indicates that Rh-negative women may have become Rh sensitized from maternal to fetal transmission of Rh-positive cells during the pregnancy that resulted in the Rh-negative female, then a fetus, and so have produced part of the 1.8% of Rh-negative women who become sensitized as primigravidas.[2] It is possible that microtransplants of maternal Rh-positive hematopoietic cells may explain sensitization despite the small quantity of maternal blood found in fetal blood at birth. More significant is what this spontaneous transplantation may mean to the future of stem cell transplantation for the treatment of thalassemia major or combined immune deficiency victims. Although it is currently difficult to obtain these chimeras even in experimental animals, those spontaneously successful human transplants provide hope that with time the process may become a therapeutic reality.

T.H. Kirschbaum, M.D.

References

1. Schroeder J: *Transplantation* 17:346, 1974.
2. Scott JR: *Obstet Gynecol* 49:9, 1977.

Clinical Experience With Preimplantation Genetic Diagnosis of Cystic Fibrosis (F508)

Ao A, Ray P, Harper J, et al (Hammersmith Hosp, London; Univ College London; Baylor College of Medicine, Houston; et al)
Prenat Diagn 16:137–142, 1996

8–7

Background.—Cystic fibrosis (CF) results from mutations in the cystic fibrosis transmembrane regulator (CFTR) gene on chromosome 7, the most frequent mutation being a 3 base pair deletion designated ΔF508. With preimplantation genetic diagnosis (PGD), embryos fertilized in vitro can now be screened for possible CF before they are implanted. An experience with the use of PGD for prenatal genetic diagnosis of the ΔF508 CF mutation is reported.

Methods.—The study included 12 couples for whom both parents had the ΔF508 deletion. Embryos were fertilized by in vitro fertilization (IVF), followed by cleavage stage biopsy on days 2 and 3. On these days, 1 or 2 cells were removed for genetic analysis by nested polymerase chain reaction and heteroduplex formation. Of 115 embryos developing to cleavage stages, successful biopsy was done in 114.

Results.—Seventy-three percent of embryos underwent successful genetic analysis. In the rest, amplification was unsuccessful, or 2 or more cells gave discordant results. One or 2 normal or carrier embryos were transferred in 15 of 18 cycles, with 5 clinical pregnancies established. The 5 singleton babies born were homozygous for the normal allele.

Conclusions.—For couples with the ΔF508 mutation, IVF and cleavage-stage biopsy can provide sufficient, unaffected embryos for uterine transfer. The 33% pregnancy rate achieved in this study is comparable to that in other IVF patients. The PGD technique may be applicable to other genetic diseases, including those with higher rates of affected embryos.

▶ The identification of the CFTR gene on chromosome 7 has made it possible, through IVF and biopsy of blastomeres before compaction, to rule out CF in pregnancies produced by couples heterozygous for the trait.[1-3] Further, this Hammersmith Hospital–based group now has sufficient experience, based on 18 cycles in 12 such couples to establish some success rates that serve as benchmarks for others. In general the techniques are the same as those described in the paper abstracted in the 1994 YEAR BOOK.[2] Starting with 243 recovered oocytes, 137 (56%) were successfully fertilized in vitro, but 22 embryos were lost at or before the 2-cell stage. This left 115 (47%) of the initial oocytes for continued study. All but 1 were successfully biopsied, approximately half contributing 2 blastomeres for PCR amplification. Amplification efficiency was 73%, leaving 83 interpretable studies or 34% of recovered ova. In the total experience of 18 IVF cycles, it was possible to identify 15 unaffected embryos, and these were transferred and resulted in 7 pregnancies (39% of embryo transfers). Two failed normal development and the 5 resulting infants have been delivered and are homozygous negative for the altered CFTR gene. No errors in diagnosis were established in this study, but the ratio of heterozygotes to homozygotes, which Mendelian laws would predict is 1, was 0.41, indicating a deficiency of heterozygotes. The authors attribute this to failure to amplify 1 of the alleles (allele drop out) in some allele pairs. This is a particular problem when more than 1 mutation involving the CFTR gene is present and the team finds it can reduce this error by modifying the denaturation temperature in PCR. This is a seminal report by this group, which stands at the forefront of this piece of selective gene identification.

T.H. Kirschbaum, M.D.

References

1. 1990 YEAR BOOK OF OBSTETRICS AND GYNECOLOGY, p 184.
2. 1994 YEAR BOOK OF OBSTETRICS AND GYNECOLOGY, pp 210–211.
3. 1995 YEAR BOOK OF OBSTETRICS AND GYNECOLOGY, pp 218–220.

Intestinal Atresia Following Intraamniotic Use of Dyes
Glüer S (Medizinische Hochschule Hannover, Germany)
Eur J Pediatr Surg 5:240–242, 1995

8–8

Background.—The use of methylene blue dye for diagnostic amniocentesis has been discouraged because of its association with jejunoileal atresia. Four cases of jejunoileal atresia after intra-amniotic injection of dye have occurred since 1991.

Case Report Summary.—The indication for amniocentesis was advanced maternal age in 3 cases and a pathologic result in a noninvasive chromosomal screening test in 1 case. Amniocentesis was performed between the 15th and 17th week of gestation in all cases. To be certain that samples of amniotic fluid were taken from both sacks, dyes were injected into the first puncture. Methylene blue dye was used as the marker in 3 cases and indigo carmine was used in 1 case. The results of amniocentesis were normal in all cases. The neonates were born between the 29th and 36th week of gestation, with birth weights of 1,120 to 2,300 g. There were no associated anomalies. Three neonates had multiple jejunoileal atresias and 1 had a single atresia. By fetus position and sex, the infant with jejunoileal atresia was identified as the one exposed to the dye in utero in all 4 cases. The dilated proximal part of the jejunum was resected and end-to-end anastomosis performed. After 12 to 17 days of total parenteral nutrition, oral feeding was initiated. All 4 of these neonates had complicated postoperative courses, with sepsis in 4, cholestasis in 1, and reoperation for postoperative ileus in 2.

Conclusions.—Although the teratogenic effect of methylene blue and indigo carmine on the small bowel is not well understood, the use of synthetic dyes in second-trimester amniocentesis should be avoided because of the association with intestinal atresia. As an alternative dye marker, a membrane-free hemolysate made from maternal blood has been proposed.

▶ Though hardly conclusive evidence establishing methylene blue or indigo carmine as a teratogen, this series of 4 case reports should provide a caution to those who use amniotic injection of these materials to ensure appropriate amniotic fluid sampling in multiple gestation. Unlike atresia of upper and lower gastrointestinal tract segments, atretic small-bowel segments often show amniotic debris distal to the point of atresia, testifying to small-bowel patency at some time in fetal life prior to an acquired bowel insult that results in atresia. Further, this Hannover pediatric surgical unit reports an increasing incidence of the defect, which parallels the increasing use of amniocentesis in Germany. Though certainly more data should be collected on this point, the authors point to the possibility that synthetic dye substances capable of injuring the small-bowel lumen during exposure to swallowed dye, prolonged by the torpid activity of fetal small bowel, should be avoided in the second trimester and some biologically derived marker material substituted for these dyes.

T.H. Kirschbaum, M.D.

Limb Defects and Chorionic Villus Sampling: Results From an International Registry, 1992–94

Froster UG, Jackson L (Universitätsspital Zürich, Switzerland; Jefferson Med College, Philadelphia)
Lancet 347:489–494, 1996   8–9

Background.—The safety of chorionic villus sampling (CVS) during pregnancy has been questioned. Several reports have described limb defects in infants exposed to this procedure. The World Health Organization (WHO) began an international registration of post–CVS limb defects in 1992 to address these concerns.

Methods.—Seventy-seven of 138,996 infants or fetuses reported to the WHO CVS Registry between May 1992 and May 1994 had limb defects. Affected infants and fetuses were evaluated using standard methods—by excluding syndromes, inherited disorders, and defects occurring in previable fetuses. Pattern analysis was used to study the limb deficiencies.

Findings.—In 64.6% of the affected infants and fetuses, defects occurred in the upper limbs. Lower limbs were affected in 12.5%. Both upper and lower limbs were affected in 20.8%. These values are consistent with limb defect distribution figures in several large population-based studies. Limb defects were transverse in 40.8% and longitudinal in 59.2%, compared with 42.7% and 57.3%, respectively, in a population not exposed to prenatal CVS.

Conclusions.—These findings do not suggest that the risk of limb defects is increased by CVS. The overall frequency and pattern distribution of limb deficiencies in the cohort studied did not differ significantly from the background population. Also, gestational age at CVS was uncorrelated with the severity of defects.

▶ This report of limb reduction defects following CVS collected from 63 European and American centers reporting to the WHO CVS Registry established in 1992 helps bring us up-to-date in this controversy.[1] Following 2 initial reports of case incidences of more than 1% among 2 series of 289 and 394 cases of CVS, 2 larger studies, one for more than 80,000 cases of CVS[2] and one in a population study of 1.2 million births,[3] yielded incidence figures of approximately 1 in 1,600 or 0.06%. In this, the largest collection of reported cases of CVS, the incidence of limb reduction defects range from 0.05% to 0.06% depending on whether simple nail defects alone were counted and whether abortion material was included. Still, occasional reports of limb defects following CVS before 8 weeks gestational age continue.[4] In this study, almost 25% of cases were excluded for inadequacies in data, and reports from multiple centers increase the chance of differences in data management and diagnostic criteria. It is impossible to prove CVS does not result in an increased incidence of limb defects, just as it is impossible to prove any negative hypothesis. Nonetheless, the preponderance of data suggests that it does not occur with increased risk. It still seems prudent to avoid CVS before complete limb differentiation at 10 weeks of gestational age.

T.H. Kirschbaum, M.D.

References

1. 1993 YEAR BOOK OF OBSTETRICS AND GYNECOLOGY, pp 185–187.
2. Kuliev AM, Modell B, Jackson L, et al: Limb abnormalities and chorionic villus sampling. *Lancet* 340:668, 1992.
3. Froster-Iskenius UG: *Teratology* 39:127, 1990.
4. Brombati B, et al: *Prenat Diagn* 12:789, 1992.

9 The Puerperium

Long-term Diabetogenic Effect of Single Pregnancy in Women With Previous Gestational Diabetes Mellitus
Peters RK, Kjos SL, Xiang A, et al (Univ of Southern California, Los Angeles)
Lancet 347:227–230, 1996   9–1

Background.—The progressive metabolic changes occurring during pregnancy lead to marked insulin resistance. However, these episodes of insulin resistance have little or no effect on the general population's risk of non-insulin-dependent diabetes mellitus (NIDDM). Women in whom gestational diabetes develops appear to have insufficient pancreatic β-cell reserves to increase insulin secretion in the presence of pregnancy-related insulin resistance. The effects of subsequent pregnancy on NIDDM risk in women with a history of gestational diabetes—and thus with a high prevalence of pancreatic β-cell dysfunction—were evaluated.

Methods.—The study sample comprised 666 Hispanic women with gestational diabetes who were seen at a county hospital high-risk family planning clinic. Each patient was followed up from the time of her last postpartum visit until her last clinic visit or until diabetes developed, as defined by the National Diabetes Data Group criteria. During follow-up, the women underwent an annual examination, which included weighing and oral glucose tolerance testing. Additional pregnancies and other risk factors for diabetes were evaluated for their long-term diabetogenic effects. The other risk factors included antepartum oral glucose tolerance, highest fasting glucose, and gestational age at diagnosis during the index pregnancy; postpartum body mass index; and glucose tolerance, weight change, breast-feeding, and contraceptive use during follow-up.

Results.—The mean duration of follow-up was 7.5 years, during which time 87 of the women completed another pregnancy. In just 7 of these women NIDDM developed immediately after the additional pregnancy. Patients with an additional pregnancy had a subsequent annual NIDDM incidence rate of 31%, compared with 12% for the cohort overall. Additional pregnancy increased the rate ratio of NIDDM to 3.34, according to proportional hazards regression analysis, compared with women without additional risk factors and after adjustment for other diabetes risk factors. The rate ratio for NIDDM also increased by 1.95 for each 10 pounds gained during follow-up, after adjustment for the additional pregnancy and other risk factors.

"

Conclusions.—In women with a history of gestational diabetes, a subsequent pregnancy more than triples the risk of developing NIDDM. This increase occurs independent of the well-recognized effects of weight gain and other risk factors. Episodes of insulin resistance may play a role in the declining β-cell function in patients at high risk of NIDDM. Intervention should focus on early identification of patients with limited β-cell reserve, before hyperglycemia develops.

▶ It has long been assumed that gestational diabetes, reverting to normal carbohydrate metabolism post partum, is a mark of a relative pancreatic β-cell deficiency in insulin production and that subsequent years, marked by aging, increased obesity, increased insulin resistance, and subsequent childbearing, have a high likelihood of resulting in fixed chemical diabetes.[1,2] This study allows the calculation of the relative impact of at least 2 of those 3 variables. The long-term follow-up involved 666 women with gestational diabetes treated for a mean duration of 22 months and as long as 7.5 years at a contraceptive, general gynecologic care clinic at Los Angeles County Women's Hospital.

Because past work from this clinic demonstrated a high rate of progression to permanent diabetes in this Hispanic population, this facilitates the establishment of statistically significant rate calculations. The key to the study is the use of proportional hazards regression analysis. This technique uses the time variable as in life-table analysis, establishing a new subset of women with a pregnancy subsequent to that first manifesting gestational diabetes, without subtraction from the entire sample. It allows confounding variables such as the rate of weight gain, age, severity of the disease, and adequacy of control to be considered as independent, time-linked variables affecting the time of diagnosis of eventual fixed diabetes.

In data collected from 1987 through the first half of 1993, 21.9% of women following gestational diabetes mellitus (GDM) had diabetes mellitus, an incidence rate of 11.9% per year. During this time, the impact of subsequent pregnancy alone was to increase the risk ratio for diabetes by 3.34 times (confidence interval, 1.80–6.19). The independent effect of weight gain of 10 pounds after the weight recorded at the first postpartum visit after the pregnancy with GDM was a risk ratio of 1.95-fold (confidence interval, 1.63–2.33) longer. This means that women with GDM should be cautioned that contraception is important in reducing the likelihood of diabetes, more so than restricting weight gain, an important covariate.

T.H. Kirschbaum, M.D.

References

1. 1992 YEAR BOOK OF OBSTETRICS AND GYNECOLOGY, p 62.
2. 1995 YEAR BOOK OF OBSTETRICS AND GYNECOLOGY, pp 228–229.

Resistance to Insulin-Mediated Glucose Uptake and Hyperinsulinemia in Women Who Had Preeclampsia During Pregnancy

Fuh MM-T, Yin C-S, Pei D, et al (Natl Defense Med Ctr, Taipei, Taiwan; Stanford Univ, Palo Alto, Calif)
Am J Hypertens 8:768–771, 1995
9–2

Background.—Patients with high blood pressure are resistant to insulin-mediated glucose uptake and are hyperinsulinemic. By examining women in whom hypertension developed during pregnancy, the potential causal relationship among insulin resistance, compensatory hyperinsulinemia, and blood pressure regulation was investigated.

Methods.—Twenty-six nulliparous women were studied approximately 8 weeks after a normal delivery. Thirteen of the group had preeclampsia diagnosed during pregnancy; the other 13 served as controls. Both groups underwent 2 tests: plasma glucose and insulin concentrations were measured before and 30, 60, 90, 120, and 180 minutes after a 75-g oral glucose load; and resistance to insulin-mediated glucose disposal was estimated by the insulin suppression test.

Results.—Plasma glucose responses were essentially identical in the 2 groups (Fig 1). However, the insulin response of the preeclamptic group was significantly greater than that of those who had a normal pregnancy. Steady-state plasma insulin concentrations during the insulin suppression test were similar in the 2 groups. However, the mean steady-state plasma glucose values were significantly higher in those with preeclampsia compared within the control group.

Conclusion.—Compared with women who had had a normal pregnancy, women who had preeclampsia during pregnancy were resistant to

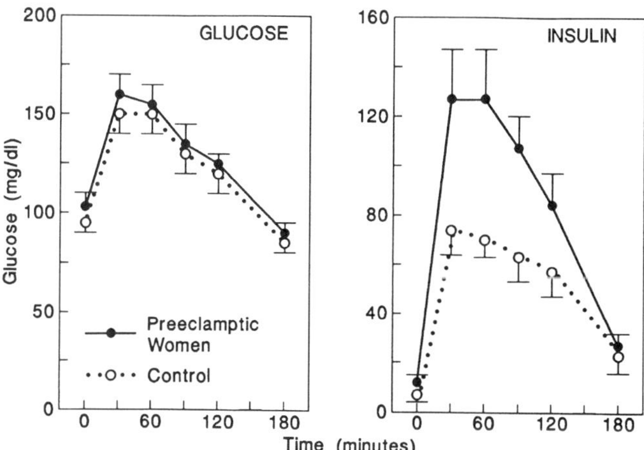

FIGURE 1.—Plasma glucose (**left**) and insulin (**right**) concentrations in response to a 75-g oral glucose challenge 2 months after delivery in patients with either a normal (*open circles*) or preeclamtic (*filled circles*) pregnancy. (Courtesy of Fuh MM-T, Yin C-S, Pei D, et al.: Resistance to Insulin-Mediated Glucose Uptake and Hyperinsulinemia in Women Who Had Pre-eclampsia During Pregnancy. *Am J Hypertens* 8:768–771, Copyright 1995 by American Journal of Hypertension, Inc.)

insulin-mediated glucose uptake and were hyperinsulemic 8 weeks after delivery. These results offer direct support for the conclusions of past studies, in which evidence of an association between high blood pressure and insulin resistance in pregnancy was based on estimates of plasma glucose and/or insulin response to a glucose challenge.

▶ Forty years ago, Dr. Richard Burt, a fine obstetrician-investigator from Bowman Gray School of Medicine, demonstrated insulin resistance and hyperinsulinemia in preeclampsia.[1] Those early observations have gained in significance and are now understood as part of the syndrome X, linking those same changes in carbohydrate metabolism to altered lipid metabolism, obesity, chronic hypertension, and arteriosclerotic heart disease.[2] This study of puerperal preeclamptic women 8 weeks after delivery shows quite nicely the presence of reactive hyperinsulinism compared with controls, likely reflecting hyperinsulinism during pregnancy. Some, but not all, women showed residual hypertension. This is not surprising since preeclamptic blood pressures may take 12 to 16 weeks to return to normal. In a few patients, an elevated steady-state plasma glucose concentration was seen. In this study, obesity was not a determinant since body mass indices showed no significant difference when comparing test and control groups. That is important because surplus body fat depositions have been linked to the production of tumor-necrotizing factor, which serves to decrease insulin sensitivity at end-organ sites. There's no longer any question that insulin resistance and hyperinsulinism, often coexisting with obesity, are part of the preeclamptic syndrome in primigravid women. Whether altered carbohydrate metabolism is caused by preeclampsia or reflects a metabolic predisposition to preeclampsia is an important question waiting to be answered.

T.H. Kirschbaum, M.D.

References

1. Burt RL: *Obstet Gynecol* 6:51, 1955; 9:310, 1957.
2. 1996 YEAR BOOK OF OBSTETRICS AND GYNECOLOGY, pp 67–68.

Maternal Thyroid Peroxidase Antibodies During Pregnancy: A Marker of Impaired Child Development?
Pop VJ, de Vries E, van Baar AL, et al (Univ of Tilburg, The Netherlands; Catharina Hosp, Eindhoven, The Netherlands; Academic Med Ctr, Amsterdam; et al)
J Clin Endocrinol Metab 80:3561–3566, 1995   9–3

Background.—In the postpartum period, thyroid dysfunction occurs in 4% to 7% and depression in 10% to 15% of women. Some evidence indicates an association between postpartum depression and thyroid dysfunction or elevated levels of thyroid peroxidase antibodies (TPO-Ab;

formerly microsomal antibodies). The effects of maternal thyroid dysfunction and depression on child development were investigated.

Methods.—During an 18-month period, 382 women were invited to participate in the study. The final analysis of data included 230 women and their children. These women were studied at 32 weeks' gestation and after delivery at 4 weeks, every 6 weeks until 34 weeks, and at 5 years. The Dutch translation of the McCarthy Scales of Children's Abilities was used to assess child development.

Results.—All the children had normal thyroid function tests on postpartum day 7; the 178 evaluated children were clinically euthyroid at school age. At 5 years after delivery, the children of the 19 women with elevated TPO-Ab at 32 weeks' gestation (and normal thyroid function) had significantly lower McCarthy Scales of Children's Abilities scores than the children of the women who were TPO-Ab–negative. The difference in extrapolated IQ scores was about 10.5 points, and the difference was significant even after correction for possible confounding variables. Extrapolated IQ scores were also lower in children whose mothers had a low education level or who had a current, past, or family history of depression.

Conclusions.—Children of women with high titers of thyroid peroxidase antibodies (and normal thyroid function) in late gestation may be at increased risk of impaired development. A larger prospective study identifying antibody-positive women in the first trimester is needed to decide whether the mothers might benefit from low doses of T_4 during early pregnancy.

▶ Readers may recognize thyroid peroxidase antibody by its former name—thyroid microsomal antibody.[1] Useful as an indicator of autoimmune thyroiditis, it is most commonly associated with postpartum clinical hyperthyroidism over the 6 to 12 weeks after delivery, with mild if any symptoms, followed by a more prolonged period of hypothyroidism lasting for as long as 6 to 9 months. Occasionally, chronic hypothyroidism follows such a sequence.[2, 3]

The usual reported incidence of postpartum immune thyroiditis is 5% to 10% among those who have previously written about the problem, and the 3% incidence of puerperal thyroid dysfunction here seems a bit low. There is no question of the relationship between puerperal thyroid dysfunction and the presence of the antibody.

The authors make 2 additional contributions to what is generally known, both using psychometrics. The incidence of postpartum depression of 12% and of depression over the 5 years after delivery of 23% seems extraordinarily high in terms of the reports of others. Second, when behavioral skills of child performance are compared between 19 children with antibody-positive mothers and 211 with antibody-negative mothers, a series of *t* tests found lower mean performance scores in those of antibody-positive mothers, except for quantitative performance and memory functions. Because thyroid function was normal in antibody-positive women with no difference in thyroid assay values from those who were antibody-negative, and because all infants had normal thyroid function at 5 days of life, it is hard to use these data to control anything in particular. Perhaps a problem lies in the use of *t* tests for differences between mean psychometric values for mothers who are antibody-positive and the 19 antibody-negative women with whom they are compared. A requirement for the use of *t* tests for evaluating differences in women is to prove, for each of the 6 tests applied to the data, that the 19 test scores have normal frequency distributions. Without that information, the reader should not accept the authors' claims to statistical significance.

T.H. Kirschbaum, M.D.

References

1. 1990 YEAR BOOK OF OBSTETRICS AND GYNECOLOGY, pp 189–190.
2. 1988 YEAR BOOK OF OBSTETRICS AND GYNECOLOGY, pp 189–191.
3. 1992 YEAR BOOK OF OBSTETRICS AND GYNECOLOGY, p 175.

Clinical Case Seminar: Lymphocytic Hypophysitis: Clinicopathological Findings
Thodou E, Asa SL, Kontogeorgos G, et al (Univ of Toronto)
J Clin Endocrinol Metab 80:2302–2311, 1995   9–4

Introduction.—Lymphocytic hypophysitis is often associated with other autoimmune disorders, such as thyroiditis, adrenalitis, atrophic gastritis, and lymphocytic parathyroiditis. The clinicopathologic findings of 16 patients with histologically proved lymphocytic adenohypophysitis were analyzed.

Results.—Fourteen of 16 patients were women. In 10 of the 14 women, illness was associated with pregnancy. Laboratory findings included 7 elevated blood hormone levels; 6 cases of hyperprolactinemia; 2 elevated T_4 levels; 1 elevated human growth hormone blood level, resulting in elevated insulin-like growth factor-1 level and a clinical picture of acromegaly; and 3 cases of hypercalcemia. In 4 patients, hyperprolactinemia was associated with pregnancy. In 2 patients, hyperthyroidism was attributed to coexisting autoimmune thyroiditis. In 3 of 4 patients with thyroid dysfunction, onset was associated with pregnancy. Of these, 2 had hypothyroidism and 2 had hyperthyroidism. In the 2 patients evaluated, tests of circulating antipituitary antibodies yielded negative results. Light microscopy showed a lymphoplasmacytic infiltrate in all patients. These infiltrates occasionally formed lymphoid follicles and were accompanied by differing numbers of neutrophils, eosinophils, and macrophages. Fourteen of 16 specimens underwent immunocytochemical analysis. In 13 of 14 specimens, immunoreactivity for growth hormone and prolactin was detected. In 5 patients, corticotropin was not identified. Evaluation of inflammatory cells showed a polyclonal population of T and B cells with positivity for LCA, L-26, UCHL, and κ- and λ-light chains, and DND 53. Electron microscopy showed adenohypophysial tissue infiltrated by inflammatory cells. These cells were mostly plasma cells, lymphocytes, macrophages, and periodically eosinophils and neutrophils.

In 2 patients, a progressive and total recovery of pituitary function was seen after transsphenoidal biopsy. Surgical intervention resulted in further deterioration of the visual field defects in 1 patient and in diabetes insipidus in another patient.

Conclusion.—Lymphocytic hypophysitis should be suspected in the differential diagnosis of pituitary masses in patients with pituitary hormone deficiency with coexisting autoimmune disorder and in pregnant and postpartum women. This diagnosis should also be considered in patients with rapidly growing pituitary masses associated with compressive effects with or without hypophysial dysfunction and patients with hyperprolactinemia that responds to bromoergocriptine therapy without an associated decrease in pituitary mass or compressive symptomatology. Patients with progressive compressive features and those in whom radiographic or neurologic deterioration is observed during conservative management with corticosteroids and hormone replacement should undergo surgical treatment. However, conservative treatment may obviate the need for surgical intervention. The diagnosis can be proved only by histologic confirmation.

▶ This uncommon syndrome appears most often in either late pregnancy or the puerperium and resembles lymphocytic thyroiditis in its pathology, time of occurrence, and tendency to spontaneously resolve. Lymphocytic hypophysitis presents most often as a pituitary mass lesion with headache and bitemporal visual field defects. Hyperprolactinemia may result from failure of tonic dopamine inhibition to act on altered pituitary. Pituitary hormone deficiencies may be global, but isolated thyroid-stimulating hormone or corticotropin deficiencies appear most commonly. In this series of 16 cases, 25% had autoimmune thyroiditis. Clinical findings in the puerperium may suggest Sheehan's syndrome, but the pituitary enlargement is useful in ruling out that diagnosis. Though autoimmunity to pituitary hormone or a structural component is certainly likely, the precise role of the variety of identified pituitary autoantibodies remains obscured. There may well be multiple discrete causes. Bromoergocryptine is effective in relieving hyperprolactinemia, but not in reducing the size of the pituitary enlarged with inflammatory infiltrate. Thyroid and adrenal hormone replacement is often needed, and its failure can lead to mortality. Transsphenoidal resection may be needed to prevent blindness or to replace other failed modes of therapy. The diagnosis of lymphocytic hypophysitis belongs in the differential appraisal of hypopituitarism, hyperprolactinemia, or hypothyroidism occurring in the puerperium.

T.H. Kirschbaum, M.D.

Infectious Morbidity, Operative Blood Loss, and Length of the Operative Procedure After Cesarean Delivery by Method of Placental Removal and Site of Uterine Repair

Magann EF, Washburne JF, Harris RL, et al (Univ of Mississippi, Jackson; Univ of Florida, Gainesville)
J Am Coll Surg 181:517–520, 1995   9–5

Background.—Prophylactic antibiotics at the time of cesarean delivery reportedly help decrease the incidence of postoperative endometriosis. The effect of uterine site repair and placental management in women treated with prophylactic antibiotics has not been investigated. The relationship between postcesarean infectious morbidity and method of placental removal and site of uterine repair therefore was prospectively investigated among women treated with prophylactic antibiotics at cesarean delivery.

Patients and Methods.—Two hundred eighty-four women who underwent cesarean delivery were randomly assigned to 1 of 4 groups based on method of placental removal and site of uterine repair. Seventy-one women were placed in each group. Group 1 patients underwent spontaneous placental removal and in situ uterine repair, group 2 had spontaneous placental removal and exteriorized uterine repair, group 3 underwent manual placental removal and in situ uterine repair, and group 4 had manual placental removal with exteriorized uterine repair.

Patients with temperatures of 100.4°F on 2 occasions separated by 6 hours and exclusive of the first 24 hours, uterine tenderness, or foul-smelling lochia received diagnoses of endometriosis. Women with postoperative endometriosis underwent antibiotic therapy until they were afebrile and asymptomatic for a period of 24 hours, after which treatment was discontinued.

Results.—Maternal age, race, parity, weight, length of time from rupture of membranes, number of vaginal examinations from rupture of membranes to cesarean delivery, and preoperative hematocrit were comparable between groups. Women in each group also had similar intraoperative uterine incisions, anesthesia, incidence of meconium-stained amniotic fluid, Apgar scores, and cord gases. The incidence of postoperative endometriosis was significantly higher among women in group 4, occurring in 45%, compared with 24% in group 1, 30% in group 2, and 18% in group 3 patients. Duration of operation and blood loss at delivery were significantly greater in group 4 patients and hospital stay was longer, compared with patients in the other 3 groups.

Conclusions.—In women receiving prophylactic antibiotics at the time of cesarean delivery, rates of infectious mortality were increased among those undergoing manual placental removal and exteriorization of the uterus for incision repair. Use of these methods also resulted in significantly longer hospital stays, with consequent increased treatment expenses.

▶ This is the latest in a series of well-conducted pieces of clinical research from this group aimed at reducing the maternal morbidity of abdominal delivery. The investigators have previously shown that in women not receiving prophylactic antibiotics, manual placental removal and exteriorization of the uterus for repair increases the incidence of endometritis, and that prophylactic antibiotics reduce the rate of endometritis after spontaneous placental removal. By this latter term, they mean removal of the placenta by uterine compression and cord traction without invading the decidua inside the uterus with the operator's hand.

Here, in a prospective, randomized, comparative study, the investigators evaluate placental and uterine management together in 284 women, administering 4 g of cefazolin within 4 hours after birth in all. They show that the antibiotic use renders exteriorization of the uterus harmless when combined with spontaneous placental expression, but they report a significantly greater risk of endometritis when manual placental removal is combined with exteriorization for repair. Exteriorization lengthens the duration of cesarean section by an average of 4–5 minutes; because blood loss was not measured and observers evidently were not blinded to management. Only the incidence of endometritis appears to be a secure piece of outcome information here. This group's work indicates a need to evaluate the values of exteriorizing the uterus for repair, especially because some have linked it to an increased incidence of symptomatic air embolization, no matter how harmless that apparently common finding usually proves to be.[1]

T.H. Kirschbaum, M.D.

Reference

1. 1995 YEAR BOOK OF OBSTETRICS AND GYNECOLOGY, pp 192–193.

Pudendal Nerve Damage Increases the Risk of Fecal Incontinence in Women With Anal Sphincter Rupture After Childbirth
Tetzschner T, Sørensen M, Rasmussen OØ, et al (Univ of Copenhagen, Glostrup and Herlev, Denmark)
Acta Obstet Gynecol Scand 74:434–440, 1995   9–6

Objective.—The causes and risk factors associated with fecal incontinence resulting from sphincter rupture during childbirth have not been investigated. Women with and without sphincter rupture after childbirth were studied to relate anorectal physiology and history of childbirth to the presence of fecal incontinence.

Methods.—Anal manometry, electromyography, and pudendal nerve terminal motor latency determinations were performed 3 to 5 days after childbirth and 3 months post partum in 94 women (71 primiparous), aged 17 to 40 years, with repaired sphincter rupture and in 19 controls.

Results.—After 3 months, 18 patients were incontinent. Although anal myography showed no differences between groups, anal manometry showed decreased resting and squeeze pressures in continent and incontinent women with sphincter rupture compared with controls after child-

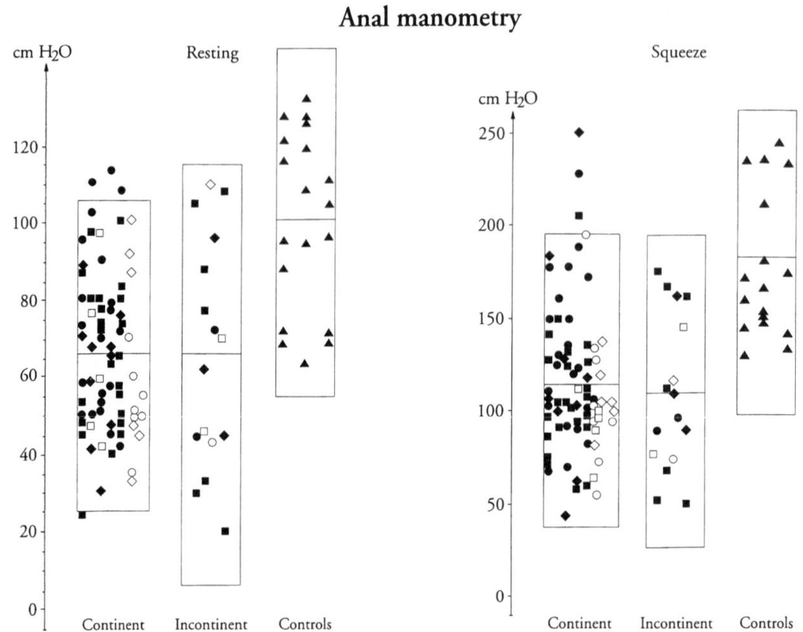

FIGURE 5.—Value of anal manometry at rest and at squeeze in cm H_2O in continent patients, incontinent patients, and controls 3 months after childbirth. The *box* represents mean ± SD. *Filled symbols* represent primiparous and *open symbols* represent multiparous patients. *Open squares* indicate total anal sphincter rupture; *open circles,* partial anal sphincter rupture; *open diamonds,* superficial anal sphincter rupture. (Courtesy of Tetzscher T, Sørensen M, Rasmussen OØ, et al.: Pudendal Nerve Damage Increases the Risk of Fecal Incontinence in Women With Anal Sphincter Rupture After Childbirth. *Acta Obstet Gynecol Scand* 74:434-440, 1995 Munksgaard International Publishers Ltd., Copenhagen, Denmark.)

birth and at 3 months (Fig 5). There was a significant increase in pudendal nerve terminal motor latencies in patients who were incontinent as compared with patients who were continent and controls. Patients with motor latencies of more than 2 ms had a significantly increased risk of incontinence as compared with patients having motor latencies of 2 ms or less. Fecal incontinence or motor latency was not related to either weight or head circumference of the child, manometric or myographic findings, use of pudendal nerve block, length of the second stage of labor, degree of rupture, or use of vacuum extraction.

Conclusion.—Anal manometry indicated the presence of sphincter function damage in both continent and incontinent women and pudendal nerve function damage in incontinent women. Because there was no clear distinction in anorectal physiologic data between incontinent and continent women, it is not possible to predict fecal incontinence.

▶ Here the question is whether the application of neurophysiologic techniques to the analysis of anal incontinence after third-degree perineal laceration or sphincterotomy has anything to offer the practicing obstetrician. The reader may wish to review the 1992 YEAR BOOK[1] and 1995 YEAR BOOK [2] this connection. The incidence of some degree of incontinence was 19% in this sample of 94 women with repaired sphincters studied 3 months post partum. That incidence is similarly reported by other authors and was larger than noted in the small control group used for comparison. The latency between pudendal nerve stimulation and muscular response indicates apparently permanent stretch injury to those largely medullated fibers but was, as in other studies, unrelated to birth weight, parity, fetal head size, pudendal nerve block, or length of the second stage of labor. Forceps were not used, and births were either spontaneous or, in 40% of the cases, by vacuum extractor. Evidence of nerve injury was sufficiently common in control women and showed such wide variability among groups that no significant differences could be discerned. Similarly, anal manometry and electromyography showed decreased function after birth and partial repair at 3 months post partum but no significant differences were seen between continent and incontinent women. Though the findings confirm the relatively high incidence of neuromuscular pelvic floor dysfunction in the puerperium, the number of factors that determine the presence of the symptom is large, and many appear to be independent of the findings of neurophysiologic investigation. In brief, the use of these techniques as currently constituted seems to have little to offer the practicing gynecologist.

T.H. Kirschbaum, M.D.

References

1. 1992 YEAR BOOK OF OBSTETRICS AND GYNECOLOGY, p 174.
2. 1995 YEAR BOOK OF OBSTETRICS AND GYNECOLOGY, pp 196–197.

10 The Newborn

Outcome of Isolated Congenital Complete Heart Block Diagnosed In Utero
Groves AMM, Allan LD, Rosenthal E (Guy's Hosp, London)
Heart 75:190–194, 1996

Background.—Recently, cardiac failure and death have been documented in fetuses with isolated congenital complete heart block diagnosed in utero. Prenatal factors in fetal heart block that might predict death in utero, the need for intervention, or the probability of the need for a pacemaker were identified.

Methods and Findings.—Thirty-six fetuses with congenital complete heart block and structurally normal hearts detected at a tertiary referral unit for fetal echocardiography between 1980 and 1993 were included in the analysis. Twenty-four fetuses survived, 11 with pacemakers; 7 died in utero; 2 died immediately after birth; 2 were aborted electively because of severe hydrops; 1 died of unrelated causes. Heart rates tended to decrease in utero and postnatally. Deteriorating cardiac function was not necessarily associated with the lowest heart rates. A poor prognosis was associated with bradycardia of less than 55 beats/min in early pregnancy or a rapid reduction in heart rate prenatally. Hydrops was also an indicator of poor prognosis, with 83% of the 12 affected fetuses dying. Nine of 10 fetuses with initial heart rates of more than 60 beats/min survived, 3 of whom needed pacing. Only 3 of 7 fetuses with initial heart rates of 50 beats/min or less survived, 2 of whom required pacing. Two fetuses had negative maternal anti-Ro antibodies. One of these died in utero, and 1 underwent heart transplantation after a pacemaker was inserted (Fig 1).

Conclusions.—The prognosis of isolated complete heart block identified in utero can be poor. Individual heart rates do not accurately predict outcomes in utero or the need for postnatal pacing. Regular, careful prenatal monitoring is required to optimize the timing of necessary interventions.

▶ Third degree heart block results in decreased fetal ventricular output due to dissociation of atrial from ventricular systole, which in turn reduces ventricular diastolic filling. Once sino-atrial node function is lost to the cardiac conducting system, the atrio ventricular node takes up pacemaker function and in those who survive a rate of 50–55 beats/min is usually

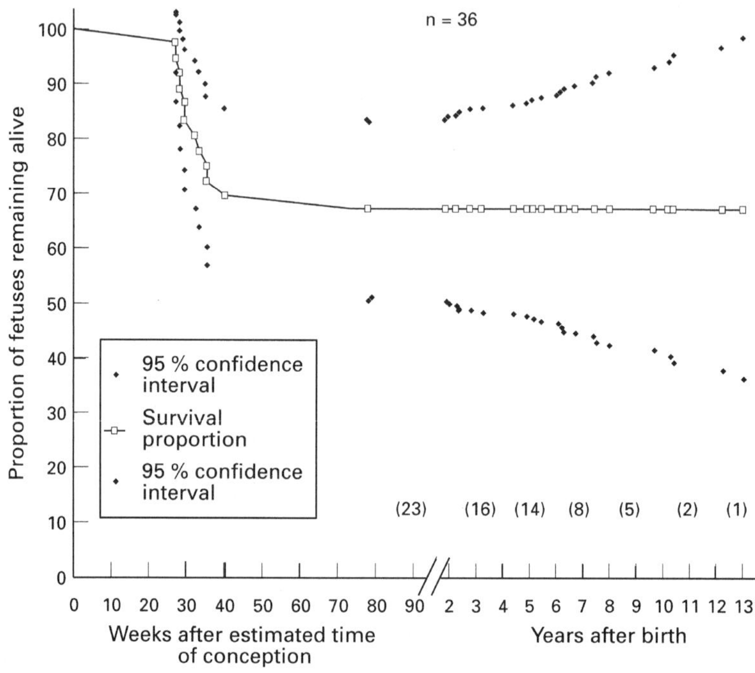

FIGURE 1.—Kaplan-Meyer survival curve for congenital complete heart block detected prenatally. This curve shows that the major attrition of patients in the prenatal series is antenatal. The noncardiac death has been excluded. There was no fetal loss before 27 weeks gestation. Numbers in parentheses are the numbers of patients alive at the follow-up interval. (Courtesy of Groves AMM, Allan LD, Rosenthal E: Outcome of isolated congenital complete heart block diagnosed in utero. *Heart* 75:190–194, 1996.)

established. If no escape rhythm emerges or if a ventricular myocardial pacemaker is established with a rate in the range of 5–40 beats/min, fetal death usually ensues. This then is a longitudinal account of fetal and infant survival in 36 fetuses, almost all with anticardiolipin antibody injury[1] who established atrioventricular nodal control of heart rate. There were 9 fetal deaths in utero and 2 induced abortions, almost all due to fetal congestive heart failure and hydrops. Follow-up was completed in 92% of newborns to 1 year of age, and in 64% to 2 years. Generally, infant survival was quite good, although nearly half of surviving newborns required external pacemakers with likely more to follow in time. This is the best data we have at this point to aid in counseling mothers of these infants. Long-term intense surveillance is certainly mandatory.

T.H. Kirschbaum, M.D.

Reference

1. 1995 Year Book of Obstetrics and Gynecology, pp 145–146.

The Natural History of Meconium Peritonitis Diagnosed In Utero

Dirkes K, Crombleholme TM, Craigo SD, et al (Tufts Univ, Boston; New England Med Ctr, Boston)
J Pediatr Surg 30:979–982, 1995   10–2

Objective.—Although obstetrical ultrasound has made it easier to diagnose meconium peritonitis in utero, there is little information about the natural history of prenatally diagnosed meconium peritonitis. Prenatally diagnosed meconium peritonitis cases were reviewed to define criteria for prenatal and postnatal management.

Methods.—Sonographic criteria for diagnosing MP were retrospectively reviewed for 9 fetuses with meconium peritonitis, between 18 and 37 weeks' gestation. Cases were divided into 2 groups: simple meconium peritonitis (SMP), or complex meconium peritonitis (CMP) (without bowel abnormalities), based on findings. Cases were followed up for 3 to 24 months.

Results.—Five fetuses received a diagnosis of SMP at 18, 23, 30, 34, and 37 weeks of gestation, and 4 received a diagnosis of CMP at 26, 31, and 37 weeks of gestation. All patients with SMP were delivered normally at term. Three had normal bowel gas patterns, and 2 had intra-abdominal calcifications. All were fed uneventfully, none had cystic fibrosis, and all are healthy at 15 months. All patients with CMP had bowel dilatation, 1 had intra-abdominal calcifications, and 2 had meconium pseudocysts, 1 with polyhydramnios and 1 with ascites. One of these patients required segmental resection and died of complications after a liver transplant, and the other patient underwent a successful resection. The 2 patients with normal bowel gas patterns were fed uneventfully.

Conclusion.—Fetal age was not correlated with outcome or severity of disease. Fetuses with CMP are at risk of bowel complications at birth, including perforation and obstruction.

▶ These 9 cases nicely illustrate the difference between MP that has occurred in utero and that which occurs in postnatal life. The latter, reflecting bowel perforation occurring after feeding has begun, is a grave complication of neonatal life and often requires laparotomy and carries a 50% to 60% risk of mortality. Many of these infants suffer from cystic fibrosis, which decreased the fluidity of bowel contents and predisposed to obstruction. Fetal intra-abdominal calcifications noted on ultrasound may represent tumor calcification, biliary or vascular lesions, all of them rare, but apparently not infrequently represent fetal bowel perforation with release of sterile meconium and spontaneous healing of the bowel defect. The prognosis is good, and the incidence of cystic fibrosis is low, variously reported as less than 10%. And in such neonates with a normal abdominal physical and x-ray exam, oral feeding should be begun. Even with evidence of dilated bowel loops and peritoneal scarring resulting in meconium pseudocysts or transient ascites during fetal life, newborn upper gastrointestinal and small-bowel follow-through may well indicate normal bowel integrity. Ultrasound is a sensitive means of detecting this abnormality in the second and third trimesters of pregnancy, and parents should be reassured that, although vigilant scrutiny of the newborn will be necessary, the prognosis for life is good and the diagnosis of cystic fibrosis is less common than in infants in whom MP occurs after birth.

T.H. Kirschbaum, M.D.

Description and Evaluation of a Program for the Early Discharge of Infants From a Neonatal Intensive Care Unit

Kotagal UR, Perlstein PH, Gamblian V, et al (Univ of Cincinnati, Ohio)
J Pediatr 127:285–290, 1995   10–3

Background.—A coalition of large Cincinnati businesses was formed to reduce the costs of employee health care insurance. This coalition caused changes in the marketplace that led to the initiation of a program in the neonatal ICU at 1 hospital to reduce costs by decreasing the length of hospital stay for high-risk infants. The clinical and financial impacts of this program were investigated.

Methods.—Data on all 257 infants dismissed from the neonatal ICU from June 1, 1993, to January 1, 1994, were included in the analysis of the early-discharge program. This information was compared with that for 477 infants discharged from April 1, 1992, to April 1, 1993, before institution of this program. No significant clinical or demographic differences were found between these 2 patient populations.

Early-Discharge Program.—A multidisciplinary team from the hospital identified ways to reduce the length of stay of infants in the neonatal ICU. The body weight guideline for discharge was dismissed. Attending physicians were asked to decrease the length of stay whenever possible without compromising patient health. Patients were discharged when the attending physician believed that they were clinically stable, free of apparent life-threatening apneic and bradycardiac episodes, able to maintain body temperature when swaddled, able to gain weight consistently with nipple feedings, and able to be discharged to a safe home environment. The safety of the home environment was determined by family screening and home visits by a neonatal ICU social worker.

Results.—After the institution of the early-discharge program, there was a significant decrease in the length of stay for each birth weight. This led to an average decrease of $10,609 in hospital charges per patient. Physician fees were also reduced. There was also a significant shift toward discharge at the lower birth weight after the institution of the early-discharge program. The early-discharge program significantly affected the resources consumed, after controlling for birth weight and month of discharge (Fig).

Conclusions.—Infants in an inner-city neonatal ICU can be discharged earlier and at lower body weights than had been previously assumed, without excessive morbidity or mortality. The ensuing reduction in hos-

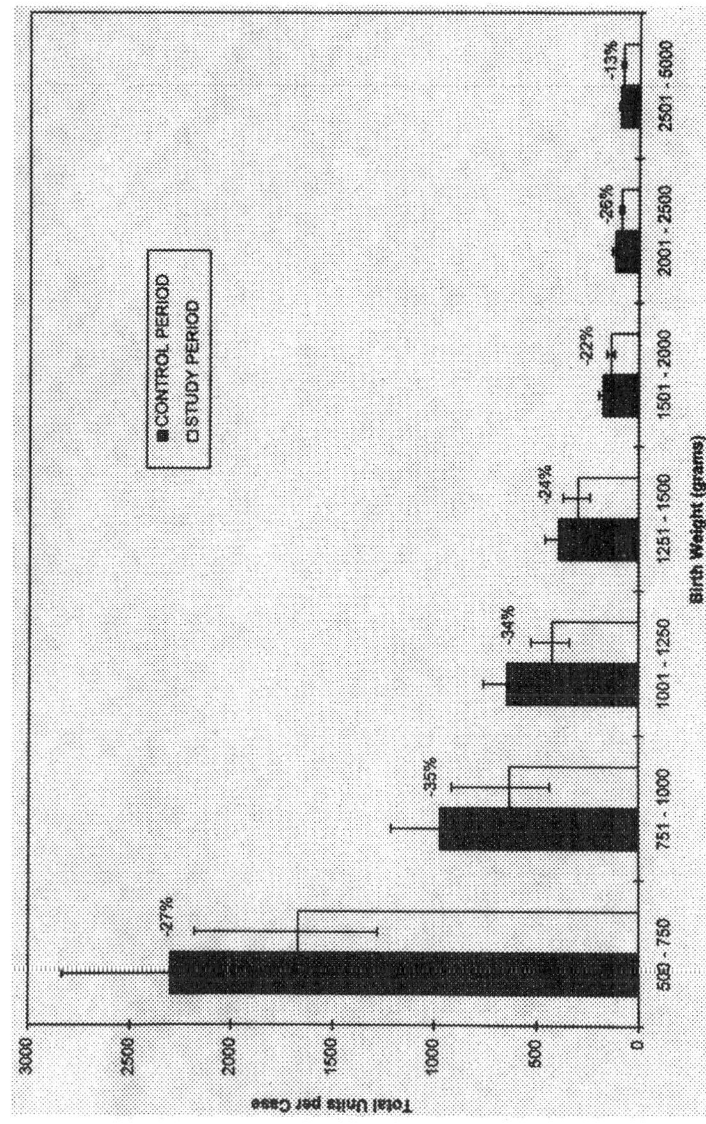

FIGURE.—Resource utilization units for infants during control and study periods stratified for birth-weight increments between 501 and 5,000 g (geometric mean with 95% confidence intervals of the mean). ($P < 0.0001$, analysis of variance), with control for birth-weight groups and month of discharge. (Courtesy of Kotagal UR, Perlstein PH, Gamblian V, et al: Description and evaluation of a program for the early discharge of infants from a neonatal intensive care unit. *J Pediatr* 127:285–290, 1995.)

pital charges was 30 times greater than the cost of the early-discharge program. The success of the program depended on the removal of body weight restrictions on discharge and provision of family support.

▶ This report from the Department of Pediatrics at the University of Cincinnati demonstrates the safety and cost savings of accelerated neonatal ICU discharge in a 1-year experience using historical controls. The impetus began with a coalition of Cincinnati employer groups seeking to reduce health care costs, acting through the managed care market, and to receive objective evaluation data for their policy decisions. Important to the success of the program was discard of an arbitrary 2.26-kg minimum weight requirement for infant hospital discharge. Instead, the group used criteria for discharge defined in terms of infant function and family support efforts. Physicians were asked to consider the clinical stability of heart and respiratory function, need for supplementary oxygen, homeothermic stability, satisfactory nutrition, and adequacy of the home environment. Most important were the designation of nurse supervisors and coordinators within the hospital, the cooperation of local home health care agencies, a system of newborn tracking, evaluatory and educational home visits prior to discharge, the evaluation of parents' competence for homecare, the access to hospital day care facilities for siblings, and the direct financial assistance if needed for family travel and communication costs. Increased hospital costs amounted to $468 per discharged baby over the 7-month interval. These support efforts were probably the most important elements of the program's economic success. The incidence of emergency room returns and readmissions was not increased in those receiving early discharge under these terms. The lesson here is that early discharge from the neonatal ICU can be safe and cost-reductive, but it takes effort and engenders additional costs for the unit to carry it out in a way that guarantees infant safety.

T.H. Kirschbaum, M.D.

Predictive Value of Early Neuroimaging, Pulsed Doppler and Neurophysiology in Full Term Infants With Hypoxic-Ischaemic Encephalopathy
Eken P, Toet MC, Groenendaal F, et al (Wilhelmina Children's Hosp, Utrecht, The Netherlands)
Arch Dis Child 73:F75–F80, 1995   10–4

Background.—Death or major neurologic sequelae are common in infants with encephalopathy, occurring in 25% to 40% of infants with moderate encephalopathy and 90% to 100% of those with severe encephalopathy. The clinical findings develop over 12–24 hours, and there are no early markers to predict which infants will have moderate or severe encephalopathy. Five different noninvasive techniques—cranial ultrasound, pulsed Doppler measurements, visual evoked potentials (VEPs), somatosensory evoked potentials (SEPs), and cerebral function monitoring (CFM)—were tested for prognostic value in full-term infants with encephalopathy.

Methods.—Thirty-four full-term infants with hypoxic-ischemic encephalopathy were studied. Within 6 hours after delivery, the infants underwent cranial ultrasound, Doppler ultrasound to measure the resistance index of the middle cerebral artery, VEPs and SEPs, and CFM recordings. The findings were analyzed to determine which test or combination of tests was most useful in predicting which infants would have a major handicap develop.

Results.—The encephalopathy was considered mild in 11 infants, moderate in 7, and severe in 16, according to Sarnat's criteria. Positive and negative predictive value were greatest—84% and 92%, respectively—for CFM. The outcome was good for infants with a continuous CFM pattern in all cases but 1. The initial CFM finding was a suppression-burst pattern in 11 infants. This changed during 24–48 hours to a continuous pattern in 4 infants, 3 of whom had a normal outcome. There were 5 infants with an isoelectric CFM, all of whom died.

Somatosensory evoked potentials had a positive predictive value of 82% and a negative predictive value of 92%. Delayed VEPs were common during the first hours of life. This finding was not associated with a poor prognosis in 5 of 14 cases and had a positive predictive value of 77%. Cranial ultrasound and Doppler resistance index measurements almost always gave normal values, so they were of no predictive help.

Conclusions.—Neurophysiologic studies performed within the first hours of life can predict which infants will have moderate-to-severe encephalopathy develop and thus are more likely to die or have neurologic sequelae. The most useful information is provided by CFM and SEPs, the findings of which could be helpful in selecting infants for treatment with neuroprotective agents.

▶ As more information has been gained about the detailed mechanics of newborn brain injury, a number of agents, among them glutamate antagonists, insulin-like growth factor I, transforming growth factor-β, free-radical antagonists, and C21 corticoids, are under evaluation as possibly effective prophylactic agents. That's the point of this study: to look for means of predicting from among term infants who appear to have suffered cerebral hypoxia and/or ischemia, those who are at high risk to suffer permanent brain injury and are therefore legitimate candidates for trials of the use of prophylactic agents.

Cranial ultrasound and Doppler velocity analysis of the middle cerebral artery done in the first 6 hours of life appear useless in this regard. On the other hand, electroneurophysiologic evaluation with amplitude-integrated electroencephalography and recording of SEPs proved to have predictive value. In general, ultrasound has proven of little use in the evaluation of these newborns and the prediction of permanent injury, and to date, early evidence of neurofunctional impairment appears to be the best means of estimating high risk of permanent injury.

T.H. Kirschbaum, M.D.

Outcome of Infants Weighing Less Than 800 Grams at Birth: 15 Years' Experience

La Pine TR, Jackson JC, Bennett FC (Univ of Utah, Salt Lake City; Univ of Washington, Seattle)
Pediatrics 96:479–483, 1995   10–5

Introduction.—Survival for extremely low birth weight (ELBW) infants has increased dramatically, to the point where 80% or more of these infants may survive. This has led to concern that increased survival may lead to an increase in various forms of major neurodevelopmental morbidity. On the other hand, some argue that aggressive, intensive care for ELBW infants leads to better survival and neurodevelopmental outcomes. Mortality and neurodevelopmental morbidity trends during a 15-year period were examined in a population of extremely premature infants.

Methods.—Three cohorts of infants with birth weights of less than 800 g were studied. Of these, 210 were admitted between 1986 and 1990, 128 were admitted between 1983 and 1985, and 95 were admitted between 1977 and 1980. The mean gestational age was 25 weeks in all 3 cohorts.

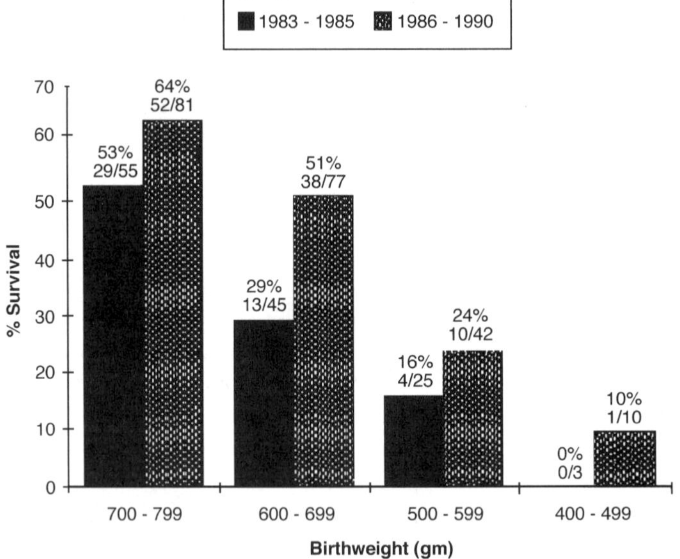

FIGURE.—Survival by birth weight subgroup of infants weighing less than 800 g in the current (1986 through 1990) and 1983 through 1985 cohorts. (Courtesy of La Pine TR, Jackson JC, Bennett FC: Outcome of Infants Weighing Less Than 800 Grams at Birth: 15 Years' Experience. Reproduced by permission of *Pediatrics,* 96:479–483, 1995.)

There were no substantive changes in the basic delivery and resuscitation policies followed during the 3 periods studied. Developmental follow-up studies were performed by a high-risk infant follow-up clinic, which used an interdisciplinary, neurodevelopmental approach to monitoring.

Results.—From 1977 to 1990, the number of ELBW infants admitted per year nearly doubled, from 24 to 42. Nursery survival improved from 20% in 1977–1980, to 36% in 1983–1985, to 49% in 1986–1990. Survival improved the most—nearly doubling from 1983–1985 to 1986–1990—for girls with birth weights of less than 700 g (Fig). In each of the 3 cohorts, girls had 20% better survival than did the boys. Major neurosensory impairments occurred in about 20% of each cohort, with boys more likely to be affected. The mean scores on cognitive testing were not significantly different between cohorts, ranging from 89 to 98.

Conclusions.—Survival for ELBW infants has been improving steadily within the last 2 decades, with no concurrent increases in neurodevelopmental morbidity. The gains have been particularly impressive for ELBW survivors with birth weights of less than 700 g. The acceptable neurodevelopmental outcomes for these tiny infants must be part of ongoing discussions about prioritization of health services, limits of care, and spending of public and private resources.

▶ This comparative review of 210 infants admitted to the University of Washington neonatal ICU from 1986 to 1990 documents the remarkable achievements that neonatologists are making in learning to care for these tiny newborns. In comparing their outcome with that for the 3 years preceding 1986, the numbers of infants weighing less than 800 g at birth has remained constant, as has the frequency distribution for each of the four 100-g intervals between 400 and 800 g, while overall survival rates have gone from 36% to 49%. Even better, extending the analysis of data back to 1970, the incidence of major neurologic deficits has remained constant at roughly 20% in this birth-weight range. Bear in mind that the short follow-up for the most recent cohort admitted from 1986 to 1990 biases the results in favor of a lower rate of CNS injury, and the 24% of survivors lost to follow-up complicates the analysis. But those things aside, here is strong evidence of improvement in the enormously intricate tasks of keeping these fragile newborns alive and intact. As always, low birth weight and male sex, both apparently independently, mitigate against intact survival.

T.H. Kirschbaum, M.D.

Dynamics of Viral Replication in Infants With Vertically Acquired Human Immunodeficiency Virus Type 1 Infection

De Rossi A, Masiero S, Giaquinto C, et al (Univ of Padova, Italy; Internatl Centre for Genetic Engineering, Trieste, Italy)
J Clin Invest 97:323–330, 1996

10–6

Introduction.—Approximately one third of children with vertical transmission of HIV-1 infection will show severe symptoms of AIDS within the first few months of life. The rest have slower disease progression, including some in whom symptoms do not develop for several years. It is important to gain information regarding the factors contributing to disease expression. Viral replication patterns early in life were studied for their contribution to disease outcome in infants with vertically acquired HIV-1 infection.

Methods.—The study included 11 infants enrolled at birth in a study of maternal-to-child HIV-1 transmission. Viral loads in plasma and HIV-1 provirus content in cells during the first few months of life were investigated using competitive reverse transcription-polymerase chain reaction for the plasma and competitive polymerase chain reaction for the cells. The HIV-1 replication findings were analyzed to determine their relationship with disease outcome.

Results.—All patients had evidence of increased viral replication during the first few weeks of life. Three separate viral replication patterns were identified. Some infants showed a rapid increase in plasma viral RNA and cell-associated proviral DNA within the first 4 to 6 weeks of life. By 2 to 3 months, these infants had reached high steady-state levels of both parameters, that is, greater than 1,000 HIV-1 copies per 10^5 peripheral blood mononuclear cells and greater than 1 million RNA copies per milliliter of plasma. All infants with this pattern had early AIDS. The second group of infants showed a similarly rapid increase in viral load at first. Subsequently, however, their viral levels declined by 2.5- to 50-fold. In the third group, the initial viral increase was more than 10 times lower. Infants with the second or third viral replication pattern had slower clinical progression of HIV-1 infection.

Conclusions.—In infants with vertically transmitted HIV-1 infection, the pattern of viral replication during the first 2 or 3 months of life is strongly predictive of evolution of HIV disease. In infants with rapid progression, the virus appears to spread rapidly—before the child can mount an immune response—and early AIDS appears to be a manifestation of the primary infection. The new findings support the theory that HIV-1 transmission in vertically infected infants occurs during late pregnancy or the intrapartum period.

▶ Human immunodeficiency virus-1 protease inhibitors, the new class of therapeutic agents active in treating this disease, function by inhibiting the generation of new intact viral particles (virions) by infected immune cells. Their ability to temporarily decrease measurable viral load to an indiscernible level and reduce symptoms and findings in many infected individuals has changed the way investigators look at this disease. Formerly, pathogenesis was thought to consist of infection followed by sequestration of dormant viral DNA, deposited by reverse transcriptase action on viral RNA, in the cells of the immune system from which it emerged years later in the form of immune suppression, opportunistic infections, and acute symptoms. Now it is clear that the virus replicates actively and continually, and it does battle with immune cells until the capacity of the immune system to replicate and contain virus adequately is ultimately lost. This new view has led to emphasis on blood virion number as the most reliable way to chart the course of the disease. Two new techniques, competitive polymerase chain reaction and competitive reverse transcription polymerase chain reaction, enable the rough quantitation of the concentration of HIV DNA proviral templates in the DNA of infected cells, and in RNA copies of that template, that is, active viral particles.

Here, these techniques are applied to the puzzle—that some infants subsequently found to be infected by their mother before birth showed neither virus nor viral antigens at birth, but nearly all were positive for both at 4 to 8 weeks of age. Three patterns of HIV-DNA and RNA changes were seen in these 11 infected infants followed up by this Padova University group. In some infants, viral and proviral replication was very rapid, with prompt decline of CD4 counts discernible in the first month of life, generally eventuating in early AIDS and infant death. In others, viremia was slower to develop, CD4 counts declined but rebounded, and the disease was indolent. An intermediate pattern also was seen. These patterns of pathogenesis strongly suggest primary infection occurring late in pregnancy, likely at about the time of birth, in HIV infection first seen in infancy and not at birth. The mechanisms that determine these differences in host response to the infection are vital, but it is uncertain still whether they are related to viral load, variable infectivity, or host response. This study re-emphasizes the value of judging prognosis in HIV infection by quantitating viral DNA and RNA copies in infected host tissue.

T.H. Kirschbaum, M.D.

Detection of Virus in Vertically Exposed HIV-antibody-negative Children
Newell M-L, Dunn D, De Maria A, et al (Inst of Child Health, London; Univ of Genoa, Italy; Univ of Padua, Italy; et al)
Lancet 347:213–215, 1996   10–7

Introduction.—Fetuses can acquire HIV infection from their HIV-infected mothers in utero or during delivery. However, cases of neonates acquiring HIV by vertical transmission with subsequently cleared infection have been reported. To investigate the frequency of HIV virus clearance, the progress of infants born to HIV-infected mothers was followed from birth.

TABLE 3.—Laboratory Data on 9 Seronegative Children Who Tested Positive by Virus Culture or Polymerase Chain Reaction on at Least 1 Sample

Child	Age (months) at loss of antibody	Number of samples in which virus detected	Test results by virus-culture/PCR (age in months)							
A	8–10	2	+/ND (1)	ND/+ (2)	ND/– (10)	–/– (13)	–/– (29)	–/ND (55)	–/ND (64)	
B	13–16	2	+/+ (3)	+/+ (6)	–/– (16)	–/– (18)	–/– (24)			
C	9–11	2	+/ND (0)	–/ND (3)	–/+ (5)	–/– (9)	–/ND (11)	–/– (15)	–/– (20)	–/– (25)
D	12–15	1	–/– (0)	+/+ (1)	–/– (4)	–/ND (6)	–/– (9)	–/– (12)	–/ND (15)	–/ND (23)
E	11–16	1	–/ND (B)	+/ND (3)	–/ND (26)	ND/– (50)				
F	7–18	1	+/ND (4)							
G	15–17	3	+/ND (3)	+/– (6)	+/+ (12)	–/– (24)	–/– (30)	–/– (45)	ND/– (47)	–/– (68) –/– (72)
H	8–11	4	+/ND (0)	–/ND (3)	–/ND (8)	+/ND (14)	+/ND (17)	–/ND (25)	ND/+ (47)	
I	5–8	2	–/ND (B)	+/ND (1)	–/ND (5)	–/ND (8)	–/ND (11)	–/ND (14) –/ND (32)	–/ND (17) +/ND (39)	–/ND (23) –/ND (56)

Abbreviations: B, birth; *ND*, not done; *PCR*, polymerase chain reaction.
(Courtesy of Newell M-L, Dunn D, De Maria A, et al.: Detection of Virus in Vertically Exposed HIV-antibody-negative Children. *Lancet*, 347:213–215, copyright by The Lancet Ltd. 1996.)

Methods.—At 4 centers participating in the European Collaborative Study, 299 infants with HIV-infected mothers, born over a 9-year period, were classified as HIV-antibody–negative. Of these, 264 were tested with virus culture or polymerase chain reaction at least once before the age of 3 months.

Results.—Of the 264 infants tested, 9 had at least 1 virus culture or polymerase chain reaction sample revealing HIV positivity, and demonstrated subsequent seroreversion (Table 3). Six infants demonstrated a pattern consistent with viral clearance, with positive virus tests early in life and later seroreversion. The other 3 infants demonstrated no clear pattern, with virus detected intermittently and later in life. All 9 infants were fed exclusively by bottle, had no HIV-related symptoms, and had received no antiviral treatment, and all but 1 were delivered vaginally.

Conclusions.—There was a 2.7% incidence of infants of HIV mothers who clear HIV or tolerate virus. In current pediatric practice, the parents of these infants are informed that their infant is HIV-negative. Further study of these infants may provide insight into the mechanisms of virus clearance and have implications for vaccine development.

▶ Although individual cases of apparently vertically infected HIV-1–positive infants spontaneously becoming HIV-negative have appeared, this is the first systematic study sufficiently large to allow rate estimates of that phenomenon. If the rate of spontaneous clearance of virus is high, estimates of vertical transmission based on viral culture and polymerase chain reaction analysis of newborn blood in the first month or 2 of life are higher than the actual rates. If newborn viral clearance takes place, as it most commonly does before 18 months of life, it indicates a possible role for passively transferred maternal antibody in the prevention of fetal infection given the presence of fetal virus. If that is not what is involved, there is an entirely new, currently unrecognized set of operations at work in the neonate that may have important implications for infected adults.

The data were derived from 4 European centers participating in the European Collaborative Study of HIV-positive pregnancy.[1] During the period from 1985 to 1994, 264 infants were tested every 3 months for 18 months or until HIV-negative, and 219 of these had at least 2 viral cultures. The crude rate for conversion of neonates initially HIV-positive both by viral culture and polymerase chain reaction was 3.4%. When corrections were made, excluding those with only 1 positive culture and estimating the likelihood of error based on the 2 positive tests occurring by random chance, the clearance rate was 2.7%. An additional finding reported gratuitously here is that of 857 infants followed for 1,700 child-years, an average of about 2 years each, none who were antibody-negative—whether or not they were originally antibody-positive—ever reverted to be antibody-positive. This suggests a low rate of horizontal transmission among those mother-infant pairs. An important study, this work will spawn a great deal of mechanistic investigation.

T.H. Kirschbaum, M.D.

Reference

1. 1993 Year Book of Obstetrics and Gynecology, pp 217–219.

Isolation of Fetal Cells From Transcervical Samples by Micromanipulation: Molecular Confirmation of Their Fetal Origin and Diagnosis of Fetal Aneuploidy
Tutschek B, Sherlock J, Halder A, et al (Univ College London)
Prenat Diagn 15:951–960, 1995   10–8

Introduction.—Recent studies have reported a noninvasive or minimally invasive procedure as a safe alternative to amniocentesis for genetic testing in the first trimester of pregnancy. The procedure involves isolating transcervical cell (TCC) samples from transcervical lavage and mucus aspirates, which contain fetal cells that can be examined by molecular analysis. A method for isolating viable fetal cells from TCC samples was tested.

Methods.—Transcervical cell samples were collected from mucus aspirates and transcervical lavages obtained from 29 women between 6 and 12 weeks' gestation who were undergoing either pregnancy termination or transcervical chorionic villus sampling. After the fetal cells were isolated from the TCC samples by micromanipulation methods, the cells were examined by dual- and triple-color fluorescent in situ hybridization (FISH) and the polymerase chain reaction. Maternal peripheral blood samples were also obtained from all patients. To confirm the findings, fetal tissue was obtained from all patients undergoing elective pregnancy termination and chorionic villus samples were obtained from patients with ongoing pregnancies who were undergoing chorionic villus sampling.

Results.—Polymerase chain reaction and FISH confirmed that 29 clumps obtained from 11 patients were of fetal origin. One case of a male triploid fetus was diagnosed by examining TCC samples obtained by mucus aspiration and lavage, and it was validated by testing clumps of fetal cells isolated by micromanipulation.

Conclusion.—The isolation of clumps of fetal cells from TCC samples and the subsequent analysis of these cells by dual- and triple-color FISH and polymerase chain reaction enables the early prenatal diagnosis of source single gene disorders without risk to mother or fetus.

▶ For nearly 20 years, this University College London group has applied recombinant DNA techniques to trophoblastic cells known to be available from the pregnant cervix.[1] One hundred forty clumps of trophoblastic cells were removed either by aspiration or lavage of the cervix before induced abortion or at the time of chorionic villus sampling at 6 to 12 weeks' gestation. In a companion paper,[2] the authors report either technique of cell collection is equally and highly efficient. For FISH, trophoblastic cell clusters are recognized and picked microscopically, subjected to a mucolytic to separate the clumps, and washed and treated with hypotonic electrolyte to produce nuclear swelling. The resulting cells are mounted on slides for hybridization with fluorescent probes to chromosomes X, Y, and 1, each exhibiting fluorescent different colors. For polymerase chain reaction, fetal cells are treated to release DNA, and polymerase chain reaction is conducted using fluorescent markers for chromosomes 21, X, and Y. A unique chromosome 21 marker that expresses the length of tandem repeats on the long arm of chromosome 21 was used with the tandem length to prove origin of the multiplied segment from 1 or both parents in a sort of DNA fingerprinting.[3]

The results with FISH are slightly less efficient than with polymerase chain reaction; the former has the advantage of clearly indicating the number of sex chromosomes or of number 21 autosomes per cell and preventing probe labeling by spermatozoa. Here, sex chromosome identity was confirmed and a triploid fetus identified. This is an important addition to the growing list of noninvasive means of fetal testing for genetic diagnosis.

T.H. Kirschbaum, M.D.

References

1. Rhine SA, Palmer CG, Thompson JF: A simple alternative to amniocentesis for first trimester prenatal diagnosis. *Birth Defects* 12:231–247, 1977.
2. Adinolfi M, Sherlock J, Tutschek B, et al: Detection of fetal cells in transcervical samples and prenatal diagnosis of chromosomal abnormalities. *Prenat Diagn* 15:943–949, 1995.
3. 1991 YEAR BOOK OF OBSTETRICS AND GYNECOLOGY, pp 154–155.

GYNECOLOGY

11 Gynecologic Urology

Female Urinary Stress Incontinence: Does It Have Familial Prevalence?
Mushkat Y, Bukovsky I, Langer R (Assaf Harofeh Med Ctr, Zerifin, Israel)
Am J Obstet Gynecol 174:617–619, 1996   11–1

Purpose.—Many different factors have been suggested to play a role in the development of stress urinary incontinence, including parity, menopause, and pelvic surgical procedures. To this list can be added a genetic defect in the connective tissue, which makes up an important part of the pelvic sensory apparatus. Clinical experience suggests that many women with stress urinary incontinence have relatives with the same problem. The possible familial prevalence of stress urinary incontinence was evaluated.

Methods.—Two hundred fifty-nine females with a diagnosis of stress urinary incontinence during a 5-year period were studied, along with a random sample of 165 women without micturition disorders. The patients were asked whether any of their first-degree relatives had the typical symptoms of stress urinary incontinence. Family members who had symptoms at least twice weekly were defined as having the condition. The patient reports were confirmed by urodynamic studies of 48 relatives said to have stress urinary incontinence.

Results.—The overall reported prevalence of stress urinary incontinence among relatives was 20% in the patient group vs. 8% in the control group. The prevalence among mothers was 35% in the patient group vs. 13% in the control group, and the prevalence among sisters was 20% in the patients vs. 7% in the controls. All 48 relatives who accepted the invitation to urodynamic investigation proved to have stress urinary incontinence.

Conclusions.—The relatives of women with stress urinary incontinence are likely to have the same disorder themselves. The mothers and sisters of affected patients are about 3 times more likely to have stress urinary incontinence than the mothers and sisters of controls. Screening relatives of women with stress urinary incontinence is likely to identify a significant number of patients who could benefit from treatment. Genetic factors may contribute to stress urinary incontinence.

▶ Stress urinary incontinence is a multifactorial problem. Anatomical defect and weakness in supporting pelvic organs play a major role in incontinence development. Childbearing is an important contributor in inadequate support and pelvic relaxation. However, pelvic relaxation and stress incontinence were observed in nulliparous women, and many multiparous women have adequate bladder control.

Recently, several publications by Ulmsten and later by Norton and by Berman demonstrated altered collagen composition in women with stress incontinence. Can this condition be hereditary or run in families? This study from Israel points to this possibility. As the authors themselves indicate, only 24% of relatives claiming incontinence responded. Probably women with less severe problems did not. Even so, the incidence of incontinence was 3 times higher in families of incontinent patients, and this is significant.

The results of this study should be kept in mind as physicians evaluate patients for incontinence. We should include questions about family members in our questionnaires. If the results of this study are confirmed by other studies, "prophylactic Kegels" may be considered for family members, who may be at risk of having pelvic relaxation and urinary incontinence develop.

A. Bergman, M.D.

Urethral Closure Pressure and Leak-Point Pressure in Incontinent Women

Sultana CJ (Univ Hosps of Cleveland, Ohio; Case Western Reserve Univ, Cleveland, Ohio)
Obstet Gynecol 86:839–842, 1995   11–2

Background.—Results from previous studies point to a relationship between a preoperative maximum urethral closure pressure of less than 20 cm H_2O and an elevated risk of failure of retropubic and needle suspension procedures in women with stress incontinence. Unlike urethral closure pressure, which has been advocated for diagnosis of incontinence in women, published data regarding Valsalva leak-point pressure measurements in adult women are limited. The association between maximum urethral closure pressure and Valsalva leak-point pressure was examined in women with genuine stress incontinence.

Patients and Methods.—Fifty-six women with GSI were studied. Multichannel urodynamic testing was used to determine maximum urethral closure pressure and vesical leak-point pressure.

Results.—Urine loss was not observed in 16 of the 56 women during attempted leak-point pressure measurements. Among the 40 women with evidence of a leak on Valsalva maneuver, a significant association between maximum urethral closure pressure and leak-point pressures was noted (Fig 1). The strongest association was observed between leak-point pressure up to 120 cm H_2O and absolute vesical pressure with Valsalva, rather than with a change in vesical pressure. The sensitivity and negative predictive value of leaking with strain for maximum urethral closure pressure of 20 cm H_2O or less was 100%, specificity was 34.7%, and positive predictive value was 25%.

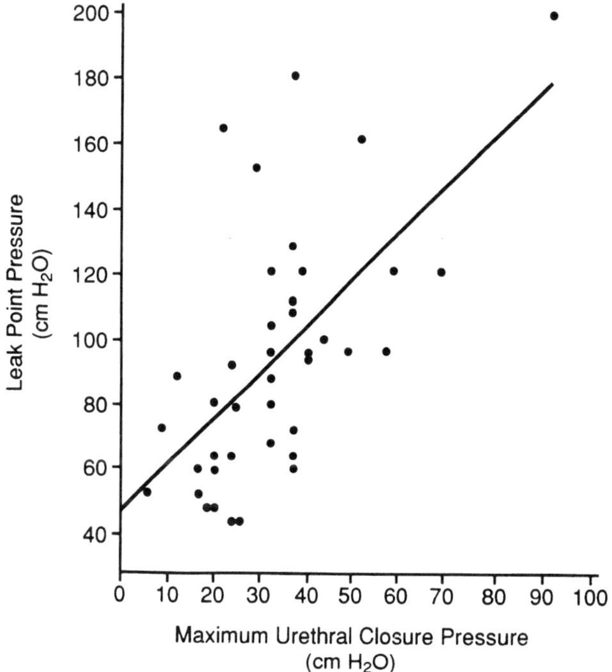

FIGURE 1.—Scatterplot of maximum urethral closure pressure vs. leak-point pressure (LPP) with regression line for predicted LPP. (Courtesy of Sultana CJ: Urethral closure pressure and leak-point pressure in incontinent women. *Obstet Gynecol* 86:839–842, 1995. Reprinted with permission from The American College of Obstetricians and Gynecologists.)

Conclusions.—The observed correlation between maximum urethral closure pressure and leak-point pressure may yield helpful information about incontinence in women. Additional studies of treatment outcomes in patients based on leak-point pressure only are recommended.

▶ One of the aims of urodynamic studies, beyond establishing diagnosis, is to identify "risk factors" for failures. Low urethral pressure (20 cm H₂O or less) has been shown, in many papers, to be associated with high failure rate of bladder neck suspensions. The problem is that, in order to detect low urethral pressure, the patient must undergo urethral pressure profile, which is still unavailable in many centers. Valsalva leak point is supposed to be another indirect predictor for success of bladder neck suspensions for stress incontinence. The test measures the pressure in the bladder (or indirectly in the abdomen) that is necessary to overcome urethral resistance and result in loss of urine. Some authors have indicated that low Valsalva leak point, i.e., loss of urine with minimal Valsalva or Valsalva of 60 cm H₂O or less, is associated with high failure rates of bladder neck suspensions. Others could not repeat these findings. Performing and measuring Valsalva leak point is simpler and easier than measuring urethral pressures, because it does not require urethral profilometry, and equipment is the same as for simple cystometry.

Does low Valsalva leak point correlate with low urethral pressure and, thus, can it serve as a screening tool to detect women who are at high risk of failing bladder neck suspension? Dr. Sultana answers positively by finding good statistical correlation between leak point and low urethral pressure. However, the clinician is interested mainly in the "high risk for failure" group, i.e., women with low urethral pressure. Is there a correlation between low urethral pressure and low leak point? Looking at Figure 1, I find women with low urethral pressure to be almost equally distributed among Valsalva leak point of less than 60 cm H_2O and more than 60 cm H_2O. In this specific group of women with stress urinary incontinence and low urethral pressure, correlation to low Valsalva leak point is not good. Urethral profilometry is unavailable for every evaluation of incontinence, and we have still to identify other risk factors for low urethral pressure.

A. Bergman, M.D.

Efficacy of Pelvic Floor Muscle Exercises in Women With Stress, Urge, and Mixed Urinary Incontinence
Nygaard IE, Kreder KJ, Lepic MM, et al (Univ of Iowa, Iowa City)
Am J Obstet Gynecol 174:120–125, 1996   11–3

Background.—The Agency for Health Care Policy and Research recommends that nonsurgical treatment be attempted in patients with urinary incontinence before resorting to surgical intervention. Pelvic muscle exercises have been found to be effective for the treatment of stress incontinence in previous studies, with reported success rates ranging from 31% to 97%. To evaluate, on the basis of intent to treat, the efficacy of a 3-month pelvic floor muscle exercise program as first-line intervention among women with stress, urge, or mixed urinary incontinence, a prospective, randomized study was performed. The ability of a specially designed audiotape to improve compliance and exercise effect also was assessed.

Patients and Methods.—Seventy-one patients evaluated in 2 tertiary care center referral clinics for urinary incontinence were enrolled in the study. Genital prolapse past the vaginal introitus was not observed in any patient. Patients were randomly assigned to pelvic floor exercise with or without the use of a 270-minute audiotape that featured technique tips, reminders, and exercise (contraction/relaxation) cues. The number of incontinent episodes, evaluated by means of a 3-day voiding diary, served as the main outcome measure.

Results.—Fifty-five women completed the entire 3-month exercise program. For all 71 participants, the mean number of incontinent episodes decreased from 3.1 to 2.3 per day. Among the 55 patients who completed the entire 3-month program, the mean number of incontinent episodes decreased from 2.6 to 1.3 per day. Six months after program completion, 10 women with stress incontinence had undergone surgical treatment. Among the 27 patients with genuine stress incontinence who were not treated surgically, 12 indicated that their improvement was good and declined further therapy. No differences in outcome or compliance were noted among women who had and had not exercised with the aid of the audiotape.

Conclusions.—Six months after completing a 3-month course of pelvic floor muscle exercises, one third of the program participants expressed satisfaction with their outcome. Use of the specially designed audiotape did not enhance the success rate or decrease the dropout rate. The exercises performed were similarly effective for all patients, regardless of urodynamic diagnosis. Additional studies are needed to determine inexpensive methods that could be used to improve the success rate of this risk-free, economical, and easy-to-provide therapy.

▶ When evaluating published results of anti-incontinence treatments, the reader should pay attention to the reported results. Although many published reports on operative procedures for stress urinary incontinence report cure and failure, or cure improvement and failure (cure is being completely dry), most reports on Kegel exercises report an improvement, or put together improvement and cure in 1 group.

This study reports improvement in more than 50% of patients. However, improvement included reduction of the number of leaking episodes from 2.6 to 1.7 for stress urinary incontinence, from 3.5 to 2.3 for detrusor instability, and from 3.9 to 3.2 for mixed incontinence. These women were not dry. They were less wet than before. In the absence of a control group (which, as Fantl et al.[1] showed, helped 25% of patients), improvement occurred in approximately 33% of patients who felt that pelvic floor training helped them to the point that they wanted to continue and wished no other treatment. For the practicing physician, this is a very important message. One in 3 women was satisfied with the results of the training program and wished not to have surgery. These numbers should be discussed with patients after a diagnosis is established and treatment plans are made.

A. Bergman, M.D.

Reference

1. Fantl JA, Wyman JF, McClish DK, et al: Efficacy of bladder training in older women with urinary incontinence. *JAMA* 265:609–613, 1991.

Long-term Effect of Pelvic Floor Muscle Exercise 5 Years After Cessation of Organized Training
Bø K, Talseth T (Norwegian Univ, Oslo; Natl Univ Hosp, Oslo, Norway)
Obstet Gynecol 87:261–265, 1996   11–4

Background.—Although studies have shown that pelvic floor muscle exercises can provide effective treatment of urinary stress incontinence, the most useful exercise regimen has been difficult to determine because of different outcome variables and differences in duration, intensity, and frequency of training. The short- and long-term effects of a 6-month intensive and structured program of pelvic floor muscle exercises were evaluated in women with demonstrable stress incontinence.

Patients and Methods.—All 23 women who had been enrolled in a structured 6-month pelvic floor muscle exercise program were evaluated 5 years after program completion. The mean age at follow-up was 50.7 years. During the 6-month exercise program, women completed 3 series of 8–12 maximum pelvic floor muscle contractions each day; they also engaged in 45 minutes of exercise with a physical therapist on a weekly basis. All patients had been on a waiting list for surgery at the time of the exercise program. At follow-up, a history by interview was obtained, and subjective rating instruments, including leakage index and social activity index, were completed. Measurements of pelvic floor muscle strength and function, urodynamic studies, and pad test with standardized bladder volume also were performed.

Results.—Three of the 23 patients had undergone surgical treatment during the 5-year period and were excluded from analysis. Of the 20 other patients, 15 did not show any visible leakage during cough, and 11 had positive closure pressure during cough. Fourteen of the 20 patients were satisfied with their condition at the 5-year follow-up and declined further treatment. Statistically significant increases in leakage index and pad test scores, but not the social activity index, were noted 5 years after completion of the organized exercise program. Sixteen patients, including 2 who had been treated surgically, continued to exercise the pelvic floor muscles at least once per week, with maintenance of pelvic muscle strength noted.

Conclusions.—Although urinary incontinence significantly increased 5 years after completion of a structured pelvic floor muscle exercise program, other outcome variables, including visible leakage and urethral closure pressure during cough and social activity index, remained stable during the follow-up period. Seventy percent of the patients not treated surgically also were satisfied with their present condition after 5 years of exercise program completion.

▶ The efficacy of Kegel exercises has been documented by many "short-term follow-up" studies. Kegel exercises, like any other muscle training program, work as long as one continues doing them. This study addresses the question of long-term efficacy of Kegel exercises. Drs. Bø and Talseth from Norway have a unique program (and a unique patient population) that is hard to compare with many programs in the United States. The program is a 6-month, intensive pelvic floor muscle exercise regimen. This is a long and intensive program. No standards have been set, so far, as to how long and intensive a program should be and how to conduct a "pelvic floor exercise program." If such standards are set in the future, the Norwegian model will no doubt be among the more intensive ones. At 5 years, 100% of women were available for clinical and urodynamic studies. Very few centers in this country can have such a motivated and compliant group of patients.

It is not surprising that in motivated women, after long and intensive training programs, 70% still continued to perform Kegel exercises 5 years after cessation of the program, and that 70% of women who continued the exercises were happy with the results.

Pelvic muscle training for treatment of stress incontinence should be a long-term commitment. When performed by motivated and committed women, a pelvic floor muscle training regimen can be an effective modality for treating urinary incontinence.

A. Bergman, M.D.

Conservative Therapy of Female Genuine Stress Incontinence With Vaginal Cones

Dellas A, Drewe J (Univ of Basle, Switzerland)
Eur J Obstet Gynecol Reprod Biol 62:213–215, 1995   11–5

Introduction.—Plevnik first used weighted vaginal cones to stimulate the pelvic floor in women with true stress urinary incontinence. Urodynamic studies were subsequently carried out before and after vaginal cone treatment in 20 parous women with genuine stress incontinence.

Methods.—The 12 postmenopausal women received estrogen. Cystometry was performed before and after 6 weeks of vaginal cone treatment. Sets of 5 cones weighing 20–100 g were available. Treatment began with the smallest cone and proceeded to the heavier ones as was possible. Cones were used at least twice a day for as long as 20 minutes.

Results.—Ten of the 20 women were cured cystometrically, and 6 others improved. In 4 cases, stress incontinence did not lessen after cone treatment. In women who became continent, the average maximum urethral closure pressure (MUCP) at rest increased from 55 to 63 cm H_2O. This parameter did not change appreciably in women who remained incontinent.

Conclusion.—Vaginal cones provide a nonsurgical means of curing mild stress urinary incontinence, particularly those with a relatively high baseline MUCP.

▶ Good results of Kegel exercise in curing stress incontinence can be expected in motivated women with relatively strong pelvic floor muscle and incontinence that is not severe. Women who responded favorably to cones (which is an indirect method of Kegel exercise) were young and had high urethral pressure and mild incontinence. Good results are not surprising, although the follow-up is short. What happens to these women in the long run and how many remain committed to the exercise program are other questions. Still, patients who are likely to respond to these exercises should be offered a trial before surgery is scheduled.

A. Bergman, M.D.

Periurethral Collagen Injections for Genuine Stress Incontinence: A 2-Year Follow-up

Monga AK, Robinson D, Stanton SL (St George's Hosp, London; Bowman Gray School of Medicine, Winston-Salem, NC)
Br J Urol 76:156–160, 1995   11–6

Objective.—Glutaraldehyde cross-linked collagen is a periurethral bulking agent purified from bovine dermal collagen. It is a biocompatible material that remains intact for about 12 weeks after being injected. The effectiveness of this material was examined in 60 women, with a mean age of 64 years, who had genuine stress incontinence. The women either were poor candidates for major surgery or had failed to respond to previous incontinence surgery.

Methods.—As many as 3 series of injections were administered under local anesthesia. A 2.5-mL volume of collagen was placed at the 3- and 9-o'clock positions until submucosal bulking was evident and the proximal urethral lumen was occluded. Women were considered to be cured when provocative cystometry failed to produce incontinence or a pad test was negative.

Results.—Thirty-four women received a single set of injections. Sixteen were treated twice, and 10, three times. Urge incontinence improved after collagen injection, but frequency, nocturia, and difficulty voiding remained unchanged. The rate of objectively assessed cure was 61% at 3 months, 54% at 1 year, and 48% at 2 years. The corresponding subjective success rates were 86%, 77%, and 68%. Neither a low urethral pressure nor decreased bladder neck mobility influenced the outcome. The chance of an objective cure at 2 years correlated with the degree of bulking achieved at the collagen injection site.

Conclusion.—Periurethral collagen injections produced lasting improvement in true stress incontinence in many of these women. It is a simple day-case procedure that may be used in frail women and those who have not done well after surgery. If injection treatment fails, other measures may be tried.

▶ Operation for recurrent stress incontinence is almost always more complicated than the first one, with a higher failure rate. In failed operations, when the bladder neck is well suspended (no bladder-base mobility), the surgeon should not perform another bladder neck suspension. Periurethral collagen injection is one of the better options for patients who failed previous operation and do not have bladder-base hypermobility. The other options for these patients are obstructive sling procedures, which are associated with high frequency of postoperative voiding difficulties and erosion of slings into the urethra, and artificial sphincters, which are technically complicated.

Periurethral collagen injection should not be considered an "easy office procedure" for stress incontinence. As opposed to other surgical procedures, periurethral collagen injection frequently has to be repeated 2 or 3 times. In this series, 43% of patients had to have multiple procedures (27%

had 2 procedures and 16% had 3 procedures) before success or failure could be determined. This series reports 2 years of follow-up; however, less than half of the patients were available for the 2-year follow-up, and results of the other half that were unavailable at 2 years cannot be assessed.

The procedure is relatively simple, short, and free of complications. The less optimistic message in this report is that cure rate declined over time, to less than 50% in 2 years. It is important to assess these patients at 5 years to see whether the trend of decline of success continues, so that we know whether we are offering only "temporary relief" to these patients.

A. Bergman, M.D.

Comparison of Anterior Colporrhaphy and Retropubic Urethropexy for Patients With Genuine Stress Urinary Incontinence

Harris RL, Yancey CA, Wiser WL, et al (Univ of Mississippi, Jackson)
Am J Obstet Gynecol 173:1671–1675, 1995   11–7

Introduction.—Genuine stress incontinence is the most common form of urinary incontinence in women. It is generally treated with surgery, most commonly with either the anterior colporrhaphy with Kelly-Kennedy plication or the retropubic urethropexy. The long-term efficacy of these 2 procedures were compared in patients with genuine stress urinary incontinence.

Methods.—The hospital records were reviewed of 56 patients treated with anterior colporrhaphy and 20 patients treated with retropubic urethropexy for genuine stress urinary incontinence over a 4-year period. Preoperative variables and evaluations were reviewed, as were postoperative voiding trial results. All patients were interviewed by telephone regarding their current state of urinary continence, which defined treatment success or failure.

Results.—At follow-up, urinary continence was reported by 46.4% of the patients who underwent anterior colporrhaphy and 75% of the patients who underwent retropubic urethropexy (Table 1). Recurrence for failures occurred at a mean of 12.4 months after anterior colporrhaphy and 13.6 months after retropubic urethropexy. The 2 groups were comparable for patient, medical, and surgical factors and for the mean duration of postoperative catheterization, but significantly more patients in the

TABLE 1.—Comparison of Incontinence Procedures

Procedure outcome	Anterior colporrhaphy (n = 56)	Retropubic urethropexy (n = 20)
Cure	26 (46.4%)	15 (75%)
Failure	30 (53.6%)	5 (25%)

Note: P < 0.037.
(Courtesy of Harris RL, Yancey CA, Wiser WL, et al: Comparison of anterior colporrhaphy and retropubic urethropexy for patients with genuine stress urinary incontinence. *Am J Obstet Gynecol* 173:1671–1675, 1995.)

anterior colporrhaphy group underwent concurrent repair of other pelvic floor defects than in the retropubic urethropexy group (93% vs. 15%).

Conclusions.—Considering only the long-term cure of genuine stress urinary incontinence, retropubic urethropexy is significantly more effective than the anterior colporrhaphy. However, severe anatomical changes may necessitate the vaginal approach or perhaps a combination of vaginal and abdominal approaches.

▶ Scientifically, this study lacks few objective criteria. Cure or failure is defined as loss of urine reported by patients in a telephone interview. Some patients may be hesitant to report failure, if they decide they do not wish to have another operation. The diagnosis was established with criteria that are less than optimal. Some patients had urodynamic testing, but others did not. Some patients had urethral pressure measured, whereas others did not. Still, the reader should appreciate that if a "mistake" was made in the methodology, it was made in both groups. The main drawback of the study is that the 2 groups are not comparable. Women with more significant pelvic relaxation had the vaginal operation, whereas women with less significant prolapse had retropubic urethropexy. Are we comparing apples to oranges?

Still, on a long-term follow-up, the abdominal retropubic procedures were significantly more successful than the vaginal ones. An interesting point is that the mean recurrence interval for failures was 12.4 months for anterior colporrhaphy and 13.6 months for abdominal retropubic procedures. The clinician should not assess results of the anti-incontinence procedure until 1 year after the operation.

A. Bergman, M.D.

Burch Colposuspension for Stress Urinary Incontinence: 5-Year Results in 153 Women

Kinn A-C (Karolinska Hosp, Stockholm; St Göran's Hosp, Stockholm; Huddinge Hosp, Stockholm)
Scand J Urol Nephrol 29:449–455, 1995   11–8

Introduction.—A variety of treatments, including bladder training pelvic floor exercises, acupuncture, electrostimulation, and various surgical techniques, have been developed to correct urinary incontinence. The efficacy of these methods must be established for both short- and long-term periods. Therefore, the efficacy of Burch colposuspension for the treatment of stress urinary incontinence was evaluated up to 5 years after surgery.

Methods.—During a 6-year period, 153 women underwent Burch colposuspension, performed by 1 urologist, for urinary stress incontinence. Preoperative evaluation included gynecologic examination, cystoscopy, and urodynamic studies. The patients underwent follow-up evaluations 2 and 24 months after surgery. At a mean of 5 years after surgery, the patients were sent a questionnaire and asked to return for a reevaluation.

Results.—Of the 153 patients, 45 had early, mostly mild, complications and 12 had late complications (after 2 months). Complete continence was reported by 88% of the patients at 2 months after the surgery, by 86% at 2 years after surgery, and by 78% of the 125 patients reevaluated at 5 years after surgery. Over time, no changes in cystometric bladder capacity and urethral closure pressure occurred. Patients with successful procedures had a 20% mean increase in urethral closure pressure, compared with a 2% mean increase in the urethral closure pressure in patients with treatment failure. Compared with the patients with successful procedures, the patients with failed procedures were older and had lower urethral closure pressures preoperatively, but no differences between these groups were found in body weight and parity.

Discussion.—The Burch procedure yields good long-term results in patients with genuine stress incontinence, but it is not suitable in patients with sphincter insufficiency caused by increased age or previous surgery. Therefore, preoperative urodynamic investigations should be performed to identify patients with low urethral closure pressure, for whom a sling urethroplasty is indicated.

▶ Here is yet another report on the long-term effect of the Burch procedure. Unlike other procedures, the failure rate of this procedure does not increase significantly over the years. The authors reported an early failure rate of 6.5%, which increased to 10.6% at 5 years. In other words, there were very few "late failures." Once the procedure works, it works over time.

An interesting point is the exclusion of patients with low urethral pressure from the "Burch group." That requires preoperative urodynamics, but if the surgeon wants to optimize the results, then this approach is recommended.

A. Bergman, M.D.

Laparoscopic Burch Bladder Neck Suspension: Early Results
Radomski SB, Herschorn S (Univ of Toronto)
J Urol 155:515–518, 1996   11–9

Background.—Although the Burch suspension provides reliable treatment for patients with stress urinary incontinence caused by hypermobility, the procedure is associated with significant morbidity and hospitalization. In an effort to reduce adverse effects and hospitalization time, the Burch suspension was performed using a laparoscopic approach. Early patient results were reported.

Patients and Methods.—Patients with bladder neck hypermobility and types 1 and 2 stress urinary incontinence were identified. Forty-six patients aged 26–70 years were considered to be candidates for a modified laparoscopic Burch bladder neck suspension, which was performed according to the method described by Tanagho using a nonabsorbable braided No. 1 suture. Before surgery, cystoscopy, multichannel urodynamics with pressure-flow studies, and measurement of Valsalva leak-point pressure were done. Early postoperative outcomes were evaluated.

Results.—Thirty-four laparoscopic Burch procedures were performed, using a transperitoneal approach in 13 patients and an extraperitoneal approach in 21 patients. The laparoscopic procedure could not be completed in 12 patients, all of whom underwent an open operation. The mean duration of surgery was 196 minutes, and the mean blood loss was 96.3 mL. Patients remained in the hospital for a mean of 3.2 days after surgery. Postoperatively, 2 patients experienced hematoma or anemia. Transient urinary retention, enterocele, and uterine prolapse also occurred in 1 patient each after surgery. Patients were followed for 12–26 months. Twenty-nine patients who had the laparoscopic Burch suspension reported that they were completely dry at a mean follow-up of 17.3 months. Only 5 patients had continued incontinence after surgery, including 3 with stress and urge incontinence, 1 with stress incontinence only, and 1 with urge incontinence only. Surgical duration and postoperative hospitalization were found to decrease with increased operative experience.

Conclusions.—The 85% cure rate noted at a mean of 17.3 months in patients undergoing the laparoscopic Burch suspension was comparable to that obtained with endoscopic and open Burch suspension procedures. Morbidity associated with the laparoscopic Burch procedure also was similar to that of endoscopic suspension, and appeared to be better than in the open Burch approach. The laparoscopic operating time was, however, longer than the other suspensions. The extraperitoneal approach can be accomplished more quickly and with less dissection, although in patients who have had previous lower abdominal surgery, the transperitoneal approach may be more suitable. Longer follow-up of patients having undergone the laparoscopic Burch suspension is currently under way.

▶ The Burch bladder suspension has been proved to be an effective procedure, with good long-term results. This study proves that the procedure can be done laparoscopically with a similar cure rate. With a follow-up of 1 year or more, 85% of the women who had the procedure were dry. These results are comparable to those of the open Burch procedure. In 12 of the 46 women, a laparoscopic operation could not be performed, but the procedure was turned into an open one.

The operating surgeon should not insist on a laparoscopic procedure at any cost, and if technical difficulty occurs, the surgeon should not hesitate to proceed with an open operation. The reported results are encouraging, although more studies with long follow-up (of at least a year) and objective evaluation are needed to confirm the efficacy of the laparoscopic Burch procedure.

A. Bergman, M.D.

Laparoscopic Colpo-Suspension
Das S, Palmer JK (Kaiser Permanente Med Ctrs, Walnut Creek and Santa Rosa, Calif)
J Urol 154:1119–1121, 1995   11–10

Objective.—A preliminary study was done in 10 women with anatomical stress incontinence to explore the feasibility of using minimally invasive laparoscopic techniques to perform colposuspension. The results were compared with those in 10 other patients having open colposuspension or the Raz vaginal needle suspension procedure.

Technique.—With the patient supine on low stirrups and the bladder catheterized, a 2-cm incision is made midway between the pubic symphysis and umbilicus. The extraperitoneal retropubic space is developed digitally and a rubber balloon placed in the space and inflated with about 1 L of saline. A laparoscopic lens in a 10-mm trocar sheath is then introduced and high-flow carbon dioxide is insufflated. Two 10-mm trocars are placed lateral to the rectus abdominis for placing dissecting instruments. The superior pubic rami and paraurethral anterior vaginal wall are dissected from overlying loose fat. A drill hole is made in the superior pubic ramus, and a bone anchor carrying a 1-0 polyester suture with cutting needle attached is hammered into the drill hole. The needle is passed twice through the dissected anterior vaginal walls and the ends are tied extracorporeally. A single suspension suture is placed on either side. The vagina is packed for 24 hours, and a Foley catheter is left in place for 48 hours.

Results.—Stress incontinence was comparably relieved early in the postoperative period in all surgical groups, but patients having the laparoscopic procedure had less pain and were hospitalized for a shorter time. In 1 patient, a diabetic, bilateral femoral neuropathy developed after prolonged abduction of the thighs. No morbidity was directly related to the use of bone anchors, and there was no evidence that the anchors migrated.

Conclusion.—Laparoscopic colposuspension is a feasible procedure for correcting stress incontinence in women, but longer-term follow-up is required.

▶ Laparoscopic surgical procedures have become more popular and eventually may replace open operations when both can achieve the same results. Operative procedures for stress incontinence are part of the same trend. The difference between operations for urinary incontinence and other gynecologic procedures is that anti-incontinence laparoscopic procedures have to prove to be effective in the long run, beyond being "doable" and safe. A number of surgical procedures for stress incontinence were "doable," safe, and even effective short-term but quite disappointing when long-term effects were studied. The Burch bladder neck suspension was found, in many studies, to have good long-term results. It is only natural that laparoscopic procedures try to be "laparoscopic Burch." The technique described by Das and Palmer is not a laparoscopic Burch. There is 1 pair of sutures on each side with bone fixation. This technique may be good, but long-term results are needed to assess its efficacy.

A. Bergman, M.D.

Continence Mechanism After Colpo-Needle Suspension for Stress Urinary Incontinence

Langer R, Tal Z, Schneider D, et al (Assaf Harofeh Med Ctr, Zerifin, Israel)
J Reprod Med 40:699–702, 1995   11–11

Background.—A new colpo-needle suspension procedure for the correction of stress urinary incontinence was previously introduced. With this new surgical technique, the abdominal ends of the sutures are attached to the fixed Cooper ligament in each side, as opposed to the loose abdominal fascia. The new procedure seems to offer better support to the bladder neck, and preliminary results with use of this technique have been promising. The mechanism by which continence is restored after the colpo-needle suspension procedure was evaluated.

Patients and Methods.—Thirty-seven women undergoing colpo-needle suspension for stress urinary incontinence during a 14-month period were studied. Preoperative urodynamic evaluations were performed, and tests were repeated at 6–12 months postoperatively. Preoperative and postoperative results were compared to determine the changes responsible for restoration of continence.

Results.—Urodynamic evaluation showed that 32 of 34 patients were dry, both subjectively and objectively, after surgery. No significant differences in values for bladder capacity, residual volume pressure increase on filling or standing, maximal urethral voiding pressure, or peak flow rates were observed between preoperative and postoperative cystometric and uroflowmetric measurements. In addition, urethral pressure profiles at rest were not significantly different in terms of urethral length or urethral pressure. The only postoperative difference was an increase in pressure. Transmission ratios were Q1, 100.3, and Q2, 100.4, on coughing and in the proximal half of the urethra, respectively.

Conclusions.—The colpo-needle suspension technique seems to ameliorate genuine stress incontinence by repositioning of the proximal urethra in the intra-abdominal pressure zone. This results in restoration of positive-pressure transmission to the proximal urethra.

▶ This is a second report on a previously published technique that combines elements of the Burch and Pereyra colposuspensions. The technique was published by the authors in 1991[1] and discussed in the 1993 YEAR BOOK OF OBSTETRICS AND GYNECOLOGY.[2] The new technique has the simplicity of the

Pereyra-type needle suspension with anchoring of sutures to a fixed structure such as Cooper's ligament rather than to the abdominal fascia.

The authors report short-term cure (6–12 months' follow-up) of 32 of 34 patients. Cure was achieved with this new technique as in Burch procedures by stabilizing the bladder base and enabling abdominal pressure to be transmitted to the urethra. This technique should offer good results on long-term follow-up, although this is still to be seen.

A. Bergman, M.D.

References

1. Caspi E, Langer R: *Br J Obstet Gynaecol* 98:1183–1184, 1991.
2. 1993 YEAR BOOK OF OBSTETRICS AND GYNECOLOGY, pp 288–289.

Long-term Follow-up Results With the Stamey Operation for Stress Incontinence of Urine
Mills R, Persad R, Ashken MH (Norfolk and Norwich Hosp, London)
Br J Urol 77:86–88, 1996   11–12

Background.—The Stamey operation, used for the treatment of stress urinary incontinence, is associated with an initial high success rate. Numerous reports also have indicated that medium-term results are comparable to those obtained using open procedures that elevate the bladder neck. In the authors' department, medium-term results have showed an objective cure rate of 75% in 100 patients. To determine longer-term results, surgical outcomes among patients with more than 10 years of follow-up were evaluated.

Patients and Methods.—Forty-one patients who had undergone the Stamey operation for treatment of clinically confirmed stress incontinence, and who had been followed for 10–14 years, were asked to participate in an interview and pad testing. Thirty of the 41 patients agreed to participate. All operations had been done by the same surgeon, and no accompanying procedures had been performed in any patient. Clinical information was collected, as were data pertaining to initial and subsequent success. Patients who were leak-free were considered cured, and those with persistent stress leaks, but to a lesser degree than before surgery, were considered improved. To minimize bias, the operating surgeon did not conduct any of the interviews. All patients were weighed, and pad tests were completed in accordance with International Continence Society guidelines.

Results.—Of 30 patients, 20 patients were initially cured, 8 experienced improvement, and 2 were without improvement. At 5 years, 16 of the initially cured patients continued to be leak-free, and 3 remained improved. By 10 years, only 10 of the initially cured patients continued to be leak-free, although 15 patients remained symptomatically improved. Pad testing showed that all 10 patients reporting complete cure were, in fact, dry. No differences in age, parity, weight at time of surgery, history of pulmonary disease, smoking, previous or subsequent hysterectomy, previous incontinence surgery, and outcome at 10 years were noted. In the 10 patients who remained symptom-free, however, mean weight change over the 10 years was 0.5 kg, compared with a 4.6-kg weight gain among the 15 who were improved and a 12.3-kg gain in the 3 who were no better after initial improvement. With the exception of recurrent stress incontinence, long-term complications were negligible, and 25 of the 28 patients who were initially cured or improved reported that they would still have the operation, knowing the outcome.

Conclusions.—The initial cure rate after the Stamey operation was 67%, which subsequently fell to 33% at 10 years. The late failures may have been associated with a postoperative weight gain. Although the long-term cure rate in patients undergoing the Stamey operation is not as favorable when compared with results obtained with open surgeries, 50% of the patients in this series remained subjectively improved, and 83% indicated that they would repeat the surgery, despite subsequent results.

▶ This is a nice report on the long-term effect of needle suspension performed by 1 surgeon. Long-term follow-up studies, using objective criteria, should be the "gold standard" in evaluating the efficacy of various surgical procedures for stress incontinence.

Most comparative studies, comparing the abdominal open approach to needle suspensions or vaginal procedures, have shown that the open abdominal procedures result in the highest cure rate. Using objective criteria, long-term (5 years or more) cure of the abdominal operations (Marshall-Marchetti-Krantz or Burch) was reported as 70% or better. Does that mean that we should not perform needle suspensions or vaginal operations? This report clearly indicates that when "cure" and "improvement" criteria are combined, 83% of patients were satisfied with their results. Patients even indicated that they would go through the operation again knowing the eventual outcome. Still, when using strict criteria of cure, only 67% were cured on initial evaluation, and that number dropped to less than half (30%) at 10 years. The Stamey operation in this report did not hold, over time, results as good as those reported by the open abdominal operation.

The needle suspensions are simpler and less morbid than the open abdominal operations. The surgeon must take into consideration the patient's medical condition and surgical risk before deciding whether to perform an open abdominal operation vs. a needle suspension, which is simpler and still results in good patient satisfaction.

A. Bergman, M.D.

Postoperative Catheterization, Urinary Retention, and Permanent Voiding Dysfunction After Polytetrafluoroethylene Suburethral Sling Placement

Weinberger MW, Ostergard DR (Univ of Wisconsin, Madison; Univ of California, Irvine)
Obstet Gynecol 87:50–54, 1996   11–13

Background.—Patients undergoing surgery for stress incontinence commonly experience postoperative delayed spontaneous voiding. The incidence of postoperative urinary retention is approximately 4% in patients who have an organic sling placed and 10% in those who have a synthetic graft.

Objectives.—To assess the incidence of associated permanent voiding dysfunction, patients with polytetrafluoroethylene suburethral slings were studied. The effects of preoperative voiding mechanism and uroflow measures on the duration of catheterization were evaluated after sling surgery.

Methods.—One hundred eight patients with genuine stress incontinence were treated with suburethral sling procedures during a 5-year period, and urodynamic and catheterization data from the medical records were reviewed. In addition, 98 patients were interviewed by telephone about incontinence, self-catheterization, and voiding symptoms at least 1 year postoperatively.

Results.—The patients had catheters in place for a mean of 11 weeks after surgery. The length of catheterization was unrelated to the preoperative uroflow measurements. Catheterization was required for a mean of 6 weeks postoperatively for patients with a preoperative detrusor contraction, compared with 15 weeks for those without this finding (Table 1). The risk of sling removal for retention was 7% vs. 33%. At follow-up, 8 patients were still performing catheterization and 14 had other problems, including the inability to urinate in an upright position and use of Credé's maneuver or double-voiding to facilitate emptying. The duration of catheterization was unrelated to ongoing voiding dysfunction. Postoperative urinary retention necessitated additional surgery in 9 women: 3

TABLE 1.—Effect of Preoperative Voiding Mechanism on Duration of
Postoperative Catheterization

	Present (*n*)	Absent (*n*)	*P*
Valsalva*	6.1 ± 8.1 (28)	7.6 ± 6.8 (42)	.20
Urethral relaxation†	6.7 ± 7.3 (62)	6.0 ± 6.9 (8)	.72
Detrusor contraction‡	6.1 ± 5.9 (65)	14.8 ± 15.4 (5)	.07

Note: Data are presented as mean weeks ± standard deviation. Data are presented for the 70 patients who urinated during the pressure-voiding study.
*Valsalva constitutes any increase in abdominal pressure during voiding.
†Urethral relaxation constitutes any decrease in urethral pressure during voiding.
‡Detrusor contraction constitutes any increase in true detrusor pressure during voiding.
(Courtesy of Weinberger MW, Ostergard DR: Postoperative catheterization, urinary retention, and permanent voiding dysfunction after polytetrafluoroethylene suburethral sling placement. *Obstet Gynecol* 87:50–54, 1996. Reprinted with permission from The American College of Obstetricians and Gynecologists.)

were still performing catheterization, 1 was using Credé's maneuver, and 1 urinated in a standing position.

Conclusions.—Many patients who have a polytetrafluoroethylene suburethral sling placed for stress incontinence will be left with permanent voiding difficulties. Furthermore, removal or revision of the sling does not necessarily restore normal voiding. The duration of postoperative catheterization is significantly related to the likelihood of restoring continence.

▶ The most common complications after sling procedures for stress incontinence are voiding difficulties and even permanent urinary retention. After such an operation, up to 15% of women need prolonged or permanent self-catheterization. The surgeon and the patient should know that they may trade one problem (incontinence) for another (retention). Still, some women may benefit from the sling procedure, e.g., women with stress incontinence, bladder base mobility, and low urethral pressure or low Valsalva leak point. These women are not ideal candidates for abdominal bladder neck suspension (Burch or Marshall-Marchetti-Krantz) or needle suspensions (Pereyra-Raz operation). When making a decision about the procedure, it is important for patients to know whether they are at high risk of postoperative urinary retention.

Weinberger and Ostergard identified a factor predicting postoperative urinary retention after sling operation: the presence or absence of bladder contraction or preoperative urodynamic voiding study. Surgery for stress urinary incontinence increases urethral resistance. Some women may have adequate preoperative urine flow and normal residual volume on preoperative voiding even if their bladder is hypotonic, just because urethral resistance is low. Postoperative urinary retention may develop in these women. Women who have adequate bladder contraction preoperatively have a detrusor that most likely will overcome resistance created by a sling, and urinary retention will be less of a problem. In this study, women who had adequate preoperative bladder contraction voided adequately after their sling, in less than half the time, than those who did not have preoperative bladder contraction. The presence or absence of bladder contraction on voiding is crucial for prediction of voiding difficulties after sling operation.

Does that mean that every woman undergoing a sling procedure needs to have full urodynamic evaluation? Probably yes. The sling operation is suited for women with stress urinary incontinence and low urethral pressure or low Valsalva leak point; these are 2 parameters detected on urodynamics. Voiding studies are another extension of urodynamic studies and an extension that, as shown in this study, cannot be ignored.

A. Bergman, M.D.

The Polypropylene Pubovaginal Sling for the Treatment of Recurrent Stress Urinary Incontinence

Morgan JE, Heritz DM, Stewart FE, et al (Univ of Toronto)
J Urol 154:1013–1015, 1995   11–14

Background.—The pubovaginal sling is an accepted procedure for recurrent urinary incontinence resulting from intrinsic sphincter deficiency or type III stress urinary incontinence. For this operation to be effective and safe, the bladder and the urethra need to be completely mobilized, with release from dense pelvic scar followed by suspension of the bladder neck from Cooper's ligaments in a mid-retropubic position. The value of a 2-team approach in the treatment of recurrent incontinence in patients with extensive pelvic scarring from previous surgery was studied.

Methods.—Eighty-eight consecutive patients undergoing treatment between 1986 and 1992 were followed up for 1 month to 7 years (mean, 4.1 years). Forty-four percent of the women were followed up for 6.6 years. An important selection criterion was the presence of a scarred, wide-open, proximal urethra or drain pipe urethra. One surgical team operated from the abdomen and the other from the vagina. The bladder neck was released from its bed of scar under direct vision, and the sling was set in place with minimal tension at the bladder neck.

Outcomes.—Seventy-five women (85.2%) were cured of stress urinary incontinence, and 9.1% were improved, with primarily urge incontinence. Five procedures (5.7%) failed. Surgical failure was significantly correlated with chronic chest disease. No major complications occurred. Postoperative urinary retention was documented in 6 patients; it was temporary in 4 of them.

Conclusions.—The 2-team approach using polypropylene mesh continues to be effective in the treatment of complicated stress urinary incontinence. The overall success rate of the pubovaginal sling procedure in this series was 85%.

▶ The question of what is the best operation for stress urinary incontinence (SUI) will continue to be asked, and the more than 100 operations designed are the proof that this is still an unresolved problem. There is no "one operation" that is good for every specific problem. Primary (not previously failed) stress incontinence with bladder-base hypermobility (anatomical defect) is best cured by most surgeons by abdominal retropubic suspension (Burch Marshall-Marchetti-Krantz type). Recurrent SUI or failures after a previous operation should be divided into "technical" and "functional" failures. Technical failures result in viable but still hypermobile urethra. These cases should be treated by repeated bladder suspension. Functional failures result in type III or intrinsic sphincteric deficiency, i.e., stem pipe "nonviable" urethra. In the absence of hypermobility, these functional failures do respond favorably to periurethral collagen injections, as well as to sling procedures. In the presence of hypermobility and intrinsic sphincteric deficiency, the sling procedure is probably the only operation to restore continence. In this difficult group, Morgan et al. report an 85% cure rate with the Marlex mesh sling. Technically it is important to release the urethra from dense pelvic scarring and to secure the sling in place with no tension at all. When done properly, the pubovaginal sling offers the best cure rate for treatment of SUI due to intrinsic sphincter deficiency and urethral hypermobility.

A. Bergman, M.D.

The Mersilene Mesh Suburethral Sling: A Clinical and Urodynamic Evaluation
Young SB, Rosenblatt PL, Pingeton DM, et al (Univ of Massachusetts, Worcester)
Am J Obstet Gynecol 173:1719–1726, 1995   11–15

Introduction.—Suburethral sling procedures may be the optimal management option for patients with primary genuine stress incontinence with chronically increased abdominal pressure and those with an increased risk of failure with standard urethropexy. Recently, suburethral sling procedures have increasingly been performed with a synthetic material, including Mersilene polyethylene. However, there is concern about increased complications with synthetic slings, including infection, prolonged urinary retention, and graft rejection. The safety and efficacy of the Mersilene mesh suburethral sling were evaluated by comparing preoperative and 1-year postoperative urodynamic studies.

Methods.—Over a 5-year period, 110 patients with genuine stress incontinence that was recurrent, associated with low-pressure urethra, or primary in association with chronically increased intra-abdominal pressure underwent Mersilene mesh suburethral sling procedures. Of these 110 patients, 91 had 1 year of follow-up and 67 had complete preoperative and 1-year postoperative urodynamic evaluations. The patients also reported voiding patterns, urinary symptoms, and the presence of incontinence before and 6 weeks after surgery.

Results.—Normal voiding occurred at a mean of 10 days after surgery, but 3 patients had long-term retention. At the 6-week examination, 19 women (17%) reported significant urgency, 11 had urge incontinence, 2 had leakage with stress, 5 had urinary frequency and nocturia, and 14 patients had had postoperative urinary tract infections. The 1-year postoperative urodynamic evaluation demonstrated an objective cure rate of 93%. There were subjective reports of complete stress continence in 95%. Physical examination revealed ascent of the anterior vaginal wall in 64% on Valsalva's maneuver and no movement in 36%. There were long-term complications in 7 patients (6%), including inadequate voiding in 3, a need for release of a midvaginal stenotic band in 1, erosion of the graft through the vaginal mucosa in 2 (which required sling removal in 1), and a persistent right groin sinus in 1 (requiring excision of the sling arm).

Conclusions.—The Mersilene mesh suburethral sling procedure resulted in a 93% objective and 95% subjective cure rate with low perioperative and postoperative morbidity and low rejection rates, indicating that the procedure is both safe and effective.

▶ Primary stress incontinence with bladder-base hypermobility (anatomical defect) and normal urethral pressure (20 cm of water or more) is best treated by bladder neck suspension. "High risk" for failure of bladder neck suspension includes previous failures and no anatomical defect, stress urinary incontinence (SUI) and low urethral pressure, chronic increased abdominal pressure and SUI, and neuropathy. These high-risk patients are better treated by bladder neck obstruction, than by suspension. Bladder neck obstruction by sling procedures is associated with a high success rate, but with complication rates that exceed those of the bladder neck suspensions.

The authors reported a 93% success rate in these high-risk patients using a Mersilene mesh suburethral sling. With this technique, the most common complications, i.e., urinary retention and erosion of the sling material into the urethra, were minimal. Only 3 of 75 patients had postoperative urinary retention, and 2 of 75 had erosion of the vaginal sling site. The high success rate and acceptable low complication rate make the Mersilene mesh sling a good option for patients who are at high risk for failure of the suspensive procedures. The authors had some exclusion criteria that a surgeon performing sling operations should keep in mind. They include perceived inability to learn self-catheterization. Postoperative voiding difficulties should be discussed with patients undergoing sling operations, which otherwise are adequate for "high-risk for failure" patients.

A. Bergman, M.D.

Postoperative Urinary Retention: Why the Patient Cannot Void
Tammela T (Tampere Univ, Finland)
Scand J Urol Nephrol 29:75–77, 1995   11–16

Background.—The incidence of postoperative urinary retention, defined as the inability to void with a full bladder, reportedly ranges from 0% to 60%. Patients undergoing general surgeries without indwelling catheters were evaluated for urinary retention over a 12-month period. A total of 5,220 operations were performed, with 124 males and 74 females subsequently affected by postoperative urinary retention. Causes of urinary retention were reviewed.

Discussion.—Pharmacologic agents used during and after surgery, including general and spinal anesthetics (halothane and bupivacaine), anticholinergic agents (atropine), opiates (morphine and pethidine), and α-adrenergic agonists (used to raise blood pressure during anesthesia and immediately postoperatively), play a role in postoperative urinary retention. Use of these drugs leads to detrusor contractility and increased bladder outlet resistance, both of which are essential to the development of urinary retention.

Other factors leading to increased outflow resistance via stimulation of α_1-receptors include postoperative pain and anxiety. Pain associated with lower abdominal and perineal regions also can impede perineal relaxation, which typically is the first step toward initiation of the micturition reflex. Edematous urethral and bladder neck tissues, especially after gynecologic surgeries, also can hinder urinary flow. Finally, overdistention of the bladder, caused by the administration of large quantities of IV fluids, has been shown in previous studies to significantly increase the risk of urinary retention after surgery. Conversely, this risk is significantly decreased when fluid administration is restricted. Patients with previous infravesical obstruction and neuropathy also are susceptible to postoperative urinary retention.

Conclusions.—Postoperative urinary retention can be caused by many different factors, most notably sedation, type of anesthesia, bladder overdistention secondary to administration of large amounts of IV fluids, and postoperative pain and anxiety. Predisposing factors also include previous infravesical obstruction and neuropathy.

▶ Postoperative urinary retention is a clinical dilemma that many gynecologists face. In the author's series, 2.9% of women had urinary retention develop after various operations. The incidence after pelvic surgery and bladder operations is much higher. The author nicely reviews causes for urinary retention such as anesthesia with halothane, spinal or epidural anesthesia, use of atropine and its derivatives or opiates, and use of α-adrenergics to increase blood pressure and bladder overdistention, which breaks the "cell-to-cell-junction," resulting in bladder hypotonicity.

The pelvic surgeon should be familiar with these factors. The reader should keep in mind that almost all these causes for retention are transient. The surgeon should leave a catheter in place and let the bladder stay contracted for as long as needed. Medications to enhance bladder contractions should not be given before 4 to 6 weeks after an operation. By that time, most bladders will resume the ability to effectively contract on their own.

A. Bergman, M.D.

Prevention of Postoperative Urinary Stress Incontinence After Surgery for Genitourinary Prolapse

Colombo M, Maggioni A, Zanetta G, et al (Univ of Milan, Italy)
Obstet Gynecol 87:266–271, 1996   11–17

Introduction.—Postoperative stress incontinence is a potential problem in women undergoing conventional vaginal repair of genitourinary prolapse. Even in continent women, the prolapse surgery should include stabilization of the bladder neck in an attempt to prevent postoperative stress incontinence. Cystopexy alone was compared with cystopexy with plication of the posterior pubourethral ligaments for the prevention of postoperative stress incontinence after prolapse surgery.

Methods.—The randomized study included 102 continent women admitted for surgical correction of severe urethrocystocele. All patients had a grade 2 or greater urethrocystocele and a negative stress test after repositioning of the prolapse. Fifty-two women were assigned to undergo cystopexy alone and 50 to have cystopexy plus posterior pubourethral ligaments plication. Six months postoperatively, the women underwent full urodynamic investigation.

Techniques.—Cystopexy is performed through a midline incision in the anterior vaginal wall. After the vaginal epithelium is separated from the underlying pubocervical fascia, 6 or 7 interrupted stitches of 2-0 braided silicone-coated polyester suture are placed in the fascia on either side of the trigone and bladder base. The sutures, each slightly more lateral than the one before, are tied to approximate and plicate the pubocervical fascia underneath the bladder. The redundant vaginal edges are then trimmed and sutured.

The procedure for plication of the posterior pubourethral ligaments starts with placement of a Kocher hemostat in the periurethral tissue 2 cm lateral on either side of the urethrovesical junction and a single mattress-type stitch of 0 polyglyconate lateral and medial to each hemostat. Once cystopexy is completed, the stitch is tied to achieve proper elevation of the urethrovesical junction. The redundant vaginal edges are studied and trimmed, without passing 1 end of the plication suture through the cut edges of the vagina. Each procedure concludes with culdeplasty and posterior colporrhaphy with perineorrhaphy.

Results.—Intermittent self-catheterization was required by 23% of patients undergoing cystopexy only (mean, 11 days) and 28% of those undergoing cystopexy plus posterior pubourethral ligaments plication (mean, 16.5 days). None of the patients in the cystopexy-only group had persistent voiding problems, compared with 10% of those undergoing posterior pubourethral ligaments plication. One patient in the latter group required urethral dilation because of complete retention of urine. One year after surgery, 8% of patients in each group had postoperative stress incontinence. Two percent of patients in each group had symptomatic detrusor instability.

Conclusions.—For women undergoing surgical repair for genitourinary prolapse, cystopexy alone reduces morbidity by encouraging resumption of spontaneous voiding and avoiding persistent voiding difficulties. Cystopexy appears to be a safe and effective treatment for severe cystourethrocele in continent patients. The addition of posterior pubourethral ligaments plication does not appear to be any more effective in preventing postoperative stress incontinence.

▶ Development of stress incontinence in a previously continent woman is a frustrating problem. Eight percent to 15% of continent women will have stress urinary incontinence after operation for pelvic relaxation. Some women may have "occult stress urinary incontinence"—stress incontinence that shows after the prolapse is reduced. This condition can be detected preoperatively by having women fill their bladder and do a stress test with reduction of prolapse (by pessary—Sims' speculum or manually). In these women, a "prophylactic" anti-incontinence procedure can be combined with repair of the prolapse.

The problem is with women with severe pelvic relaxation and no "occult stress incontinence." These women will not lose urine on a stress test done with reduction of prolapse, and their sphincter weakness may be detected only on urodynamic studies. Unfortunately, urodynamic studies cannot be done for every woman with pelvic relaxation. To overcome this problem, some authors suggested doing a "prophylactic" Kelly procedure for every woman with significant prolapse. The authors of this study demonstrated that doing a prophylactic anti-incontinence procedure was not beneficial and only created a problem of postoperative voiding difficulties.

A logical preoperative clinical approach for women with no stress incontinence and significant pelvic relaxation is to fill the bladder and do a stress test with reduction of prolapse. If loss of urine occurs, these women need some evaluation and an anti-incontinence procedure if the bladder is stable. If no loss of urine occurs, a urethral cough profile is helpful and an anti-incontinence procedure only if the sphincter is weak. Doing a prophylactic anti-incontinence procedure on all women with significant pelvic relaxation offers no benefits and may cause problems.

A. Bergman, M.D.

12 Infection

Open Study of Topical 0.025% Tretinoin in the Treatment of Vulvar Lichen Sclerosus: One Year of Therapy
Virgili A, Corazza M, Bianchi A, et al (Università di Ferrara, Italy)
J Reprod Med 40:614–618, 1995

12–1

Introduction.—Lichen sclerosus (LS) is a chronic inflammatory and degenerative disorder of the vulvar skin that is seen mainly in middle-aged and elderly women. Those affected have itching, burning, and dyspareunia.

Objective.—The value of treatment with tretinoin (all-*trans*-retinoic acid), a topical retinoid, was examined in 22 women with histologically documented LS of the vulva. The patients, with an average age of 59.5 years, had had LS for nearly 6 years on average.

Treatment.—A 0.025% tretinoin cream was applied daily 5 days a week to the vulvar lesion and gently rubbed in.

Results.—Pruritus, burning, and dyspareunia resolved in approximately 75% of the patients. Hyperkeratosis and lesions resulting from scratching resolved in a large majority of those affected, but vulvar fibrosis and sclerosis did not improve. Histopathologic study confirmed that hyperkeratosis consistently lessened and that atrophy and basal cell degeneration improved significantly. Sclerosis and inflammatory infiltration were relatively resistant to treatment. All 13 patients followed up 4–13 months after treatment ended were asymptomatic. Treatment was generally well tolerated. Erythema resolved in a few days when treatment was suspended and steroid substituted for a few days.

Conclusion.—These preliminary findings suggest that topical tretinoin is an effective treatment for LS of the vulva.

▶ Lichen sclerosus is a chronic inflammatory degenerative disease of the vulva that affects postmenopausal women and causes pruritus and dyspareunia. The etiology of this condition is unknown, and treatment usually consists of topical testosterone or corticosteroids. The results of this study indicate that topical use of a retinoid, 0.025% tretinoin, for 5 days each week for 1 year caused substantial improvement in the symptoms and histologic changes of this lesion. Clinicians may wish to try this agent, which is mainly used for the treatment of photodamaged skin, for patients with symptomatic LS.

D.R. Mishell, Jr., M.D.

Evaluation of a Rapid Diagnostic Test for Bacterial Vaginosis

O'Dowd TC, West RR, Winterburn PJ, et al (Trinity College, Dublin; Univ of Wales, Cardiff; College of Cardiff, Wales)
Br J Obstet Gynaecol 103:366–370, 1996   12–2

Background.—Bacterial vaginosis, a common condition, is underdiagnosed. An effective diagnostic test for bacterial vaginosis should yield results during consultation; be valid, reproducible, sensitive, and specific; require minimal instrumentation and technical training; and be inexpensive. A newly developed diagnostic test based on the concentrations of the diamines putrescine and cadaverine, which are significantly increased in bacterial vaginosis, meets these criteria. This new test was evaluated.

Methods.—Women seeing a general practitioner because of vaginal symptoms, undergoing cervical smears in a family planning clinic, and invited for health checks were studied. The new diamine test was compared with microbiological culture for *Gardnerella vaginalis,* clue cells, and the amine test.

Findings.—Two hundred twenty-nine vaginal swabs were assayed quantitatively. The new test's sensitivity was 86% and specificity was 81% compared with microbiologic culture of *G. vaginalis.* Compared with clue cell results, the new test was 97% sensitive and 83% specific. Compared with the amine test, the diamine test had a sensitivity and specificity of 94% and 84%, respectively. In all 3 comparisons, the new test's false-positive rates were 19%, 17%, and 16%, respectively.

Conclusions.—The new diamine test is accurate, sensitive, specific, and quick and easy to perform. The technology and chemicals required are relatively inexpensive. The new test is as valid as other tests but is less subjective and simpler to execute. It is available for commercial development in a 1-minute low-technology version that can be done alongside the patient.

▶ Because bacterial vaginosis is such a common cause of symptomatic vaginitis, it would be most helpful to have an easily performed, inexpensive laboratory test to establish the diagnosis of this condition. The test described in this report seems to have good sensitivity and acceptable specificity for the diagnosis of bacterial vaginitis. It would be helpful for the practicing clinician to have such a test for office use. Hopefully, this test will become available shortly.

D.R. Mishell, Jr., M.D.

Treatment of Bacterial Vaginosis: A Comparison of Oral Metronidazole, Metronidazole Vaginal Gel, and Clindamycin Vaginal Cream

Ferris DG, Litaker MS, Woodward L, et al (Med College of Georgia, Augusta)
J Fam Pract 41:443–449, 1995   12–3

Introduction.—Several treatment options are currently recommended for bacterial vaginosis. The efficacy and treatment complications of oral metronidazole, metronidazole vaginal gel, and clindamycin vaginal cream were compared in patients with bacterial vaginosis, using clinical and laboratory evaluations plus a new DNA probe test.

Methods.—A total of 101 women with bacterial vaginosis were randomly assigned to treatment with either oral metronidazole, 500 mg, twice a day for 1 week; 0.75% metronidazole vaginal gel, 5 g, twice a day for 5 days; or 2% clindamycin phosphate vaginal cream, 5 g, once a day for 7 days. Bacterial vaginosis was defined as the presence of clue cells in the vaginal specimen plus at least 2 of the following clinical findings: vaginal discharge, vaginal pH greater than 4.5, or a positive amine test. Alternatively, a positive DNA probe test result for *Gardnerella vaginalis* and a pH greater than 4.5 defined bacterial vaginosis. The patients were followed up 7 to 14 days after treatment was initiated, with reexamination, vaginal specimen testing, and a questionnaire addressing satisfaction with the treatment. The DNA probe test was used to detect persistent G. *vaginalis* as well as *Trichomonas vaginalis*, and *Candida* species.

Results.—Of the 72 evaluable patients, 19 received oral metronidazole, 24 received metronidazole vaginal gel, and 29 received clindamycin vaginal cream. There were no significant differences in cure rates: 86.2% for clindamycin vaginal cream, 75% for metronidazole vaginal gel, and 84.2% for oral metronidazole. No significant differences were found in patient reports of symptoms after therapy in the 3 groups; symptoms persisted in only 18%. After treatment, vulvovaginal candidiasis occurred in 12.5% of the oral metronidazole group, 14.8% of the clindamycin vaginal cream group, and 30.4% of the metronidazole vaginal gel group, reflecting nonsignificant differences. Most patients were satisfied with their treatment, but the 2 intravaginal products were associated with more reports of higher satisfaction.

Conclusions.—There were no significant differences in the short-term efficacy of the 3 treatment options. However, the intravaginal products produced greater patient satisfaction. Further investigation is needed to determine long-term cure rates with the different treatment agents.

▶ This is the first comparative trial to test the 3 most widely used therapeutic regimens to treat the most common cause of vaginitis in young women, bacterial vaginosis. The results show similar cure rates with the 3 types of treatment, all of which are recommended by the Centers for Disease Control and Prevention for the treatment of bacterial vaginosis. The DNA probe used in this study is a combination of nucleic acid probes that can identify each of the 3 most common causes of vaginitis: *G. vaginalis, T. vaginalis,* and *Candida* species. Use of this probe should enable clinicians to detect the cause and treatment of vaginitis without the necessity of performing wet mounts.

D.R. Mishell, Jr., M.D.

Ligase Chain Reaction for Detection of *Neisseria gonorrhoeae* in Urogenital Swabs

Ching S, Lee H, Hook EW III, et al (Abbott Labs, Abbott Park, Ill; Univ of Alabama, Birmingham; Case Western Reserve Univ, Cleveland, Ohio; et al)
J Clin Microbiol 33:3111–3114, 1995   12–4

Introduction.—Currently, gonorrhea is definitively diagnosed by culture on selective medium, which reportedly is 80% to 95% sensitive. The use of DNA amplification methods offers a means of eliminating problems related to specimen collection and transport, which may lessen sensitivity. A ligase chain reaction (LCR) DNA amplification assay was used to detect *Neisseria gonorrhoeae* in swab specimens from the female endocervix and the male urethra.

Methods.—Specimens were collected with sterile swabs from patients at 3 geographically disparate sites in the United States. The results of a 4-hour LCR-based assay were compared with those achieved by culture on selective medium. Discordant findings were evaluated by another LCR assay based on *N. gonorrhoeae*–specific pilin probe sets. The study assessed 1,539 endocervical and 808 male urethral specimens.

Results.—Thirty-three specimens were LCR-positive but culture-negative, and the reverse was the case for 7 specimens. The initial LCR assay was 97% sensitive and 98% specific compared with culture. The specific LCR assay confirmed that 18 of the 23 discordant endocervical specimens initially found to be LCR-positive actually were positive. All initially LCR-negative discordant specimens from both sites were confirmed as positive using the *N. gonorrhoeae*–specific assay. The final sensitivity of the LCR assay for endocervical specimens was 97% (compared with 84% for culture) and its specificity was 99.6%. The positive predictive value was 96% and the negative predictive value was 99.8%.

Conclusions.—The specific LCR assay is more sensitive than culture for detecting *N. gonorrhoeae* in endocervical specimens. It also accurately detects infection in swab specimens from the male urethra. This method is highly specific and should prove useful in screening populations with a low prevalence of gonorrheal infection.

▶ The LCR assay for the detection of *Chlamydia trachomatis* has been shown to be a highly sensitive and specific method and is now being used with increasing frequency in various clinical settings. The development of an LCR assay that is highly sensitive and specific for the gonorrhoeae organism will allow laboratories to utilize the LCR assay to help establish whether a patient is infected with either of the most common sexually transmitted organisms that can cause salpingitis and tubal infertility. The finding that about 1 of 6 women infected with *N. gonorrhoeae* did not have the organism identified on Gram's stain or routine culture indicates that the LCR assay should be used to help establish whether a woman has been infected with *N. gonorrhoeae.* The development of these LCR assays is a true advance in the ability to determine whether an individual woman is actually infected with either chlamydia or gonorrhoeae.

D.R. Mishell, Jr., M.D.

The Vaginal Introitus: A Novel Site for *Chlamydia trachomatis* Testing in Women

Wiesenfeld HC, Heine RP, Rideout A, et al (Univ of Pittsburgh, Pa)
Am J Obstet Gynecol 174:1542–1546, 1996

12–5

Background.—The identification of *Chlamydia trachomatis* has been done by tissue culture or antigen detection methods. Recently, the polymerase chain reaction (PCR) has been used to diagnose *C. trachomatis*. Because of the limitations of urine testing by DNA amplification methods and the need for noninvasive sampling procedures, the vaginal introitus was evaluated as a sampling site for *C. trachomatis* testing.

Methods.—Three hundred women attending a sexually transmitted diseases clinic were studied. Swabs were obtained from the vaginal introitus and tested using PCR. Two hundred women also self-collected an additional introitus swab and provided a urine sample for PCR testing.

Findings.—Vaginal introitus swabs obtained by health care providers had a sensitivity of 92% in the detection of urogenital *C. trachomatis*, which is more sensitive than PCR, culture, or enzyme immunoassay of the cervix or urethra. Polymerase chain reaction testing of swabs collected by the patients had an 81% sensitivity. The sensitivity of urine sample testing by PCR was 73% (Table 2).

Conclusions.—Obtaining samples from the vaginal introitus for *C. trachomatis* testing by PCR is highly effective. Sampling by patients and health care providers were both as effective as commonly used diagnostic tests requiring vaginal speculum examination.

▶ Polymerase chain reaction testing is becoming the diagnostic test of choice to detect the presence of *C. trachomatis* in the lower genital tract of

TABLE 2.—Detection of *Chlamydia trachomatis* at Various Sites, Including Self-collected Introital Swabs and Urine Samples (n = 200, Total Infected = 26)

Test	Confirmed positive	Sensitivity (%)	Specificity (%)
Cervix			
PCR	22	85	99
Culture	21	81	100
Urethra			
PCR	18	69	100
Culture	12	46	100
Introitus PCR			
Self	21	81	100
HCP	24	92	100
Urine	19	73	100

Abbreviations: PCR, polymerase chain reaction; HCP, health care personnel.
(Courtesy of Wiesenfeld HC, Heine RP, Rideout A, et al: The vaginal introitus: A novel site for *Chlamydia trachomatis* testing in women. *Am J Obstet Gynecol* 174:1542–1546, 1996.)

women. If a woman is symptomatic and has a vaginal speculum examination, a sample of endocervical mucus and urethral cells can be obtained for PCR testing. However, it is difficult to perform speculum examinations among a group of asymptomatic women, especially adolescents. The results of this study indicate that when women place swabs into their own vagina for a few minutes, sufficient cellular material can be obtained to yield a high level of sensitivity and specificity for the diagnosis of *C. trachomatis.* Thus, this method can be used for screening populations of asymptomatic young women to help detect and treat this common sexually transmitted pathogen.

D.R. Mishell, Jr., M.D.

Detection of *Chlamydia trachomatis* Infection in Urine Samples From Men and Women by Ligase Chain Reaction
van Doornum GJJ, Buimer M, Prins M, et al (Municipal Health Service of Amsterdam; Probe Diagnostic Venture, Chicago)
J Clin Microbiol 33:2042–2047, 1995   12–6

Introduction.—*Chlamydia trachomatis* infection in women may be asymptomatic, which hinders the effectiveness of efforts to combat this sexually transmitted disease. Some sensitive, reliable, and inexpensive test for *C. trachomatis* that can be performed in easily obtained specimens is needed. The use of a ligase chain reaction (LCR)–based assay was tested for the detection of *C. trachomatis* infection in urine samples from women and men.

Methods.—The study took place in an Amsterdam clinic for sexually transmitted diseases. An LCR-based assay with plasmid primers was used to test urine specimens for *C. trachomatis* infection. A retrospective study was first performed in a large sample of heterosexual men and women who had participated in a prospective study of human papillomavirus infection. In a subsequent cross-sectional study, the results of LCR-plasmid analysis of urine samples from 237 women and 258 men were compared with the cell culture results in urethral and cervical specimens from women and urethral specimens from men.

Results.—In the cross-sectional study, 15 cervical specimens (6%) from women were culture-positive for *C. trachomatis.* Twenty-five urine specimens (11%) from women were positive on the plasmid-LCR assay. Thirteen of these specimens were from women with positive cervical cultures. Of the 12 LCR-positive specimens from culture-negative women, 9 were positive on a second LCR assay using primers based on chromosomal DNA. Twenty-four urethral specimens (9%) from men were culture-positive. Twenty-five male urine specimens were LCR-positive, and 20 of them were from culture-positive men. The second LCR confirmed the results of all 5 LCR-positive urine samples from culture-positive men.

Compared with cell culture, plasmid-LCR testing of urine samples from men was 83% sensitive and 98% specific. Sensitivity improved to 86% and specificity to 100% after discordant samples were resolved. In women, plasmid-LCR testing of cervical and urine specimens had a sensitivity of 93% and 87%, compared with cervical cell culture. These values improved to 96% and 93%, respectively, after resolution of discordant samples.

Conclusions.—The plasmid-LCR–based assay used is a convenient test for *C. trachomatis* infection in urine samples from men and women. The ability to test urine samples from women avoids the need to collect cervical specimens. The plasmid-LCR assay detects considerably more true positive cases than does cell culture.

▶ This is another of several recent reports that indicate that assays of urine samples using the polymerase chain reaction as well as LCR are reliable, sensitive, and convenient methods to detect the presence of *C. trachomatis.* As 6 of the 33 infertile women had negative urine assays and positive cervical swab assays and 5 women had positive urine assays but negative cervical swab assays, it may be best to assay both a urine sample and material obtained by a cervical swab to increase the sensitivity of the assay.

D.R. Mishell, Jr., M.D.

Chlamydial Cervicitis and Urethritis: Single Dose Treatment Compared With Doxycycline for Seven Days in Community Based Practises

Thorpe EM Jr, Stamm WE, Hook EW III, et al (Univ of Tennessee, Memphis; Univ of Washington, Seattle; Univ of Alabama, Birmingham; et al)
Genitourin Med 72:93–97, 1996
12–7

Background.—The effective treatment of chlamydial infections is hindered by the need for patients to take multidose therapy for 7 days or more, usually consisting of antibiotics with some gastrointestinal (GI) effects. Azithromycin, an azalide antibiotic, has a minimum inhibitory concentration (MIC) of 0.03–0.25 mg/L against *Chlamydia trachomatis*, achieves high intracellular concentrations, and has a tissue bioavailability and half-life ranging from 2 to 4 days. The safety and efficacy of one 1-g oral dosage of azithromycin was compared with doxycycline, 100 mg every 12 hours for 7 days, in patients with uncomplicated urogenital chlamydial infection.

Methods and Findings.—Five hundred ninety-seven patients enrolled at 40 U.S. sites were included in the randomized, unblinded, comparative study. Sixty-one percent of the patients given azithromycin and 60% given doxycycline were asymptomatic within 1 week after the first dose. At 2 weeks, these proportions were 86% and 83%, respectively. Bacteriologic eradication was documented in 97% of the azithromycin group and 99% of the doxycycline group. Forty-one percent of women receiving azithromycin and 37% receiving doxycycline had at least 1 adverse event, mostly involving the GI tract. The most common azithromycin-related adverse events were nausea and diarrhea. Nausea was reported by 22% of patients given doxycycline, compared with 16% of those given azithromycin. Dizziness occurred in 2% of the azithromycin group and in 1% of the doxycycline group.

Conclusions.—A single 1-g oral dose of azithromycin is as effective as standard doxycycline therapy in patients with uncomplicated chlamydial cervicitis and urethritis. Adverse effects were approximately twice as common as previously reported for both agents.

▶ This large multicenter study was performed at sites providing regular clinical care, and the results agree with those of earlier studies performed in academic university-based centers. Although 1 g of azithromycin is more expensive than 200 µg of doxycycline given for 7 days, patient compliance is likely to be better with the single dose than with the 7-day treatment regimen. When treating an asymptomatic sexual partner or when giving a single injection of ceftriaxone to treat a concurrent gonococcal infection, the advantage of giving a single dose of therapy instead of multiple doses is probably most beneficial.

D.R. Mishell, Jr., M.D.

13 Endocrinology

Variability of Day 3 Follicle-stimulating Hormone Levels in Eumenorrheic Women
Brown JR, Liu H-C, Sewitch KF, et al (New York Hosp–Cornell Med Ctr)
J Reprod Med 40:620–624, 1995   13–1

Objective.—The variability of early follicular (cycle day 3) concentrations of follicle-stimulating hormone (FSH) and estradiol (E_2) was studied prospectively in 48 women aged 22–48 years who had regular menstrual cycles lasting 21–35 days.

Methods.—Sera were sampled on cycle day 3 for up to 10 cycles, and in 1 cycle consecutive samples were drawn on cycle days 2, 3, and 4. Day-3 results were available for an average of 4½ cycles per individual. Both FSH and E_2 were estimated by radioimmunoassay. All women were studied within a 1-year period.

Findings.—Women aged 40 years and older had higher average day-3 FSH levels than did younger participants. In women younger than age 40 years, most day-3 FSH values were less than 15 mIU/mL, and nearly all estimates were less than 20 mIU/mL. Levels were more evenly distributed in older women. Of 33 younger women having multiple day-3 estimates, 5 had subsequent levels of 20 mIU/mL or higher. Older women were likelier to have multiple day-3 FSH values exceeding 25 mIU/mL. There was no clear age trend for E_2 levels except for relatively high levels in the 2 women aged 45 years and older, who also had markedly increased FSH levels. Levels of FSH varied less than E_2 levels on cycle day 3 and also when consecutive day-2 to day-4 samples were analyzed.

Implications.—In women younger than 40 years of age, an FSH level less than 20 mIU/mL on cycle day 3 is highly predictive that subsequent values obtained in the following year also will be normal. Estimates of FSH made on cycle day 2 or 4 are acceptably reliable, but E_2 estimates are more variable.

▶ Elevation of FSH levels on day 3 of the menstrual cycle is associated with an extremely low pregnancy rate when in vitro fertilization is performed in that cycle. Thus, an elevated day-3 FSH level has been shown to indicate that the ova released from the ovary, even if fertilized, are unlikely to result in an ongoing pregnancy. For this reason, many clinicians, including myself, are measuring FSH on day 3 of the cycle as part of the initial infertility examination, especially if the woman is older than 35 years. If the day-3 FSH level remains elevated in subsequent cycles, the chances of producing a viable pregnancy with any type of infertility treatment, including controlled ovarian hyperstimulation and intrauterine insemination or an assisted reproductive technique, are extremely unlikely, and the couple should be counseled accordingly. The results of this study indicate that if initially normal, serial day-3 FSH levels should be obtained in several cycles if the infertile woman is older than 40 years, but not younger than that age, and that values on days 2 or 4 of the cycle are usually similar to those on day 3.

D.R. Mishell, Jr., M.D.

Polycystic Ovary Syndrome: The Spectrum of the Disorder in 1741 Patients

Balen AH, Conway GS, Kaltsas G, et al (Univ College London Med School)
Hum Reprod 10:2107–2111, 1995   13–2

Background.—Because of the different criteria used to define polycystic ovary syndrome (PCOS), its diagnosis is controversial. In the United Kingdom, polycystic ovaries identified on ultrasound scans are generally

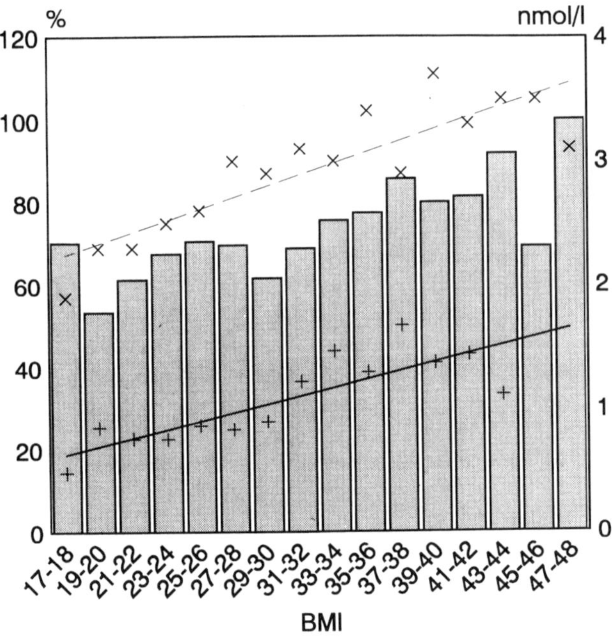

FIGURE 3.—Relationship between body mass index (*BMI*) and the rates of hirsutism and serum testosterone concentration. (Courtesy of Balen AH, Conway GS, Kaltsas G, et al: Polycystic ovary syndrome: The spectrum of the disorder in 1741 patients. *Hum Reprod* 10:2107–2111, 1995. By permission of Oxford University Press.)

accepted to be the unifying diagnostic criterion. The largest series of patients with PCOS reported to date was analyzed to provide a reference for the spectrum of this disorder and to highlight the features of ultrasound morphology with endocrine parameters.

Methods and Findings.—All 1,741 women studied had polycystic ovaries on ultrasonography and symptoms of the syndrome. Thirty-eight percent were overweight, 39.8% had increased serum levels of luteinizing hormone (LH), and 28.9% had elevated serum testosterone levels. Forty-seven percent had oligomenorrhea; 29.7%, a normal menstrual cycle; 19.2%, amenorrhea; 2.7%, polymenorrhea; and 1.4%, menorrhagia. Hirsutism was noted in 66.2% of the patients. It was mild in 20.6%, moderate in 40.7%, and severe in 4.9%. Thirty-five percent of the patients had acne, and 2.5% had acanthosis nigricans. Obesity was associated with hirsutism, increased serum testosterone levels (Fig 3), and greater rates of infertility and cycle disturbance. Infertility and cycle disturbance rates also increased with serum LH levels exceeding 10 IU/L. An increased risk of hirsutism, infertility, and cycle disturbance was associated with rising serum testosterone levels. Ovarian volume was associated with serum testosterone levels, LH, and body mass index. Body mass index was also related to uterine area.

Conclusions.—Overweight women who lose weight can expect symptomatic improvement. Increased LH concentration is correlated with infertility; thus, treatment should be selected accordingly. If the serum testosterone level exceeds 4.8 nmol/L, other causes of hyperandrogenism should be ruled out.

▶ There is disagreement regarding the criteria used for the diagnosis of the PCOS. In Britain, the diagnosis is usually made when more than 10 small follicles, less than 8 mm in diameter, are visualized in an ovary at the time of sonographic examination in a woman with at least 1 of the symptoms of PCOS: menstrual irregularity, infertility, or hyperandrogenism. In the United States, the diagnosis is usually made by the presence of the endocrinologic abnormalities of the syndrome: elevated serum LH and/or testosterone levels together with anovulation.

In this large study, the presence of obesity was directly correlated with a higher incidence of infertility, menstrual irregularity, and hirsutism. Therefore, women with PCOS and these symptoms who are obese should be told that weight reduction by means of caloric restriction and exercise will result in improvement of their abnormal symptoms. As an elevated LH concentration is associated with infertility, the authors suggest that suppression of LH by a gonadotropin-releasing hormone agonist or partial ovarian destruction may improve fecundability. Studies need to be undertaken to provide data to support this suggestion, because such data do not currently exist.

D.R. Mishell, Jr., M.D.

Optimal Use of Hormone Determinations in the Biochemical Diagnosis of the Polycystic Ovary Syndrome

Koskinen P, Erkkola R, Penttilä T-A, et al (Turku Univ, Finland)
Fertil Steril 65:517–522, 1996

13–3

Background.—Traditionally, the diagnosis of polycystic ovary syndrome (PCOS) has been based on the presence of clinical symptoms, such as oligomenorrhea, infertility, hirsutism, and obesity, and polycystic ovaries confirmed histologically after laparotomy. This syndrome is associated with a broad range of clinical and biochemical features. An array of hormone measurements was used in an attempt to improve the biochemical diagnosis of PCOS.

Methods.—Fifty-four oligomenorrheic women with PCOS diagnosed by ovarian ultrasound and 29 healthy women with regular menstrual cycles and normal ovarian morphology were included in the retrospective clinical study. All were attending an outpatient clinic of reproductive endocrinology at a teaching hospital in Finland. Serum concentrations of luteinizing

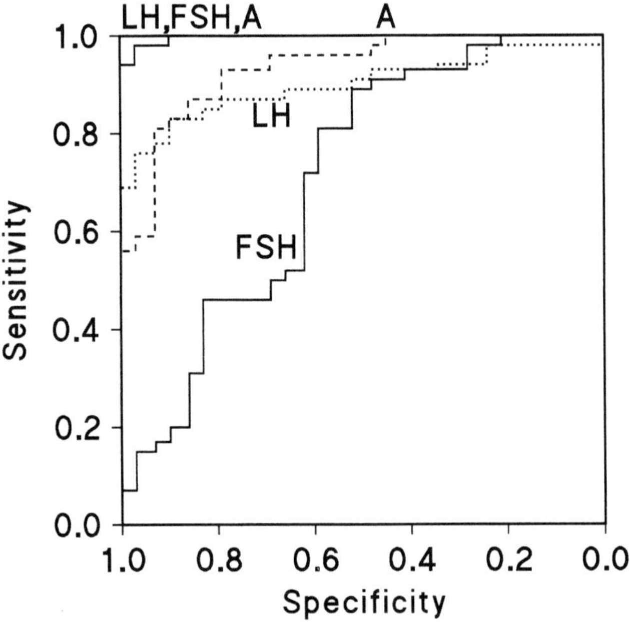

FIGURE 2.—Receiver operator characteristic (*ROC*) curves for luteinizing hormone (*LH*), follicle-stimulating hormone (*FSH*), and androstenedione (*A*) alone, and for the estimated probability level of polycystic ovary syndrome as determined by the levels of LH, FSH, and A. The areas under the ROC curves (± SE) were 0.897 ± 0.034, 0.699 ± 0.064, 0.933 ± 0.027, and 0.997 ± 0.003, respectively. The area under the ROC curve of 1.0 denotes no overlapping and the area under the ROC curve of 0.5 denotes no discrimination between the 2 groups. (From Koskinen P, Erkkola R, Penttilä T-A, et al: Optimal use of hormone determinations in the biochemical diagnosis of the polycystic ovary syndrome. *Fertil Steril* 65:517–522, 1996. Reproduced with permission of the publisher, the American Society for Reproductive Medicine [formerly The American Fertility Society].)

hormone (LH), follicle-stimulating hormone (FSH), androstenedione, testosterone, and sex hormone–binding globulin were measured.

Findings.—The most useful hormonal analytes were LH, FSH, and androstenedione when used in combination. This combination had a diagnostic sensitivity of 98%, a specificity of 93%, and an overall concordance of 96%. The degree of discrimination of each analyte used alone was lower (Fig 2).

Conclusions.—The use of LH, FSH, and androstenedione in combination can effectively distinguish women with PCOS from healthy women. Thus, with appropriate combinations of data, diagnostic usefulness is enhanced.

▶ The use of transvaginal sonography has enabled the diagnosis of polycystic ovaries to be easily made. The usual sonographic criteria for the diagnosis of polycystic ovaries are 10 or more small subcortical follicles between 2 and 10 mm in diameter and an increased amount of ovarian stroma. Many normally cycling women as well as anovulatory women have polycystic ovaries without any symptoms or endocrinologic changes consistent with hyperandrogenism. To establish the diagnosis of PCOS, some evidence of hyperandrogenism needs to be present. This study indicates that the diagnosis is best made by the finding of an elevated LH level, a low FSH level, and an elevated androstenedione level. When a combination of these findings was present, the diagnosis of PCOS could be made with a sensitivity of 98% and a specificity of 93%. Thus, clinicians can use the combination of the sonographic and hormonal findings to establish the diagnosis of PCOS with a high degree of reliability.

D.R. Mishell, Jr., M.D.

Carotid Atherosclerosis in Women with Polycystic Ovary Syndrome: Initial Results From a Case-Control Study
Guzick DS, Talbott EO, Sutton-Tyrrell K, et al (Univ of Pittsburgh, Pa)
Am J Obstet Gynecol 174:1224–1232, 1996   13–4

Background.—Women with polycystic ovary syndrome (PCOS) have characteristics that may increase the risk of atherosclerosis. Carotid ultrasonography scanning was used to assess subclinical measures of atherosclerosis in such patients.

Methods.—Sixteen premenopausal women aged 40 years or older with a history of clinical PCOS were studied. All had current serum total testosterone concentrations of 2 mol/L or more. Sixteen age-matched cycling women comprised a control group. Carotid scanning was performed, and intima-media thickness and plaque in the groups were compared. Atherosclerosis risk factors, such as body mass index and fasting insulin and lipid concentrations, were also compared.

Findings.—Women with PCOS had significantly greater mean intima-media thickness than control subjects. Evidence of plaque on ultrasound was found in 31.3% of the patients and 12.5% of control subjects (a nonsignificant difference). In univariate regressions of intima-media thickness, coefficients for insulin, total cholesterol, low-density lipoprotein cholesterol, and body mass index were significant. Total cholesterol and low-density lipoprotein both remained significant when included in the model with PCOS. However, insulin and body mass index did not remain significant, indicating possible covariance with PCOS.

Conclusions.—Women with PCOS seem to have an increased risk of subclinical atherosclerosis in their 40s. However, the small sample size in this study is a major limitation. In a larger sample, PCOS, body mass index, and insulin may be found to be independent predictors of intima-media thickness.

▶ The results of this small case-control study indicate that the presence of PCOS may be a risk factor for the acceleration of atherosclerosis in women. Earlier studies have shown that the presence of PCOS is an independent risk factor for the development of diabetes mellitus and hypertension in older age. In addition, if untreated with progestins PCOS is also a risk factor for the development of endometrial cancer. For all these reasons, women with this syndrome should be treated with long-term low androgenic oral contraceptive formulations. The increased concentrations of sex hormone–binding globulin associated with ingestion of these agents bind the excessive amounts of androgen produced by these abnormal ovaries and hopefully will reduce the risk of atherosclerosis as well as endometrial cancer developing.

D.R. Mishell, Jr., M.D.

A Contribution to the Classification of Cases of Non-classic 21-Hydroxylase-Deficient Congenital Adrenal Hyperplasia

Phocas I, Chryssikopoulos A, Sarandakou A, et al (Athens Univ, Greece)
Gynecol Endocrinol 9:229–238, 1995   13–5

Objective.—An endocrinologic study was undertaken in an attempt to distinguish patients with the nonclassic form of 21α-hydroxylase–deficient congenital adrenal hyperplasia (CAH) and heterozygous carriers from other individuals initially seen with hyperandrogenemia. Forty-five young women with symptoms of polycystic ovary syndrome were studied along with 21 family members, 12 of whom were men.

Findings.—Cluster analysis distinguished 4 groups consisting, respectively, of 3, 11, 36, and 16 individuals. The proportion of patients with elevated levels of 17-hydroxyprogesterone (17-OHP) ranged from 100% in group I to zero in group IV. The proportion of patients with high plasma cortisol levels increased in the same direction. Hyperprolactinemia was most prevalent in patients in group IV. All 3 individuals in group I had skin changes, obesity, and premature pubarche, and the single female in this group was amenorrheic. Obesity and clinical signs of hyperandrogenemia were more variable in the other groups. The response of 17-OHP to adrenocorticotropin hormone (ACTH) injection was more marked and occurred more rapidly in groups III and IV than in the other individuals. HLA typing showed that patients in group 1 were 21α-hydroxylase–deficient; patients in group II had a homozygous haplotype; patients in group III were heterozygous; and patients in group IV did not have 21α-hydroxylase deficiency.

Conclusion.—Women who are seen with hirsutism and/or menstrual irregularity should undergo ACTH stimulation testing so that nonclassic CAH caused by 21α-hydroxylase deficiency may be recognized.

▶ When the onset of symptoms of hyperandrogenism and menstrual irregularity occurs during a woman's early postadolescent years, it can be caused by polycystic ovarian syndrome (PCOS), idiopathic hirsutism, or late-onset 21-hydroxylase deficiency, also called nonclassic CAH. Late-onset CAH is an autosomal recessive disorder, the frequency and severity of which vary among different ethnic groups. Because the treatment and genetic counseling of individuals with late-onset CAH differ from those with PCOS or other causes of hyperandrogenism, it is important to establish the diagnosis.

The results of this study indicate that with ACTH testing it is possible to differentiate the severe, mild, and minimal forms of late-onset CAH from hyperandrogenism without this metabolic disorder. It is important to note that some individuals with minimal forms of late-onset CAH have normal blood levels of 17-OHP. Thus, the finding of normal levels of this hormone does not rule out the existence of this genetic disorder.

D.R. Mishell, Jr., M.D.

14 Menopause

Characterization of Reproductive Hormonal Dynamics in the Perimenopause
Santoro N, Brown JR, Adel T, et al (Univ of Medicine and Dentistry of New Jersey, Newark)
J Clin Endocrinol Metab 81:1495–1501, 1996   14–1

Background.—During the perimenopausal period, ovarian hormone secretion varies, which leads to some controversies in medical management. Reproductive hormone secretion during the perimenopause was evaluated in a longitudinal study.

Methods.—First-morning urine specimens were collected from 6 cycling women, aged 47 years and older, for 6 months. Another 5 women of older reproductive age, 43–47 years, were studied with daily urine and serum sampling for a single menstrual cycle. The urine samples were tested for luteinizing hormone (LH), follicle-stimulating hormone (FSH), estrone conjugates, and pregnanediol glucuronide and normalized for creatinine (Cr). Three comparison groups were studied as well: 11 normally cycling women of reproductive age (i.e., 19–38 years); 5 women with known premature ovarian failure; and 5 women, 54 years of age and older, who were at least 1 year postmenopausal.

Results.—Cycles were shorter in perimenopausal women than in mid-reproductive-aged women because of an attenuated follicular phase (Fig 1). Estrone conjugate excretion was also greater in the perimenopausal women, including follicular and luteal phase estrone excretion. Pregnanediol excretion was significantly decreased in the luteal phase in perimenopausal women. The perimenopausal women had increased gonadotropin concentrations, particularly FSH and particularly in the early follicular phase. They also had a lesser increase in LH. The 2 groups showed identical correlation coefficients between serum and urinary gonadotropin and sex steroid levels.

Most cycles in the perimenopausal women were ovulatory. There were clear increases in estrone and surges in LH, although with periods of tonically increased gonadotropin concentrations and persistently low estrone excretion (Table 1). These changes became more prominent as menopause drew nearer. Two perimenopausal women, who became amenorrheic within 2 years after the study, had amenorrheic periods lasting up to

"

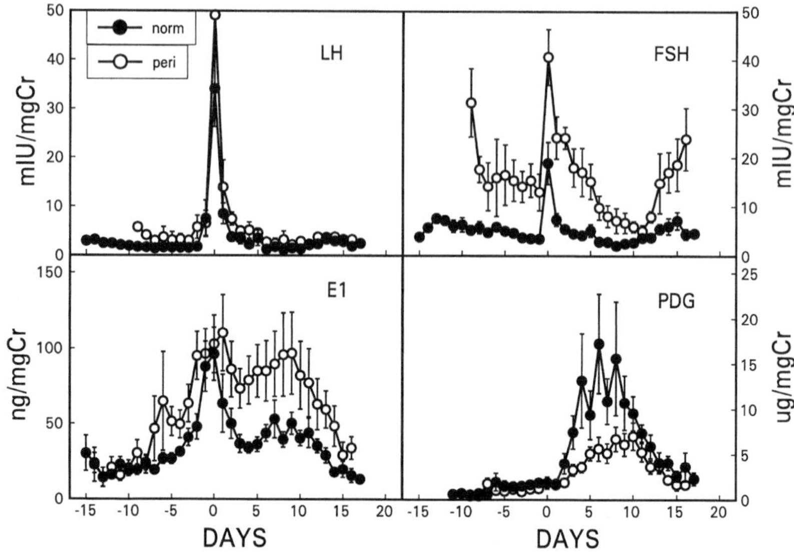

FIGURE 1.—Mean ± SEM daily urinary gonadotropin and sex steroid excretion patterns in 11 perimenopausal women, aged 43–52 years (*open circles*), compared with those in 11 midreproductive-aged women (*closed circles*). Data are standardized to day 0, the putative day of ovulation. *Abbreviation:* E_1, estrone conjugates. (Courtesy of Santoro N, Brown JR, Adel T, et al: Characterization of reproductive hormonal dynamics in the perimenopause. *J Clin Endocrinol Metab* 81:1495–1501, 1996. Copyright The Endocrine Society.)

3 months during the study. Their hormone excretion during these times was the same as in postmenopausal women.

Conclusions.—Perimenopausal women have alterations in ovarian function. These changes—including hyperestrogenism, hypergonadotropism, and decreased luteal phase progesterone excretion—start as early as 43

TABLE 1.—Comparison of Hormonal Parameters by Group

	PERI	Young	Premature	Menopause
Mean estrone (ng/mg Cr)	13–135*	23–60	4–44	3–6
Peak estrone (ng/mg Cr)	47–278	58–237	—†	—
Integrated pregnanediol (μg/mg Cr · luteal phase)	1.0–8.4*	1.6–12.7	—	—
Mean FSH (IU/g Cr)	4–32‡	3–7	36–82	24–85
Mean LH (IU/g Cr)	1.4–6.8§	1.1–4.2	5.5–23.8	4.3–14.8

Note: Ranges of hormonal values are shown.

Abbreviations: PERI, perimenopausal controls (n = 11); *Young,* youthful controls, aged 19–38 years (n = 11); *Premature,* women with premature menopause, (n = 5); *Menopause,* age appropriately menopausal women (n = 5).

*P < 0.02 vs. younger women.

†A line in lieu of data indicates that insufficient observations were available for a comparison.

‡P < 0.02 vs. young, premature, and menopausal women.

§P < 0.05 vs. young, premature, and menopausal women.

(Courtesy of Santoro N, Brown JR, Adel T, et al: Characterization of reproductive hormonal dynamics in the perimenopause. *J Clin Endocrinol Metab* 81:1495–1501, 1996. Copyright The Endocrine Society.)

years of age and may play a role in the high rate of gynecologic morbidity during perimenopause. The process of menopause is not smooth and steady; rather, different types of ovulatory and anovulatory activity eventually give way to a permanent hypergonadotropic hypoestrogenic amenorrhea.

▶ A great amount of attention is currently being given to the endocrinologic and morphologic alterations that occur in the female reproductive tract during the years immediately before menopause, which is called the perimenopause. It has been well established that during ovulatory perimenopausal cycles the menstrual cycle length decreases by a few days due to a shortened follicular phase. It was previously believed that during this short follicular phase circulating estradiol concentrations were less than they had been earlier in life and FSH concentrations were increased.

The results of this study indicate that during the ovulatory cycles of perimenopausal women the amount of urinary estrone conjugates are actually increased together with increased amounts of FSH and, to a lesser extent, LH. Urinary pregnanediol glucuronide excretion was significantly decreased. When menses fail to occur for a few months during this transition, estrone concentrations decrease to the postmenopausal range. During this time of life, growth of uterine leiomyomas and episodes of dysfunctional uterine bleeding are common and frequently result in a hysterectomy being performed. The high concentrations of estrogen and low concentrations of progesterone can also cause endometrial hyperplasia. Because of the changes in sex steroid hormone concentrations at this time of life, it is beneficial to treat women in whom abnormal bleeding develops with oral contraceptives to produce regular cyclic bleeding episodes and avoid the need for hysterectomy.

D.R. Mishell, Jr., M.D.

Family History as a Predictor of Early Menopause
Cramer DW, Xu H, Harlow BL (Brigham and Women's Hosp, Boston)
Fertil Steril 64:740–745, 1995   14–2

Introduction.—Less than 10% of women go through menopause before 46 years of age. Case studies suggest that such early menopause may have a genetic basis. Family history was evaluated as a potential predictor of early menopause in a case-control study.

Methods.—Epidemiologic data on family history and other factors were gathered from 344 women with early menopause. The women represented about 10% of respondents to a previously reported cross-sectional survey. All had undergone menopause before the age of 47 years; the average age at menopause was 42 years. The findings were compared with those for 344 randomly selected, age-matched women who had a normal age at menopause or had not yet stopped menstruating.

TABLE 1.—Odds Ratio for Early Menopause by Family History of Early Menopause

Family history of early menopause	Case (n = 344)	Control (n = 344)	Odds ratio*
None	215	313	1.0
Any†	129	31	6.1 (4.0 to 9.3)
Single relative			
Paternal, 2nd degree	2	0	—‡
Maternal, 2nd degree	10	6	2.4 (0.9 to 6.8)‡
Mother	58	17	5.0 (2.8 to 8.8)§
Sister	25	4	9.1 (3.1 to 26.5)§
Multiple relatives	34	4	12.4 (4.4 to 34.2)§

*95% confidence interval in parentheses.
†Defined as a natural menopause before age 46 years in a mother, sister, aunt, or grandmother.
‡P (chi-square) = 0.09.
§P < 0.001.
(Courtesy of Cramer DW, Xu H, Harlow BL: Family history as a predictor of early menopause. *Fertil Steril* 64:740–745, 1995. Reproduced with permission of the publisher, the American Society for Reproductive Medicine [formerly The American Fertility Society].)

Results.—Women with early menopause were no more likely than controls to report an excess of medical events in their family history. However, 38% of women in the case group reported having at least 1 female relative with menopause before 46 years of age, compared with just 9% of women in the control group. Therefore, the odds ratio for early menopause associated with a family history of early menopause was 6.1. Odds ratios for early menopause were 5 in women with an affected mother, 9.1 in those with an affected sister, and 12.4 in those with multiple affected relatives (Table 1). The risk of early menopause was significantly associated with family history even with adjustment for potential confounders, such as education, smoking, and estimated number of ovulatory cycles.

Conclusions.—Early menopause appears to be 6 times more likely in women with a family history of early menopause. This association is likely to have a genetic basis, and few cases of early menopause appear to be passed on through paternal lines. The strongest associations are noted for women undergoing menopause before age 40 years and those with an affected sister or multiple relatives. For a woman whose sister or mother underwent menopause before age 46 years, the likelihood of early menopause increases from 5% to 25%.

▶ The age at which menopause occurs is genetically determined and is not altered by the number of times a woman ovulates in her lifetime. The only environmental factor, aside from therapeutic toxins such as irradiation and chemotherapy, known to alter the age of menopause is cigarette smoking, which hastens the onset of menopause by about 2 years. Premature ovarian failure, defined as menopause at younger than the age of 40, occurs in about 1% of women in the United States, and about 10% undergo menopause before age 46. It is likely that genetic abnormalities on the long and short arm of the X chromosome are the cause of early menopause and that these genetic abnormalities can be transmitted to female offspring.

D.R. Mishell, Jr., M.D.

Possible Acceleration of Age Effects on Cognition Following Menopause

Halbreich U, Lumley LA, Palter S, et al (State Univ of New York, Buffalo)
J Psychiatr Res 29:153–163, 1995   14–3

Background.—Many cognitive functions deteriorate with advancing age. Possible differences in declining cognitive functions between women of reproductive age and postmenopausal women were investigated.

Methods.—Thirty-three postmenopausal women, aged 41 to 59 years, were compared with 24 premenopausal women, aged 21 to 47 years. All had been healthy physically and mentally for at least 2 years before study participation. The battery of tests administered included the Simulated Driving Reaction Time test, the Leeds Psychomotor Test Battery, Crawford's Small Parts Dexterity Test, the Trails A and B Tracking Time tests, the Booklet Category Test, the Benton Visual Retention Test, the Digit Symbol Substitution Test, the Bushke Selective Reminding Procedure, and the Gestalt Completion Test.

Findings.—Age and performance were significantly correlated on the Simulated Driving Reaction Time test in postmenopausal women only (Fig 1). Similarly, the association between age and recognition on the Leeds test was significantly only in postmenopausal women. However, menopause-related acceleration in the decline of performance was not observed on all tests. Performance on the Gestalt Completion Test was significantly asso-

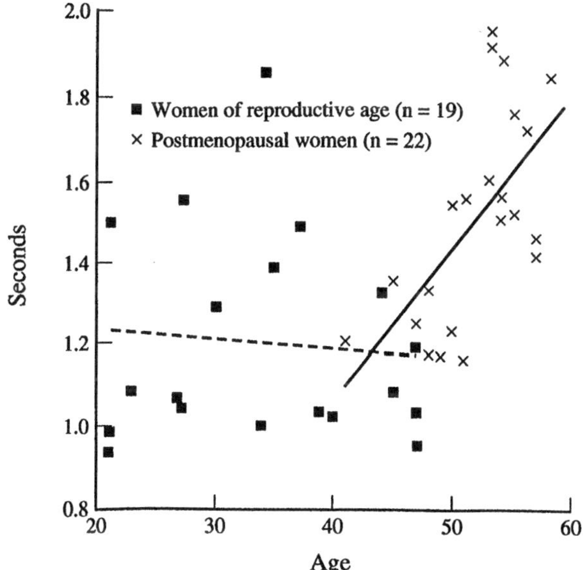

FIGURE 1.—Association between performance on driving simulation test and age. (Reprinted from Halbreich U, Lumley LA, Palter S, et al: Possible acceleration of age effects on cognition following menopause. *J Psychiatr Res* 29:153–163, Copyright 1995, with kind permission from Elsevier Science Ltd, The Boulevard, Langford Lane, Kidlington 0X5 1GB, UK.)

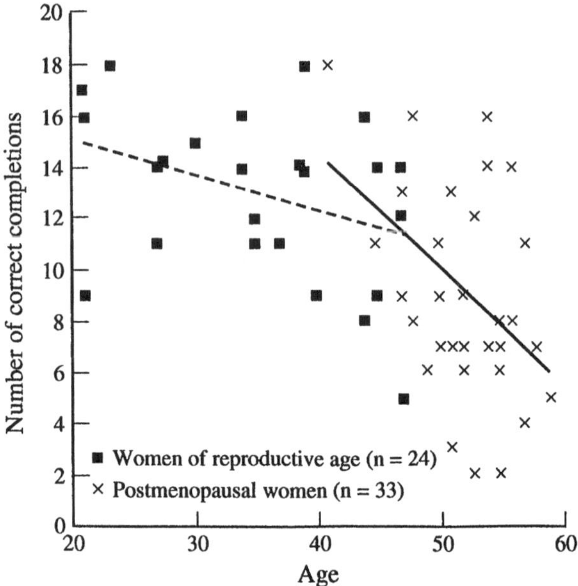

FIGURE 3.—Association between performance on Gestalt Completion Test and age. (Reprinted from Halbreich U, Lumley LA, Palter S, et al: Possible acceleration of age effects on cognition following menopause. *J Psychiatr Res* 29:153–163, Copyright 1995, with kind permission from Elsevier Science Ltd, The Boulevard, Langford Lane, Kidlington 0X5 1GB, UK.)

ciated with age in the 2 groups combined (Fig 3). Significant correlations between age and performance in the combined group only were also noted for the Crawford Manual Dexterity Test I and II, the Booklet Category Test, the Digit Symbol Substitution Test, the Trails A and B tests, and the Benton Visual Retention Test.

Conclusions.—On certain cognitive tests, such as driving simulation, reaction time, and some visuospatial tasks, deterioration of function is significantly accelerated after menopause. This acceleration may be associated with a lack of gonadal hormones or other factors associated with reproduction that might have a protective effect against age-related deterioration in some cognitive functions in women.

▶ Evidence is accumulating that estrogen affects CNS function and that estrogen deficiency is a risk factor for Alzheimer's disease. The results of this study indicate that there is a rapid increase in the amount of deterioration of certain cognitive functions after menopause. It is likely that estrogen deficiency contributes to this deterioration. Previous studies have reported that estrogen replacement improves tests of cognitive function and short-term memory in postmenopausal women. If verified by additional studies, improvement in memory and cognitive function may prove to be another major benefit of providing estrogen replacement postmenopausally.

D.R. Mishell, Jr., M.D.

Effects of Hormone Replacement Therapy on Weight, Body Composition, Fat Distribution, and Food Intake in Early Postmenopausal Women: A Prospective Study
Reubinoff BE, Stein P, Wurtman J, et al (Hebrew Univ, Jerusalem; Massachusetts Inst of Technology, Cambridge, Mass)
Fertil Steril 64:963–968, 1995
14--4

Background.—Many studies have established the efficacy of postmenopausal hormone replacement therapy (HRT) in maintaining bone mass, but the effect of HRT on fat mass and fat distribution is not known. Because obesity is an important risk factor for various medical conditions, the influence of HRT on weight gain needs to be elucidated. Therefore, the effect of HRT on weight, fat mass, fat distribution, and food intake was studied prospectively in early postmenopausal women.

Methods.—Seventy-five healthy women who had experienced menopause 2 to 3 years previously and had no history of treatment with gonadal hormones or medication influencing body weight or composition were studied, including 42 women who were treated with continuous daily oral estrogen and progestin (group A) and 33 women who were eligible for HRT therapy but refused it (group B). The patients were examined at baseline and after 12 months. Examinations included anthropometric measurements and a questionnaire addressing food intake, food choices, activity levels, and smoking.

Results.—Sixty-three women completed the 1-year study. At baseline, there were no significant differences between the 2 groups in examination findings. Weight and proportional body fat increased significantly during the study period in both groups, with no significant differences between the 2 groups. There was a significant difference between the groups in the waist-to-hip girth ratio, which increased significantly during the year in the control group and did not change significantly in the HRT group (Table 2). Food intake and food choices did not change significantly during the study period in either group.

TABLE 2.—Anthropometric Measurements of Women Who Used Hormone Replacement Therapy (HRT) and Among Controls Who Received No Hormone Replacement Therapy

	HRT		Control	
	Baseline	*1 year*	*Baseline*	*1 year*
Weight (kg)	73.22 ± 1.76	75.57 ± 1.12*	71.45 ± 3.11	73.51 ± 1.23*
BMI (kg/m²)	27.14 ± 0.58	27.85 ± 0.41*	25.8 ± 0.92	26.41 ± 0.49*
% body fat	30.80 ± 0.88	32.97 ± 0.67*	29.28 ± 1.16	31.1 ± 0.56*
Waist-to-hip ratio	0.82 ± 0.01	0.83 ± 0.01	0.80 ± 0.01	0.85 ± 0.01*

Note: Values are means ± SE.
*Significant difference ($P \leq 0.05$) between baseline measurements and 1 year later.
Abbreviation: BMI, body mass index.
(From Reubinoff BE, Stein P, Wurtman J, et al: Effects of hormone replacement therapy on weight, body composition, fat distribution, and food intake in early postmenopausal women: A prospective study. *Fertil Steril* 64:963–968, 1995. Reproduced with permission of the publisher, the American Society for Reproductive Medicine [formerly The American Fertility Society].)

Conclusions.—Hormone replacement therapy neither increased nor prevented weight gain and increased fat mass associated with early postmenopause. However, it did prevent the shift from peripheral to central fat distribution, suggesting that combined estrogen and progestin may preserve a gynoid, as opposed to android, fat distribution pattern. Because increased abdominal fat is a recognized cardiovascular risk factor, part of the protective influence of HRT on cardiovascular disease may be related to its prevention of this postmenopausal shift in fat distribution.

Changes in Energy Balance and Body Composition at Menopause: A Controlled Longitudinal Study

Poehlman ET, Toth MJ, Gardner AW (Univ of Maryland, Baltimore)
Ann Intern Med 123:673–675, 1995   14–5

Background.—Physiologic changes of menopause include decreases in resting metabolic rate and in fat-free body mass. Longitudinal changes in resting metabolic rate, body composition, and physical activity were followed up in a group of women, half of whom underwent menopause during the study period.

Methods.—At the start and end of a 6-year period, 35 women underwent measurement of resting metabolic rate, body fat mass, and plasma glucose and insulin levels. Food intake and amount of leisure physical activity were determined. Eighteen of the women had undergone menopause in the 6 years. None had received hormone replacement therapy.

Results.—The postmenopausal women experienced significantly larger decreases in fat-free mass, resting metabolic rate, and leisure physical

TABLE 1.—Longitudal Changes in 18 Women Who Experienced Menopause and in 17 Women Who Remained Premenopausal

	Values at Baseline Examination		Change at Follow-up Examination	
Variable	*Women Who Remained Premenopausal*	*Women Who Experienced Menopause*	*Women Who Remained Premenopausal*	*Women Who Experienced Menopause*
Age, *y*	45 ± 2	46 ± 2	6 ± 2	6 ± 2
Weight, *kg*	62 ± 3	63 ± 2	−1.0 ± 1	0.5 ± 1.1
Fat-free mass, *kg*	46 ± 3	46 ± 4	−0.5 ± 0.5	−3.0 ± 1.1*
Fat mass, *kg*	16 ± 2	17 ± 3	1.0 ± 1.5	2.5 ± 2*
Resting metabolic rate, *kcal/d*	1501 ± 120	1530 ± 135	−8.0 ± 17	−103 ± 55*
Leisure time activity, *kcal/d*	425 ± 116	416 ± 121	64 ± 60	−127 ± 79*
Peak oxygen consumption, *L/min*	2.1 ± 0.7	2.1 ± 0.6	−0.2 ± 0.2	−0.2 ± 0.3
Fasting insulin level, *pmol/L*	85 ± 10	90 ± 11	−2.0 ± 5	11 ± 9*
Fasting glucose level, *mmol/L*	5.8 ± 0.3	5.7 ± 0.2	0.02 ± 0.02	0.01 ± 0.02
Energy intake, *kcal/d*	2232 ± 115	2285 ± 127	110 ± 98	117 ± 100
Waist-to-hip ratio	0.77 ± 0.06	0.78 ± 0.07	0.01 ± 0.01	0.04 ± 0.01*

Note: Values are means ± standard deviation.
*Denotes a significant menopause-related effect ($P \leq 0.001$), that is, the change in women during natural menopause was greater than the change in women who remained premenopausal.
(Courtesy of Poehlman ET, Toth MJ, Gardner AW: Changes in energy balance and body composition at menopause: A controlled longitudinal study. *Ann Intern Med* 123:673–675, 1995.)

activity than those still premenopausal. Postmenopausal women gained significantly more fat mass than premenopausal women (Table 1). Postmenopausal women also had higher fasting insulin levels and waist-to-hip ratios. Body weight, fasting glucose levels, energy intake, and peak oxygen consumption were not affected.

Conclusion.—Menopause is associated with several metabolic changes that could increase women's metabolic and cardiovascular risk profiles.

▶ The results of these 2 longitudinal studies (Abstracts 14–4 and 14–5) indicate that after menopause there is an increase in total body fat and a shift of the fat deposition from peripheral sites to the abdomen, with a resultant greater waist-to-hip ratio. This shift of fat distribution from a gynecoid to android type has been considered to be a risk factor for the development of cardiovascular disease. Ingestion of estrogen-progestin hormone replacement has no effect on total body weight or total body fat but prevents the shift of body fat from peripheral sites to the abdomen. This effect may be an additional mechanism whereby hormone replacement reduces the risk of cardiovascular disease in postmenopausal women.

D.R. Mishell, Jr., M.D.

Hormone Replacement Therapy, Hormone Levels, and Lipoprotein Cholesterol Concentrations in Elderly Women
Paganini-Hill A, Dworsky R, Krauss RM (Univ of Southern California, Laguna Hills, Los Angeles; Univ of California, Berkeley)
Am J Obstet Gynecol 174:897–902, 1996   14–6

Objective.—The benefits of estrogen replacement therapy in reducing cardiovascular disease risk may be related to changes in serum lipoprotein concentrations in estrogen users, including an increase in high-density lipoprotein (HDL) cholesterol and a reduction in low-density lipoprotein (LDL) cholesterol. However, the effects of combined estrogen-progestin formulations on the lipid profile are unknown. The links between hormone replacement therapy, hormone concentrations, and lipid and lipoprotein cholesterol concentrations in elderly women were studied.

Methods.—The cross-sectional study included 292 independent-living elderly white women (average age, 76 years). All were residents of an upper middle-class retirement community. One hundred seventy of the women had never taken hormone replacement therapy, 84 were taking unopposed estrogen replacement therapy, and 38 were taking combination hormone replacement therapy. The 3 groups were compared for possible differences in lipid and lipoprotein cholesterol concentrations.

Results.—The 3 groups were similar in height, weight, exercise, and alcohol use. Women who used estrogen, alone or in combination with progestin, had lower total and LDL cholesterol and higher HDL cholesterol, with no significant differences in triglyceride levels. The lipid concentrations were similar between the 2 hormone replacement therapy

TABLE 2.—Mean ± SEM of Lipid and Lipoprotein Cholesterol and Hormone Levels by Use of Hormone Replacement Therapy

	Never used HRT	Unopposed ERT	Combination HRT	Significance
Triglycerides	127 ± 4.5	130 ± 7.4	129 ± 12.1	
Total cholesterol	232 ± 3.2	218 ± 4.0	219 ± 6.4	$p=0.02$
LDL cholesterol	147 ± 2.9	124 ± 3.7	128 ± 5.9	$p<0.0001$
HDL cholesterol	60 ± 1.2	68 ± 1.8	69 ± 3.1	$p=0.0001$
HDL$_2$	33 ± 1.0	39 ± 1.7	41 ± 2.8	$p=0.0003$
HDL$_{2a}$	15 ± 0.3	18 ± 0.6	18 ± 0.8	$p<0.0001$
HDL$_{2b}$	18 ± 0.8	21 ± 1.2	24 ± 2.2	$p=0.004$
HDL$_3$	28 ± 0.4	30 ± 0.7	27 ± 1.1	$p=0.01$
HDL$_{3a}$	17 ± 0.3	18 ± 0.4	17 ± 0.6	$p=0.01$
HDL$_{3b}$	7.7 ± 0.1	8.2 ± 0.3	7.2 ± 0.4	
HDL$_{3c}$	3.3 ± 0.1	3.4 ± 0.1	2.7 ± 0.2	$p=0.03$
Hormone levels*				
Progesterone	30 ± 2.3	28 ± 2.5	26 ± 1.3	
Estrone	3.1 ± .14	8.9 ± 1.3	7.5 ± .92	$p<0.0001$
Estradiol	0.64 ± .03	2.6 ± .85	1.7 ± .28	$p<0.0001$
Steroid hormone-binding				
globulin	1.5 ± .12	2.3 ± .22	2.8 ± .22	$p<0.0001$

*Hormone levels were measured on 101 individuals: 35 never users of hormone replacement therapy, 33 using unopposed estrogen replacement therapy, and 33 using combination hormone replacement therapy.

Abbreviations: HRT, hormone replacement therapy; *ERT,* estrogen replacement therapy.

(Courtesy of Paganini-Hill A, Dworsky R, Krauss RM: Hormone replacement therapy, hormone levels, and lipoprotein cholesterol concentrations in elderly women. *Am J Obstet Gynecol* 174:897–902, 1996.)

groups and significantly different from the non–hormone replacement therapy group. Hormone replacement therapy was associated with significantly higher HDL$_2$ subfractions; HDL$_3$ subfractions tended to be lower in the women using combination hormone replacement therapy. Women taking hormone replacement therapy also had higher concentrations of estrone, estradiol, and steroid hormone-binding globulin than the nonusers (Table 2). On examination of specific preparations used, the dose of medroxyprogesterone acetate had no consistent effect on lipid profile. However, the dose of conjugated equine estrogen was negatively correlated with total and LDL cholesterol and positively correlated with HDL and HDL subfractions.

Conclusions.—Elderly women taking estrogen replacement therapy have a more favorable lipid profile than those who are not taking hormone therapy. Estrogen replacement therapy reduces total cholesterol, mainly through a decrease in LDL cholesterol, and increases HDL cholesterol. This study found no differences in lipoprotein cholesterol concentrations between women taking unopposed estrogen replacement therapy vs. combination hormone replacement therapy.

▶ Almost all the epidemiologic studies showing a protective effect of estrogen replacement therapy on cardiovascular disease have studied women using estrogens without the addition of a progestin. The effect of combination therapy on this major cause of female mortality was thus undetermined. The results of this cross-sectional study indicate that overall ingestion of a progestin together with estrogen in a group of older women does not alter the beneficial effect of estrogen alone on the lipid profile. Whether progestins have an adverse effect on other mechanisms whereby estrogen causes cardiovascular protection, such as coronary artery blood flow as well as on cardiovascular events, remains to be determined.

D.R. Mishell, Jr., M.D.

Long-term Postmenopausal Hormone Use, Obesity, and Fat Distribution in Older Women

Kritz-Silverstein D, Barrett-Connor E (Univ of California, San Diego)
JAMA 275:46–49, 1996   14–7

Purpose.—The effects of postmenopausal estrogen use on obesity and fat distribution are unclear. Some studies have found that estrogen users have lower self-reported body mass index (BMI), but others have found that estrogen is associated with greater weight gain or has no effect on weight. The relationship between long-term hormone replacement therapy and measures of obesity and body composition was assessed.

Patients and Methods.—The 15-year prospective, cross-section cohort study included 671 women aged 65–94 years at their most recent follow-up. The average age was 61 years at baseline and 73 years at follow-up. One hundred ninety-four women had never used hormone replacement therapy, 146 had used it continuously from baseline to follow-up, and 331 had used it intermittently. Most women who had taken hormone replacement therapy used unopposed conjugated equine estrogen, with less than one fifth having ever used a progestin. Ninety-nine percent had used conjugated estrogen. The mean duration of hormone use among continuous users was 26 years.

The difference in BMI from baseline to follow-up was calculated. Waist and hip circumferences and bioelectric impedance were measured at follow-up only.

Results.—The 3 groups were not significantly different in any of the follow-up measures of obesity, fat distribution, or body composition at follow-up, after adjustment for age and baseline BMI. The women who used hormones intermittently and continuously were not significantly different in follow-up BMI, change in BMI and weight from baseline to follow-up, waist-hip ratio, or fat mass, after adjustment for covariates. The results were the same on exclusion of women with a history of progestin use. Obesity and body composition were also unrelated to the number of years of hormone use or the dose of estrogen.

Conclusions.—Long-term use of hormone replacement therapy appears to have no effect on fat mass among older women. The weight gain and central obesity that commonly occur after menopause are neither caused nor prevented by taking estrogen either on a continuous or an intermittent basis. Women who use hormone replacement therapy tend to be leaner when they first start taking estrogen.

▶ As women become older, they gain weight and have more central obesity. The results of this large longitudinal study indicate that the use of estrogen replacement therapy after menopause does not alter the amount of body weight gain or degree of central obesity that occurs postmenopausally. Many women who take estrogen replacement postmenopausally believe that the hormones cause them to gain weight and therefore wish to discontinue their use. This study indicates that the weight gain is not caused by the exogenous hormones, and women receiving or considering use of estrogen replacement therapy should be so informed.

D.R. Mishell, Jr., M.D.

Age at Menopause as a Risk Factor for Cardiovascular Mortality

van der Schouw YT, van der Graaf Y, Steyerberg EW, et al (Utrecht Univ, The Netherlands; Erasmus Univ, Rotterdam, The Netherlands; Academic Hosp, Utrecht, The Netherlands)
Lancet 347:714–718, 1996

14–8

Background.—Estrogen deficiency after menopause may lead to an increased risk of cardiovascular disease. However, previous studies have been inconclusive, largely because of short postmenopausal follow-up periods. The link between age at menopause and cardiovascular mortality was investigated in a study with a median follow-up of 16 years.

Methods.—The research subjects came from a cohort of 12,115 postmenopausal women living in 1 Dutch city between 1974 and 1977. The analysis included 1,199 women who went through menopause during follow-up, which lasted from 1 to 20 years. The women were followed up through regular screening visits, at which information on menopausal status, age at menopause, medication use, cardiovascular risk factors, and indicators of ovarian function was obtained. The link between age at menopause and total cardiovascular mortality was analyzed, with information on deaths obtained from the research subjects' family physicians.

Results.—The women in the various strata of age at menopause (which ranged from 39 years and younger to 55 years and older) were similar in the baseline characteristics. Risk of cardiovascular mortality was significantly increased for women with early menopause (Fig). Women with menopause at age 40–44 had a 5.7% annual hazard of cardiovascular death at age 70, compared with 4.3% for those with menopause at age 55 or older. Each 1-year delay in menopause carried a 2% decrease in the annual hazard of cardiovascular death. Age at menopause had a reasonably linear effect on cardiovascular mortality—the effects of a 1-year delay were approximately the same at age 50 as at age 40. Age at menopause clearly affected cardiovascular mortality at age 65; however, by age 80 this effect had disappeared.

Conclusions.—Early menopause is associated with an increased risk of cardiovascular mortality. Early menopause is an independent risk factor for cardiovascular mortality, and seems to play a more important role at younger biological ages. Age at menopause has no effect on cardiovascular mortality for women who have undergone hysterectomy and an increased

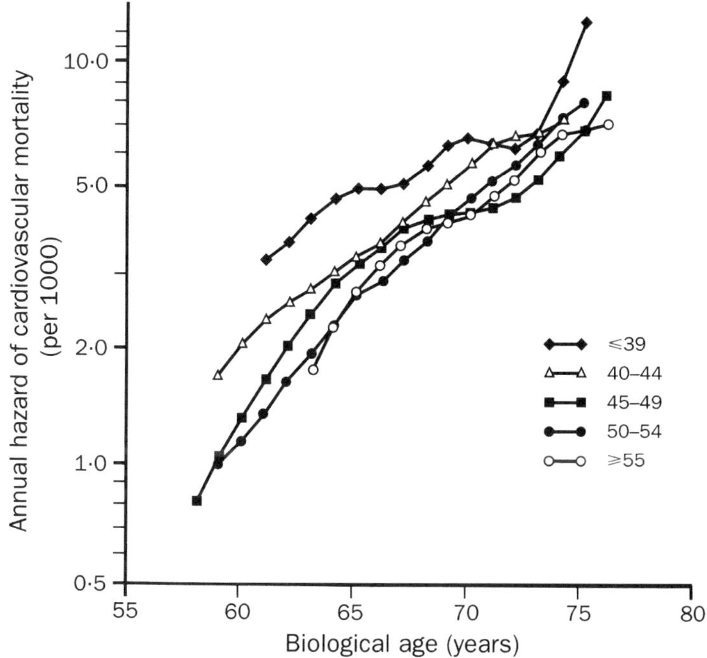

FIGURE.—Annual hazard of cardiovascular mortality (logarithmic scale) in relation to age at menopause. For proportional hazards, the lines should be parallel. (Courtesy of van der Schouw YT, van der Graaf Y, Steyerberg EW, et al: Age at menopause as a risk factor for cardiovascular mortality. *Lancet* 347:714–718, copyright by The Lancet Ltd. 1996.)

effect for those who have had oophorectomy. The impact of smoking on cardiovascular mortality is strong enough to eliminate the effects of early menopause.

▶ There have been no prospective randomized clinical trials demonstrating that exogenous estrogen replacement therapy (ERT) given to postmenopausal women reduces the risk of cardiovascular disease. However, a meta-analysis of 31 observational studies has shown that postmenopausal women taking ERT have only half the risk of having a myocardial infarction that women not taking ERT have. In addition to providing a favorable lipid profile, there are several other mechanisms whereby exogenous estrogen prevents acceleration of coronary artery atherosclerosis. The results of this study indicate that endogenous estrogen is also protective against cardiovascular disease because women with early menopause have a significantly greater risk of cardiovascular death between the ages of 60 and 75 years than women who become menopausal after age 50. Thus, women who became menopausal younger than age 45 should be particularly encouraged to ingest ERT.

D.R. Mishell, Jr., M.D.

Carotid Plaque Regression on Oestrogen Replacement: A Pilot Study

Akkad A, Hartshorne T, Bell PRF, et al (Univ of Leicester, England)
Eur J Vasc Endovasc Surg 11:347–348, 1996   14–9

Background.—Animal studies suggest that estrogen treatment can prevent or even reverse atheroma formation. The effects of estrogen replacement therapy on carotid plaques were evaluated in menopausal women.

Methods.—The pilot study included 17 women with natural or surgical menopause and known carotid plaque disease. All underwent duplex ultrasound scanning of the carotid arteries before and after 3 and 6 months of unopposed estrogen replacement therapy. Measurements included intimal thickness, plaque length, and plaque thickness.

Results.—Follow-up data were obtained on 22 carotid plaques. Nonsignificant reductions of 5% after 3 months of estrogen treatment and 6% after 6 months of treatment were seen in mean intimal thickness. However, plaque length was decreased significantly, by 8% at 3 months and 28% at 6 months. Plaque thickness was significantly decreased, by 18% at 6 months.

Conclusions.—Estrogen replacement therapy may be associated with carotid plaque regression in menopausal women. The results of this pilot study are consistent with the findings of previous studies in animals.

▶ The results of this study indicate that unopposed orally administered estrogen can cause a significant reduction in the size of atheromatous plaques in the carotid arteries of postmenopausal women with existing carotid artery atherosclerosis. These findings, although preliminary, support the use of postmenopausal estrogen replacement in women who have clinical evidence of atherosclerosis. Sullivan has shown that, among a group of women with moderate to severe coronary atherosclerosis, the 10-year survival rate is significantly greater if they take estrogen replacement than if they do not do so.[1] Estrogen replacement should be given to postmenopausal women with angina, or those who have had a myocardial infarction or stroke, to reduce the extent of their existing atherosclerosis.

D.R. Mishell, Jr., M.D.

Reference

1. Sullivan JM, Vander Zwaag R, Hughes JP, et al: Estrogen replacement and coronary artery disease: Effect on survival in postmenopausal women. *Arch Intern Med* 150:2557–2562, 1990.

Estrogen Replacement Therapy and Progression of Intimal-Medial Thickness in the Carotid Arteries of Postmenopausal Women
Espeland MA, for the ACAPS Investigators (Bowman Gray School of Medicine, Winston-Salem, NC; Univ of Tennessee, Memphis; Univ of Kentucky, Lexington; et al)
Am J Epidemiol 142:1011–1019, 1995   14–10

Background.—Epidemiologic evidence suggests that estrogen replacement therapy (ERT) is an effective means of preventing deaths from cardiovascular disease in postmenopausal women. Angiographic studies indicate that ERT may prevent atherosclerotic disease. Manolio et al. recently described an inverse relationship between ERT and the intimal-medial thickness (IMT) of the carotid artery wall.

Objective and Methods.—Ultrasound estimates of carotid IMT were related to the use of ERT by women enrolled in the Asymptomatic Carotid Artery Progression Study, a randomized, placebo-controlled trial. Lovastatin and warfarin were administered separately and in combination to 186 postmenopausal women. Ultrasound studies were done twice before randomization and then every 6 months for 2½ to 3 years.

Results.—Women currently using ERT had relatively high plasma triglyceride and high-density lipoprotein cholesterol levels, and lower levels of low-density lipoprotein cholesterol. Users were evenly distributed between the arms of the study. The low-density lipoprotein cholesterol levels decreased substantially in lovastatin-treated women. Among placebo recipients, mean IMT tended to increase gradually in women not using estrogen but decreased slightly in users of ERT (Fig 1). The difference appeared unrelated to changes in lipoprotein levels. Lovastatin therapy was associated with declining IMT, and ERT had little added effect on IMT in these women.

Conclusion.—In postmenopausal women who are not receiving lipid-lowering agents, ERT may stop or even reverse the progression of carotid artery narrowing.

▶ A large body of evidence indicates that use of ERT by postmenopausal women reduces the risk of cardiovascular disease. These data indicate that use of ERT halts or even reverses the progression of carotid artery intimal wall thickness over time among postmenopausal women by direct action on the vessels. The mechanism whereby estrogen causes this antiatherosclerotic effect is independent of its effect on lipoprotein concentrations. This effect is most likely induced by several modalities including inhibition of low-density lipoprotein oxidation, which suppresses cholesterol deposits on the arteries, increasing arterial blood flow; and by modulating the degree of vascular reactivity to constricting agents.

D.R. Mishell, Jr., M.D.

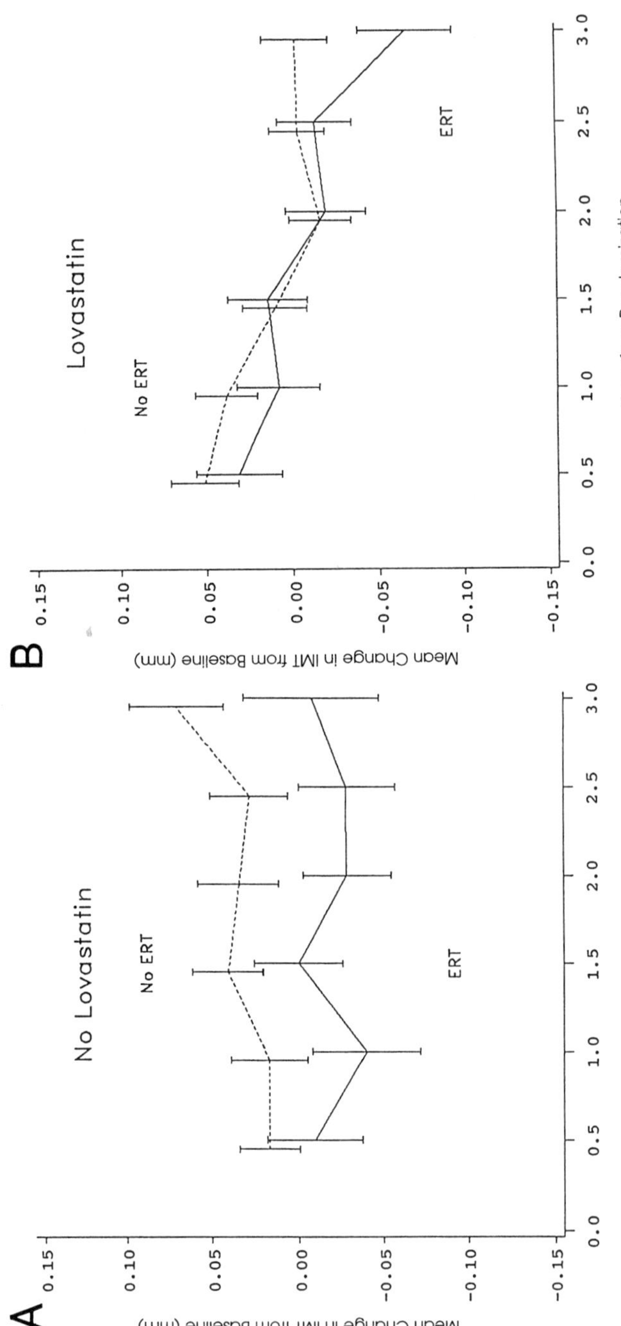

FIGURE 1.—Mean changes (± SEs) from baseline of average intimal-medial thickness (*IMT*) for participating Asymptomatic Carotid Atherosclerosis Progression Study women grouped by reported use of estrogen replacement therapy (*ERT*) and lovastatin randomization assignment and based on 1989–1993 data. (Courtesy of Espeland MA, for the ACAPS Investigators: Estrogen replacement therapy and progression of intimal-medial thickness in the carotid arteries of postmenopausal women. *Am J Epidemiol* 142:1011–1019, 1995.)

Postmenopausal Hormone Use and Risk of Large-bowel Cancer

Newcomb PA, Storer BE (Univ of Wisconsin, Madison)
J Natl Cancer Inst 87:1067–1071, 1995

14–11

Background.—The production of secondary bile acids is thought to promote colon carcinogenesis. Because progestins and exogenous estrogens may reduce the production of these acids, women receiving hormone replacement therapy (HRT) might lessen their risk for large-bowel cancer. Clear evidence for such an effect is lacking, however. To investigate the potentially important relationship between HRT and colon and rectal cancer risk, a case-control study was conducted.

Methods.—Patients considered for the study were all Wisconsin women with a new diagnosis of cancer of the colon or rectum who were younger than 75 years of age at diagnosis and whose cases had been reported to a statewide cancer registry from 1990 through 1991. The final case group included 694 postmenopausal women, 480 who had received a diagnosis of colon cancer and 214 who had received a diagnosis of rectal cancer. Controls were 1,622 women randomly selected from a list of licensed drivers and a roster of Medicare beneficiaries in Wisconsin. Telephone interviews were conducted to obtain information on medical history, postmenopausal HRT use, and family history.

Results.—The risk for colon cancer developing was about 30% lower among women who reported ever using HRT, compared with women who never used HRT. Recent use only, not former use, was associated with reduced risk. Risk reduction was similar for estrogen-only users and for women who took estrogen and progestin (Table 2). Hormone use, whether at any time or recently, had no effect on the risk of rectal cancer. There was a trend for an inverse association between decreasing time since the last use of HRT and the risk for colon cancer, but not for rectal cancer. The inverse association between HRT and cancer risk appeared to be strongest among

TABLE 2.—Relative Risks (RR) of Colon and Rectal Cancers According to Use of Hormone Replacement Therapy (HRT)

Use of HRT*	No. of controls	Colon cancer		Rectal Cancer	
		No. of cases	RR† (95% CI)	No. of cases	RR† (95% CI)
Ever	541	113	0.73 (0.56–0.94)	65	1.17 (0.83–1.63)
Former	273	78	0.85 (0.63–1.15)	45	1.32 (0.90–1.92)
Recent‡	268	35	0.54 (0.36–0.81)	20	0.91 (0.54–1.55)
Estrogen only	171	24	0.54 (0.34–0.88)	12	0.90 (0.46–1.76)
Estrogen and progestin	62	11	0.54 (0.28–1.05)	8	1.13 (0.51–2.50)
Never	1044	357	1.00	142	1.00

*The type of HRT (i.e., estrogen only or estrogen and progestin) could not be determined for 35 patients.

†Relative risks adjusted for age, use of sigmoidoscopy screening, family history of large-bowel cancer, body mass index, and intake of beer or hard liquor.

‡Within year before the diagnosis or reference date.

Abbreviation: CI, confidence interval.

(Courtesy of Newcomb PA, Storer BE: Postmenopausal hormone use and risk of large-bowel cancer. *J Natl Cancer Inst* 87:1067–1071, 1995.)

women at lower absolute risk of disease, particularly among those with leaner body mass.

Conclusion.—A significant reduction in colon cancer incidence was found among postmenopausal women who used HRT. The reduction was about 30% for ever use and 46% for recent use. No association was observed between HRT and rectal cancer. Because adenocarcinoma of the large bowel is among the most common cancers in Western populations, the finding of a reduced risk for women taking postmenopausal hormones may have important public health implications.

▶ The results of this study indicate that the use of postmenopausal estrogen replacement, with or without the use of progestins, is associated with a significantly reduced risk for the development of colon cancer. A decreased risk of colon cancer with postmenopausal estrogen use has also been observed in 5 other studies published since 1991. It has been hypothesized that increased concentration of bile acids may stimulate carcinogens in the colon, and exogenous estrogen may reduce the amount of bile acids synthesized or secreted. Asymptomatic postmenopausal women should be informed of these data to assist them in their decision as to whether to use long-term estrogen replacement.

D.R. Mishell, Jr., M.D.

Hormonal Replacement Therapy and Morbidity and Mortality in a Prospective Study of Postmenopausal Women
Folsom AR, Mink PJ, Sellers TA, et al (Univ of Minnesota, Minneapolis)
Am J Public Health 85:1128–1132, 1995   14–12

Introduction.—The risks and benefits of hormone replacement therapy remain controversial in the absence of large-scale, randomized clinical trial data. The association of hormone replacement therapy and mortality and the incidence of several diseases was assessed in more than 40,000 postmenopausal women who were participating in the Iowa Women's Health Study.

Methods.—A mailed questionnaire sought information on current and past hormone replacement therapy, prevalent diseases, anthropometric data, and other risk factors. Also determined were disease end points from 1986 to 1991. Site-specific cancer incidence and deaths were determined by health registries, and the incidence of fractures was determined by self-report. Data were not available on the proportion of women using progestins in combination with estrogen. It is estimated from the questionnaires that no more than 20% of current users and fewer former users took combination hormone replacement therapy. Analyses were confined to postmenopausal women with hormone replacement therapy data.

Results.—Women currently using hormone replacement therapy were most likely to be young, alcohol drinkers, married, nonobese, and nondiabetic. Compared with nonusers, women with current hormone replace-

TABLE 3.—Multivariate-Adjusted Relative Risks (RR) and 95% Confidence Intervals (CI) of Death or Disease Over 6 Years in Relation to Duration of Hormone Replacement Therapy (HRT)

| | RR (95% CI) by Baseline HRT Status* | | |
End Point	Current ≤ 5 y	Current > 5 y	P Trend
	Mortality		
All causes†	0.85 (0.62, 1.15)	0.77 (0.61, 0.96)	.02
All causes† with exclusions§	0.90 (0.61, 1.34)	0.96 (0.73, 1.25)	.73
Coronary heart disease†	0.64 (0.28, 1.44)	0.80 (0.48, 1.31)	.36
Coronary heart disease† with exclusions§	0.57 (0.18, 1.79)	0.90 (0.47, 1.72)	.75
Stroke†	2.08 (0.74, 5.82)	1.05 (0.41, 2.64)	.92
Other Cardiovascular disease†	0.71 (0.22, 2.25)	0.33 (0.10, 1.03)	.06
Cancer‡	0.75 (0.48, 1.17)	0.79 (0.58, 1.08)	.14
Cancer‡ with exclusions§	0.84 (0.47, 1.50)	1.17 (0.83, 1.67)	.37
Other causes†	0.99 (0.50, 1.95)	0.86 (0.52, 1.42)	.56
	Incidence		
Any cancer‡	1.01 (0.80, 1.29)	1.02 (0.86, 1.21)	.85
Endometrial cancer‡	1.82 (0.74, 4.49)	7.37 (4.28, 12.67)	<.001
Breast cancer‡	1.45 (1.03, 2.06)	1.21 (0.92, 1.60)	.18
Colon cancer‡	0.31 (0.10, 0.98)	0.92 (0.57, 1.50)	.74
Other cancer‡	0.90 (0.62, 1.30)	0.78 (0.59, 1.03)	.08
Fracture (any)‡	0.81 (0.67, 0.98)	0.75 (0.65, 0.86)	<.001
Hip fracture‡	0.74 (0.33, 1.68)	0.47 (0.24, 0.91)	.03

*Reference category for RR is those who never used HRT (RR, 1).

†Adjusted for age (continuous), marital status (currently married, not married), physical activity level (low, medium, high), alcohol use (0, less than 4, or more than 4 g/day), pack-years of smoking (0,1–19, 20–39, 40 or more), body mass index (quartiles), waist-hip ratio (quartiles), hypertension (yes, no), and diabetes (yes, no).

‡Adjusted for age, marital status, physical activity level, alcohol use, smoking, body mass index, waist-hip ratio, and parity (nulliparous, first birth at age younger than 30 years, first birth at 30 years or older).

§Excluding women with baseline cancer and heart disease.

(Courtesy of Folsom AR, Mink PJ, Sellers TA, et al: Hormonal replacement therapy and morbidity and mortality in a prospective study of postmenopausal women. *Am J Public Health* 85:1128–1132, Copyright 1995 by the American Public Health Association.)

ment therapy had a relative risk of death of about 0.75 and former users had a relative risk of death of 1. An appreciable reduction in coronary heart disease was observed for current and former hormone replacement therapy users. No association was observed between hormone replacement therapy and stroke mortality. Other cardiovascular deaths were also reduced substantially in former and current hormone replacement users. The total cancer mortality was reduced by 20% in current hormone replacement therapy users, but it was slightly elevated in former users. The overall cancer incidence was not considered to be related to hormone replacement therapy use. In women with intact uteri, the endometrial cancer incidence was elevated threefold to fourfold in current hormone replacement therapy users and about 1.5-fold in former users. The breast cancer incidence was nearly 20% greater in current users, not a significant difference. Colon cancer was inversely associated with hormone replacement therapy use. All other cancers had a somewhat reduced risk in current users. The incidence of fractures was substantially reduced in current users and slightly elevated in former users. The number of hip fractures in current users was about half that of nonusers. Compared with never users, current users of hormone replacement therapy were projected to have 22 fewer deaths, for every 10,000 person-years of observation. With the exception of endometrial cancer and fractures, long-term hormone replacement therapy did not appear to confer a benefit over short-term therapy (Table 3).

Conclusions.—The use of hormone replacement therapy has positive and negative physiologic effects. When clinical trial data are available within the next 10 years, they will give more conclusive information on the risks and benefits of this treatment approach.

▶ The results of this very large cohort study are in agreement with those from previous epidemiologic studies. Women using hormone replacement have a lower incidence of overall mortality, coronary heart disease, and fractures than do postmenopausal women not taking hormone replacement. Despite the fact that the risk of endometrial cancer developing was increased threefold to fourfold, the overall risk of cancer among women using estrogen replacement was not changed, mainly because of a reduction in the risk of colon cancer developing. Although this was not a prospective clinical trial, the results should be made available to women considering the use of estrogen replacement, because data from a large clinical trial, the Women's Health Initiative, will not become available for at least 10 years.

D.R. Mishell, Jr., M.D.

Reduced Mortality Associated With Long-term Postmenopausal Estrogen Therapy
Ettinger B, Friedman GD, Bush T, et al (Kaiser Permanente Med Care Program, Oakland, Calif; Univ of Maryland, Baltimore)
Obstet Gynecol 87:6–12, 1996   14–13

Background.—Considerable controversy still exists regarding the relative risks and benefits of postmenopausal estrogen replacement therapy (ERT). Many of the studies have been limited by having no data on the duration of use or dosage, studying the effects of relatively short-term use, and including relatively young patients. To examine the hypothesis that increasing age and use would increase both the risks and benefits of ERT, the effects of ERT were studied in a cohort of women with well-defined and prolonged postmenopausal estrogen use.

Methods.—A group of 232 women were identified who had been born between 1900 and 1915, had begun to use at least 0.3 mg of conjugated estrogens within 3 years of menopause, and had used ERT for at least 5 years. A control group was identified of 222 age-matched women who had not used estrogen or had used it for less than 1 year. Their medical records were reviewed to identify demographic data and health risk factors. In those who died during the study period (1980–1993), the cause of death was determined. Age-specific mortality was compared in the 2 cohorts and calculated by duration, recency, and dosage of estrogen use. Mortality also was adjusted for mortality risk factors.

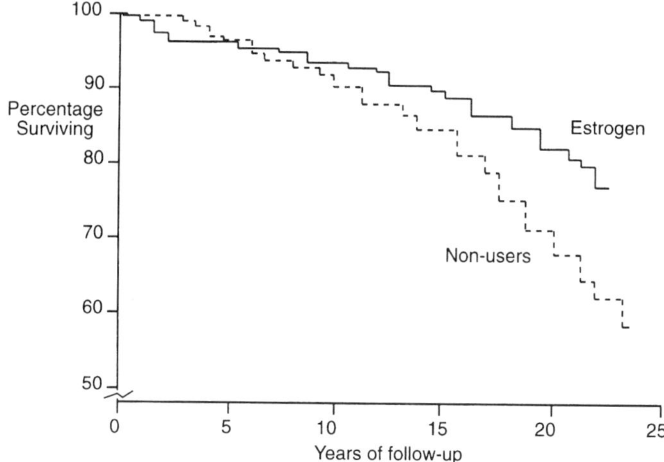

FIGURE 1.—All-cause mortality in postmenopausal women using estrogen vs. that in matched controls. (Courtesy of Ettinger B, Friedman GD, Bush T, et al: Reduced mortality associated with long-term postmenopausal estrogen therapy. *Obstet Gynecol* 87:6–12, 1996. Reprinted with permission from the American College of Obstetricians and Gynecologists.)

Results.—The 2 groups had similar demographic profiles. The estrogen users were followed up for a mean of 26.8 years, had a mean age in 1993 of 77.6 years, and had used estrogen for a mean of 17.1 years. The nonusers were followed up for a mean of 17.9 years and had a mean age of 77.4 years. The survival benefit in the estrogen users increased significantly with age (Fig 1, Table 3).

TABLE 3.—Age-Specific All-Cause Mortality Rates and Rate Ratios

Age (y)	Mortality rate/1000 person-years		Mortality rate ratio	95% CI
	Nonuser (N = 222)	Estrogen user (N = 232)		
50–59	2.1 (1/478)*	6.2 (3/485)	2.96	0.31–28.43
60–69	7.3 (14/1930)	6.1 (12/1973)	0.84	0.39–1.81
70–79	34.7 (57/1641)	16.7 (30/1793)	0.48	0.31–.75
≥ 80	47.5 (15/316)	22.0 (8/364)	0.46	0.20–1.09
Total	19.6 (87/4365)	11.2 (53/4615)	0.56†	0.40–0.79†

*Number of deaths per person-years of observation.
†Age-adjusted relative risk using Mantel-Haenszel method.
Abbreviation: CI, confidence interval.
(Courtesy of Ettinger B, Friedman GD, Bush T, et al: Reduced mortality associated with long-term postmenopausal estrogen therapy. *Obstet Gynecol* 87:6–12, 1996. Reprinted with permission from The American College of Obstetricians and Gynecologists.)

Overall, there was a 46% reduction in age-adjusted mortality risk in the ERT group. The relative risk of mortality was 0.48 with at least 15 years of use and 0.69 with less than 15 years of use. Relative risks were 0.48 for current use, 0.18 for recent use, and 0.55 for remote use. The relative mortality risk was lowest in patients using the lowest dosage; no association with mortality risk was found at the highest dosage. Most of the increased survival was related to the reduced mortality from coronary heart disease and cardiovascular disease. No statistically significant differences were found between the 2 groups in mortality from cancer or other causes, although there was a general trend toward lower mortality in the users group.

Conclusions.—Long-term estrogen use in aging women was associated with significantly reduced all-cause mortality, which was primarily a result of reduced mortality from coronary heart disease and cardiovascular disease. The survival benefit of estrogen use increased with age and with the duration and recency of use, although the benefit continued for several years after the discontinuation of long-term use. The survival benefits of estrogen use were substantial even after adjustment for health risk factors.

▶ Although this study, like all other studies of the effect of postmenopausal estrogen use on cardiovascular disease and mortality, was not a randomized, prospective, clinical trial, the women who took estrogen replacement for a long duration and those who did not were demographically similar. The significant decrease in mortality from all causes and particularly from cardiovascular disease among the estrogen users provides additional evidence that use of estrogen postmenopausally lengthens a woman's life span, if estrogen therapy is initiated within a few years of the menopause and is continued for many years.

These data were derived from a group of women who nearly always took estrogen without a progestin. Data regarding overall mortality and cardiovascular disease among women taking estrogen and progestins will not be available for several years, but low-dose progestin therapy in combination with estrogen appears to have little impact on cardiovascular risk markers. It is interesting that only 1 of the 232 long-term estrogen users in this study died of endometrial cancer. The endometrial cancer associated with unopposed estrogen replacement is nearly always cured by hysterectomy.

D.R. Mishell, Jr., M.D.

Can Women With Systemic Lupus Erythematosus Safely Use Exogenous Estrogens?

Buyon JP, Kalunian KC, Skovron ML, et al (New York Univ; Univ of California, Los Angeles; Johns Hopkins Univ, Baltimore, Md; et al)
J Clin Rheumatol 1:205–212, 1995   14–14

Introduction.—It is commonly believed that oral contraceptives and estrogen replacement therapy can induce increased disease activity in patients with systemic lupus erythematosus (SLE). To investigate the validity of this belief, information was collected on the past and present use of oral contraceptives and estrogen replacement therapy among women with SLE, as well as any adverse effects from their use.

Methods.—A total of 404 women with SLE seen at 5 medical centers were surveyed. A questionnaire, which gathered information on demographics, age at diagnosis of SLE, history of exogenous estrogen use, side effects, and disease activity, was completed during interviews either during a clinical visit or by telephone. A substudy at 1 site compared the use of oral contraceptives in 160 patients with SLE with that in 133 healthy women of similar age and ethnicity. A second substudy at another site focused on the history of estrogen replacement therapy among 94 postmenopausal patients with SLE.

Results.—Of the 404 women with SLE, 224 (55%) had ever taken oral contraceptives for a mean duration of 42.4 months. Fifty-one (13%) women were taking oral contraceptives when SLE was diagnosed, and 55 (14%) used oral contraceptives after the diagnosis of SLE. Of the 173 women younger than age 36 years, 10.4% were currently taking oral contraceptives. Only 7 of the 55 patients (13%) who took oral contraceptives after SLE was diagnosed had an increase in disease activity. The comparison of oral contraceptive use among women with and without SLE showed that women with SLE were significantly less likely than healthy women to be currently using oral contraceptives. Of the 94 postmenopausal patients, 59% had ever taken estrogen therapy, and 51% initiated or remained taking estrogen therapy after SLE was diagnosed. Only 8% of the patients taking estrogen replacement therapy after SLE was diagnosed had increased disease activity.

Conclusions.—Exogenous estrogen therapy is well tolerated by both premenopausal and postmenopausal patients. This finding should be validated with prospective studies and may change standard prescribing practices for women with SLE.

▶ Although there are theoretical reasons why exogenous estrogen administration to women with SLE may produce exacerbations of the disease, there are very few studies of the relation between exogenous estrogen and SLE. The few studies published to date suggest that use of either oral contraceptives or estrogen replacement does not increase the incidence of exacerbations of SLE compared with nonestrogen users. The fact that in this descriptive study, only 13% of the oral contraceptive users and 8% of the estrogen replacement users had exacerbations of SLE indicates that exogenous estrogens are tolerated by the great majority of women with SLE and that they may take either agent under medical supervision.

D.R. Mishell, Jr., M.D.

Menopause, Postmenopausal Estrogen Preparations, and the Risk of Adult-onset Asthma: A Prospective Cohort Study

Troisi RJ, Speizer FE, Willett WC, et al (Harvard Med School, Boston; Harvard School of Public Health, Boston)
Am J Respir Crit Care Med 152:1183–1188, 1995

14–15

Objective.—Because there is considerable evidence that hormonal factors contribute to asthma, the development of adult-onset asthma was related to menopausal status and the use of exogenous hormones in women 34–68 years of age enrolled in the prospective Nurses' Health Study (NHS).

Study Population.—An initial population of 121,700 female nurses aged 30–55 years entered the NHS in 1976. In 1980, 41,202 premenopausal women and 23,035 postmenopausal women were available for analysis. In the subsequent 10 years, there were nearly 600,000 person-years of follow-up. There were 404 new cases of asthma in premenopausal women and 322 in postmenopausal women during 10 years of follow-up.

Correlations.—Naturally menopausal women who had not used hormones since menopause had a relative risk (RR) of 0.65 of asthma developing compared with premenopausal women. For those who had ever used hormones, the RR was 0.77. The time since menopause was not a factor when adjusting for age at diagnosis. Naturally menopausal women who currently used hormones had an age-adjusted RR of 1.50 compared with those never using hormones (Table 3). Past users remained at increased risk for several years after ceasing to use hormones. The age-adjusted risk of asthma was related to the current dose of conjugated estrogens (Fig 1). Women who had used oral contraception in the past had an age-adjusted RR of 1.25.

Conclusion.—Some postmenopausal women may be at a moderately elevated risk for asthma developing when using high doses of estrogen for an extended time.

TABLE 3.—Relative Risk (95% Confidence Interval [CI]) for Postmenopausal Hormone Use and Asthma, Stratified by Type of Menopause, Assessed in 1980 and Updated Every 2 Years

	Never	Current	Past
Natural menopause:			
No. of cases	116	25	50
No. of person-years	139,347	20,095	41,395
Relative risk	1.0	1.50	1.52
(95% CI)		(0.98–2.30)	(1.08–2.13)
Surgical menopause			
No. of cases	28	55	48
No. of person-years	21,482	36,852	36,523
Relative risk	1.0	1.14	1.03
(95% CI)		(0.71–1.83)	(0.65–1.64)

(Courtesy of Troisi RJ, Speizer FE, Willett WC, et al: *Am J Respir Crit Care Med* 152:1183–1188, 1995.)

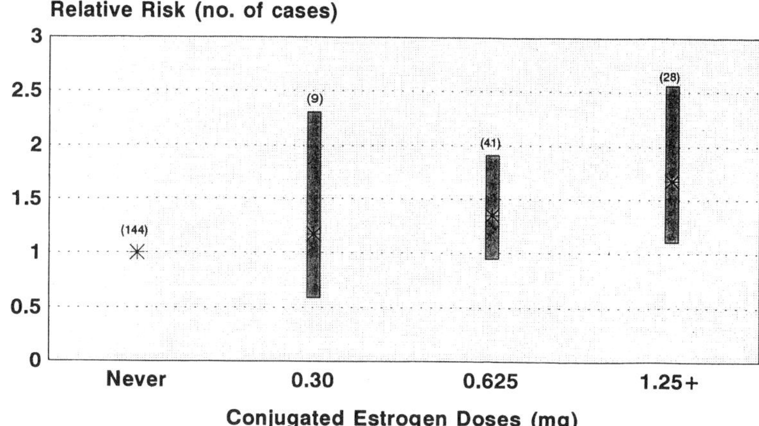

Test for trend includes never users; p=0.007.

FIGURE 1.—Age-adjusted relative risk (95% confidence interval) for dose of conjugated estrogens and asthma among current users. Test for trend includes never users; $P = 0.007$. (Courtesy of Troisi RJ, Speizer FE, Willett WC, et al: *Am J Respir Crit Care Med* 152:1183–1188, 1995.)

▶ This is the first epidemiologic study to suggest that postmenopausal hormone use is associated with an increased incidence of the initial diagnosis of asthma. Since this is an observational study, not a clinical trial, a causal relation between postmenopausal hormone replacement and the onset of asthma cannot be established. However, that the risk of asthma developing increased with increasing dosage and duration of estrogen use suggests that the association is causal. Additional studies are needed to further clarify the relation between postmenopausal estrogen replacement and the development of bronchial asthma.

D.R. Mishell, Jr., M.D.

Postmenopausal Osteoporosis: Patient Choices and Outcomes
Cosman F, Nieves J, Walliser J, et al (Helen Hayes Hosp, West Haverstraw, NY; Columbia Univ, New York)
Maturitas 22:137–143, 1995

14–16

Background.—Only estrogen and subcutaneously administered salmon calcitonin are currently approved in the United States as drug therapies for the treatment of osteoporosis. Another agent, oral etidronate, has been shown to be effective in increasing spinal bone mass in osteoporotic women, but has not yet gained Food and Drug Administration approval for this purpose. The appeal, efficacy, and tolerability of etidronate, estrogen, and subcutaneous calcitonin for the treatment of osteoporosis were compared in a nonrandomized, open-label trial.

Methods.—Women, aged 50–80 years, with postmenopausal osteoporosis were treated for 2 years with their choice of intermittent oral etidronate

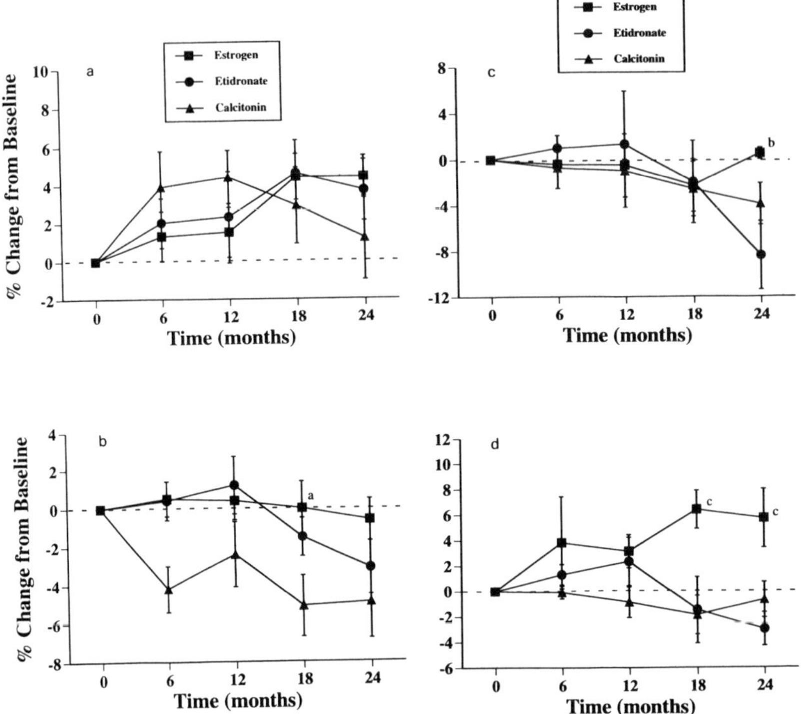

FIGURE 1.—Changes in bone mineral density (as percentage from baseline) over 2 years during treatment with antiresorptive therapy. *Squares* indicate estrogen treated; *circles*, etidronate-treated; *triangles*, calcitonin-treated. **A**, lumbar spine. **B**, femoral neck. **C**, distal forearm. **D**, proximal forearm. Significance values are shown only for differences among groups. [a]$P < 0.03$ compared with percentage change in calcitonin group. [b]$P < 0.04$ compared with percentage change in etidronate group. [a]$P < 0.01$ compared with percentage change in etidronate and calcitonin groups. (Reprinted from *Maturitas* Vol 22, Cosman F, Nieves J, Walliser J, et al: Postmenopausal osteoporosis: Patient choices and outcomes, pp 137-143, Copyright 1995, with kind permission from Elsevier Science Ireland Ltd., Bay 15K, Shannon Industrial Estate, Co. Clare, Ireland.)

(2 weeks of therapy with 11–13 weeks of no therapy), estrogen, or subcutaneous calcitonin (daily or on alternate days). All patients were instructed to take calcium and multivitamin supplements and to exercise at least 3 times per week. Bone density measurements were obtained at baseline and every 6 months.

Results.—Of the 52 patients, 21 chose treatment with estrogen, 20 chose treatment with etidronate, and 11 chose treatment with self-injected calcitonin. All 3 therapies resulted in increased lumbar spine bone mineral density (BMD), with mean 2-year increments of 4.4% with estrogen, 3.7% with etidronate, and 1.2% with calcitonin. The BMD in the femoral neck of the hip did not change in the estrogen group but decreased significantly with etidronate (3.1%) and calcitonin (4.9%). There was no change in the BMD of the distal forearm in the estrogen group, but it decreased significantly in the etidronate (more than 8%) and the calcitonin (3.9%) groups.

In the proximal forearm, BMD increased by 5.7% in the estrogen group but decreased by 3% in the etidronate group and by 0.6% in the calcitonin group (Fig 1). All 3 therapies were well tolerated.

Conclusions.—Estrogen, etidronate, and calcitonin all induced small increments in spinal BMD, but only estrogen was effective at maintaining or increasing bone mass in the peripheral skeleton. The bone loss in the hip and forearm seen in the etidronate and calcitonin groups was similar to that expected in osteoporotic patients with no treatment. Therefore, etidronate or calcitonin therapy may not provide as much protection as does estrogen against limb fractures.

▶ Although this study was not randomized, the results indicate that estrogen is superior to calcitonin and etidronate for prevention of postmenopausal bone loss in the hip and forearm. The 3 agents had a similar level of effectiveness for prevention of spinal bone loss. Calcitonin has the additional disadvantages of increased cost, need for frequent subcutaneous injection, and high incidence of nausea, whereas etidronate is not approved for the treatment of existing osteoporosis. Now that another bisphosphonate, alendronate, has recently been approved for the treatment of osteoporosis, this agent should be used to prevent bone loss for those women who have contraindications to or do not wish to take estrogen replacement therapy.

D.R. Mishell, Jr., M.D.

Applications of an Enzyme Immunoassay for a New Marker of Bone Resorption (CrossLaps): Follow-up on Hormone Replacement Therapy and Osteoporosis Risk Assessment

Bonde M, Qvist P, Fledelius C, et al (Osteometer A/S, Rodovre, Denmark; Ctr for Clinical and Basic Research, Ballerup, Denmark)
J Clin Endocrinol Metab 80:864–868, 1995   14–17

Background.—Increased attention has been given to identifying a specific marker for bone resorption, given its direct association with bone loss. Although urinary excretions of calcium and hydroxyproline have been used as indices of bone resorption, neither is specific for bone metabolism. More recently, the pyridinium cross-links in free- and peptide-bound forms have been introduced as markers of bone resorption, and commercially available immunoassays are currently being evaluated. The recently developed CrossLaps enzyme-linked immunosorbent immunoassay (ELISA), which measures degradation products of type I collagen in urine, was evaluated. Considering that more than 90% of the organic matrix of bone consists of type I collagen, the CrossLaps immunoassay may be a potential specific marker of bone resorption.

Patients and Methods.—Serum and urine samples obtained from 104 healthy premenopausal women and 180 healthy postmenopausal women were evaluated. Longitudinal serum and urine samples from 80 randomly selected women after 1 year of hormone replacement therapy and 35 randomly selected women after 1 year of placebo therapy were also assessed. Correlations between values obtained in the ELISA and in pyridinoline by high-pressure liquid chromatography were analyzed after correcting for creatinine.

Results.—A high correlation (0.77; $n = 81$) between values obtained in the CrossLaps ELISA and pyridinoline on high-pressure liquid chromatography was noted. Compared with the premenopausal group, among the postmenopausal women, the following values were increased: CrossLaps, 71%; hydroxyproline, 23%; osteocalcin, 52%; pyridinoline, 31%; and deoxypyridinoline, 50%. Compared with the placebo group, in women undergoing hormone replacement therapy, a highly significant decrease in the CrossLaps values (60.7%) was observed after 12 months. The spontaneous bone loss in the untreated women was assessed by repeat forearm bone mass measurements over 24 months. Baseline CrossLaps ELISA values were associated with the rate of loss, with a highly significant r value of -0.61 noted.

Conclusions.—The CrossLaps ELISA is a sensitive marker for changes in bone turnover that occur at menopause and during hormone replacement therapy. The correlation between the values obtained using this newly developed ELISA procedure and the rate of bone loss also indicate that CrossLaps may be useful for assessing the risk of postmenopausal osteoporosis.

Comparison of Markers for Bone Formation and Resorption in Premenopausal and Postmenopausal Subjects, and Osteoporosis Patients
Kushida K, Takahashi M, Kawana K, et al (Hamamatsu Univ, Japan)
J Clin Endocrinol Metab 80:2447–2450, 1995   14–18

Background.—For many years, alkaline phosphatase and urinary hydroxyproline were the only 2 bone metabolic markers in clinical use. More recently, bone gla protein, also called osteocalcin, was found to reflect osteoblastic activity. Novel markers related to collagen molecules have recently been developed. Pyridinoline and deoxypyridinoline are mature cross-links synthesized by the posttranslational modification of collagen molecules. Pyridinoline, deoxypyridinoline, and carboxy-terminal telopeptide of type I collagen (ICTP), including those cross-links, are excreted through collagen degradation at the time of bone resorption. Thus, bone resorption may be reflected by pyridinoline, deoxypyridinoline, and ICTP.

Methods and Findings.—Bone formation markers alkaline phosphatase, bone gla protein, and carboxy-terminal propeptide of type I collagen (PICP) were compared with bone resorption markers ICTP, pyridinoline, and deoxypyridinoline to determine whether they reflected the effects of aging and menopause in 95 healthy premenopausal and 66 healthy postmenopausal women. All markers but ICTP increased significantly with age in these patients. Postmenopausal women had significantly greater alkaline phosphatase, bone gla protein, PICP, pyridinoline, and deoxypyridinoline

TABLE 2.—Characteristics of the Patient Groups and the Values (Mean ± Standard Error) of 6 Markers in 3 Groups

	PRE (n = 95)	POST (n = 66)	VX (n = 29)
Age (mean ± SE)	39.7 ± 0.7	57.7 ± 0.6	77.8 ± 1.6
Range	30–53	50–69	55–91
Menopause	Pre	Post	Post
Alp (mKat/L)	2.0 ± 0.1	3.2 ± 0.1*	3.6 ± 0.3*
BGP (ng/ml)	4.8 ± 0.3	8.4 ± 0.5*	6.4 ± 1.0†
PICP (mg/mL)	92.3 ± 2.6	118.1 ± 6.2‡	155.1 ± 20.7*†
ICTP (mg/mL)	2.9 ± 0.1	3.1 ± 0.2	9.4 ± 1.8‡§
Pyr (nmol/mmol creatine)	21.4 ± 0.7	31.8 ± 1.4‡	73.0 ± 10.0*§
Dpyr (nmol/mmol creatinine)	4.0 ± 0.2	6.6 ± 0.4‖	13.6 ± 1.8*§

*$P < 0.001$ vs. premenopausal (PRE) group.
†$P < 0.05$ vs. postmenopausal (POST) group.
‡$P < 0.05$ vs. premenopausal group.
§$P < 0.001$ vs. postmenopausal group.
‖$P < 0.01$ vs. premenopausal group.
Abbreviation: VX, vertebral osteoporotic group.
(Courtesy of Kushida K, Takahashi M, Kawana K, et al: *J Clin Endocrinol Metab* 80:2447–2450, 1995.)

than did premenopausal women (Table 2). Premenopausal women in their 50s already had significantly increased bone gla protein, pyridinoline, and deoxypyridinoline compared with premenopausal women in their 30s and 40s. The discriminatory power of the 6 markers was determined in postmenopausal women and patients with osteoporosis by calculating the z scores against the premenopausal group. The bone resorption marker z scores were substantially greater than those of the bone formation markers in patients with osteoporosis. The z scores of bone resorption markers were comparable to those of bone formation markers in postmenopausal women.

Conclusions.—Alkaline phosphatase, bone gla protein, PICP, pyridinoline, and deoxypyridinoline were useful markers of postmenopausal status. Bone resorption markers were increased more than formation markers in patients with vertebral osteoporosis. Bone turnover in patients with osteoporosis was more uncoupled than in postmenopausal women.

▶ It would be very useful to have a substance that could be measured in blood or urine that would be a sensitive indicator of the magnitude of bone loss and thus the likelihood of osteoporosis developing. Measurement of serum alkaline phosphatase and urinary hydroxyproline has been used for several years to reflect the degree of bone formation or bone resorption but is too insensitive to be used as a marker for the low rate of bone loss that occurs with osteoporosis. The new markers that reflect the amount of collagen degradation measured in these studies appear to be more sensitive indicators of the development of osteoporosis. If measurement of these markers becomes generally available, it could be used in place of serial measurement of bone mass to determine whether a postmenopausal woman is likely to have osteoporosis develop. If the markers indicate that substantial bone loss is occurring, the woman should be strongly advised to use therapy to prevent osteoporotic fractures.

D.R. Mishell, Jr., M.D.

Alendronate Treatment of the Postmenopausal Osteoporotic Woman: Effect of Multiple Dosages on Bone Mass and Bone Remodeling
Chesnut CH III, McClung MR, Ensrud KE, et al (Univ of Washington, Seattle; Providence Med Ctr, Portland, Ore; Univ of Minnesota, Minneapolis; et al)
Am J Med 99:144–152, 1995   14–19

Background.—The group of compounds known as bisphosphonates has been proposed as a means to treat postmenopausal women who have osteoporosis. Although the bisphosphonate etidronate has received growing attention, the geminal aminobisphosphonate alendronate provides 100- to 500-fold more potent inhibition in comparison, and it is also a highly selective inhibitor of resorption with no detrimental effects on mineralization. The effects of alendronate sodium on bone mass and markers of bone remodeling were examined in a multicenter, randomized, double-blind, placebo-controlled study.

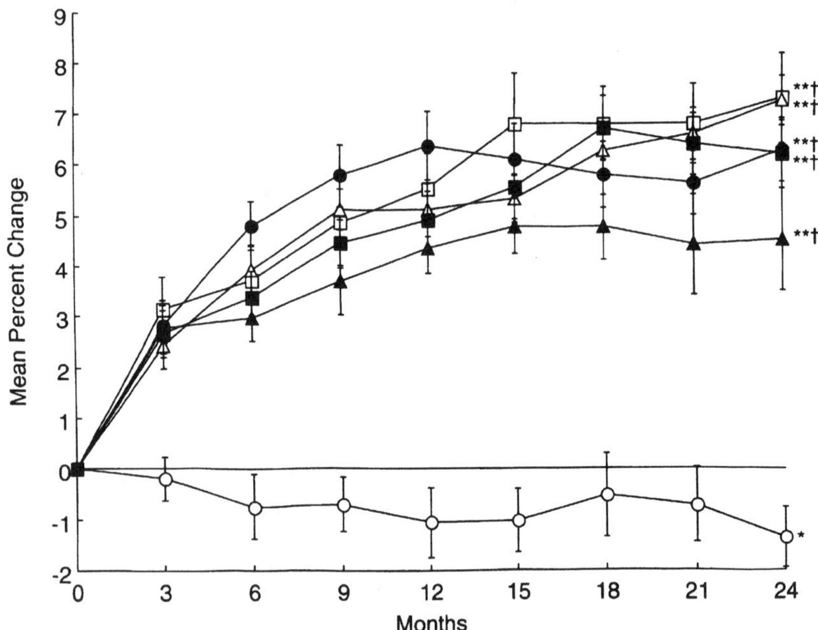

FIGURE 1.—Mean (± standard error of the mean) changes in bone mineral density of the spine in postmenopausal women, as measured by dual-energy x-ray absorptiometry, in placebo (*open circles*), 5-mg (*open squares*), 10-mg (*open triangles*), 20-mg/placebo (*filled circles*), 40-mg/placebo (*filled squares*), and 40/2.5-mg (*filled trianges*) treatment groups. *P* < 0.05, **P* < 0.01, both compared with baseline; †*P* < 0.001, alendronate-treated groups vs. placebo. (Reprinted by permission of the publisher from Chesnut CH III, McClung MR, Ensrud KE, et al: *Am J Med* 99:144–152, Copyright 1995 by Excerpta Medica, Inc.)

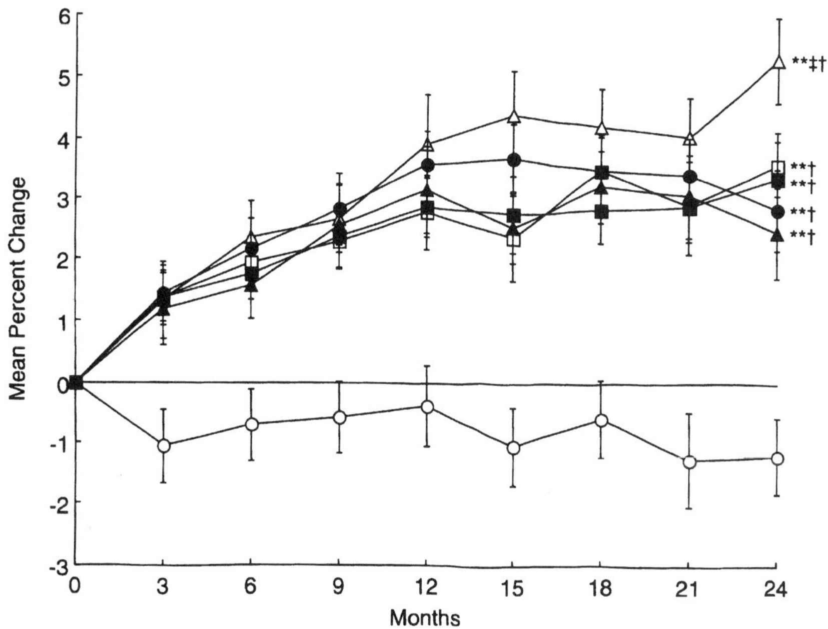

FIGURE 2.—Mean (± standard error of the mean) changes in bone mineral density of the total hip in postmenopausal women, as measured by dual-energy x-ray absorptiometry, in placebo (*open circles*), 5-mg (*open squares*), 10-mg (*open triangles*), 20-mg/placebo (*filled circles*), 40-mg/placebo (*filled squares*), and 40/2.5-mg (*filled triangles*) treatment groups. **$P < 0.01$, compared with baseline; †$P < 0.001$, alendronate-treated groups vs. placebo; ‡$P < 0.006$ to $P = 0.046$, 10-mg group vs. other treatment groups. (Reprinted by permission of the publisher from Chesnut CH III, McClung MR, Ensrud KE, et al: *Am J Med* 99:144–152, Copyright 1995 by Excerpta Medica, Inc.)

Patients and Methods.—One hundred eighty-eight postmenopausal women from 7 participating centers were enrolled in this 24-month study. The patients ranged in age from 42 to 75 years. All women had low bone mineral density (BMD) of the lumbar spine, and all were randomly assigned to 1 of 6 treatment groups. These included placebo for 24 months, 5–10 mg of alendronate for 24 months, 20 or 40 mg of alendronate for 12 months followed by placebo for 12 months, or 40 mg of alendronate for 3 months followed by 2.5 mg for 21 months. All women also received 500 mg of elemental calcium per day as calcium carbonate.

Results.—Significant reductions in markers of bone resorption and formation were observed with all doses of alendronate. In addition, significant increases in bone mass at the lumbar spine, hip, and total body were also noted in patients receiving alendronate. In contrast, decreases in bone mass were observed at each site in patients given placebo; these decreases were significant at the lumbar spine (Figs 1 and 2). Among women given 10 mg of alendronate, the mean urinary deoxypyridinoline/creatinine decreased by 47% at 3 months and the mean serum osteocalcin decreased by 53% at 6 months. Within the 24-month period, the mean changes in BMD with 10 mg of alendronate were +7.21% for the lumbar spine, +5.27% for total hip, and +2.53% for the total body. Corresponding figures among patients receiving placebo treatment were -1.35%, -1.2%, and -0.31% at each of the 3 sites. During the second year of the study, progressive increases in BMD were noted in the lumbar spines and hips of women given 10 mg of alendronate.

Conclusions.—Alendronate reduces markers of bone remodeling and significantly increases BMD at the lumbar spine, hip, and total body. This agent is well tolerated at daily doses of 5–10 mg and provides effective treatment for postmenopausal women with osteoporosis.

▶ Currently, 3 agents are available to prevent the increased bone resorption that normally occurs after the menopause: estrogen, calcitonin, and etidronate. None of these 3 agents causes a progressive increase in BMD as was observed during 2 years of treatment with the well-tolerated bisphosphonate, alendronate. Postmenopausal estrogen replacement prevents bone loss and reduces the incidence of osteoporosis and fracture of the hip and spine. It has many other health benefits as well. Therefore, estrogen replacement should be the primary method to prevent postmenopausal osteoporosis. However, if women have contraindications to estrogen replacement or initially seek medical care with established osteoporosis, use of alendronate may be the best treatment.

D.R. Mishell, Jr., M.D.

Effects of Oral Alendronate and Intranasal Salmon Calcitonin on Bone Mass and Biochemical Markers of Bone Turnover in Postmenopausal Women With Osteoporosis
Adami S, Passeri M, Ortolani S, et al (Univ of Verona, Italy; Univ of Parma, Italy; Ospedale San Luca, Milano, Italy: et al)
Bone 17:383–390, 1995   14–20

Background.—Alendronate is a bisphosphonate that suppresses osteoclastic bone resorption during the remodeling process. It is not known to influence osteoblastic bone formation, and it does not impede bone mineralization when given in therapeutic doses. The drug may lessen the amount of bone resorbed to below the amount formed, with a net increase in bone mass and strength resulting.

Objective.—The efficacy and safety of oral alendronate were examined in comparison to intranasal salmon calcitonin in 286 women aged 48–76 years from 9 clinical centers who were at least 2 years past their natural menopause.

Methods.—In all cases, the initial lumbar spinal bone mineral density (BMD) was more than 2 SD below the average for young premenopausal women. Alendronate was given in daily doses of 10 and 20 mg, and salmon calcitonin was given intranasally in a daily dose of 100 IU. Bone mineral density was measured in the lumbar spine and hip at 6-month intervals by dual-energy x-ray absorptiometry.

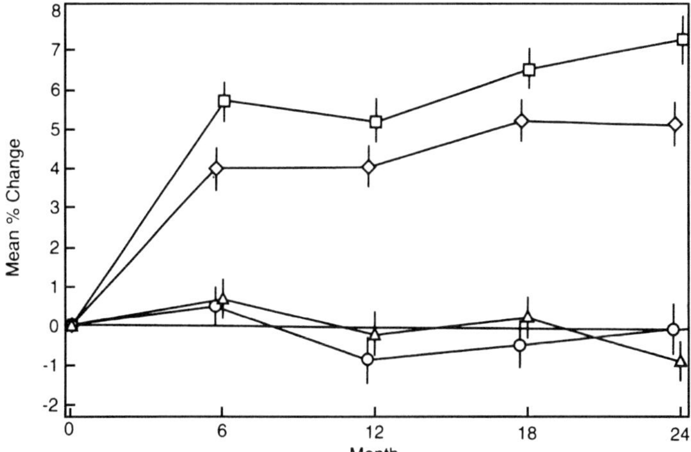

FIGURE 1.—Lumbar spine bone mineral density (*BMD*). Mean percentage changes (standard error) in BMD with placebo (*circle*); alendronate, 10 mg (*diamond*); alendronate, 20 mg (*square*); intranasal salmon calcitonin, 100 IU (*triangle*), baseline to 24 months. (Reprinted from *Bone*, Vol. 17, Adami S, Passeri M, Ortolani S, et al: Effects of oral alendronate and intranasal salmon calcitonin on bone mass and biochemical markers of bone turnover in postmenopausal women with osteoporosis, pp 383–390, Copyright 1995, with kind permission from Elsevier Science Ltd, The Boulevard, Langford Lane, Kidlington 0X5 1GB, UK.)

Effects on Bone.—The 10- and 20-mg doses of alendronate increased spinal bone mass by 5.2% and 7.3%, respectively, after 2 years, compared with in placebo recipients (Fig 1). Most of the gain in bone mass occurred in the first year of treatment. Bone mineral density deceased by 0.8% on

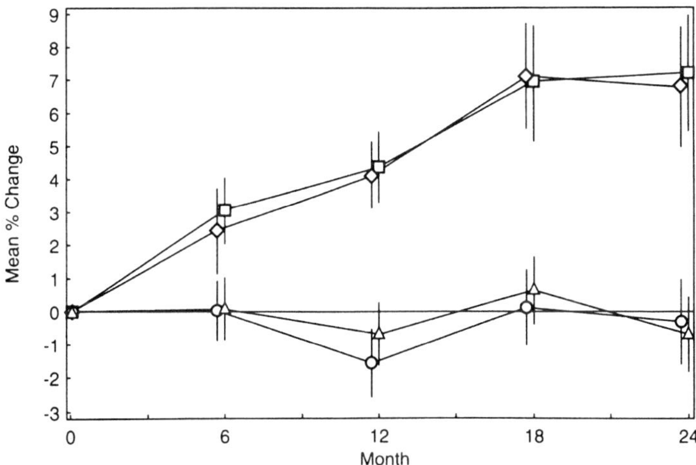

FIGURE 3.—Trochanter bone mineral density (*BMD*). Mean percentage changes (standard error) in BMD with placebo (*circle*); alendronate, 10 mg (*diamond*); alendronate, 20 mg (*square*); intranasal salmon calcitonin, 100 IU (*triangle*), baseline to 24 months. (Reprinted from *Bone*, Vol. 17, Adami S, Passeri M, Ortolani S, et al: Effects of oral alendronate and intranasal salmon calcitonin on bone mass and biochemical markers of bone turnover in postmenopausal women with osteoporosis, pp 383–390, Copyright 1995, with kind permission from Elsevier Science Ltd, The Boulevard, Langford Lane, Kidlington 0X5 1GB, UK.)

average in women given calcitonin. Alendronate treatment increased BMD in the femoral neck by 1% to 2% and in the trochanter by as much as 7.2% (Fig 3). Calcitonin was relatively ineffective.

Biochemistry.—Alendronate significantly decreased the urinary excretion of deoxypyridinoline, a marker of bone resorption, but calcitonin had no such effect. Alendronate also reduced the serum alkaline phosphatase and osteocalcin levels—both markers of bone formation.

Tolerance.—Active treatment was not associated with a significant risk of side effects. Gastrointestinal effects were essentially as frequent in placebo recipients. Alendronate did not alter the blood pressure, heart rate, or body size.

Conclusion.—Oral alendronate therapy is a safe means of promoting increased bone mass in postmenopausal women.

▶ The potent bisphosphonate, alendronate, has recently been approved for marketing in the United States. The results of this 2-year study indicate that a daily dose of 10 mg of this agent is well tolerated and increases bone mass in both trabecular (lumbar spine) and cortical (femoral neck) bone. Although data regarding the incidence of reduction of fracture incidences with this agent are not yet available, the increase in bone density is substantial and most likely will decrease the incidence of fractures in women who already have osteoporosis. This agent can also be used by women without osteoporosis who are at risk for osteoporotic fractures and do not wish to use estrogen replacement or have contraindications to its use.

D.R. Mishell, Jr., M.D.

Effects of Hormone Replacement Therapy on Endometrial Histology in Postmenopausal Women: The Postmenopausal Estrogen/Progestin Interventions (PEPI) Trial
The Writing Group for the PEPI Trial (Natl Heart, Lung, and Blood Inst, Bethesda, Md)
JAMA 275:370–375, 1996   14–21

Background.—Although many researchers have studied endometrial changes in postmenopausal women given estrogen plus progestin (E + P), methodological problems make the findings of this research difficult to interpret. To further assess the effect of hormone replacement treatments on the endometrium, data from the Postmenopausal Estrogen/Progestin Interventions Trial, a double-masked, placebo-controlled, 3-year follow-up trial, were studied.

Methods.—Five hundred ninety-six women randomly assigned to 1 of 3 E + P regimens, estrogen only, or placebo in the Postmenopausal Estrogen/ Progestin Interventions Trial were included in the current study. The patients were aged 45–64 years, and all had a uterus. The active treatments given were 28-day cycles of 0.625 mg/day of conjugated equine estrogens (CEE), 0.625 mg/day of CEE plus 10 mg/day of medroxyprogesterone acetate (MPA) for the first 12 days, 0.625 mg/day of CEE plus 2.5 mg/day

TABLE 2.—Summary of Endometrial Biopsy Changes Since Normal Baseline to Most Extreme Abnormal Results, by Treatment Regimen

Result	Treatment Regimen					Total, No. (%)
	Placebo	CEE Only	CEE + MPA (cyc)	CEE + MPA (con)	CEE + MP	
Normal*	116	45	112	119	114	506 (84.9)
Simple (cystic) hyperplasia†	1	33	4	1	5	44 (7.4)
Complex (adenomatous) hyperplasia†	1	27	2	0	0	30 (5.0)
Atypia†	0	14	0	0	1	15 (2.5)
Adenocarcinoma	1	0	0	0	0	1 (0.2)
Total	119	119	118	120	120	596 (100)

Note: Includes 30 cases in which the diagnosis was assigned by the local gynecologist because the local, central, and arbiter pathologists gave different options.

*P = 0.16 (normal vs. abnormal) for placebo compared with conjugated equine estrogens (*CEE*) + medroxyprogesterone acetate (*MPA*), (*cyc*), CEE + MPA (*con*), and CEE + micronized progesterone (*MP*).

†P < 0.001 for placebo compared with CEE only.

(Courtesy of The Writing Group for the PEPI Trial: Effects of hormone replacement therapy on endometrial histology in postmenopausal women: The Postmenopausal Estrogen/Progestin Interventions (PEPI) trial. *JAMA* 275:370–375. Copyright 1996, American Medical Association.)

of MPA, or 0.625 mg/day of CEE plus 200 mg/day of micronized progesterone for the first 12 days. Annual assessments included a pelvic examination, a Papanicolaou test, and an endometrial biopsy.

Findings.—During follow-up, simple hyperplasia developed in 27.7% of women given estrogen alone and in 0.8% of those receiving placebo; complex hyperplasia developed in 22.7% vs. 0.8%, and atypical hyperplasia developed in 11.8% vs. 0% (Table 2). The rates of hyperplasia among women given an E + P regimen were similar to those among women given placebo. Women receiving only estrogens had a higher number of unscheduled biopsies and curettages than women given placebo or 1 of the E + P regimens. Study medications were discontinued in all 45 women with complex or atypical hyperplasia. The biopsy findings of 34 of 36 these women normalized after progestin treatment was initiated. Dilatation and curettage was performed in 2 women and hysterectomy in 8, with or without previous medical treatment. One patient refused further biopsies. In 1 woman in the placebo group, adenocarcinoma of the endometrium developed.

Conclusions.—Daily CEE administration at a dose of 0.625 mg appears to increase the occurrence of endometrial hyperplasia. The addition of cyclic or continuous MPA or cyclic micronized progesterone to CEE treatment protects the endometrium from these hyperplastic changes.

▶ Several interesting findings come from this randomized, prospective, clinical trial comparing the effects on endometrial histology of daily estrogen alone, sequential progestin and estrogen, and continuous progestin and estrogen with that of placebo. The incidence of endometrial hyperplasia was very high in the women receiving daily doses of CEE, with nearly two thirds of the women having some type of hyperplasia. In contrast, the risk of having endometrial hyperplasia develop was very low in the women receiving MPA either cyclically or continuously.

It is interesting that the incidence of hyperplasia was higher in the women receiving a high dose of progestin intermittently—6 of 118 (5%)—than in those receiving a low dose of progestin daily—1 of 120 (0.8%)—together with a daily dose of estrogen. Because approximately 80% of the women receiving progestin cyclically have withdrawal bleeding after its use, whereas most women receiving a low dose of progestin daily have little bleeding after the first few months of therapy, the latter regimen should be preferable in women who have a uterus. For women without a uterus who cannot tolerate the adverse symptoms associated with progestin therapy, use of estrogen alone is preferable to withholding all forms of estrogen replacement.

Even though the incidence of hyperplasia is high, it can be detected by serial endometrial biopsies or measuring the endometrial thickness sonographically. In my practice I use a regimen of estrone sulfate, 0.625 mg 5 days a week with 2 days of no therapy. With this low dose of an estrogen with a shorter half-life than CEE and interrupted instead of continuous therapy, none of a small series of women have yet had endometrial hyperplasia develop after several years of treatment.

D.R. Mishell, Jr., M.D.

Long-term Hormone Replacement Therapy and Risk of Breast Cancer in Postmenopausal Women

Newcomb PA, Longnecker MP, Storer BE, et al (Univ of Wisconsin, Madison; Univ of California, Los Angeles; Univ of Chicago; et al)
Am J Epidemiol 142:788–795, 1995
14–22

Introduction.—Although endogenous estrogens appear to be important in the genesis or promotion of breast cancer, there is no clear evidence that exogenous hormones play a similar role. However, some studies have reported a modest association between breast cancer and long-term hormone replacement therapy (HRT). The breast cancer risks associated with postmenopausal HRT (with either unopposed estrogen or progestin and estrogen) were examined in a large, multicenter, case-control study.

Methods.—All women younger than 75 years of age with newly diagnosed invasive breast cancer were identified in state cancer registries in Wisconsin, western Massachusetts, Maine, and New Hampshire between 1989 and 1991, providing data for 6,888 cases. Controls were randomly selected from lists of licensed drivers and from lists of Medicare beneficiaries. Cases and controls were interviewed by telephone to gather data about potential risk factors for breast cancer, including use of exogenous hormones. Analysis was limited to the data on postmenopausal women, which included 3,130 cases and 3,698 controls.

Results.—Hormone replacement therapy had been used by 36% of the cases and 38% of the controls. Only 15% had used combined estrogen and progestin regimens. There were no significant differences in the risk of breast cancer between those who had ever used HRT and those who had never used HRT, either estrogen alone or combination therapy. There was no significant increase in the relative risk of breast cancer among women who had used HRT for at least 15 years (1.11 overall and 1.02 for women who had used only estrogen) (Table 3). Among recent users of hormones, the relative risk was slightly decreased (0.87). Risk was not altered by age, history of benign breast disease, family history of breast cancer, alcohol consumption, body mass index, preparation used, or type of menopause.

Discussion.—The use of postmenopausal HRT does not increase the risk of breast cancer, even among long-term users. The large sample size and null association among all subgroups, duration categories, and use patterns testify to the robustness of the findings.

▶ Several meta-analyses have demonstrated that there is no change in the risk of breast cancer with *ever* use of postmenopausal estrogen replacement therapy (ERT). Uncertainty exists, however, regarding the relation between *long-term* use of ERT and the risk of breast cancer developing. Some studies, particularly from Europe, with long-term use of high-dose synthetic estrogens, have shown an increased risk of breast cancer. Other studies, including this one, have found that the risk is not increased with long-term ERT. There have been no randomized, clinical trials to investigate the relation between breast cancer and ERT. Therefore, it is necessary to rely on the data

TABLE 3.—Estimated Relative Risk (RR) of Breast Cancer According to Duration of Use of Hormone Replacement Therapy (HRT), 1989–1991

Duration of use (years)	All HRT users			Users of estrogen only			Users of estrogen and progestin			Women with natural menopause only (all users)		
	No. of cases	No. of controls	RR* (95% CI)	No. of cases	No. of controls	RR* 95% CI	No. of cases	No. of controls	RR* (95% CI)	No. of cases	No. of controls	RR* (95% CI)
Never use	2,207	2,574	1.00	2,207	2,574	1.00	2,207	2,574	1.00	1,961	2,324	1.00
<2	288	363	1.02 (0.85–1.21)	144	207	0.88 (0.69–1.11)	44	52	0.95 (0.61–1.48)	218	257	1.05 (0.86–1.29)
2–4	230	261	1.09 (0.89–1.33)	144	160	1.12 (0.87–1.44)	38	42	1.12 (0.69–1.83)	154	175	1.09 (0.86–1.38)
5–9	156	196	1.02 (0.81–1.30)	104	153	0.90 (0.68–1.18)	31	29	1.23 (0.71–2.13)	99	113	1.08 (0.80–1.44)
10–14	99	132	0.99 (0.74–1.32)	73	108	0.93 (0.67–1.29)	10	19	0.55 (0.24–1.27)	52	61	1.12 (0.75–1.66)
≥15	150	172	1.11 (0.87–1.43)	122	155	1.02 (0.78–1.34)	15	15	1.05 (0.49–2.25)	75	94	0.96 (0.69–1.35)
p trend (categorical)	0.44			0.87			0.94			0.59		
Trend per year			1.00 (0.99–1.01)			1.00 (0.99–1.01)			1.00 (0.97–1.03)			1.00 (0.99–1.01)
p trend (per year)	0.83			0.52			0.99			0.99		

*Adjusted for age, state of residence, type of menopause, time since menopause, age at menarche, age at first full-term pregnancy, history of benign breast disease, body mass index, family history of breast cancer, alcohol consumption, and education.

Abbreviation: CI, confidence interval.

(Courtesy of Newcomb PA, Longnecker MP, Storer BE, et al: Long-term hormone replacement therapy and risk of breast cancer in postmenopausal women. *Am J Epidemiol* 142:788–795, 1995.)

of observational studies such as this one and 2 other recently published reports to determine whether long-term use of conjugated equine estrogen (CEE), the estrogen most commonly used in the United States, affects the risk of breast cancer. The other reports, 1 from Boston and 1 from Washington State, indicated that there is either no increased risk or only minimally increased risk of breast cancer with long-term ERT. The advantages of this study, which show no increased risk with long-term ERT, include its extremely large size, the fact that it was restricted to postmenopausal women, and that various high-risk subgroups were analyzed. The results should help reassure women about the lack of a proven increased risk of breast cancer with either current or long-term use of CEE.

D.R. Mishell, Jr., M.D.

The Short Term Effects of Tamoxifen on Bone Turnover in Older Women

Kenny AM, Prestwood KM, Pilbeam CC, et al (Univ of Nebraska, Omaha; Univ of Connecticut, Farmington)
J Clin Endocrinol Metab 80:3287–3291, 1995   14–23

Background.—In women in early postmenopause, tamoxifen (TAM) therapy has been found to maintain or increase bone density and may also decrease bone turnover. The effects of TAM on bone turnover and lipid profiles were studied in healthy women in late postmenopause.

Methods.—Eleven women without systemic disease or endocrine disorders and no history of osteoporotic fracture or excessively reduced bone mineral density who had not used estrogen or androgen therapy within the preceding 3 months were given 20 mg of TAM per day for 10 weeks. Before treatment, dietary intake was analyzed and calcium and vitamin D supplements were given to ensure standardized intake. Twice at baseline and once in weeks 9 and 10 of therapy, blood and 2-hour urine samples were obtained and analyzed for markers of bone formation and resorption and lipid profiles.

Results.—The 10 women who completed the study had a mean age of 75 years, with an average of 25 years since menopause. None had taken supplemental estrogen for the preceding 20 years. The markers of bone resorption generally decreased during therapy and increased toward baseline levels after therapy. The changes were significant for deoxypyridinoline and pyridinoline, whereas hydroxyproline and urinary calcium excretion changed by less than 10% (Fig 1). The markers of bone formation similarly decreased during therapy and returned toward baseline after therapy, although, in contrast with osteocalcin and total alkaline phosphatase, bone-specific alkaline phosphatase only showed a partial return and type I procollagen peptide remained low after therapy. The markers of resorption and the markers of formation correlated significantly. During therapy, ionized calcium and phosphorus decreased, parathyroid hormone increased, and vitamin D levels did not change. There were significant decreases in cholesterol and low-density lipoprotein levels, but triglyceride and high-density lipoprotein levels were not affected.

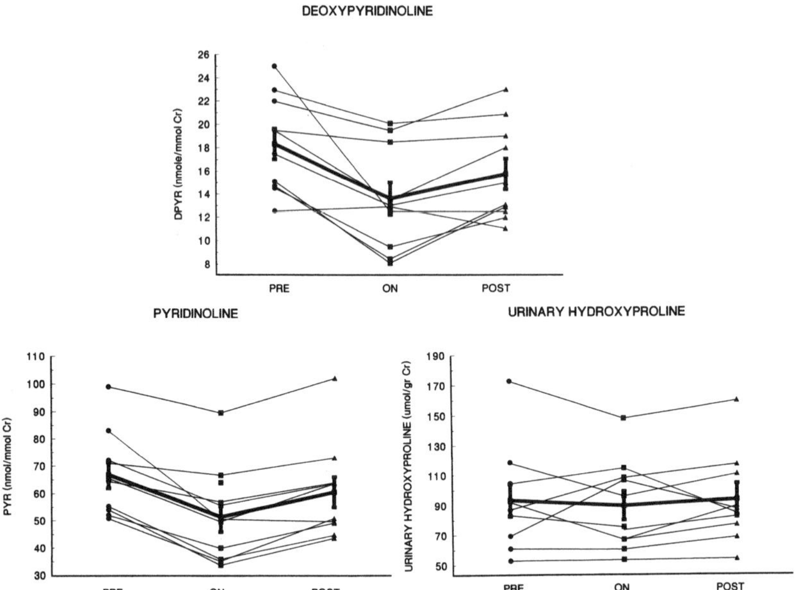

FIGURE 1.—Response of bone resorption markers to a 10-week course of tamoxifen treatment in older women. The *bold lines* represent the mean, and the *vertical lines* represent the SEM for each marker. The *thinner lines* represent changes in each marker for individual women. (Courtesy of Kenny AM, Prestwood KM, Pilbeam CC, et al: The short-term effects of tamoxifen on bone turnover in older women. *J Clin Endocrinol Metab* 80:3287–3291, 1995. © The Endocrine Society.)

Conclusions.—Short-term TAM therapy reduces bone turnover in healthy postmenopausal women older than age 70 years. The changes are similar, though smaller, to the changes seen with short-term estrogen treatment. Because pyridinoline and deoxypyridinoline, but not hydroxyproline and urinary calcium, showed significant changes during therapy, pyridinium cross-links may be a more sensitive marker of bone resorption.

The Effect of the Anti-estrogen Tamoxifen on Cardiovascular Risk Factors in Normal Postmenopausal Women

Grey AB, Stapleton JP, Evans MC, et al (Univ of Auckland, New Zealand)
J Clin Endocrinol Metab 80:3191–3195, 1995   14–24

Background.—Treatment with tamoxifen in women with breast cancer has been associated with a reduced risk of recurrent breast cancer, cardiovascular disease, and osteoporosis, but these effects have not been studied in healthy women. To assess the potential of tamoxifen therapy for reducing cardiovascular risk in normal women, the impact of 2 years of treatment was studied on major cardiovascular risk factors: serum lipids, fibrinogen, and body composition.

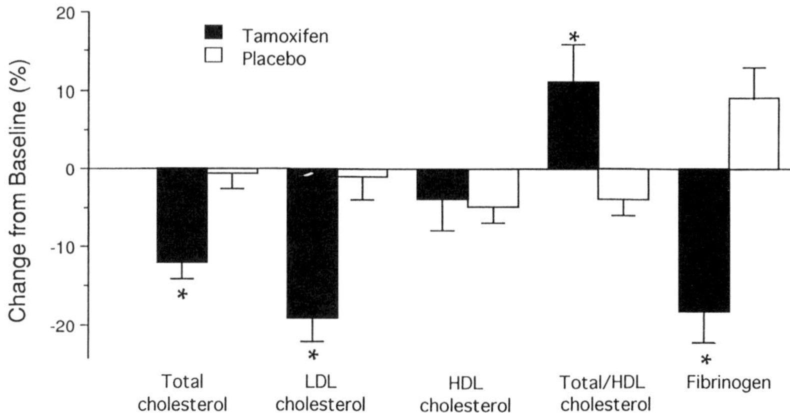

FIGURE 1.—Percentage change from baseline in serum lipids and fibrinogen after 2 years of tamoxifen or placebo therapy in normal postmenopausal women. *Horizontal bars* indicate SEM. *$P < 0.001$ vs. placebo. *Abbreviations: LDL,* low-density lipoprotein; *HDL,* high-density lipoprotein. (Courtesy of Grey AB, Stapleton JP, Evans MC, et al: The effect of the anti-estrogen tamoxifen on cardiovascular risk factors in normal postmenopausal women. *J Clin Endocrinol Metab* 80:3191–3195, 1995. © The Endocrine Society.)

Methods.—Fifty-seven healthy women at least 36 months postmenopausal were randomly assigned to receive either tamoxifen or placebo daily for 2 years. Forty-six completed the trial. At baseline, 6 months, and 2 years, blood specimens were obtained and analyzed for the serum lipid profile and fibrinogen concentration. Regional fat distribution was determined by calculating the ratio of android (waist) to gynoid (thigh) fat, as measured by dual-energy x-ray absorptiometry.

Results.—There were no significant differences between the groups in the studied variables at baseline. After treatment, the tamoxifen group had significantly lower levels of total cholesterol (12% fall), low-density lipoprotein cholesterol (19%), ratio of total cholesterol to high-density lipoprotein (HDL) cholesterol (11%), and fibrinogen (18%) (Fig 1). The 2 groups had no significant differences in the levels of HDL cholesterol, HDL cholesterol subfractions, triglycerides, or glucose. The tamoxifen group also demonstrated a trend toward a higher apolipoprotein A1 level. Both groups showed an increased ratio of android to gynoid fat, which was not altered by tamoxifen treatment.

Conclusions.—Tamoxifen treatment of normal postmenopausal women produces favorable changes in the levels of serum lipids and fibrinogen, which can substantially reduce the risk of cardiovascular disease.

▶ Tamoxifen is a nonsteroidal weak estrogen similar in structure to clomiphene citrate. Both agents bind to estrogen receptors and thus have an antiestrogenic action on certain target tissues by preventing the endogenous estrogens to bind to these receptors and produce an estrogenic effect. However, on other target organs, TAM has a direct estrogenic effect. Thus, although TAM has an antiestrogenic effect on the breast and the vagina, it has an estrogenic effect on the endometrium as well as on bone metabolism and cholesterol synthesis. Therefore, if a woman with a history of breast cancer does not wish to take postmenopausal estrogen replacement, if she takes TAM, she may still have a reduction in risk of osteoporotic fracture and cardiovascular disease. The magnitude of this reduction in risk remains to be defined by additional studies but is probably less than that of estrogen replacement therapy.

D.R. Mishell, Jr., M.D.

15 Infertility

Estimates of Human Fertility and Pregnancy Loss
Zinaman MJ, O'Connor J, Clegg ED, et al (Georgetown Univ, Washington, DC; US Environmental Protection Agency, Washington, DC; Loyola Univ, Maywood, Ill; et al)
Fertil Steril 65:503–509, 1996

15–1

Purpose.—It is difficult to establish fertility rates in presumably fertile populations. The results depend largely on the method used to estimate pregnancy loss rates. Fertility and pregnancy wastage rates in a presumably fertile population were prospectively studied.

Methods.—The study included 200 couples who stopped using contraception in an effort to become pregnant. The women were between age 21 and 37 years and had regular menstrual cycles; the men were between age 21 and 60 years. Most of the couples were nulliparous, and 60% had stopped using contraception within 1 month of enrolling in the study. Couples with known risk factors for infertility were excluded. The couples were counseled on coital timing and frequency and followed up for 12 months. For the first 3 months, the women kept detailed menstrual calendars and collected first morning urine specimens for testing of human chorionic gonadotropin (hCG). Thereafter, hCG testing was done only if menses was delayed, so occult pregnancies were not detected.

Results.—One hundred ninety-two couples completed the study. Pregnancy occurred within 1 year in 72% of nulliparous women and 88% of parous women. The conception rate in couples who completed the study was 82%. Of the original 200 couples, 30% conceived during the first cycle. In the remaining couples, conception rates were 30% during the second cycle and 17% during the third cycle; pregnancy rates tended to decrease thereafter. The cumulative pregnancy rate was 50% by 2 cycles and 65% by 4 cycles. Thirteen percent of pregnancies were detected only by hCG assay. Pregnancy loss rate was 32% in cycle 1, 29% in cycle 2, and 33% in cycle 3. Occult pregnancy accounted for 37%, 58%, and 20% of these losses, respectively, or 42% of pregnancy losses occurring in the first 3 cycles.

Conclusions.—In presumably fertile couples stopping contraception, the fertility rate is approximately 30% for the first 2 cycles, decreasing thereafter. Almost 20% of such couples will fail to conceive, even after 12 complete cycles. The number of occult pregnancies in presumably fertile couples is small, but it makes a substantial contribution to the pregnancy loss rate. Approximately 30% of all detectable conceptions are pregnancy losses.

▶ This interesting study supplies more information about normal human fecundity. If occult pregnancies are included in conception rates, it seems that among a group of presumably fertile couples who have midcycle coitus, there is a maximum rate of conception of 30%. The rate of clinical pregnancies among fertile couples attempting to conceive reaches 50% in 30 months and 75% in 6 months. Thus, one fourth of presumably normal fertile couples will not have evidence of a clinical pregnancy after 6 months trying to conceive.

D.R. Mishell, Jr., M.D.

Background Pregnancy Rates in an Infertile Population
Gleicher N, VanderLaan B, Pratt D, et al (Blue Cross Blue Shield of Illinois, Chicago; Ctr for Human Reproduction, Chicago)
Hum Reprod 11:1011–1012, 1996   15–2

Background.—A spontaneous background pregnancy rate can be detected, even in patient populations that are obviously infertile. To understand the effectiveness of infertility treatment, this rate should be studied in patient populations who are receiving attention from an infertility care provider but who are not in an active treatment cycle. Such a population was studied to determine the true spontaneous background pregnancy rate in infertile couples.

Methods.—The data were drawn from the 1,016 new infertility couples treated by the Center for Human Reproduction, Chicago, in 1994. The analysis included 5,541 months in which the women were receiving no cycle stimulation or cycle monitoring, only passive cycle monitoring, or gonadotropin-releasing hormone analogue (GnRHa) suppression. These accounted for 61% of the total treatment months during 1994. The rate of pregnancies occurring during these months was evaluated.

Results.—There were 112 clinical pregnancies in 5,541 months, for a spontaneous background pregnancy rate of 2.02%. Excluding pregnancies that occurred in GnRHa downregulated cycles, the monthly pregnancy rate was 1.83%. Further analysis of HMO patients who were to receive all of their infertility care at the study center revealed a background pregnancy rate of 2.21%.

Conclusions.—The spontaneous background pregnancy rate among couples receiving infertility treatment is approximately 2%. Thus, the cumulative clinical conception rate after 12 months in this patient population is approximately 20%. These and other recent results have important implications for evaluating the cost-effectiveness of infertility treatment.

▶ Unless anovulation, tubal blockage, or severe abnormalities in the semen analysis exist, the infertile couple has some degree of subfertility and conception can occur without therapy. The normal rate of human fecundability is approximately 20% per ovulatory cycle with midcycle coitus. The results of this study indicate that in the infertile population, without the abnormalities listed, which make conception impossible, the fecundability rate per cycle is reduced to approximately 2%. This incidence will be reduced to a greater extent when the woman is older than age 35 or the duration of infertility exceeds 3 years. To increase fecundability rates in these couples, use of controlled ovarian hyperstimulation and timed intrauterine insemination should increase their fecundability rate to approximately 15% per cycle.

D.R. Mishell, Jr., M.D.

Timing of Sexual Intercourse in Relation to Ovulation: Effects on the Probability of Conception, Survival of the Pregnancy, and Sex of the Baby
Wilcox AJ, Weinberg CR, Baird DD (Natl Inst of Environmental Health Sciences, Research Triangle Park, NC)
N Engl J Med 333:1517–1521, 1995   15–3

Objective.—It is agreed that conception must take place near the time of ovulation, but the precise timing and duration of fertility remain uncertain. For this reason, the timing of intercourse was monitored in 221 healthy women who were planning to conceive.

Methods.—Daily first morning urine specimens were collected from the time the participants stopped using birth control and were analyzed for estrogen and progesterone metabolites (Fig 1). Specimens were collected up to week 8 of clinical pregnancy or for up to 6 months. A total of 625 ovulatory cycles in 217 women were available for analysis.

Findings.—Without exception, conception was associated with at least one episode of intercourse in the 6-day period ending on the day of ovulation. None of 31 cycles lacking intercourse during this time resulted in conception. When intercourse took place only once during the 6-day period, it most commonly was on the day of ovulation. The chance of conception decreased substantially with intercourse less often than every other day during the 6-day period. Only 6% of conceptions were definitively related to fertilization by sperm that were 3 or more days old. No particular pattern of intercourse could be related to the sex of infants (Fig 4).

Implications.—The fertile period of the cycle lasts approximately 6 days and ends on the day of ovulation. These findings do not support limiting the frequency of intercourse to achieve pregnancy. Deliberately timing intercourse for the day of ovulation will not aid sex selection.

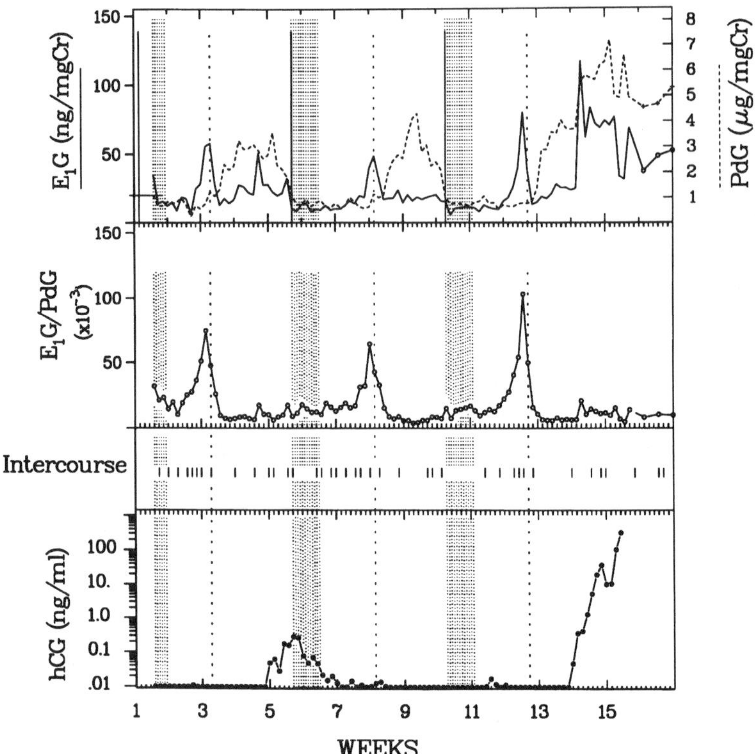

FIGURE 1.—Serial urinary hormone values in a woman trying to conceive. The *shaded bars* show days of menstrual bleeding. The estimated days of ovulation, based on an algorithm, are indicated by the *dotted lines*. In the **top panel**, values are provided for estrone 3-glucuronide (E_1G) (*solid line*) and pregnanediol 3-glucuronide (*PdG*) (*dashed line*), adjusted for the creatinine concentration. The **second panel from the top** shows the ratio of estrone 3-glucuronide to pregnanediol 3-glucuronide. Days on which sexual intercourse occurred are shown in the **third panel** by tick marks. The **bottom panel** shows the urinary concentration of human chorionic gonadotropin (*hCG*). (Reprinted with permission from The American College of Obstetricians and Gynecologists [*Obstetrics and Gynecology*, 1995, Vol. 86, pp 520–528.)]

▶ The results of this study provide additional data to confirm the long-standing belief that the duration of time after vaginal insemination whereby spermatozoa can fertilize the human ovum is much longer than the amount of time after ovulation during which the human egg is capable of being fertilized by spermatozoa. In this study, if sexual intercourse occurred on the estimated day of ovulation or 1 or 2 days before ovulation, the conception rate was about 35%. If insemination occurred 3 to 5 days before ovulation, the conception rate varied from 8% to 13%. If vaginal insemination occurred more than 5 days prior to ovulation or on any day after ovulation, pregnancy did not occur. Thus, these data provide additional evidence to substantiate the current practice for subfertile couples seeking to become pregnant to use tests that measure urinary luteinizing hormone, which peaks prior to ovulation, to determine the optimal time for sexual intercourse or intrauterine insemination. For couples who wish to use natural methods of family

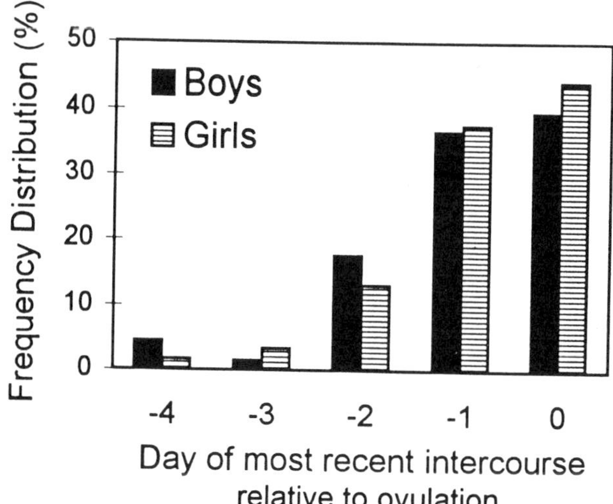

FIGURE 4.—Frequency distribution of live-born boys and girls, according to the time of the most recent instance of sexual intercourse before ovulation during the cycle when conception occurred. *Zero* denotes the day of ovulation. (Reprinted with permission from The American College of Obstetricians and Gynecologists [*Obstetrics and Gynecology*, 1995, Vol. 86, pp 520–528].)

planning to avoid pregnancy, once ovulation has occurred, as documented by a substantial rise in basal body temperature, sexual intercourse can ensue without the likelihood of conception occurring.

D.R. Mishell, Jr., M.D.

Weight Loss Results in Significant Improvement in Pregnancy and Ovulation Rates in Anovulatory Obese Women

Clark AM, Ledger W, Galletly C, et al (Univ of Adelaide, Australia; Queen Elizabeth Hosp, Woodville, Australia)
Hum Reprod 10:2705–2712, 1995

15–4

Objective.—Few studies have investigated the effects of weight loss in infertile women who have and do not have polycystic ovary syndrome (PCOS). Thus, the effects of a weight-loss program on fertility in anovulatory, obese, infertile women were prospectively evaluated. A low-technology, inexpensive group weight-loss program, consisting of dietary, exercise, and behavioral interventions, was used.

Patients and Methods.—Thirty women who had been infertile for more than 2 years were invited to enroll in the study; 18 agreed to participate. All women were anovulatory, were resistant to previous clomiphene treatment, had a body mass index of 30 kg/m² or greater, had patent fallopian tubes, and were prepared to refrain from standard medical infertility treatments for 6 months. During the 6-month study period, women attended weekly 2-hour group sessions. The first hour was devoted to low-impact aerobic exercise and the second hour to seminar discussions about diet and nutrition, abnormal eating behaviors, and obesity-related endocrine effects. Ovulation and pregnancy rates were evaluated after program completion.

Results.—Five of the 18 women dropped out of the exercise program and were included for comparison purposes. Women who completed the entire 6-month program lost significantly more weight during the study period than those who failed to complete the program (mean, 6.3 kg vs. 1.4 kg). Twelve of the 13 women completing the exercise program also were ovulating spontaneously at the end of 6 months, compared with none of the patients in the dropout group. Time taken to become ovulatory was similar between the 8 women with PCOS and the 5 women without PCOS in the exercise group, at 3.8 months for the former group vs 3.3 months for the latter group. Within 4 months of starting the program, 92% of the women were ovulatory, despite a mean weight loss of only 4.3 kg at that time. One year after program completion, 11 of the exercise-group patients had conceived, with spontaneous conception occurring more often in women with PCOS (75% of this group conceived vs. 25% in those without PCOS). All 5 women who had dropped out of the program failed to conceive spontaneously during or after treatment. Follow-up of the 12 women who had declined to participate in the study when initially asked showed that only 1 pregnancy had occurred on subsequent treatment cycles over the ensuing 18 months.

Conclusions.—A group-oriented exercise, dietary, and behavioral program can dramatically improve ovulation and pregnancy rates among obese, infertile women, thereby decreasing the need for high-technology medical treatment. The program described is less costly compared with standard forms of therapy, and it may potentially improve long-term physical and psychological well-being.

▶ Although this study was not a prospective, randomized, controlled trial, the results indicate that substantial weight loss among obese, infertile women was associated with a very high return of ovulatory cycles and spontaneous pregnancy. In obese, anovulatory, infertile women with and without PCOS who fail to ovulate with clomiphene citrate, it would appear therapeutically, emotionally, and financially preferable to treat with a standard weight reduction program for 6 months. This would be better than using human menopausal gonadotropin therapy with or without a gonadotropin-releasing agonist. The latter treatment requires frequent monitoring, is very expensive, and has the risk of causing ovarian hyperstimulation.

D.R. Mishell, Jr., M.D.

Smoking Reduces Fecundity: A European Multicenter Study on Infertility and Subfecundity

Bolumar F, Olsen J, Boldsen J, et al (Univ of Alicante, Spain; Aarhus Univ, Denmark)
Am J Epidemiol 143:578–587, 1996

15–5

Purpose.—Most but not all studies have suggested that smoking reduces fecundity. Most of these studies have failed to control for potential confounders, however. Particularly in Europe, smoking cessation is often not a part of the clinical management of couples who are infertile. Data from a large infertility study were used to examine the effects of smoking on fecundity.

Methods.—The study used data from the European Study of Infertility and Subfecundity, in which the time to pregnancy was used as the main estimator of the subjects' fecundability and fecundity. The study included randomly selected, population-based samples of women aged 25–44 years and pregnancy-based samples of women recruited during prenatal care visits. The population sample included 6,630 women, and the pregnancy sample had 4,035 women. The units of analysis in these samples were the couple and the pregnancy, respectively; the subjects were drawn from 10 European regions. Most of the data were collected by personal interview and included information on smoking in relation to the period in which the couple started cohabiting in order to conceive.

Results.—In the population sample, the link between smoking by women and subfecundity was consistent within and across countries. This was true for both the first pregnancy (odds ratio 1.7 for women at the highest level of smoking exposure) and most recent waiting time to pregnancy (odds ratio 1.6). The results were comparable in the pregnancy sample. Smoking by men was unrelated to fecundity, either in terms of the first pregnancy or the most recent waiting time. For smokers, the fecundity distribution tended to shift toward longer waiting times, although there was no change in the shape of the distribution. The link between smoking and fecundity was most strongly confounded by past oral contraceptive use and frequency of intercourse.

Conclusions.—This large and detailed analysis suggests that smoking by women seems to reduce fecundity. Women who are having trouble conceiving are well advised to quit smoking. Fecundity for former smokers is similar to that of nonsmokers.

▶ There have been several prior studies that have found that women who smoke cigarettes and wish to become pregnant take a longer time to conceive than women of similar age who do not smoke. In this study, the median time until conception occurred was 2.6 months for nonsmokers and 3.9 months for women who smoked more than 10 cigarettes a day. Thus, the detailed data on fecundity from this large study performed in several countries substantiate the adverse effect of cigarette smoking on human conception. In this study, former smokers had a waiting time to conception similar to that of nonsmokers. Therefore, if the woman in an infertile couple smokes cigarettes, she should be strongly advised to stop smoking.

D.R. Mishell, Jr., M.D.

Vaginal Douching and Reduced Fertility
Baird DD, Weinberg CR, Voigt LF, et al (Natl Inst of Environmental Health Sciences, Research Triangle Park, NC; Univ of Washington, Seattle)
Am J Public Health 86:844–850, 1996   15–6

Background.—In one national survey, 37% of American women of childbearing age reported douching. Eighteen percent douched at least once a week. However, this common practice may have adverse effects. It

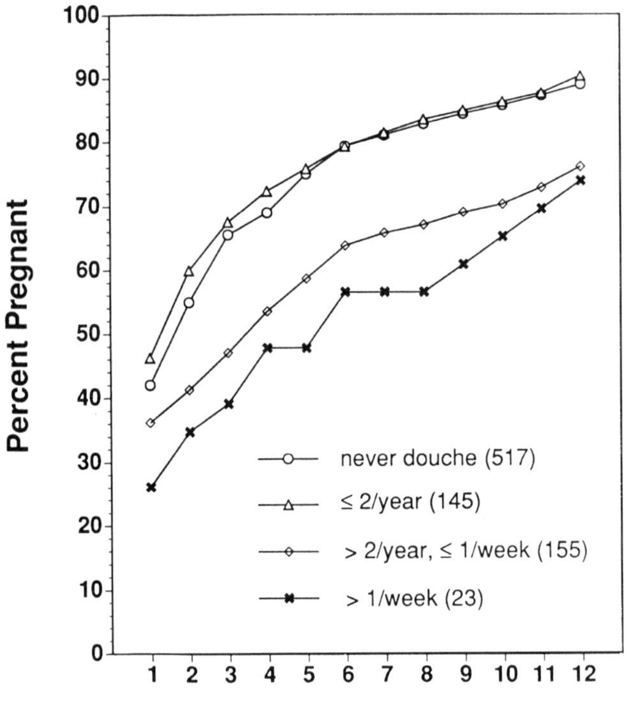

FIGURE 1.—Unadjusted cumulative percentage pregnant each month for women in 4 groups determined by their frequency of douching. (Courtesy of Baird DD, Weinberg CR, Voigt LF, et al: Vaginal douching and reduced fertility. *Am J Public Health* 86:844–850, copyright 1996, American Public Health Association.)

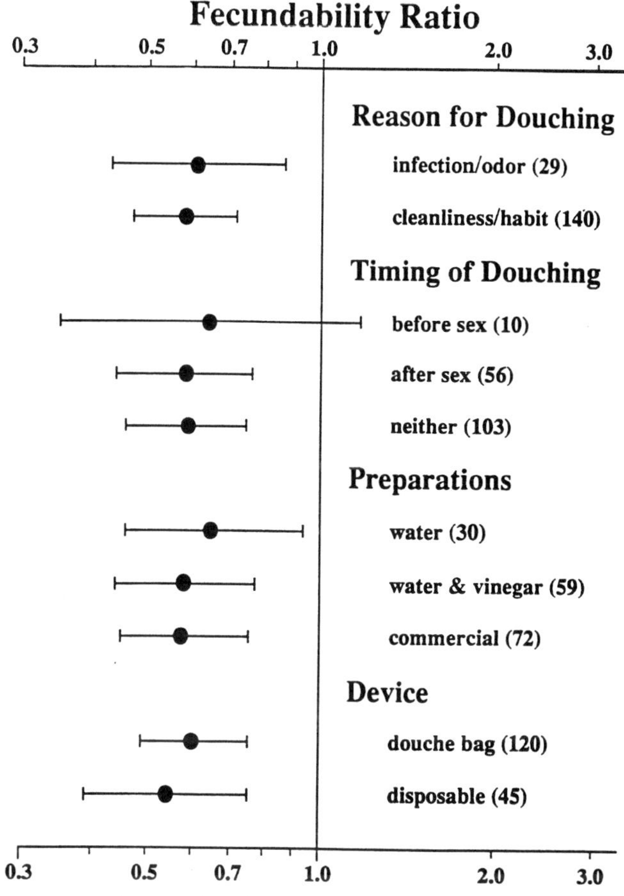

FIGURE 2.—Adjusted fecundability ratios (with 95% confidence intervals) for groups of women with different douching habits. The numbers in parentheses represent the number of douchers in each group. The comparison group in all cases was nondouchers. (Courtesy of Baird DD, Weinberg CR, Voigt LF, et al: Vaginal douching and reduced fertility. *Am J Public Health* 86:844–850, copyright 1996, American Public Health Association.)

has been associated with an increased risk of chlamydia infection, pelvic inflammatory disease, and ectopic pregnancy. The relationship between vaginal douching and fertility was investigated.

Methods.—To avoid problems inherent in studying patients who are infertile, the fertility of douchers and nondouchers was compared by collecting data on the number of months parous women required to become pregnant. This method was expected to underestimate the effect of douching on fertility because women who were sterile were excluded. Eight hundred forty women participated.

Findings.—Compared with nondouchers, douchers were 30% less likely to become pregnant each month they tried to conceive. This association persisted after adjustment for covariates and was not explained by douching for medical reasons. The reduction in fertility was unassociated with the type of douching preparation used. Monthly fertility was reduced by 50% among women 18–24 years of age, 29% among those 25–29 years of age, and 6% among those 30–39 years of age. These age differences were significant (Figs 1 and 2).

Conclusions.—In this series, douching was associated with decreased fertility. Additional research is needed to determine whether this relationship is causal and, if so, the degree to which pelvic infection mediates it.

▶ In prior epidemiologic studies, the environmental factors of cigarette smoking and caffeine ingestion have each been shown to independently decrease female fecundability. The data in this study indicate that vaginal douching with any liquid material also reduces fecundability, especially in women of young reproductive age. Thus, the woman in an infertile couple should be advised to stop smoking, stop drinking caffeinated beverages, and avoid vaginal douching.

D.R. Mishell, Jr., M.D.

Effect of Laparoscopic Ovarian Electrocautery on Ovarian Response and Outcome of Treatment With Gonadotropins in Clomiphene Citrate-Resistant Patients With Polycystic Ovary Syndrome

Farhi J, Soule S, Jacobs HS (Univ College London)
Fertil Steril 64:930–935, 1995

15–7

Study Group.—Forty-three women with polycystic ovary syndrome (PCOS) underwent ovarian electrocautery treatment by the laparoscopic approach. Twenty-two of them subsequently presented for further treatment. The patients, whose average age was 31 years, had been infertile for 4 years on average. Infertility was primary in 15 cases and secondary in 7. The women were followed up for 26 months on average after electrocautery. At the time of the procedure, all of them were oligomenorrheic or amenorrheic. All patients had failed to ovulate when given clomiphene and, in some cases, human menopausal gonadotropin (hMG) or follicle-stimulating hormone (FSH).

Management.—Hydrotubation was done with methylene blue before applying unipolar cautery at 4 points on each ovary. Regardless of the status of menstrual function, women who failed to conceive within 6 months of electrocautery received hMG or FSH.

Results.—Normal menstrual cycles returned in 41% of patients after electrocautery treatment. The overall results were significantly improved compared to previous gonadotropin therapy. Doses of both hMG and FSH were reduced after electrocautery. No hormonal differences were apparent between the women who responded and those who did not, either at baseline or after electrocautery. One of 3 women having a "second look" laparoscopy because of continued infertility was found to have adhesions and occlusion of both tubes.

Conclusions.—Infertile women with PCOS become more sensitive to gonadotropin therapy following laparoscopic ovarian electrocautery. This procedure may prove more effective than medical treatment alone in some clomiphene-resistant patients.

Laser Vaporization of the Ovarian Surface in Polycystic Ovary Disease Results in Reduced Ovarian Hyperstimulation and Improved Pregnancy Rates

Fukaya T, Murakami T, Tamura M, et al (Tohoku Univ, Sendai, Japan)
Am J Obstet Gynecol 173:119–125, 1995

15–8

Background.—The incidence of polycystic ovary disease is high among infertile women with anovulation. Treatment of this disease generally consists of clomiphene citrate, human menopausal gonadotropin (hMG), or human chorionic gonadotropin. Successful treatment outcomes can, however, be difficult to achieve, because of the ovarian hyperstimulation syndrome, particularly with hMG stimulation. The effect of laser vaporization on patients with polycystic ovary disease who were not ovulating spontaneously and who could not undergo successful ovarian stimulation because of severe ovarian hyperstimulation syndrome was studied.

Patients and Methods.—Twenty-six infertile women with polycystic ovary disease who had ovarian hyperstimulation caused by stimulation with hMG and who had failed to conceive were studied. Twenty to 30 vaporizations were performed with potassium titanyl phosphate and Nd:YAG laser. Treatment with either clomiphene citrate or hMG was administered to patients not ovulating spontaneously after vaporization.

Results.—Spontaneous ovulation occurred in 6 patients (23%) after laser vaporization. Of the other 20 patients, 3 were given clomiphene citrate and 17 received hMG for ovulation induction. In all patients, the stimulation regimen was completed without the occurrence of severe ovarian hyperstimulation syndrome. Clinical pregnancy occurred in 19 of the 26 patients, for a pregnancy rate per patient of 73%. Of these, 5 conceived after a spontaneous ovulation, 2 after ovulation induction with clomiphene citrate, and 12 after stimulation with hMG.

Conclusions.—Laser vaporization appears to aid in the prevention of ovarian hyperstimulation syndrome, and it helps improve pregnancy outcome in patients with polycystic ovary disease who have had ovarian hyperstimulation syndrome. Ovulation stimulation was, however, required in approximately 77% of the patients after vaporization. This may be because the benefits of laser treatment become less effective with time.

▶ The ovarian hyperstimulation syndrome (OHSS) is an iatrogenic condition produced by exogenous ovarian stimulation that results in perfusion of fluid from the vascular to the extracellular compartment with resultant hemoconcentration. Serious complications, including venous thrombosis, renal failure, and adult respiratory distress syndrome, can occur. Use of hMG to induce ovulation in women with polycystic ovarian syndrome (PCOS) is associated with appreciable risk of OHSS developing. In this study, women with PCOS who had previously had OHSS develop with hMG treatment before multiple laser vaporization of the ovarian surface either ovulated spontaneously after such treatment or did not have moderate or severe OHSS develop with use of hMG after laser vaporization. If women with anovulation due to PCOS fail to ovulate after use of clomiphene citrate, it may be better to use multiple laser or coagulation treatment of the ovarian surface instead of treating them with hMG to reduce the risk of OHSS.

D.R. Mishell, Jr., M.D.

Randomized Comparison of Ovulation Induction With and Without Intrauterine Insemination in the Treatment of Unexplained Infertility

Chung CC, Fleming R, Jamieson ME, et al (Royal Infirmary, Glasgow, Scotland)
Hum Reprod 10:3139–3141, 1995   15–9

Background.—In patients with unexplained infertility, ovulation induction alone has not significantly improved pregnancy rates. The results obtained with intrauterine insemination (IUI) have been contradictory. Therefore, cycle fecundity in patients with unexplained infertility was compared in those managed with ovulation induction combined with either timed intercourse (TI) or IUI in a prospective, randomized study.

Methods.—One hundred women in couples with unexplained infertility received ovulation induction and were randomly assigned to either IUI or TI for up to 3 cycles. The ovulation induction protocol for all patients involved continuous gonadotropin-releasing hormone analogue to sup-

TABLE 3.—The Outcome of Pregnancies in the 2 Treatment Groups

	TI (*n* = 50)	IUI (*n* = 50)
Cycles with hCG (*n*)	130	110
Conception cycles (*n*)	10	24*
Pregnancies per cycle (%)	7.7	21.8*
Patients pregnant (*n*)	9	21*
Pregnancies per patient (%)	18	42*
Miscarriage in first trimester (*n*)	1	3
Ectopic (*n*)	0	1
Singleton (*n*)	8	17
Twin (*n*)	1	2
Higher order (*n*)	0	1
Total delivered (*n*)	9	20

Note: The 2 treatment groups were treated with ovulation induction with timed intercourse *(TI)* or intrauterine insemination *(IUI).*
*Significantly different from corresponding TI value (*P* < 0.05).
Abbreviation: hCG, human chorionic gonadotropin.
(Courtesy of Chung CC, Fleming R, Jamieson ME, et al: Randomized comparison of ovulation induction with and without intrauterine insemination in the treatment of unexplained infertility. *Hum Reprod* 10:3139–3141, 1995, by permission of Oxford University Press.)

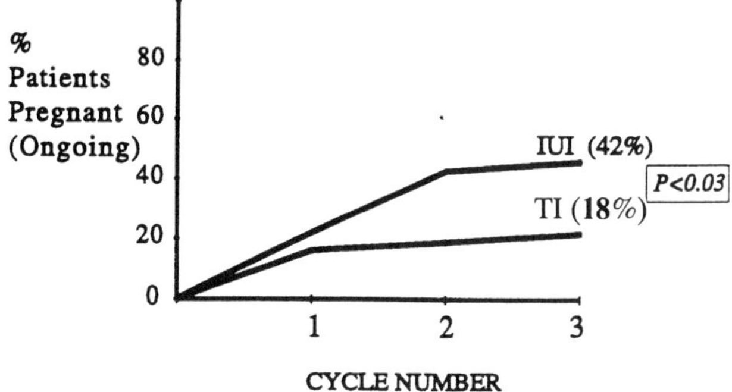

FIGURE 1.—Cumulative pregnancy profiles for patients in 2 treatment groups: intrauterine insemination (*IUI*) and timed intercourse (*TI*); there were initially 50 patients in each group. (Courtesy of Chung CC, Fleming R, Jamieson ME, et al: Randomized comparison of ovulation induction with and without intrauterine insemination in the treatment of unexplained infertility. *Hum Reprod* 10:3139–3141, 1995, by permission of Oxford University Press.)

press endogenous gonadotrophin secretion, exogenous follicle-stimulating hormone to stimulate follicular growth, and human chorionic gonadotrophin (hCG) given when there were fewer than 4 mature follicles and plasma estradiol levels were between 925 and 9,250 pmol/L. Timed intercourse was recommended between 24 and 48 hours after hCG administration. Intrauterine insemination was performed 36 to 48 hours after hCG administration, using spermatozoa prepared with the swim-up technique.

Results.—The 2 groups were comparable in age, infertility duration, follicular phase follicle-stimulating hormone levels, and semen analysis findings. The groups had similar responses to ovulation induction, with comparable duration, estradiol levels, and numbers of mature follicles. The IUI group had a significantly higher pregnancy rate per cycle and per patient than the TI group (Table 3). The groups had comparable pregnancy outcomes. An ongoing pregnancy was achieved by 42% of the patients in the IUI group and 20% of the patients in the TI group, a significant difference (Fig 1).

Conclusions.—Ovulation induction combined with IUI resulted in significantly higher fecundity than ovulation induction combined with TI, suggesting that ovulation induction with IUI is an effective therapeutic approach for couples with unexplained infertility.

▶ This study indicates that when couples with unexplained infertility are treated with controlled ovarian hyperstimulation, with use of a gonadotropin-releasing hormone agonist and follicle-stimulating hormone and IUI, with motile sperm separated by the swim-up technique, fecundability rates of about 20% per cycle can be achieved. This high conception rate was significantly better than the 8% pregnancy rate per cycle achieved with ovarian hyperstimulation and TI. Ovarian stimulation with a gonadotropin-releasing hormone agonist and follicle-stimulating hormone is much more expensive than use of clomiphene citrate and has not been shown to have higher pregnancy rates than with clomiphene citrate in any randomized clinical trial. Therefore, initial therapy of unexplained infertility should be 100 mg of clomiphene citrate daily beginning on cycle day 2, followed by IUI motile sperm separated by swim-up or Percoll gradient.

D.R. Mishell, Jr., M.D.

Minimal Stimulation Achieves Pregnancy Rates Comparable to Human Menopausal Gonadotropins in the Treatment of Infertility

Lu PY, Lee SH, Chen ALJ, et al (Mayo Clinic and Found, Rochester, Minn)
Fertil Steril 65:583–587, 1996
15–10

Background.—The efficacy of controlled ovarian hyperstimulation in the treatment of nonovulatory infertility has been established. Clomiphene citrate (CC) is typically the first agent used for ovarian stimulation because it is fairly inexpensive and easy to administer. Women who fail to become ovulatory on this regimen generally progress to more aggressive ovarian stimulation with human menopausal gonadotropin (hMG). A new "minimal stimulation" protocol for controlled ovarian hyperstimulation, consisting of combined CC and hMG treatment, has been developed. This approach helps curtail costs by decreasing the total amount of hMG needed in an ovarian stimulation cycle, without compromising treatment efficacy. Preliminary experience with minimal stimulation in a patient population not undergoing in vitro fertilization was reviewed.

Patients and Methods.—During a 3-year period, patients scheduled for controlled ovarian hyperstimulation in conjunction with timed intercourse or intrauterine insemination were offered the choice of minimal stimulation or conventional hMG. Most women had failed to respond to previous CC treatment and were ready to progress to more aggressive therapy. Patients selecting the minimal stimulation protocol received 100 mg of CC per day orally for 5 days (cycle days 3 through 7), after which a single injection of 150 IU of hMG was given on cycle day 9. Transvaginal ultrasound was done on cycle day 12 to evaluate follicle growth. Delivery of 10,000 IU of IM human chorionic gonadotropin was timed to occur with the appearance of a lead mean follicle diameter of 20 mm.

Women choosing the hMG protocol received daily doses ranging from 75 to 600 units, with dosage adjustments and timing of human chorionic gonadotropin administration based on transvaginal ultrasound or serum E_2 findings or both.

Patients undergoing minimal stimulation therapy who responded with fewer than 2 dominant follicles (less than 20 mm in diameter), who had a thin endometrium, or who had not become pregnant after 3 or 4 cycles were switched to the hMG protocol.

Results.—Two hundred thirty-two women completed 549 ovarian stimulation cycles and were evaluated. One hundred six cycles of minimal stimulation were completed by 61 women, and 443 cycles of hMG were completed by 183 patients. Although treatment assignments were not

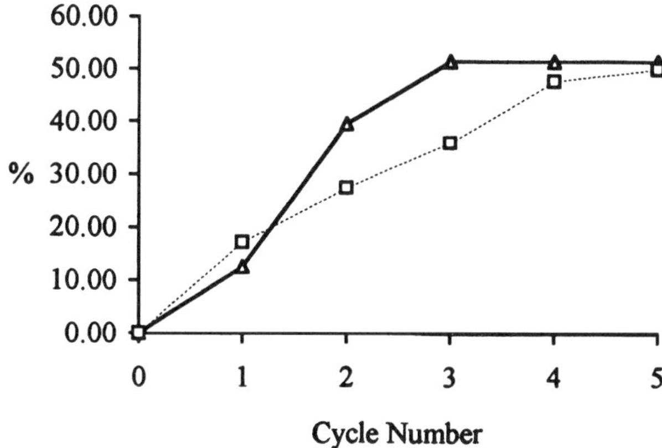

FIGURE 1.—Cumulative pregnancy rates of minimal stimulation and human menopausal gonado-tropins treatment groups expressed as percentages. Pregnancy rates are based on the cycles of women who initially started each treatment. Data do not include the subsequent treatment cycles after switching from 1 protocol to the other. *Triangles*, no significant difference between treatments; *squares*, human meno-pausal gonadotropin. (Courtesy of Lu PY, Lee SH, Chen ALJ, et al: Minimal stimulation achieves pregnancy rates comparable to human menopausal gonadotropins in the treatment of infertility *Fertil Steril* 65:583–587, 1996. Reproduced with permission of the publisher, the American Society for Reproductive Medicine [formerly The American Fertility Society].)

randomized, multivariate analysis did not identify any significant differences between treatment groups. The mean number of days to human chorionic gonadotropin was 10.2 for the minimal stimulation group and 8.6 for the hMG group. The cumulative pregnancy rates were not significantly different between groups over 5 cycles (Fig 1). A 33% miscarriage rate was noted for women in the hMG group, a finding consistent with previous studies. The 4.6% miscarriage rate in women receiving combined treatment was less than rates reported for CC or hMG, however.

Nine women completing a total of 20 minimal stimulation cycles failed to conceive and were switched to the hMG protocol. A cumulative total of 13 additional hMG cycles were performed in this subgroup, with 3 clinical pregnancies resulting after the first hMG cycle. This finding indicates that hMG may still be effective in women who fail to respond to minimal stimulation.

The total number of hMG ampules required for treatment was significantly different between groups, with 2.0 ampules needed for minimal stimulation vs. 16.8 for hMG. The mean medication cost for minimal stimulation was $257, compared with $1,215 for hMG.

Conclusions.—In this patient population, minimal stimulation proved to be as effective as hMG therapy for treatment of infertility. The clinical pregnancy rates were comparable between treatment groups, but medication costs were considerably lower with minimal stimulation. Minimal stimulation therefore should be considered in nonovulatory patients before progression to more aggressive hMG therapy.

▶ Currently, if an infertile couple does not have evidence of tubal blockage in the female partner or severe abnormalities of the semen analysis in the male partner, the most effective treatment is controlled ovarian hyperstimulation of the female partner followed by periovulatory intrauterine insemination of motile sperm separated by swim-up or Percoll gradient. Because no randomized trials have compared pregnancy rates when controlled ovarian hyperstimulation is performed with CC with those when hMG is used, and because both agents significantly improve fecundability about threefold, most clinicians initiate controlled ovarian hyperstimulation with CC. Clomiphene citrate is less expensive and requires less monitoring than hMG. If conception does not occur after 4 cycles of controlled ovarian hyperstimulation, with CC and intrauterine insemination, controlled ovarian hyperstimulation with hMG for a few additional cycles is then usually performed. Human menopausal gonadotropin is expensive and requires frequent monitoring to reduce the incidence of multiple gestations and ovarian hyperstimulation.

This study suggests that if pregnancy does not occur with the use of CC and intrauterine insemination alone, it may be preferable and just as effective to try a few cycles of CC followed by a single injection of hMG. The latter regimen is safer and less expensive and has a lower rate of spontaneous abortion than when hMG is given without previous treatment with CC.

D.R. Mishell, Jr., M.D.

The Efficacy of Immunotherapy in Patients Who Underwent Superovulation With Intrauterine Insemination

Kim CH, Cho YK, Mok JE (Univ of Ulsan, Seoul, Korea)
Fertil Steril 65:133–138, 1996   15–11

Background.—Of the many factors that have an impact on implantation, embryo-associated immunosuppressor factor and placenta protein 14 have been shown to modulate the immune response before implantation. They may encourage implantation by reducing the maternal immune response to the fetal allograft. Other studies have documented decreased immune responsiveness in pregnancy. It was therefore hypothesized that immunotherapy with corticosteroids can enhance the effects of superovulation with in utero implantation (IUI) in infertile patients. The hypothesis was tested in patients with ovulatory or unexplained infertility.

Methods.—During a 10-month period, 91 patients with ovulatory infertility (but without polycystic ovary syndrome or hyperandrogenism) and 78 patients with unexplained infertility who were undergoing superovulation with IUI were randomly assigned to receive or not receive corticosteroid treatment. Superovulation was induced with gonadotropin-releasing hormone agonist, with human menopausal gonadotropin and/or human follicle-stimulating hormone started on day 3 and human chorionic gonadotropin used to induce follicular maturation. Within 36–40 hours after human chorionic gonadotropin was given, the IUI procedure was performed. In the corticosteroid groups, prednisolone was begun on day 2 of the menstrual cycle at a daily oral dose of 10 mg until the day before

IUI, then increased to 60 mg for 4 days after IUI (Fig 1). On the day superovulation was begun, blood was drawn and analyzed for detection of antinuclear antibody, lupus anticoagulant, anticardiolipin antibody, anti–double-stranded DNA antibody, and antiribonucleoprotein antibody.

Results.—In the corticosteroid group, 45 patients with ovulatory infertility underwent 72 cycles of superovulation with IUI, and 38 patients with unexplained infertility underwent 75 cycles. In the control group, 46 patients with ovulatory infertility underwent 66 IUI cycles, and 40 patients with unexplained infertility underwent 75 cycles. The patients with unexplained infertility had a significantly higher prevalence of autoantibodies than did the patients with ovulatory infertility (20.5% vs. 3.3%). Among patients with ovulatory infertility, there was a higher, though not statistically significantly higher, pregnancy rate per cycle in the corticosteroid group than in the control group (38.9% vs. 33.3%). Among patients with unexplained infertility, the pregnancy rate per cycle was significantly higher in the corticosteroid group than in the control group (45.3% vs. 29.3%) (Table 3). No significant differences were found among the groups in spontaneous abortion or multiple pregnancy rates.

Conclusions.—Because there is a higher prevalence of antibodies in patients with unexplained infertility, immune function abnormalities may play a role in the infertility in these patients. Corticosteroids, which modulate abnormal immune function, could improve the pregnancy rate in these patients who undergo superovulation with IUI.

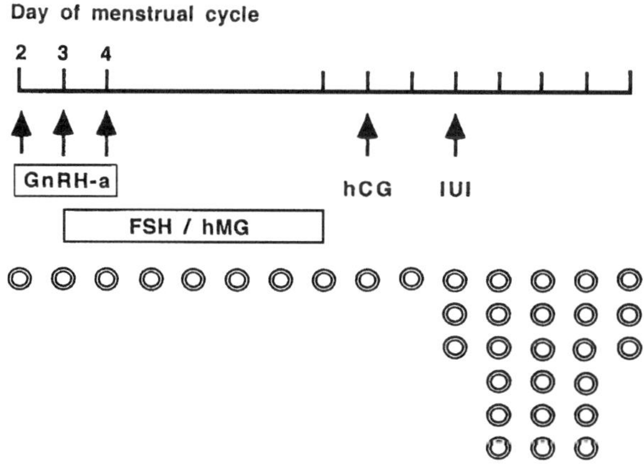

FIGURE 1.—Schematic representation of the immunotherapy protocol in superovulation with intrauterine insemination (*IUI*) cycle. Ultrashort protocol of gonadotropin-releasing hormone agonist (*GnRH-a*) was used for superovulation. *Abbreviations: hCG*, human chorionic gonadotropin; *FSH/hMG*, follicle-stimulating hormone/human menopausal gonadotropin. (Courtesy of Kim CH, Cho YK, Mok JE: The efficacy of immunotherapy in patients who underwent superovulation with intrauterine insemination. *Fertil Steril* 65:133–138, 1996. Reproduced with permission of the publisher, the American Society for Reproductive Medicine [formerly The American Fertility Society].)

TABLE 3.—Comparison of Pregnancy Outcome Between Treatment and Control Groups

	Ovulatory infertility		Unexplained infertility	
	Treatment	Control	Treatment	Control
No. of patients	45	46	38	40
No. of cycles	72	66	75	75
No. of clinical pregnancies*	28 (38.9)	22 (33.3)	34 (45.3)†	22 (29.3)
Abortion‡	4 (14.3)	3 (13.6)	6 (17.6)	3 (13.6)
Ectopic‡	0	1 (4.5)	0	0
Ongoing†	24 (85.7)	18 (81.8)	28 (82.4)	19 (86.4)
Multiple pregnancies‡	5 (17.9)	3 (13.6)	6 (17.6)	2 (9.1)
Twin	4	2	5	2
Triplet	1	0	1	0

*Values in parentheses are percentages per cycle.
†$P < 0.05$ vs. control in unexplained infertility group.
‡Values in parentheses are percentages per clinical pregnancy.
(Courtesy of Kim CH, Cho YK, Mok JE: The efficacy of immunotherapy in patients who underwent superovulation with intrauterine insemination. *Fertil Steril* 65:133–138, 1996. Reproduced with permission of the publisher, the American Society for Reproductive Medicine [formerly The American Fertility Society].)

▶ The cycle fecundability rate in this report in both the groups treated with corticosteroids and not receiving corticosteroid treatment are much higher than the rates reported by other clinics for both ovulatory and unexplained infertility. Therefore, the results of this study need to be confirmed in other clinics. If confirmed, the results would indicate that the addition of corticosteroid therapy to ovarian hyperstimulation and IUI would increase the chances of pregnancy when treating couples with unexplained infertility. However, confirmatory studies are essential before adding corticosteroids to regimens for women treated with ovulation-inducing agents and IUI.

D.R. Mishell, Jr., M.D.

A New System for Fallopian Tube Sperm Perfusion Leads to Pregnancy Rates Twice as High as Standard Intrauterine Insemination

Fanchin R, Hazout A, Olivennes F, et al (Hôpital Antoine Béclère, Clamart, France)
Fertil Steril 64:505–510, 1995

15–12

Background.—To overcome the limitations of standard intrauterine insemination (IUI), several investigators have focused on new IUI methods that can ensure the presence of higher sperm densities in the fallopian tubes at the time of ovulation. One device specifically adapted for fallopian tube sperm perfusion—the Fallopian Sperm Transfer (FAST) System—was tested.

Methods.—Seventy-four infertile women, aged 20 to 38 years, were enrolled in a prospective, randomized comparison of fallopian tube sperm perfusion using the FAST System and standard IUI. The patients underwent 100 cycles of controlled ovarian hyperstimulation between December 1993 and May 1994. Exclusion criteria were obstructed or severely damaged fallopian tubes, E_2 levels per mature follicle of less than 250 pg/mL on the day of human chorionic gonadotropin administration, spontaneous luteinizing hormone surge, and marked sperm abnormalities. Three types of ovarian stimulation protocols were used to achieve controlled ovarian hyperstimulation: clomiphene citrate and human menopausal gonadotropin (hMG) in 35 patients, hMG alone in 35, and gonadotropin-releasing hormone agonist, follicle-stimulating hormone, and hMG in 30. Thirty-six hours after hCG was administered, 50 patients were assigned to IUI (group A) and 50 to fallopian tube sperm perfusion (group B). The FAST System ensures a good cervical seal and allows a pressurized injection of 4 mL of sperm suspension.

Findings.—Ten clinical pregnancies occurred in group A (20% per cycle). Seven of these pregnancies were ongoing. Twenty clinical pregnancies occurred in group B (40% per cycle). Seventeen (34%) were ongoing. The group B rate was significantly higher than the group A rate. The 2 groups were comparable in the prevalence of twin and 3 or more sac pregnancies. None of the patients experienced moderate or severe ovarian hyperstimulation syndrome.

Conclusions.—The pregnancy rates associated with fallopian tube sperm perfusion are significantly better than those obtained with standard IUI. The FAST System is not invasive or traumatic. None of the patients had cervical bleeding, vasovagal episodes, or pelvic infections after this new procedure.

A Randomized Prospective Comparison Between Intrauterine Insemination and Fallopian Sperm Perfusion for the Treatment of Infertility
Karande VC, Levrant S, Rao R, et al (Ctr for Human Reproduction, Chicago; Found for Reproductive Medicine, Chicago)
Fertil Steril 64:638–640, 1995   15–13

Introduction.—Previous reports suggested that fallopian tube sperm perfusion resulted in higher pregnancy rates than did intrauterine inseminations, now considered standard treatment in infertility therapy. In intrauterine inseminations, pretreated semen is concentrated in a small volume and deposited into the uterine cavity by catheter. With fallopian tube sperm perfusion, the sperm is diluted in a larger volume of media. To determine whether fallopian tube sperm perfusion resulted in higher pregnancy rates than did intrauterine inseminations, a prospective, randomized study was conducted.

Methods.—Consecutive infertile women had ovulation induction with clomiphene citrate or gonadotropins. On 2 consecutive days after human chorionic gonadotropin administration, 120 women received intrauterine inseminations and 120 women had fallopian tube sperm perfusion. Semen for both procedures had 3 routine sperm washes. During fallopian tube sperm perfusion, the sperm was suspended in 4 mL of media, whereas for the intrauterine insemination the sperm volume was less than 0.5 mL. The fallopian tube sperm perfusion was carried out over 4 minutes, whereas the intrauterine insemination was conducted by the rapid plunger action of a syringe.

Results.—Consecutive ovarian stimulation cycles were performed in 240 women. In the intrauterine insemination group, 44 had received clomiphene citrate and 76 had received gonadotropin. In the fallopian tube sperm perfusion group, 44 had received clomiphene citrate and 76 had received gonadotropin. The pregnancy rate for both groups was 10.8%. When compared for ovulation induction methods, the pregnancy rates were also similar. Women receiving clomiphene citrate had a pregnancy rate of 6.8% for the intrauterine insemination group and 9.1% for the fallopian tube sperm perfusion group. Gonadotropins resulted in a pregnancy rate of 13.2% for the intrauterine insemination group and 11.8% for the fallopian tube sperm perfusion group.

Conclusion.—The fallopian tube sperm perfusion has no advantage over intrauterine insemination. Fallopian tube sperm perfusion is also more time consuming and costly because of the increased media use and should not replace intrauterine insemination.

▶ The techniques of controlled ovarian hyperstimulation (COH) and intrauterine insemination (IUI) are being used very frequently for the treatment of unexplained infertility as well as in couples with a mild degree of sperm abnormalities and tubal damage. Most reports indicate that these techniques result in cycle fecundability rates of 10% to 15%. The results of these studies (Abstracts 15–12 and 15–13) indicate that insemination of a greater volume of sperm suspension in order to place a portion of the sperm directly into the oviduct does not result in increased pregnancy rates unless some technique is used to create a cervical seal so that most of the inseminated fluid is directed toward the oviduct. In the study by Fanchin et al., gonadotropins were used to stimulate the ovaries, with a high incidence of multiple pregnancy. Other studies need to be undertaken using the system that creates a cervical seal in which clomiphene is used to stimulate the ovaries in order to determine whether cycle fecundability can be increased with this simple method of hyperstimulation combined with IUI. The cervical seal technique is promising, and if found by others to be more effective than routine IUI, it deserves increased use for the treatment of the infertile couple.

D.R. Mishell, Jr., M.D.

Clomiphene Citrate With Intrauterine Insemination: Is It Effective Therapy in Women Above the Age of 35 Years?

Agarwal SK, Buyalos RP (Univ of California, Los Angeles)
Fertil Steril 65:759–763, 1996

15–14

Background.—Clomiphene citrate (CC) with intrauterine insemination (IUI) is being used more often for couples with infertility of various causes. Because reproductive capacity is profoundly reduced in women older than 35 years, the effects of female age on CC with IUI were assessed. Specifically, the age at which clinical pregnancy rates (PRs) with this treatment decrease most rapidly was determined, and the efficacy of this treatment was compared between patients with ovulatory and anovulatory infertility.

Methods and Findings.—Two hundred ninety women (age range, 22–48 years) were included in the study. Data were collected on a total of 664 CC with IUI cycles. Compared with women aged 35 and younger, women older than 35 had markedly reduced cumulative and clinical PRs. These parameters did not differ significantly in groups with ovulatory and anovulatory infertility. Most pregnancies occurred within the first 4 treatment cycles, regardless of age or infertility diagnosis (Fig 1).

Conclusions.—Clomiphene citrate with IUI treatment yields markedly reduced PRs in women older than 35 years. Thus, clinicians should consider using other treatments that may initially seem more expensive but are ultimately more effective. The most cost-effective treatment for infertile women older than 35 years requires further study.

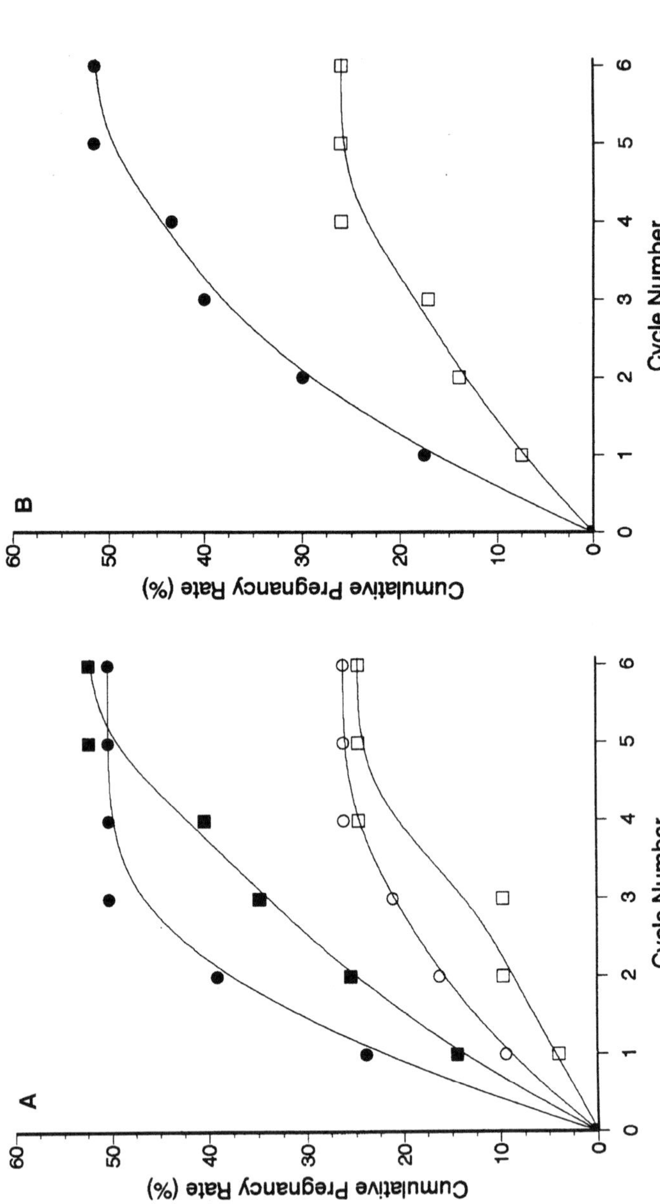

FIGURE 1.—Cumulative PRs by Kaplan Meier life-table analysis for 290 infertile couples undergoing CC with IUI therapy stratified by the age of the female partner. A *solid circles*, ≤30 years; *solid squares*, 31–35 years; *open circles*, 36–40 years; *open squares*, ≥41 years. B, *solid circles*, ≤35 years; *open squares*, ≥36 years. *Abbreviations: PR*, pregnancy rate; *CC*, clomiphene citrate; *IUI*, intrauterine insemination. (Courtesy of Agarwal SK, Buyalos RP: Clomiphene citrate with intrauterine insemination: Is it effective therapy in women above the age of 35 years? *Fertil Steril* 65:759–763, 1996. Reproduced with permission of the publisher, the American Society for Reproductive Medicine [formerly the American Fertility Society].)

Ovulation Induction Combined With Intrauterine Insemination in Women 40 Years of Age and Older: Is It Worthwhile?

Corsan G, Trias A, Trout S, et al (UMDNJ-Robert Wood Johnson Med School, New Brunswick, NJ; Centro Medico Docente La Trinidad, Venezuela)
Hum Reprod 11:1109–1112, 1996
15–15

Objective.—To identify patients who might benefit from intrauterine insemination, data from a trial of ovulation induction with intrauterine insemination in subfertile women 40 years and older were reviewed.

Background.—Fertility in women decreases with age. Many women in Western countries delay reproduction until they are in their 30s and 40s. There is increasing interest in fertility treatment of these women. Many women do not have access to in vitro fertilization/embryo transfer or gamete intrafallopian transfer because of financial reasons. Also, some women may not be interested in these methods. Ovulation induction with intrauterine insemination may be an alternative treatment or a preliminary treatment to the 2 methods mentioned above. There is little information on this method in women aged 40 years or older.

Methods.—Patients older than 40 years of age undergoing ovulation induction with intrauterine insemination were identified. Couples were infertile for at least 1 year; diagnoses included unexplained infertility, American Fertility Society stage I–II endometriosis, male factor infertility, cervical factor infertility, and ovulatory dysfunction. Ovulation induction protocols involved sequential clomiphene citrate, human menopausal gonadotropin (hMG), human chorionic gonadotropin or daily hMG followed by human chorionic gonadotropin, or follicle-stimulating hormone at an individualized dose. Sperm preparations were washed and intrauterine insemination was performed 36 hours after ovulation induction.

Results.—A total of 168 women between 40 and 47 years of age underwent 469 cycles of ovulation induction with intrauterine insemination. A second group of 180 women younger than 40 years underwent 210 cycles of ovulation induction with intrauterine insemination. In the first group, 34 pregnancies occurred. The pregnancy loss rate was 34.4%. The ongoing/delivered pregnancy rate was 4.47% per initiated cycle and 5.22% per completed cycle. The multiple gestation rate was 9.38% (Table 1). In the second group, there were 35 pregnancies and 1 ectopic gestation. The pregnancy loss rate was 17.14%. The ongoing/delivered pregnancy rate was 13.8% per initiated cycle and 14.9% per completed cycle. The multiple gestation rate was 17.14% (Table 1). In women older than age 42 years, there were no deliveries from the 136 cycles performed.

Conclusions.—These findings confirm the low probability of a live birth resulting from ovulation induction with intrauterine insemination in women 40 or older. No ongoing viable pregnancies occurred in women older than 42 years of age. The live birth rate was 9.63% per initiated cycle in women 40 years of age, 5.2% per initiated cycle in women 41 years of age, and 2.38% per initiated cycle in women 42 years of age. It is unlikely

TABLE 1.—Outcome of Ovulation Induction With Intrauterine Insemination Treatment in Women Aged ≥ 40 Years (Group A) and < 40 Years (Group B)

	Group A	Group B	P value
Clinical pregnancy rate per completed cycle (%)	6.96	17.95	0.0005
Cancellation rate (%)	14.30	7.14	0.01
Abortion rate (%)	34.40	17.14	NS
Multiple gestation rate (%)	9.38	17.14	NS

Abbreviation: NS, not significant

(Courtesy of Corsan G, Trias A, Trout S, et al: Ovulation induction combined with intrauterine insemination in women 40 years of age and older: Is it worthwhile? *Hum Reprod* 11:1109–1112, 1996, by permission of Oxford University Press.)

that this method of assisted reproduction will result in a viable birth in women 43 years or older. Therefore, such women should consider adoption or egg donation. In women between 40 and 42 years of age, it may be reasonable to attempt a short trial of ovulation induction with intrauterine insemination; this could be attempted before in vitro fertilization/embryo transfer or gamete intrafallopian transfer.

▶ After a woman reaches age 31 her fecundability rate steadily decreases as she becomes older. Furthermore, after age 35 the incidence of spontaneous abortion steadily increases with increasing maternal age. In economically advanced societies many women are delaying the initiation of childbearing until the fourth decade of life, thereby increasing their chance of being infertile. The initial treatment for the infertile couple, when the woman ovulates regularly and has at least 1 patent oviduct and the man has an adequate number of motile sperm, is superovulation followed by timed intrauterine insemination. These techniques are much less costly and less complicated than those of assisted reproductive technology. The results of these 2 studies indicate that whether superovulation is performed, fecundability rates decrease markedly when the woman becomes older than age 35 when clomiphene is used, or age 40 when hMG is used. It is interesting that in both studies the pregnancy rate per cycle in women older than 40 years was approximately 5% whether they were treated with clomiphene citrate or hMG. The pregnancy rate in women younger than 35 or 40 in the 2 studies was approximately 15%, similar to the pregnancy rates reported in other studies in which superovulation and intrauterine insemination has been used to treat couples with unexplained infertility. This information should be used to counsel couples with no known cause of infertility about their likelihood of becoming pregnant with superovulation and intrauterine insemination at different ages.

D.R. Mishell, Jr., M.D.

The Age-related Decline in Female Fecundity: A Quantitative Controlled Study of Implanting Capacity and Survival of Individual Embryos After In Vitro Fertilization

Hull MGR, Fleming CF, Hughes AO, et al (Univ of Bristol, England)
Fertil Steril 65:783–790, 1996

15–16

Objective.—In both sexes, fecundity (defined as the monthly chance of conception) decreases with advancing age. In women, the reason for the age-related reduction in fecundity is now thought to be a decrease in the embryo's ability to implant, which results from a decrease in oocyte quality. The effects of the woman's age on the rate of embryo implantation were studied in infertile couples.

Methods.—The study was done at the University of Bristol IVF Service, British United Provident Association Hospital from 1990 to 1993 and included all couples undergoing their first cycle of in vitro fertilization (IVF) who reached the oocyte recovery phase. All of the women had a normal uterus and normal ovulatory menstrual cycles, and all men had favorable sperm function. The rates per embryo of implantation and birth were analyzed in terms of the woman's age, which was used as a relative indicator of natural fertility. A total of 572 couples were considered in 5-year age strata.

Results.—Women older than 40 years had only a slight decrease in the number of embryos per transfer. However, the rates of pregnancy and birth per transfer decreased significantly with increasing age, as did the implantation rate and the "live baby rate" per embryo transfer. These worsening outcomes were most apparent in women older than 40 years; the progressive increase in miscarriage rate had a major impact on the eventual birth rate. The reduction in implantation rates was greater for women aged 35–39 years who had less than 4 embryos implanted and for all women older than 40 years, including those with more embryos transferred.

Conclusions.—In couples treated for infertility, the embryo implantation and birth rates decrease significantly with the woman's advancing age. Older women have impaired ovarian responsiveness to stimulation, suggesting a premature reduction in ovarian capacity of follicle numbers, which is independently related to impaired oocyte quality. The implantation rate per embryo decreases gradually after age 30. After age 40, the chances of successful birth is reduced by more than two thirds because of the high miscarriage rate.

▶ The results of this study indicate that the decrease in fecundity that occurs in women after age 30 is due in part to the fact that the implanting ability of each embryo decreases gradually after this age. After age 40, the implanting ability of the embryo as well as the rate of spontaneous abortion both increase markedly. This information should be used to help counsel all women who wish to have children that they should not delay initial attempts to become pregnant until they are older than age 35 because the rates of infertility will increase markedly after this age.

D.R. Mishell, Jr., M.D.

Gamete Intra-Fallopian Transfer or In-Vitro Fertilization After Failed Ovarian Stimulation and Intrauterine Insemination in Unexplained Infertility?

Ranieri M, Beckett VA, Marchant S, et al (Univ College, London)
Hum Reprod 10:2023–2026, 1995

15–17

Background.—Deciding on treatment for patients with unexplained infertility who do not conceive with ovarian stimulation and intrauterine insemination (IUI) is difficult. Gamete intrafallopian transfer (GIFT) and in vitro fertilization (IVF)/embryo transfer were compared prospectively in patients with unexplained infertility and at least 3 failed cycles of ovarian stimulation and IUI.

Methods and Findings.—Sixty-nine couples with primary unexplained infertility and at least 3 previous failed cycles of gonadotrophin ovarian stimulation and IUI were assigned randomly to GIFT or IVF/embryo transfer. Of the 34 patients undergoing IVF, 25 received 3 embryos, 7 received 2, and 2 received 1. All 35 patients undergoing GIFT had 3 oocytes transferred. The groups had comparable fertilization rates. Significantly more embryos implanted per embryo transfer in the IVF group than per oocyte transferred in the GIFT group. However, the difference in clinical pregnancy rate was nonsignificant. The patients undergoing IVF had a significantly greater twin pregnancy rate than did those undergoing GIFT. Pregnancy outcomes in the 2 groups were comparable. Although the

TABLE 1.—Results of Gamete Intrafallopian Transfer (GIFT) and In Vitro Fertilization (IVF) in Couples With Unexplained Infertility at Their First Attempt After Previous Failure of Ovarian Stimulation and Intrauterine Insemination

	Gift (n = 35)		*IVF (n = 34)*		
	Number	*Mean/rate*	*Number*	*Mean/rate*	*P value**
Age (years)		32.8 (±3.2)		31.9 (±3.7)	0.3
Retrieved oocytes	275	7.8 (±2.8)	231	6.8 (±2.7)	0.1
Transferred oocytes (GIFT) or embryos (IVF)	105	3.0 (±0.1)	91	2.7 (±0.1)	0.001
Inseminated oocytes	170	4.8 (±2.7)	231	6.8 (±2.7)	0.005
Oocytes fertilized in vitro (%)	96	57	135	58	0.8
Pregnancies (%)	12	34	17	50	0.28
Implanted embryos (%)	14	13	26	29	0.01
Twin pregnancies (%)	2	17	9	53	0.005
Delivered (%)	9	75	16	94	0.1

*$*P < 0.05$ was considered statistically significant.
(Courtesy of Ranieri M, Beckett VA, Marchant S, et al: Gamete intra-fallopian transfer or in-vitro fertilization after failed ovarian stimulation and intrauterine insemination in unexplained infertility? *Hum Reprod* 10:2023–2026, 1995. By permission of Oxford University Press.)

IVF and GIFT pregnancy delivery rates were 94% and 75%, respectively, the difference was nonsignificant (Table 1).

Conclusions.—In these couples with unexplained infertility and failed ovarian stimulation and IUI, the clinical pregnancy rate after GIFT was 34% and after IVF/embryo transfer it was 50%. Thus, these procedures still offer hope to such patients.

▶ Evidence is accumulating that the optimal initial treatment for couples with unexplained infertility (those women with patent oviducts who ovulate and whose male partner has an adequate number of motile sperm) is controlled ovarian hyperstimulation (COH) and IUI. Cycle fecundability rates with this treatment are generally reported to range between 10% and 20%. If the couple does not conceive with several cycles of this therapy, and they wish to undergo assisted reproduction, the results of this study indicate that satisfactory and comparable pregnancy rates are achieved with both GIFT and IVF. Because IVF is less invasive than GIFT, and the problem of infertility may be due to failure of fertilization, IVF should be the assisted reproductive technique that is recommended to couples with unexplained infertility who fail to conceive with several cycles of COH and IUI.

D.R. Mishell, Jr., M.D.

Results of IVF in Patients With Endometriosis: The Severity of the Disease Does Not Affect Outcome, or the Incidence of Miscarriage
Geber S, Paraschos T, Atkinson G, et al (Royal Postgraduate Med School, London)
Hum Reprod 10:1507–1511, 1995   15–18

Purpose.—Previous reports have suggested that the outcomes of in vitro fertilization (IVF) for patients with endometriosis are influenced by the stage of endometriosis. Patients with more severe disease are believed to have a higher IVF failure rate, and women treated for endometriosis are believed to have a higher miscarriage rate. The results of IVF in patients with endometriosis were assessed.

Methods.—One hundred forty patients with endometriosis who underwent IVF were studied. None received any treatment during or after diagnostic laparoscopy, which was performed 2 to 4 years before IVF was attempted. The patients underwent a total of 182 cycles of IVF with gonadotropin-releasing hormone analogues. Patients with endometriosis only and those with endometriosis with associated severe tubal disease were considered separately. The results of the patients with endometriosis only were compared with those of 3 other groups of patients: 44 couples with male-factor infertility only, 161 couples with unexplained infertility, and 3 couples with tubal-factor infertility only.

Results.—No differences were found between groups in the number of oocytes retrieved. The fertilization rate was significantly lower only for the couples with male-factor infertility; all other groups had comparable fertilization rates. The groups were comparable in the number of transferred embryos and implantation rates. The pregnancy rates per transfer were 39% in couples with male-factor infertility, 48% in those with unexplained infertility, 45% in those with tubal-factor infertility, and 40% in those with endometriosis only.

Within the endometriosis group, there were 100 cycles in patients with revised American Fertility Society stage I–II endometriosis and 29 in those with revised American Fertility Society stage III–IV endometriosis. Although the stage III–IV patients had a greater fertilization rate, number of embryos, and transfer rate per cycle, the difference was not significant. The implantation rate and overall pregnancy rate per transfer were also non-significantly higher in the stage III–IV group.

Conclusions.—The largest study to date of IVF in patients with endometriosis suggests that the results are similar to those of other patients. The presence or degree of endometriosis does not appear to affect pregnancy outcomes, including the pregnancy rate or the incidence of spontaneous abortion. In contrast to previous reports, this study found no cases of miscarriage in patients with endometriosis.

▶ This very large study of couples undergoing IVF indicates that neither the presence of endometriosis nor the severity of endometriosis affects the pregnancy rate after IVF treatment when compared with the rate among couples with tubal disease or unexplained infertility. These findings suggest that the presence of endometriosis does not cause problems of fertilization or implantation or increase the rate of abortion. Endometriosis is probably a result of infertility and repeated episodes of retrograde menstruation but does not cause infertility unless it produces tubal adhesions or endometriomas that interfere with ovum pickup.

D.R. Mishell, Jr., M.D.

Pregnancies and Births Resulting From In Vitro Fertilization: French National Registry, Analysis of Data 1986 to 1990
FIVNAT (French In Vitro National) (Universitaire de Bicêtre, France)
Fertil Steril 64:746–756, 1995   15–19

Background.—Any assessment of the cost-benefit ratio of in vitro fertilization (IVF) must include the evaluation criteria of pregnancy outcome and infant characteristics. In 1986, a French collaborative survey began collecting individual data about patients undergoing assisted reproductive technology techniques. These data were used to examine the outcomes of pregnancy and birth after IVF.

Methods.—The analysis included prospective registry data on each recovery attempt performed at most French IVF centers since 1986. Up to 1990, the registry received more than 76,000 IVF cycle forms and about 8,000 obstetric and pediatric forms regarding all assisted reproductive technology techniques. This report included IVF pregnancies and resulting newborns only, excluding thawed embryo transfers. A total of 7,024 clinical pregnancies, 5,371 deliveries, and 6,879 newborns were analyzed (Table 1).

Results.—Miscarriage occurred in 18% of clinical pregnancies and ectopic pregnancy in 6%. The multiple delivery rate increased from 20% in 1986 to 29% in 1990. Nearly half of the infants were the result of multiple pregnancies; 34% were twins and 10% were triplets. Preeclampsia occurred in 6% of pregnancies and diabetes in 1%. The rate of induced labor increased 3% during the study. Ninety-two percent of singleton pregnancies had a cephalic presentation. Although 57% of deliveries were vaginal, 13% required forceps. One third of cesarean sections were performed before labor. Eighty-eight percent of multiple pregnancies were delivered by cesarean section, mainly for prophylactic reasons. Just 39% of births were uncomplicated vaginal deliveries; the rate was lower for multiple pregnancies.

Twenty-nine percent of the infants were born prematurely, even more for multiple pregnancies. Multifetal pregnancies were unassociated with variation in the sex ratio. The overall mean Apgar score was 9, with less than one third of the infants being underweight. Ninety-four percent of infants were in good health, with no complications or malformations, at birth. The perinatal mortality was 27% and was higher for multiple births.

The congenital malformation rate was 2.8% (1.2% major and 1.6% minor) with no change from 1986 to 1990. The malformation rate was 3.3% when interrupted pregnancies were included. The most common major malformations in live-born infants were cardiopathies. Twelve infants had chromosomal defects, including 7 with Down's syndrome. Down's syndrome accounted for 3.4% of malformations in live-born infants and 8.2% of malformations when interrupted pregnancies were included.

TABLE 1.—Outcomes of Clinical Pregnancies From 1986 to 1990

| | Clinical pregnancies | Miscarriages* | | Ectopic pregnancies*† | Voluntary abortions* | Therapeutic abortions* | Deliveries *‡ |
		Early, <12 weeks of amenorrhea	Late, > 12 weeks of amenorrhea <6th month				
1986	665	93 (14.0)	16 (2.4)	48 (7.2)	0	0	508 (76.4)
1987	1,455	233 (16.0)	51 (3.5)	92 (6.3)	0	5 (0.3)	1,074 (73.9)
1988	1,397	199 (14.2)	33 (2.4)	83 (5.9)	2 (0.1)	7 (0.5)	1,073 (76.9)
1989	1,617	250 (15.5)	39 (2.4)	82 (5.1)	1 (0.1)	7 (0.4)	1,238 (76.6)
1990	1,890	262 (13.9)	60 (3.2)	78 (4.1)	2 (0.1)	10 (0.5)	1,478 (78.2)
Total	7,024	1,037 (14.8)	199 (2.8)	383 (5.4)	5 (0.1)	29 (0.4)	5,371 (76.5)

Note: Clinical pregnancies are defined as the detection of a gestational sac by ultrasound or a very high level of human chorionic gonadotropin (greater than 1,000 mIU/mL [conversion factor to SI unit, 1]).

*Values are number of incidences with percentages in parentheses.

†In addition, 21 ectopic pregnancies associated with an intrauterine pregnancy (i.e., heterotopic pregnancies) are included among "Deliveries"; thus, the total percentage of both ectopic and heterotopic pregnancies was 5.8% of the clinical pregnancies and 7.5% of the deliveries.

‡Includes simple deliveries and heterotopic pregnancies (*n* = 21), or therapeutic abortion (*n* = 1), terminated with deliveries.

(Courtesy of FIVNAT [French In Vitro National]: Pregnancies and births resulting from in vitro fertilization: French National Registry, analysis of data 1986 to 1990. *Fertil Steril* 64:746–756, 1995. Reproduced with permission of the publisher, the American Society for Reproductive Medicine [formerly The American Fertility Society].)

Conclusions.—In the French experience, more than three fourths of clinical pregnancies induced by IVF resulted in a delivery. Rates of ectopic pregnancy, prematurity, stillbirth, and perinatal mortality all were higher with IVF than in the general population. However, for singleton IVF pregnancies, stillbirth and perinatal mortality rates were similar to those of the general population. Malformations appear to be no more common after IVF than after natural conception.

▶ It is estimated that, to date, more than 100,000 children have been born throughout the world as a result of IVF or other assisted reproductive techniques. The data reported from this large French study are in agreement with surveys of pregnancy outcome after assisted reproductive techniques obtained in other countries. The data regarding a similar prevalence of congenital malformations after assisted reproduction and natural conception are reassuring. However, the higher rates of spontaneous abortion, ectopic pregnancy, multiple gestation, preterm birth, and perinatal mortality with assisted reproduction remain problems caused by this expensive method of human procreation.

D.R. Mishell, Jr., M.D.

Cumulative Pregnancy Rate Following In-Vitro Fertilization: The Significance of Age and Infertility Aetiology
Dor J, Seidman DS, Ben-Shlomo I, et al (Tel Aviv Univ, Israel; Golda Med Centre, Petach Tikva, Israel)
Hum Reprod 11:425–428, 1996   15–20

Background.—In vitro fertilization (IVF) is now the standard treatment for infertile couples who have failed to conceive by all previous treatment modalities as well as for those with tubal obstruction. In a retrospective life-table analysis of 1 entire computerized database from 1984 through 1992, the effects of different variables on cumulative pregnancy rates (PRs) in IVF treatments were studied.

Methods.—Nine hundred fifty-one couples with infertility of various causes underwent 2,252 consecutive treatment cycles. The maximum number of treatments per couple was 10.

Findings.—Clinical PRs per cycle remained similar in the first 6 cycles, attaining a 56% cumulative PR. In the next 3 cycles, the PR dropped significantly from a mean of 9.3% to 2.4% per cycle. After 9 cycles, the cumulative PR was 63% (Fig 1). Women aged 40 years or older were significantly less likely to conceive with repeated cycles compared with women aged 35–39 years and women aged 34 years or younger (Fig 2). There were no cumulative PR differences among groups with tubal, anovulatory, or unexplained infertility.

Conclusions.—The cumulative PR after IVF treatments increases constantly in the first 6 cycles, then levels off. Women aged 40 years or older are also less likely to conceive than women aged 39 years and younger.

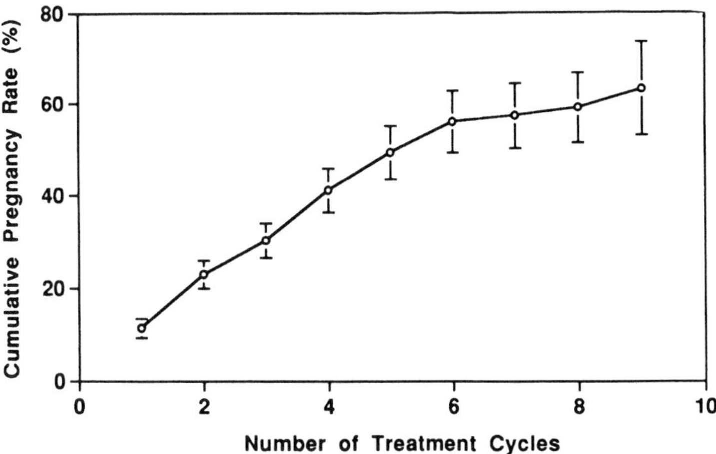

FIGURE 1.—Overall cumulative pregnancy rate in IVF treatment (with 95% confidence interval). (Courtesy of Dor J, Seidman DS, Ben-Shlomo I, et al: Cumulative pregnancy rate following in-vitro fertilization: The significance of age and infertility aetiology. *Hum Reprod* 11:425–428, 1996 by permission of Oxford University Press.)

▶ Women in Israel can have up to 8 IVF procedures performed with government financial support. Therefore, the data in this study are less likely to be influenced by cost considerations than would occur in the United States. The cumulative pregnancy rate after 6 cycles of IVF is probably greater today than that found in this study, which was initiated in 1984, because of

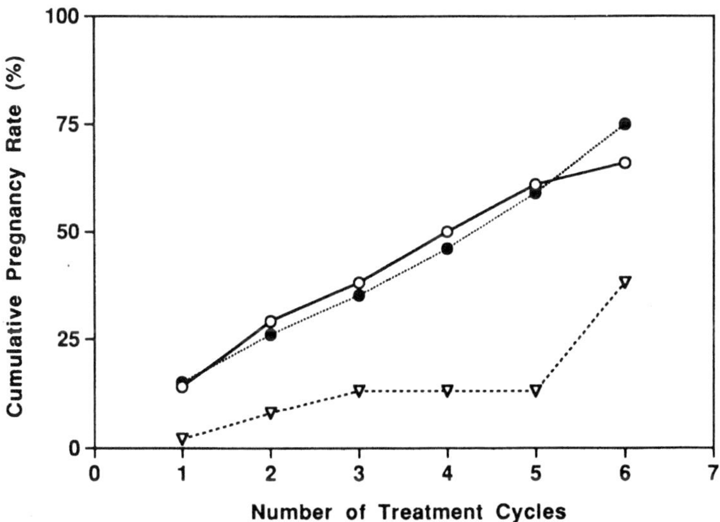

FIGURE 2.—Cumulative pregnancy rate in in vitro fertilization by age of the patients. *Open triangles,* ≥ 40 years; *closed circles,* ≤ 39 years; *open circles,* ≤ 34 years. (Courtesy of Dor J, Seidman DS, Ben-Shlomo I, et al: Cumulative pregnancy rate following in-vitro fertilization: The significance of age and infertility aetiology. *Hum Reprod* 11:425–428, 1996, by permission of Oxford University Press.)

advances in technology. Nevertheless, that pregnancy rates do not increase markedly after 6 cycles of treatment and that pregnancy rates are similar in the 35–39 year age group and those women younger than age 35 are interesting findings that are probably still valid.

D.R. Mishell, Jr., M.D.

Gamete Intrafallopian Transfer: Prospective Randomized Comparison Between Hysteroscopic and Laparoscopic Transfer Techniques

Seracchioli R, Fabbri R, Porcu E, et al (Univ of Bologna, Italy)
Fertil Steril 64:355–359, 1995   15–21

Background.—At 1 center, hysteroscopy is preferred as an alternative to the traditional gamete intrafallopian transfer (GIFT) by laparoscopy. The efficacies of hysteroscopy and laparoscopy were prospectively compared in a randomized study of patients undergoing GIFT.

Methods.—One hundred thirty-three couples with tubal patency documented at a previous diagnostic laparoscopy were enrolled. Fifty-seven were randomly assigned to hysteroscopic GIFT and 60 to laparoscopic GIFT. All women were younger than age 38 years. The duration of infertility was 3 years or longer. Laparoscopic GIFT was done with patients under general anesthesia 34 to 36 hours after human chorionic gonadotropin administration. Transvaginal ultrasound-guided retrievals were scheduled 34 to 36 hours after administration of human chorionic gonadotropin in hysteroscopic GIFT. In both techniques, 2 to 4 mature oocytes with 200,000 to 300,000 motile spermatozoa were transferred.

Findings.—In the hysteroscopic group, 547 oocytes were recovered and 205 mature oocytes transferred, compared with 522 recovered and 229 transferred in the laparoscopic group. No complications occurred during or just after either procedure. The mean duration of the procedures,

TABLE 3.—Pregnancy Outcome of Hysteroscopic Gamete Intrafallopian Transfer (GIFT) and Laparoscopic GIFT

	Group 1 Hysteroscopic GIFT (n = 57)	Group 2 Laparoscopic GIFT (n = 60)
No. of clinical pregnancies	17 (29.8)	26 (43.3)
No. of singletons (%)	15 (88.2)	21 (80.7)
No. of twins (%)	2 (11.7)	4 (17.3)
No. of triplets (%)	0 (0)	1 (3.8)
No. of deliveries (%)	11 (64.7)	17 (65.3)
No. of ongoing pregnancies (%)	2 (11.7)	4 (15.3)
No. of miscarriages (%)	4 (23.5)	5 (19.2)
No. of ectopic pregnancies (%)	0 (0)	1 (3.8)
Implantation rate	9.2	14

Note: Values in parentheses are percentages.
(Courtesy of Seracchioli R, Fabbri R, Porcu E, et al: Giamete intrafallopian transfer: Prospective randomized comparison between hysteroscopic and laparoscopic transfer techniques. *Fertil Steril* 64:355–359, 1995. Reproduced with permission of the publisher, the American Society for Reproductive Medicine [formerly The American Fertility Society].)

including ultrasound-guided oocyte recovery, was 28 minutes in the hysteroscopic group and 33 minutes in the laparoscopic group. Patients undergoing hysteroscopic GIFT were discharged after 3 hours, whereas those undergoing laparoscopic GIFT were hospitalized for 24 hours. The pregnancy rate in the hysteroscopic group was 29.8% and the implantation rate was 9%. These rates were not significantly different from those in the laparoscopic group: 43.3% for pregnancy and 14% for implantation (Table 3).

Conclusions.—Hysteroscopic GIFT is a safe procedure that can be done quickly and easily. Because it requires no hospitalization, general anesthesia, or operating room, costs are reduced and psychophysical involvement is low.

▶ Even though the pregnancy rate with hysteroscopic GIFT was only 30% compared with 43% with laparoscopic GIFT, it appears that the cost savings of the former technique make it an attractive alternative to the latter. Hysteroscopic GIFT can be performed in an office setting and does not require the use of an operating room or general anesthesia, as does laparoscopic GIFT. Further experience with transfer of sperm and eggs into the oviduct transcervically instead of transperitoneally is certainly warranted as hysteroscopic transfer appears to be safe and effective.

D.R. Mishell, Jr., M.D.

Breast and Ovarian Cancer Incidence After Infertility and In Vitro Fertilisation
Venn A, Watson L, Lumley J, et al (La Trobe Univ, Carlton, Australia; Natl Perinatal Epidemiology Unit, Oxford, England; Anti-Cancer Council of Victoria, Carlton, Australia; et al)
Lancet 346:995–1000, 1995   15–22

Background.—Some recent studies have suggested that exposure to fertility drugs may be correlated with an increased risk of ovarian cancer. Studies of cancer in women experiencing infertility have been hampered by low statistical power and inability to distinguish between the effects of fertility drug exposure and the effects of the underlying ovulation disorder. Studying cancer incidence in women having undergone in vitro fertilization (IVF) allows this distinction because most patients exposed to ovarian stimulation for IVF do not have abnormal ovulatory patterns. The incidence of cancer in a cohort of women referred for IVF was analyzed in an effort to determine whether cancer risk is increased by exposure to fertility drugs.

Methods.—The records of 10,358 women referred for IVF over a 14-year period were evaluated. Ovarian stimulation (to produce multiple folliculogenesis) was performed in 5,564 women; the other 4,794 women were either untreated or underwent natural cycle treatment without fertility drug exposure. Follow-up duration ranged from 1 to 15 years. Record linkage with data from population-based cancer registries was used to identify women with cancer.

Results.—Invasive ovarian cancer developed in 6 women; invasive breast cancer developed in 34. The expected numbers of cases of cancer as determined by application of age-standardized general population rates were compared with the statistics from the cohort, resulting in a 0.89 standardized incidence ratio (SIR) for breast cancer in the exposed group and a 0.98 SIR for breast cancer in the unexposed group. Women exposed to fertility drugs showed a 1.70 SIR for ovarian cancer; unexposed women showed an SIR of 1.62. The incidence of cancers among women exposed to fertility drugs were also compared as to number of IVF cycles. Risk of cancer did not appear to increase in association with greater exposure to stimulated treatment cycles. The rate of all cancers among the cohort did not differ significantly from that of the general population. After adjustment for age and infertility type, treated women showed a relative risk of breast cancer of 1.11 relative to untreated women and a relative risk of ovarian cancer of 1.45 relative to untreated women (Table 4). Risks of ovarian cancer and body of uterus cancer were increased in women with unexplained infertility relative to those with known causes of infertility, independent of IVF exposure. The combined group of treated and untreated women showed an increased risk of cancer of the body of the uterus.

Conclusions.—The incidence of breast cancer in women treated with fertility drugs for IVF was not significantly greater than either that of women referred for IVF but not treated or that of the general population. The incidence of body of uterus cancer appeared higher in the cohort, but this could be an artifact of the increased gynecologic surveillance of

---

TABLE 4.—For Various Cancers, Relative Risk (RR) Estimates for IVF Exposure Adjusted for Age and Infertility Type, and Relative Risk Estimates for Unexplained Infertility vs. Known Causes of Infertility, Adjusted for Age and IVF Exposure

	RR adj	95% CI	p
Breast cancer			
IVF exposure	1.11	0.56–2.20	0.8
Unexplained infertility	0.77	0.19–3.10	0.7
Ovarian cancer			
IVF exposure	1.45	0.28–7.55	0.7
Unexplained infertility	19.19	2.23–165	0.007
Cancer of body of uterus			
IVF exposure	0.65	0.11–3.94	0.6
Unexplained infertility	6.34	1.06–38.0	0.04
All cancers			
IVR exposure	0.96	0.62–1.47	0.8
Unexplained infertility	2.01	0.84–4.78	0.11

Abbreviations: IVF, in vitro fertilization; *CI,* confidence interval.

(Courtesy of Venn A, Watson L, Lumley J, et al: Breast and ovarian cancer incidence after infertility and in vitro fertilization. *Lancet* 346:995–1000, 1995. © by The Lancet Ltd. 1995.)

women experiencing infertility. Little evidence existed to establish a link between fertility drug use and incidence of ovarian cancer. However, this study was limited by the rarity of ovarian cancer and the relatively short follow-up period. Lack of reliable information regarding parity is also a limitation because nulliparity, which is likely to be more prevalent among women in the cohort than among the general population, is a risk factor for several cancers.

▶ The risk of ovarian cancer developing in women is inversely associated with parity. The risk is also reduced by the use of oral contraceptives, with the extent of the reduction in risk directly related to the duration of oral contraceptive use. Therefore, it has been hypothesized that the risk of ovarian cancer developing is directly related to the number of times a woman ovulates in her lifetime. There has been a suggestion that administration of ovulation-inducing agents to anovulatory women may increase their risk of ovarian cancer developing, but there are no definitive studies to support this assumption. Infertile women undergoing IVF usually ovulate regularly and are nulliparous. The results of this study indicate that with only a few years of follow-up, there is little evidence that administration of agents that induce multiple ovulations increase the risk of a woman having either ovarian cancer or breast cancer develop. Obviously, further studies, with a longer follow-up until the age when ovarian cancer becomes more common, are needed to determine whether the use of agents that induce multiple ovulations in ovulatory women affect their risk for any type of cancer developing.

D.R. Mishell, Jr., M.D.

Intracytoplasmic Sperm Injection Facilitates Fertilization Even in the Most Severe Forms of Male Infertility: Pregnancy Outcome Correlates With Maternal Age and Number of Eggs Available
Sherins RJ, Calvo LP, Thorsell LP, et al (Genetics & IVF Inst, Fairfax, Va)
Fertil Steril 64:369–375, 1995   15–23

Introduction.—For the most severe forms of male infertility, intracytoplasmic sperm injection offers a new therapy. In infertile couples with severe male infertility, the fertilization and pregnancy rates were prospectively evaluated after intracytoplasmic sperm injection.

Methods.—In 190 couples who did not respond to conventional in vitro fertilization, a series of 229 consecutive in vitro fertilization cycles was studied using intracytoplasmic sperm injection, using only the husband's sperm, as the only method of egg micromanipulation. The median age of the women was 35 years (range, 23–48 years) and the median age of the men was 38 years (range, 27–65 years). There was no waiting list or other type of patient prioritization. Using gonadotropin-releasing hormone analogue with gonadotropins, multiple follicular development was induced. Under transvaginal ultrasound guidance 34 to 35 hours after injection of

10,000 IU of human chorionic gonadotropin, follicles were aspirated. The intracytoplasmic sperm injection was performed, and 4 hours after oocyte retrieval, a single motile sperm was injected into each egg.

Results.—Embryo transfers resulted from 206 cycles with 52 pregnancies initiated, giving an overall pregnancy rate of about 25% per transfer. Clinical pregnancies resulted in 38 of 52 (18% per transfer) having established gestational sacs, that were ongoing more than 12 weeks, or that were delivered. Even in older women, pregnancies were achieved; however, pregnancies were more readily established in younger women. The fertilization rate was slightly affected by the severity of semen abnormality; however, a greatly decreased frequency of embryo formation was associated with actual necrospermia. Fewer than 100 viable sperm in the ejaculate resulted in pregnancy in some cases. In the oldest age group, the fertilization rate was 36%, whereas in the youngest group it was 50%.

Discussion.—For severe male infertility, intracytoplasmic sperm injection is a powerful new treatment, often succeeding with sperm incapable of zona penetration or egg fusion. Now the main determinants of success in treating male infertility are egg number and probably egg quality. Fertilization rates were far better than expected with intracytoplasmic sperm injection than with conventional in vitro fertilization. A sperm concentration less than 2 million sperm per milliliter of semen is an indicator for intracytoplasmic sperm injection, as well as semen samples with nearly all sperm having a poor acrosome reaction. More studies are needed to develop criteria for initial treatment by intracytoplasmic sperm injection.

▶ Before the development of intracytoplasmic sperm injection (ICSI), the presence of severe sperm abnormalities was associated with the worst prognosis for conception among infertile couples. Although ICSI is an expensive, meticulous technique, the results achieved in the treatment of severe sperm abnormalities are truly remarkable. Questions remain as to whether ICSI should be tried before or after an attempt of regular in vitro fertilization if abnormalities of sperm number and function exist. Also to be determined is the magnitude of sperm abnormalities, which indicates that the initial fertilization attempt should be performed by ICSI. These authors suggest that a sperm concentration of less than 2 million sperm per milliliter of semen is an indication for ICSI, as well as those semen samples with nearly all sperm having a poor acrosome reaction. More studies are needed to develop criteria for initial treatment by ICSI.

D.R. Mishell, Jr., M.D.

Intracytoplasmic Sperm Injection: Achievement of High Pregnancy Rates in Couples With Severe Male Factor Infertility Is Dependent Primarily Upon Female and Not Male Factors
Oehninger S, Maloney M, Veeck L, et al (Jones Inst for Reproductive Medicine, Norfolk, Va)
Fertil Steril 64:977–981, 1995

15–24

Objective.—Factors influencing the outcome of intracytoplasmic sperm injection (ICSI) were examined in a prospective series of 92 consecutive couples with severe male-factor infertility who underwent a total of 102 cycles of in vitro fertilization (IVF) augmented with ICSI. In 50 cases at least one previous attempt at fertilizing mature preovulatory oocytes had failed. In the other 42 cases, sperm parameters were unsuitable for conventional IVF.

Findings.—The diploid fertilization rate for 1,163 preovulatory oocytes was 61%, and the cleavage rate was 99%. Normal fertilization was achieved in 97% of treatment cycles. An average of 4 embryos were transferred per cycle. The clinical implantation rate was 12%, and the clinical pregnancy rate per transfer was 32%. Twenty-six ongoing pregnancies were achieved in 97 transfers. They included 8 twin and 4 triplet gestations. No basic sperm parameters significantly influenced fertilization or pregnancy rates after ICSI. Women who became pregnant had an average age of 34 years, compared to 36 years for those who did not conceive. Age was significantly related to both the basal serum follicle-stimulating hormone level and the outcome of pregnancy.

Conclusions.—Female factors are the chief determinant of the outcome following IVF with ICSI. Intracytoplasmic sperm injection is a promising approach to couples with male infertility resistant to conventional IVF.

Is Intracytoplasmic Sperm Injection (ICSI) a Safe Procedure? What Do We Learn From Early Pregnancy Data About ICSI?
Govaerts I, Koenig I, Van den Bergh M, et al (CUB Erasme, Brussels, Belgium)
Hum Reprod 11:440–443, 1996

15–25

Background.—The safety of intracytoplasmic sperm injection (ICSI) has been questioned. Severely infertile men have an increased incidence of genetic abnormalities, and conventional semen parameters do not yield data about the quality of spermatozoa DNA. Also, injecting the spermatozoa directly into the oocyte bypasses the natural selection processes mediated by the egg envelope. Pregnancy loss before 12 weeks' gestation is thought to be a good indicator of embryo toxicity and genetic abnormalities. The safety of ICSI was studied by comparing early data on ICSI and in vitro fertilization (IVF) pregnancies.

Methods and Findings.—Fifty ICSI and 226 IVF pregnancies were compared in the first 9 weeks after theoretical last menstrual period. Patients

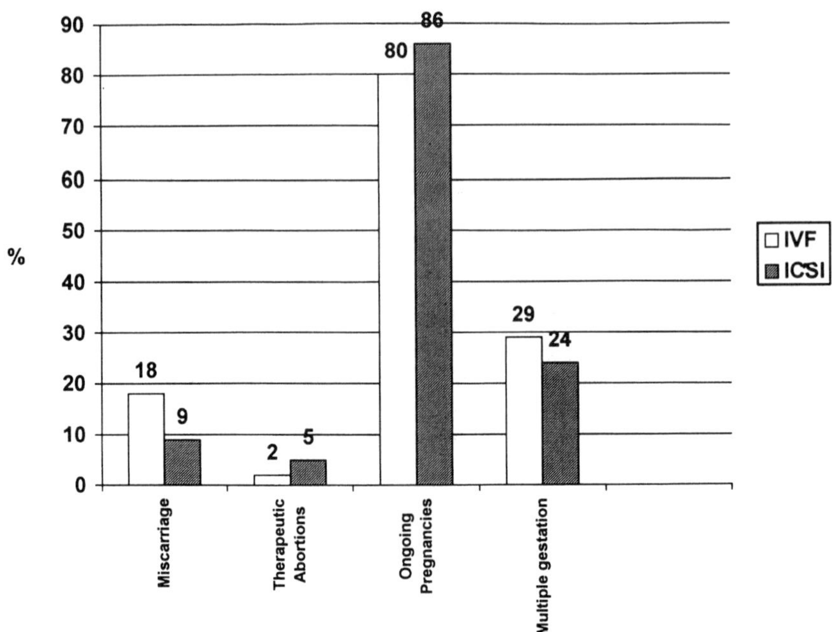

FIGURE 1.—The outcome of ICSI and IVF pregnancies. The outcome of 187 IVF pregnancies is compared with 42 ICSI pregnancies, including miscarriages, therapeutic abortions, ongoing pregnancies, and multiple gestations. Biochemical pregnancies are excluded. *Abbreviations: IVF,* in vitro fertilization; *ICSI,* intracytoplasmic sperm injection. (Courtesy of Govaerts I, Koenig I, Van den Bergh M, et al: Is intracytoplasmic sperm injection (ICSI) a safe procedure? What do we learn from early pregnancy data about ICSI? *Hum Reprod* 11:440–443, 1996, by permission of Oxford University Press.)

undergoing ICSI were significantly younger (mean age, 31 years) than those having IVF (mean age, 33 years), although infertility duration was similar. Miscarriage and multiple gestation rates were both 24% after ICSI, compared with 32% and 29%, respectively, after IVF. These differences were nonsignificant. The groups had similar probabilities of intrauterine sac arrest—16% after ICSI and 25% after IVF. The groups also had comparable mean plasma hormonal levels beginning on day 11 after oocyte retrieval. At 7 weeks, all ICSI and IVF pregnancies showed embryonic cardiac activity (Fig 1).

Conclusions.—The risk of miscarriage in women becoming pregnant after ICSI and IVF is comparable. These first-trimester data suggest that the ICSI procedure is safe. The prevalence of congenital malformations, however, is slightly higher after ICSI.

Comparisons of Pregnancy Loss Patterns After Intracytoplasmic Sperm Injection and Other Assisted Reproductive Technologies

Coulam CB, Dorfmann A, Opsahl MS, et al (Genetics & IVF Inst, Fairfax, Va)
Fertil Steril 65:1157–1162, 1996
15–26

Background.—The best available treatment for severe male infertility is in vitro fertilization with intracytoplasmic sperm injection (ICSI), but there are concerns about the potential for a high pregnancy loss rate with this technique. Pregnancy loss rates of ICSI and other assisted reproductive techniques were compared.

Methods.—Pregnancy outcomes were compared among 4 groups of infertile couples: 136 who had undergone ICSI, 71 who had in vitro fertilization (IVF), 35 who had received donor oocytes, and 19 who had undergone frozen-thawed embryo transfer.

Results.—The total pregnancy loss rate in ICSI couples was 47%, with a preclinical loss rate of 26% and a clinical loss rate of 21%. The pregnancy loss rate in this group was unrelated to the various semen categories (Fig 1). The risk of preclinical pregnancy loss increased along with the female partner's age. There was no difference in the frequency of preclini-

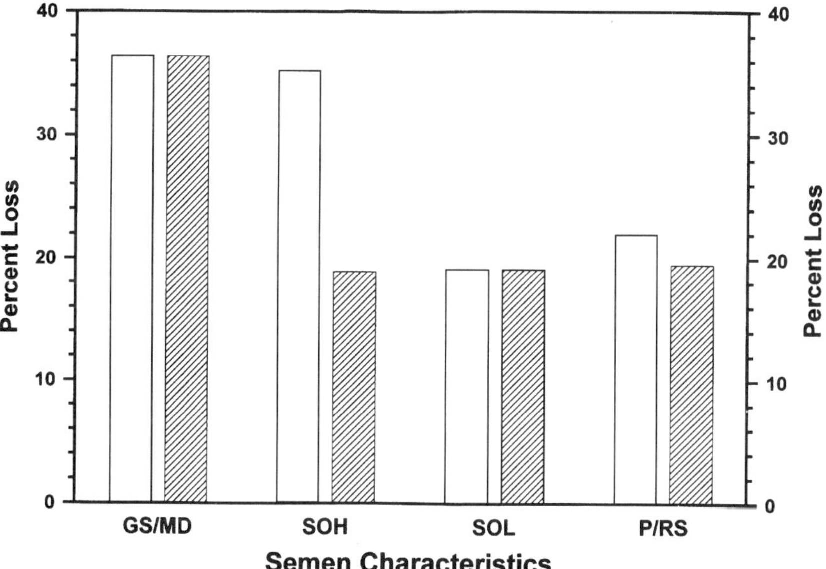

FIGURE 1.—Percentage of preclinical (*open box*) and clinical (*shaded box*) pregnancy loss rates with 4 categories of semen quality. *Abbreviations: G S/MD,* good semen or sperm with isolated morphological defects; *SOH,* suboptimal semen with sperm densities > 20 × 10^6/mL; *SOL,* suboptimal semen with sperm concentrations 5.9 × 10^6/mL; *P/RS,* poor semen with sperm concentration 0.1 to 4.9 × 10^6/mL; and rare sperm with < 0.1 × 10^6/mL sperm. No differences between preclinical and clinical pregnancy losses among semen categories (χ^2, 6.81, *P,* 0.33, power, 44%). (Courtesy of Coulam CB, Dorfmann A, Opsahl MS, et al: Comparisons of pregnancy loss patterns after intracytoplasmic sperm injection and other assisted reproductive technnologies. *Fertil Steril* 65:1157–1162, 1996. Reproduced with permission of the publisher, the American Society for Reproductive Medicine [formerly The American Fertility Society].)

cal pregnancy loss between ICSI and conventional IVF. However, the preclinical pregnancy loss rate was significantly lower with donor oocyte cycles. The clinical pregnancy loss rates were similar in all 4 groups, and there were no differences in the frequency of karyotypic abnormalities.

Conclusions.—The pregnancy outcomes after ICSI are similar to the outcomes from other assisted reproduction techniques. There is no increase in the preclinical or clinical pregnancy loss rate with ICSI, nor is there any difference in the risk of karyotypic abnormalities, despite the fact that ICSI bypasses the process of natural selection of sperm.

▶ Among all the causes of infertility, male-factor infertility was previously associated with the worst prognosis for conception. With the development and widespread use of ICSI, treatment of this cause of infertility now has one of the most favorable prognoses. There have been concerns that because the process of natural selection of sperm by the egg's membrane is bypassed, more genetically abnormal embryos may be formed. The results of these 2 studies indicate that the rates of pregnancy loss and abnormal pregnancies were not significantly different when the results of conceptions occurring after ICSI were compared with those of standard IVF, even with different types of semen abnormalities.

D.R. Mishell, Jr., M.D.

16 Contraception

Venous Thromboembolic Disease and Combined Oral Contraceptives: Results of International Multicentre Case-Control Study
Poulter NR, for the World Health Organization Collaborative Study of Cardiovascular Disease and Steroid Hormone Contraception (Univ College London)
Lancet 346:1575–1582, 1995

16–1

Introduction.—The formulation and use of oral contraceptives (OCs) have changed since previous studies of the OC-associated risk of venous thromboembolism (VTE). Also, the results obtained in European and U.S. studies do not necessarily apply to populations with different rates of and risk factors for VTE. Data from a case-control study of stroke, acute myocardial infarction, and VTE in Africa, Asia, Europe, and Latin America were used to assess the association between current OC use and risk of a first VTE.

Methods.—The hospital-based study was conducted in 21 centers in 17 countries. The patients were women in their twenties through forties who had been admitted to the hospital with a discharge diagnosis of deep venous thrombosis (DVT), pulmonary embolism, or both. Each case of DVT or pulmonary embolism was categorized as definite or probable, based on the clinical and radiologic findings. The controls were women admitted to the same hospital with a diagnosis considered to be unrelated to OC use. Cases and controls were evaluated in a standardized interview.

Results.—One thousand eleven women with DVT and 206 with pulmonary embolism were recruited into the study. Forty-two percent of those with DVT and 25% of those with pulmonary embolism were confirmed by definitive investigations, and more than 80% of both case types were categorized as definite or probable. The analysis included a total of 1,143 cases and 2,998 matched controls. European cases were better educated and more likely to have had hypertension during pregnancy than their controls. Cases in the developing countries were more likely than their controls to have had 1 or more live births and to have a previous history of high blood pressure and rheumatic heart disease.

Crude odds ratios of VTE in European women and women in developing countries were 2.32 and 33.0, respectively, for a history of rheumatic heart disease; 2.70 and 4.61 for body mass index greater than 30 kg/m^2 vs. 20 kg/m^2 or less; 2.65 and 3.81 for a history of varicose veins; 2.59 and 1.22 for moderate smoking; 1.66 and 1.16 for hypertension during pregnancy; and 0.95 and 1.82 for a history of high blood pressure. Europe and all 3 regions of the developing world showed an increased overall odds ratio for VTE associated with current OC users, compared with nonusers and never-users (Table 3). The risk estimates—about 4.2 in Europe and 3.3 in the developing world—were not significantly altered by duration of current and lifetime use.

Risk increased significantly with increasing body mass index. The increased risk was apparent within 4 months of the start of OC use and resolved within 3 months of stopping. Although risk estimates were similar for OCs containing low vs. higher estrogen doses, the risks associated with first- and second-generation progestogens were somewhat greater when used in combination with a higher dose of estrogen. Risks were higher for women whose OC contained third-generation progestogens—which are only given with low-dose estrogen—than for those receiving first- and second-generation progestogens. The odds ratio of VTE was greater for European women who used other progestogens combined with a low-dose estrogen.

Conclusions.—In the developing world as in Europe, OC use is associated with an increased risk of VTE. The overall OC-related risk estimates are lower than in most previous studies of nonfatal idiopathic VTE. The only confounder is a history of hypertension in pregnancy among Euro-

TABLE 3.—Odds Ratios (OR) of Venous Thromboembolism in Relation to Combined Oral Contraceptive Use by Region, With Nonuser or Never User as Reference Group

Region	Type of user	Cases	Controls	Crude OR (95% CI)
Relative to nonusers				
Europe	Nonuser	168	688	1.00
	User	265	356	3.95 (2.96–5.28)*
Developing countries	Nonuser	505	1715	1.00
	User	205	239	3.25 (2.59–4.08)
Africa	Nonuser	107	338	1.00
	User	46	69	2.14 (1.37–3.36)
Asia	Nonuser	56	228	1.00
	User	26	16	7.30 (3.39–15.72)
Latin American	Nonuser	342	1149	1.00
	User	133	154	3.37 (2.53–4.48)
Relative to never users				
Europe	Never	53	204	1.00
	Past	115	484	0.84 (0.58–1.24)
	Current	265	356	3.53 (2.39–5.21)
Developing countries	Never	320	1068	1.00
	Past	185	647	1.00 (0.80–1.24)†
	Current	205	239	3.25 (2.54–4.14)‡

*Adjusted odds ratio is 4.15 (3.09–5.57) adjusted for hypertension in pregnancy excluding 3 cases (users) and 1 control (nonuser) with unknown hypertension in pregnancy.

†Adjusted odds ratio is 0.93 (0.74–1.17).

‡Adjusted odds ratio is 3.08 (2.40–3.96) adjusted for number of live births (0. 1–2, 3 or more).

(Courtesy of Poulter NR, for the World Health Organization Collaborative Study of Cardiovascular Disease and Steroid Hormone Contraception: Venous thromboembolic disease and combined oral contraceptives: Results of international multicentre case-control study. *Lancet* 346: 1575–1582, 1995. © by The Lancet Ltd. 1995.)

pean women; the only other VTE risk factors are history of varicose veins, body mass index greater than 25 kg/m², and history of rheumatic heart disease.

Effect of Different Progestagens in Low Oestrogen Oral Contraceptives on Venous Thromboembolic Disease
Meirik O, for the World Health Organization Collaborative Study of Cardiovascular Disease and Steroid Hormone Contraception (World Health Organization, Geneva)
Lancet 346:1582–1588, 1995

16–2

Introduction.—A previous report of increased risk of venous thromboembolism (VTE) associated with the use of oral contraceptives (OCs), especially with the use of third-generation OCs, prompted further analysis to evaluate the risk of VTE associated with the use of low-estrogen OCs containing levonorgestrel or the newer third-generation progestogens, desogestrel or gestodene.

Methods.—Case-control data from 10 centers were analyzed, involving 829 patients with VTE, 2,135 controls matched for age and hospital, and 506 community controls. Risk of VTE was calculated for current users of third-generation desogestrel (further classified by dose), gestodene, and norgestimate, as compared with risk in nonusers and in current users of levonorgestrel or norgestimate OCs in combination with less than 35 μg of ethinyl estradiol.

Results.—Patients with VTE tended to have a higher body mass index (BMI), more live births, and a history of hypertension outside or during pregnancy. The risk of VTE was 7.6 among users of desogestrel combined with 30 μg of ethinyl estradiol and 38.2 among users of desogestrel combined with 20 μg of ethinyl estradiol, compared with nonusers. The risk of VTE among current users of desogestrel and gestodene was 2.6 times higher than the risks among levonorgestrel users, which was not significantly altered after controlling for BMI. Increasing BMI increased the risk of VTE among nonusers and among levonorgestrel users but not among desogestrel and gestodene users. The risk estimates were higher when compared with community than with hospital controls.

Conclusions.—The risk of VTE was significantly increased in users of second-generation combined OCs containing levonorgestrel, compared with nonusers, and was significantly further increased in users of OCs containing the third-generation progestogens. However, it is possible that the differences in risk can be attributed to chance, confounding, or bias. Therefore, these results must be confirmed with other studies.

Risk of Idiopathic Cardiovascular Death and Nonfatal Venous Thromboembolism in Women Using Oral Contraceptives With Differing Progestogen Components

Jick H, Jick SS, Gurewich V, et al (Boston Univ)
Lancet 346:1589–1593, 1995

16–3

Objectives.—There is public concern in the United Kingdom about the possible risks of cardiovascular illness associated with the use of combined oral contraceptives (OCs) containing the progestogens desogestrel and gestodene. This issue was addressed in 2 studies using data from the United Kingdom General Practice Research Database. The first study looked at the risk of unexpected cardiovascular death in otherwise healthy women who used OCs containing less than 35 µg of ethinyl estradiol plus levonorgestrel, desogestrel, or gestodene. The second study investigated the risks of nonfatal venous thromboembolism associated with the same 3 OCs.

Methods.—The General Practice Research Database included more than 4 million people in the United Kingdom whose general practitioners provide computerized data for research purposes. These records were reviewed to identify otherwise healthy women younger than age 40 years who received prescriptions for the defined OCs in 1991 or later. The first study analyzed all such women who died of pulmonary embolism, stroke, myocardial infarction, sudden death, or cardiac arrest. The second study included women with a diagnosis of nonfatal deep venous thrombosis, pulmonary embolism, or both. In the latter study, each case was classified as "confirmed" or "possible" according to the results of objective diagnostic tests. Potential confounders were evaluated in a nested case-control analysis.

Results.—The first study identified 15 unexpected, idiopathic cardiovascular deaths. Estimated incidence rates for the various progestogen components were 4.3/100,000 for levonorgestrel, 1.5/100,000 for desogestrel,

TABLE 3.—Results of Cohort Analysis on Risk of Nonfatal Venous Thromboembolism (VTE) (Study 2)

Progestagens	*Women with VTE*	*Woman-years at risk*	*Crude risk per 100,000 (95% CI)*	*Adjusted RR (95% CI)*
Levonorgestrel*	23	143 255	16.1 (10.7, 24.1)	1.0
Desogestrel	30	102 270	29.3 (20.5, 41.9)	1.9† (1.1–3.2)
Gestodene	22	78 363	28.1 (18.5, 42.5)	1.8† (1.0–3.2)
Past use	5	130 590	3.8 (1.6, 9.0)	0.2 (0.1–0.6)

*Reference group.
†Adjusted for age and calendar time.
Abbreviations: RR, relative risk; *CI*, confidence interval.
(Courtesy of Jick H, Jick SS, Gurewich V, et al: Risk of idiopathic cardiovascular death and nonfatal venous thromboembolism in women using oral contraceptives with differing progestagen components. *Lancet* 346:1589–1593, 1995. © by The Lancet Ltd. 1995.)

TABLE 5.—Distribution of Oral Contraceptive Exposure in Cases and Controls

Progestogens	Cases	Controls	Adjusted RR* (95% cl)
All cases and controls			
Levonorgestrel†	23	141	1.0
Desogestrel	30	91	2.2 (1.1, 4.4)
Gestodene	22	68	2.1 (1.0, 4.4)
Confirmed cases and their controls			
Levonorgestrel†	17	101	1.0
Desogestrel and gestodene	31	101	2.2 (1.0, 4.7)
Possible cases and controls			
Levonorgestrel†	6	40	1.0
Desogestrel and gestodene	21	58	2.2 (0.7, 7.3)

Note: Controls matched to cases by age, practice, and index date of case.
*Adjusted for smoking and body mass index.
†Reference group.
Abbreviations: RR, relative risk; *CI,* confidence interval.
(Courtesy of Jick H, Jick SS, Gurewich V, et al: Risk of idiopathic cardiovascular death and nonfatal venous thromboembolism in women using oral contraceptives with differing progestogen components. *Lancet* 346:1589–1593, 1995. © by The Lancet Ltd. 1995.)

and 4.8/100,000 for gestodene. Age- and year-adjusted relative risks, compared with levonorgestrel, were 0.5 for desogestrel and 1.4 for gestodene.

Of the 80 cases of nonfatal venous thromboembolism identified in the second study, 64% were classified as confirmed and 36% as possible. Forty-two were deep venous thrombosis and 38 were pulmonary embolus. Crude incidence rate estimates were 16.1/100,000 for levonorgestrel, 29.3/ 100,000 for desogestrel, 28.1/100,000 for gestodene, and 3.8/100,000 for past users. Age- and year-adjusted relative risks, again compared with levonorgestrel, were 1.9 for desogestrel and 1.8 for gestodene (Table 3).

In the case-control analysis, estimated relative risks on unadjusted matched analysis were 2.3 for both desogestrel and gestodene (Table 5). Crude relative risk estimates for women who used desogestrel with 20 and 30 μg of ethinyl estradiol were 2.7 vs. 1.9, compared with those who used levonorgestrel.

Conclusions.—Women using OCs containing levonorgestrel, desogestrel, or gestodene are at low and similar risk of idiopathic cardiovascular death. Risk could be higher for women who use the newer OCs for 6 months or fewer, but this could be a chance finding. The risk of nonfatal venous thromboembolism appears to be about twice as high for women who use OCs containing desogestrel or gestodene than for women who use OCs containing levonorgestrel. The results of this community-based study are similar to those of a World Health Organization Study that used hospital-based controls.

Enhancement by Factor V Leiden Mutation of Risk of Deep-vein Thrombosis Associated With Oral Contraceptives Containing a Third-generation Progestagen

Bloemenkamp KWM, Rosendaal FR, Helmerhorst FM, et al (Univ Hosp Leiden, The Netherlands; Univ of Amsterdam)
Lancet 346:1593–1596, 1995   16–4

Objective.—Third-generation progestogens were introduced into oral contraceptives (OCs) in the hope of reducing the associated risk of cardiovascular diseases. So far, no clinical studies have demonstrated any such reduction. Prompted by concerns about the safety of the new low-dose OCs, data from a previous case-control study were analyzed to assess the associated risk of deep venous thrombosis (DVT).

Methods.—The original study included 474 consecutive patients with a first episode of proven DVT, each of whom was matched for age and sex to a healthy control. The new analysis included 126 premenopausal women from among the cases. These women were not pregnant or in the puerperium at the time of their thrombosis; they had not had a recent miscarriage or used injectable estrogens. The risk of DVT associated with the use of an OC containing a third-generation progestogen was assessed, compared with the use of older OCs. The effects of other factors—including family history of thrombosis, previous pregnancy, age, and the thrombogenic factor V Leiden mutation—were evaluated as well.

Results.—Relative risks (RR) ranged from 2.2 to 3.8 for most types of OC. The exception was the desogestrel-containing monophasic OC, which had a RR of 8.7. No conclusions could be drawn about women using contraceptives containing gestodene or norgestimate. Among women using an OC containing 30 µg of ethinyl estradiol, the risk was 2.2-fold higher when the progestogen was desogestrel vs. levonorgestrel. For women receiving 30 µg of ethinyl estradiol plus desogestrel, the age-adjusted RR compared with all other types of OC use was 2.3. Relative risk associated with a family history of thrombosis was 2.9. When the analysis was restricted to patients and controls with a positive family history, age-adjusted RR was 7.2 for women who used a desogestrel-containing OC and 3.9 for those who used a levonorgestrel-containing product. Corresponding RRs among women with a negative family history were 8.0 and 3.3.

In a logistic model that included age, factor V Leiden mutation, and family history, the RRs associated with OC use were virtually unchanged. This included the twofold increase in risk with desogestrel-containing OCs vs. levonorgestrel-containing OCs. Pregnancy history had no effect on the risk estimates. The risk associated with desogestrel-containing OCs was higher for women in their teens than for those in their early twenties. The baseline risk was elevated eightfold in women who carried the factor V Leiden mutation. The RR of 6.0 produced a much greater overall effect in women who were positive for the factor V mutation than in those who were negative for it, RR 9.2. Thus, a factor V carrier who used a desogestrel-containing OC would be at almost 50 times greater risk for DVT than a woman negative for factor V who did not use OCs. Compared with 30 μg of ethinyl estradiol OCs with levonorgestrel, the risk associated with desogestrel-containing OCs was 3.5 times higher among factor V–positive women vs. just 2.1 times higher in women negative for factor V.

Conclusions.—The new low-dose OCs with a third-generation progestogen appear to significantly increase the risk of DVT, compared with older OC formulations. The presence of factor V Leiden mutation and a positive family history of venous thrombosis further enhance this effect of OCs. Adjustment for pregnancy history does not appear to affect the risk estimates.

Third Generation Oral Contraceptives and Risk of Myocardial Infarction: An International Case-Control Study
Lewis MA, for the Transnational Research Group on Oral Contraceptives and the Health of Young Women (Potsdam Inst of Pharmacoepidemiology and Technology Assessment, Germany)
BMJ 312:88–90, 1996   16–5

Background.—The third-generation combined oral contraceptives contain the progestogens desogestrel and gestodene. Three matched case-control studies—assessing the outcomes of venous thromboembolism, myocardial infarction, and ischemic stroke—are being conducted to examine the safety of these agents. Initial results of the study assessing the relationship of second- and third-generation oral contraceptives with myocardial infarction in young women were assessed.

Methods.—Women aged 16 to 45 years were recruited at 16 centers in 5 European countries. The analysis included 153 women with myocardial infarction and 498 controls. At least 3 controls were selected per case, at least 1 from a hospital and at least 1 from the community.

Results.—A comparison of current use of third-generation vs. second-generation oral contraceptives as risk factors for myocardial infarction yielded an odds ratio of 0.36 (Table 1). On comparison of third-generation oral contraceptives use in those with no previous oral contraceptive use, the odds ratio was 0.3. The odds ratio estimate for third- vs. second-generation products increased to 0.45 when 3 countries with small sample sizes were excluded. On matched analyses, odds ratios were 3.1 for second-generation and 1.2 for third-generation products vs. no oral contraceptive use. The odds ratio for myocardial infarction rose to 10.1 when current smoking was adjusted for oral contraceptive use: 3.1 for women who used third-generation products, 11.1 for those who used second-generation products, and 7.7 for those who were not currently using oral contraceptives. If all users switched from second- to third-generation oral contraceptives, the result would be 12 fewer deaths per year from myocardial infarction in England and Wales and 46 fewer such deaths per year in Germany.

TABLE 1.—Odds Ratios for Risk of Myocardial Infarction for Current Use of Different Types of Oral Contraceptives: Principal Results of Transnational Study

Comparison	Odds ratio (95% confidence interval)	P value	No exposed cases; No exposed controls
All cases (n=153)			
All controls (n = 498)			
Third generation *v* second generation products	0.36 (0.1 to 1.2)	0.1	6; 34
Third generation products *v* no current use	1.1 (0.4 to 3.4)	0.9	6; 34
Second generation products *v* no current use	3.1 (1.5 to 6.3)	0.003	23; 45
Hospital controls (n = 210)			
Third generation *v* second generation products	0.91 (0.2 to 4.6)	0.9	6; 11
Third generation products *v* no current use	1.9 (0.4 to 8.7)	0.4	6; 11
Second generation products *v* no current use	2.0 (0.8 to 4.9)	0.1	23; 26
Community controls (n = 288)			
Third generation *v* second generation products	0.25 (0.1 to 1.0)	0.05	6; 23
Third generation products *v* no current use	0.9 (0.3 to 3.0)	0.8	6; 23
Second generation products *v* no current use	3.5 (1.5 to 8.6)	0.005	23; 19

Note: Adjusted for center, age, body mass index, smoking, alcohol intake, and duration of exposure to oral contraceptives before current contraceptive.

(Courtesy of Lewis MA, for the Transnational Research Group on Oral Contraceptives and the Health of Young Women: Third generation oral contraceptives and risk of myocardial infarction: An international case-control study. *BMJ* 312:88–90, 1996.)

Conclusions.—Using third-generation rather than second-generation oral contraceptives may reduce the risk of myocardial infarction by twofold to fourfold, the results suggest. This benefit of third-generation products may offset the increased risk of venous thromboembolism. The findings underscore the need to consider all known risks and benefits when making decisions about oral contraceptive use. No oral contraceptive product carries as great a risk of heart attack as smoking or pregnancy does.

Third Generation Oral Contraceptives and Risk of Venous Thromboembolic Disorders: An International Case-Control Study

Spitzer WO, for the Transnational Research Group on Oral Contraceptives and the Health of Young Women (Potsdam Inst of Pharmacoepidemiology and Technology Assessment, Germany)
BMJ 312:83–88, 1996   16–6

Introduction.—There is concern about the possible increased risk of venous thromboembolism in women using oral contraceptives containing desogestrel or gestodene. Preliminary results of an international study of venous thromboembolism risk associated with the use of combined oral contraceptives containing third-generation progestogens were reported.

TABLE 3.—Odds Ratios of Venous Thromboembolism for Current Use of Different Groups of Oral Contraceptives

	United Kingdom			Germany			Total		
Comparison	No of cases exposed (n= 282)	No of controls exposed n= 1048)	Odds ratio (95% confidence interval)*	No of cases exposed (n= 189)	No of controls exposed n= 724)	Odds ratio (95% confidence interval)*	No of cases exposed (n= 471)	No of controls exposed (n= 1772)	Odds ratio (95% confidence interval)*
All oral contraceptives† v									
no current use	167	411	3.4 (2.4 to 4.9)	146	333	5.5 (3.5 to 8.7)	313	744	4.0 (3.1 to 5.3)
First generation products‡ v									
no current use	1	3	2.0 (0.2 to 20.8)	38	56	8.3 (4.5 to 15.2)	37	59	5.7 (3.4 to 9.4)
Second generation products‡ v									
no current use	64	189	3.0 (1.9 to 4.5)	68	213	3.7 (2.2 to 6.2)	132	402	3.2 (2.3 to 4.3)
Third generation products‡ v									
no current use	98	197	4.4 (3.0 to 6.6)	29	52	6.7 (3.4 to 13.0)	127	249	4.8 (3.4 to 6.7)
Products containing levonorgestrel v									
no current use	37	131	2.5 (1.5 to 4.0)	52	180	3.4 (2.0 to 5.7)	89	311	3.0 (2.0 to 3.9)
Third generation products v									
second generation products‡	98	197	1.5 (1.0 to 2.2)	29	52	1.8 (1.0 to 3.3)	127	249	1.5 (1.1 to 2.1)
Products containing gestodene v									
second generation products‡	45	101	1.4 (0.9 to 2.3)	10	11	2.6 (1.0 to 7.2)	55	112	1.5 (1.0 to 2.2)
Products containing desogestrel v									
second generation products‡	53	96	1.6 (1.0 to 2.5)	12	25	1.5 (0.8 to 3.1)	72	137	1.5 (1.1 to 2.2)

*Adjusted for linear age, smoking, alcohol use, study center, body mass index, and duration of exposure to oral contraceptives used before current contraceptive.

†Including progesterone-only oral contraceptives.

‡Users of progesterone-only oral contraceptives (17 cases and 34 controls) were not classified as users of first-, second-, or third-generation products. Thus, rows and columns do not necessarily add up. Including them as third- or second-generation products makes no meaningful difference to odds ratios.

(Courtesy of Spitzer WO, for the Transnational Research Group on Oral Contraceptives and the Health of Young Women: Third generation oral contraceptives and risk of venous thromboembolic disorders: An international case-control study. *BMJ* 312:83–88, 1996.)

Methods.—The study was 1 of 3 simultaneous case-control studies performed to examine the outcomes of deep venous thrombosis and pulmonary embolism, arterial thrombotic stroke, and myocardial infarction. Research subjects were recruited at 16 centers in 5 European countries. All cases with venous thromboembolism were identified in the hospital and matched to 3 controls, including at least 1 community control and 1 hospital control. Women who had used oral contraceptives within 3 months before the event were considered current users. Eighteen cases and 28 controls used oral contraceptive products containing norgestimate, which were classified among the second-generation products. Data were gathered by personal interview. This preliminary report was based mainly on data from the United Kingdom and Germany.

Results.—The analysis included 471 cases and 1,772 controls, 789 from the hospital and 983 from the community. Current use of any oral contraceptive product was linked to a fourfold increase in relative risk of venous thromboembolism. Odds ratios were 1.5 for third- vs. second-generation oral contraceptive use and 3.2 for use of either category of oral contraceptives vs. no current oral contraceptive use (Table 3). There was no significant difference between third-generation products containing gestodene vs. desogestrel. In a further analysis including first-time users only, the odds ratio for use of third- vs. second-generation products was 2.7. This ratio declined to 1.4 when the analysis was restricted to women who had previously used an oral contraceptive.

Conclusions.—The use of third-generation as opposed to second-generation oral contraceptives is weakly associated with an increased risk of venous thromboembolism. The odds ratio for this association is 1.5. Even if this association is not a causal one, the possible increase in risk must be taken seriously. The resulting increase in risk of death from venous thromboembolism may be on the order of 6 per million per year in the United Kingdom. There are many potential sources of bias in the reported analysis, including diagnostic bias, referral bias, prescribing bias, and attrition.

▶ The results of these 6 epidemiologic studies (Abstracts 16–1 to 16–6) relating the risk of venous thromboembolism (VTE) and oral contraceptives performed by 4 different groups of investigators in several different population groups are remarkably consistent. The findings indicate that use of all low estrogen (less than 50 µg) dose OCs is associated with about a fourfold increased relative risk of VTE developing compared with non-OC use. This increased relative risk is estimated to result in about 10 to 15 episodes of VTE per 100,000 woman-years of use of low estrogen dose OCs compared with about 4 episodes per 100,000 woman-years among women of similar age who are not pregnant who are not using OCs. Among pregnant and postpartum women, the estimated risk of VTE is about 60 per 100,000 woman-years. The major new finding of these studies is that use of low estrogen dose OCs containing desogestrel or gestodene is associated with about a twofold increased risk of VTE compared with use of levonorgestrel compounds with the same amount of estrogen. Because each study was observational and not a prospective clinical trial, there can be 2 explanations for this finding. The increased risk of VTE with the newer OC formulations containing desogestrel or gestodene could be causally related to a thrombotic effect on these progestins, or the findings could be due to selection bias that resulted in a group of women at higher risk for VTE being prescribed these newer formulations. The similarity of results of several different studies as well as retention of statistical significance after adjustment for potentially confounding factors are indicators that the findings are most likely causally related to the progestins themselves and not due to chance or bias. On the other hand, several factors suggest that the findings are due to selection bias. First, there is no biological basis for the findings. Ingestion of pharmacologic amounts of ethinyl estradiol induces an increase in several clotting parameters that produce hypercoaguability, and the degree of increase is directly related to the dose of ethinyl estradiol ingested. Thus, there is a biological reason for the increased risk of venous thrombosis associated with high-dose estrogen formulations. However, no differences in the type or amount of change in these clotting parameters have been reported when comparing women ingesting formulations containing gestodene and desogestrel with those ingesting formulations containing the same amount of ethinyl estradiol and either norethindrone or levonorgestrel. Second, the increased risk of VTE with the newer progestins could be due to the facts that they were marketed as safer and were preferentially prescribed to women with risk factors for VTE such as obesity, i.e., there was a prescribing bias. In addition, women with adverse symptoms such as headache or dizziness while taking the older formulations could have been switched to the newer ones. Another reason is that the risk of VTE could be greater in recent OC users than in longer users, and the women taking levonorgestrel compounds could have taken them for several years before the studies were initiated. Thus, the entire elevated risk with the newer formulations could be due to selection bias, not a causal relation. The same selection bias could be the cause of the decreased risk of cardiovascular deaths and acute myocardial infarction associated with use of the newer formulations, as was reported in 2 of these papers. Because it is possible that the results could have a causal basis, however, it might be prudent to no longer prescribe OCs containing desogestrel or gestodene to women with risk factors for VTE such as obesity, varicose veins, and family history of VTE. However, it would also be prudent to selectively prescribe these agents for women at risk for myocardial infarction, such as cigarette smokers and women with dyslipidemias and hypertension.

The risk of VTE with formulations containing the other third-generation progestin, norgestimate, was either not separately investigated in these studies or was not found to be associated with an increased risk of VTE, except in the transnational study. Therefore, these studies do not indicate that prescribing practices for norgestimate containing OC formulations should be changed at this time.

D.R. Mishell, Jr., M.D.

Thrombotic Risk Factors and Oral Contraception

Bokarewa MI, Falk G, Sten-Linder M, et al (Karolinska Inst/Hosp, Stockholm)
J Lab Clin Med 126:294–298, 1995   16–7

Introduction.—Oral contraception is an established risk factor for thrombosis. Recent studies have shown that patients with thromboembolic disease have a high incidence of elevated levels of antibodies to anionic phospholipids (PLa) and of activated protein C (APC) resistance. The occurrence of APC resistance and elevated PLa levels was investigated in women in whom thromboembolic disease developed while taking oral contraceptives, and the findings were compared with those in women who had never used oral contraceptives or had used them without vascular complications occurring.

Methods.—Eighty-one women with a history of thrombotic events were divided into 3 groups: those who had a thrombotic event while taking oral contraceptives (29 patients), those who had a history of oral contraceptive use but had a thrombotic event in another risk situation (33 patients), and those with no history of oral contraceptive use (19 patients). Blood samples were obtained from all patients and were analyzed for APC resistance, both with an activated partial thromboplastin time–based assay and with a polymerase chain reaction to detect the mutation in the coagulation factor V gene, and for PLa levels, as determined by levels of lupus anticoagulant activity, protein C activity, and protein S activity.

Results.—There were no significant differences in the 3 groups in the prevalence of a family history of thrombosis, age at the first thrombotic episode, or time since the first thrombotic episode. There was APC resistance in 27% of the women overall, with a varying incidence in the different groups. The proportion of patients with APC resistance was significantly lower among the women who had their first thrombotic event while taking oral contraceptives than in the other 2 groups. There was a correlation between the incidence of APC resistance and recurrent thrombosis. The mutation causing APC resistance was found in 40% of the study population, with a similar distribution in the 3 groups. The levels of PLa were comparable in the 3 groups, and elevated levels occurred concurrently with APC resistance in 12% of the patients.

Conclusions.—The occurrence of the factor V mutation was relatively increased in relation to the incidence of APC resistance in women with a history of thrombosis during oral contraception use, suggesting that APC response may be variably manifested in women with the factor V mutation. Therefore, both the clotting determination of APC response and detection of the mutation in the factor V gene should be used to determine the thrombotic risk in patients using oral contraceptives.

▶ The relation of the hereditary disorder of APC resistance to the risk of a thrombotic event developing has been extensively studied in the past few years since the existence of APC resistance was first described in 1993. In contrast to the uncommon inherited disorders of antithrombin III, protein C, and protein S deficiency, APC resistance occurs in 3% to 5% of Northern European populations and is present in as many as 50% of individuals with thrombotic events. Unfortunately, a control group of women without thrombosis was not included in this study. Nevertheless, that antiphospholipid antibodies, as well as the genetic mutation associated with APC resistance, was found in a similar high proportion of women in whom thrombosis developed while using and not using oral contraceptives indicates that although each of these 2 factors is a risk marker for thrombosis, oral contraceptive use may not increase the risk of thrombosis in women with either factor. When investigating whether APC resistance is present, it may be better to measure the genetic marker instead of the activated partial thromboplastin time because abnormalities of the latter were not present as frequently in oral contraceptive users who had thrombosis.

D.R. Mishell, Jr., M.D.

Resistance to Activated Protein C in Healthy Women Taking Oral Contraceptives
Olivieri O, Friso S, Manzato F, et al (Univ of Verona, Italy; Univ of Ferrara, Italy)
Br J Haematol 91:465–470, 1995   16–8

Background.—The most common laboratory abnormality found in patients with deep venous thrombosis is resistance to activated protein C (APC). At least 1 in 5 individuals with APC resistance do not carry the so-called Leiden factor V mutation, suggesting that other mutations or acquired factors may interfere with APC. Women taking oral contraceptives (OCs) reportedly are at increased risk of venous thrombosis.

Objective.—Coagulation parameters and sensitivity to APC were determined in 50 healthy women aged 18–41 years who were taking a low-dose estrogen-progestogen OC and 50 others not taking an OC.

Findings.—There were slight but nevertheless significant procoagulative changes in the women using OCs, including an increased level of fibrinogen and shortened coagulation times. The mean APC sensitivity ratio (APC-SR) was significantly lower in OC users than in controls (Fig 1). A decreased APC-SR was the only thrombotic marker that was significantly more prevalent in OC users (Table 2). All but 1 of 8 women with a low APC-SR were OC users. Two of these 8 women were heterozygous for the factor V Leiden mutation. Two women without the mutation discontinued OC use, and both regained a normal APC-SR.

Implications.—Oral contraceptive use may be associated with resistance to APC, increasing the risk of venous thrombosis. All women taking an estrogen-progestogen OC should be screened for APC resistance.

▶ Since the entity of APC resistance was first described in 1993, there has been a steadily increasing amount of information about this condition that enhances the risk of a thrombotic event developing. Activated protein C

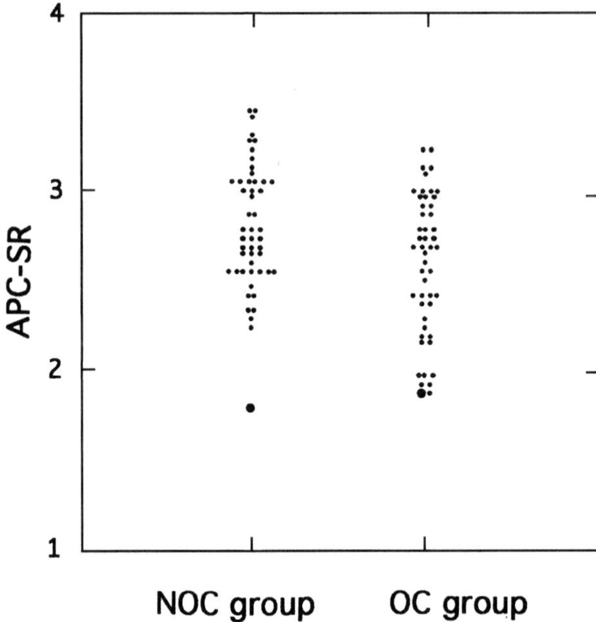

FIGURE 1.—Distribution of activated protein C sensitivity ratio (*APC-SR*) in women not taking oral contraceptives (*OCs*) (*NOC group*) and those taking OCs (OC group). The *large symbols* indicate individuals heterozygous for the factor V Leiden mutation. (Courtesy of Olivieri O, Friso S, Manzato F, et al: *Br J Haematol* 91:465–470, 1995. Published by Blackwell Science Ltd.)

normally inactivates the clotting factors, Va and VIIIa, causing a prolongation of the activated partial thromboplastin time (APTT) in vitro. When APC resistance is present, the APTT is only prolonged a short time after the addition of APC to the plasma sample. It was initially postulated that APC resistance was only caused by a certain genetic mutation, the Leiden factor V mutation. However, it is now known that as many as 20% of individuals with APC resistance do not have this genetic mutation.[1]

The results of this study indicate that ingestion of OCs may cause a temporary increase in APC resistance. This change may produce venous

TABLE 2.—Prevalence of Thrombophilic Markers

Thrombotic markers	Total subjects (n = 100)	Non-OC users (n = 50)	OC users (n = 50)	χ_2*
APC-R sensitivity ratio ≤2 (prevalence)	8 (8%)	1 (2%)	7 (14%)	< 0·05
At III deficiency value < 80 U/dl (prevalence)	0 (—)	0 (—)	0 (—)	—
Protein C deficiency value < 70 U/dl (prevalence)	3 (3%)	2 (4%)	1 (2%)	N.S.
Protein S deficiency value < 60 U/dl (prevalence)	3 (3%)	1 (2%)	2 (4%)	N.S.
LAC positivity (prevalence)	2 (2%)	0 (—)	2 (4%)	N.S.

*Comparison between those not using oral contraceptives (*OCs*) and OC users.
Abbreviations: APC-R, activated protein C resistance; *LAC*, lupus anticoagulant activity.
(Courtesy of Olivieri O, Friso S, Manzato F, et al: *Br J Haematol* 91:465–470, 1995. Published by Blackwell Science Ltd.)

thrombosis in women taking OCs. More studies of this alteration in clotting factors and OC use are warranted to verify this finding and to determine whether it is caused by the estrogen or progestin component of the formulation. If resistance APC is due to the progestin, whether it is only associated with certain of these compounds needs to be determined as well.

D.R. Mishell, Jr., M.D.

Reference

1. *Focus & Opinion: Obstetrics and Gynecology,* Vol. 1, No. 6, p 464.

Stroke in Users of Low-dose Oral Contraceptives
Petitti DB, Sidney S, Bernstein A, et al (Kaiser Permanente Med Care Program, Southern California, Pasadena; Kaiser Permanente Med Care Program, Northern California, Oakland)
N Engl J Med 335:8–15, 1996   16–9

Background.—In previous research, the use of oral contraceptives (OCs) has been associated with an increased risk of stroke. However, that research studied only OCs containing more estrogen than is now generally used. The relationship between stroke and OC use was examined in a large HMO in which high-estrogen OCs were rarely used.

Methods.—The population-based, case-control study included female patients (age range, 15–44 years) who had and had not experienced strokes, fatal and nonfatal. Data on the use of OCs were gathered in interviews.

Findings.—Four hundred eight strokes occurred among 1.1 million women during 3.6 million woman-years, for an incidence of 11.3 strokes per 100,000 woman-years. Two hundred ninety-five women with stroke and their matched control subjects were interviewed. Compared with former users and women who had never used OCs, current OC users had an odds ratio of 1.18 for ischemic stroke, after adjustment for other risk factors for stroke. The adjusted odds ratio was 1.14 for hemorrhagic stroke. Current OC use and smoking interacted positively to affect hemorrhagic stroke risk (Table 4).

Conclusions.—Overall, current low-estrogen OC use does not seem to increase the risk of hemorrhagic stroke. This study confirms that the incidence of stroke among young women is low.

▶ In the 1960s, soon after their introduction, high estrogen dose oral contraceptive formulations were found to be causally linked to venous thromboembolism. In the 1970s, reports were published showing that women ingesting these high steroid dose formulations also were at an increased relative risk of having stroke and myocardial infarction develop. Subsequent studies showed that the increased risk of myocardial infarction was only significantly increased among women older than 35 years who also smoked

TABLE 4.—Adjusted Odds Ratios for Ischemic Infarction and Hemorrhagic Stroke, According to Oral Contraceptive Use*

VARIABLE	ISCHEMIC INFARCTION†			HEMORRHAGIC STROKE‡		
	NO. OF WOMEN WITH STROKE	NO. OF MATCHED CONTROLS	OR (95% CI)	NO. OF WOMEN WITH STROKE	NO. OF MATCHED CONTROLS	OR (95% CI)
Current use vs. non-current use						
Current use	17	43	1.18 (0.54–2.59)	21	50	1.14 (0.60–2.16)
Noncurrent use§	125	335	1.00	127	346	1.00
Current use vs. past use and no use¶						
Current use	14	43	0.65 (0.25–1.70)	14	50	1.02 (0.37–2.82)
Past use	82	271	0.49 (0.25–0.98)	81	272	0.89 (0.41–1.91)
No use§	28	64	1.00	14	74	1.00
Any use vs. no use¶						
Any use	96	314	0.52 (0.27–1.00)	95	322	0.91 (0.43–1.93)
No use§	28	64	1.00	14	74	1.00

Abbreviations: OR, odds ratio; *CI,* confidence interval.
*Women with missing values not included. Current use denotes use in the month before the index date. Noncurrent use includes past use and no use.
†Odds ratios have been adjusted for the presence or absence of treated hypertension, the presence or absence of treated diabetes, smoking status, race or ethnic group, and body-mass index.
‡Odds ratios have been adjusted for the presence or absence of treated hypertension, the presence or absence of treated diabetes, smoking status, race or ethnic group.
§Reference category.
¶Women for whom proxy respondents were interviewed have been excluded.
(Reprinted by permission of *The New England Journal of Medicine* from Petitti DB, Sidney S, Bernstein A, et al: Stroke in users of low-dose oral contraceptives. *N Engl J Med* 335:8–15, Copyright 1996, Massachusetts Medical Society.)

and ingested high-dose formulations. It was also shown that the cause of the myocardial infarction in oral contraceptive users was due to arterial thrombosis, not accelerated atherosclerosis, brought about by the thrombophilic effect of the estrogenic component. The magnitude of the thrombophilic effect, as well as the extent of risk of venous thrombophlebitis, were both found to be directly correlated to the amount of estrogen in the formulation. Data regarding the risk of stroke with oral contraceptive use are less clear. Some studies show an increased risk of only thrombotic stroke, whereas others found an increased risk of only hemorrhagic stroke. The effect of age, smoking, and existing hypertension on the risk of stroke with oral contraceptive use is also not well defined, perhaps because these factors affect the risk of hemorrhagic and thrombotic stroke differently. The results of this large case-control study, which indicate no significant increase in risk of either thrombotic or hemorrhagic stroke among women using low estrogen dose oral contraceptives and a low overall incidence of these events among women of reproductive age, are very reassuring.

D.R. Mishell, Jr., M.D.

Breast Cancer and Hormonal Contraceptives: Collaborative Reanalysis of Individual Data on 53 297 Women With Breast Cancer and 100 239 Women Without Breast Cancer From 54 Epidemiological Studies
Collaborative Group on Hormonal Factors in Breast Cancer (Emory Univ, Atlanta, Ga; Johns Hopkins Univ, Baltimore, Md; Univ of Queensland, Australia; et al)
Lancet 347:1713–1727, 1996   16–10

Background.—Female sex hormones have been widely used as contraceptives. A number of epidemiologic studies have evaluated a possible association between hormonal contraceptive use and breast cancer. To collect, analyze, and publish all the data regarding the effect of hormonal contraceptives on breast cancer risk, the Collaborative Group on Hormonal Factors in Breast Cancer was formed.

Methods.—Epidemiologic studies, including both prospective and case-control studies related to the effect of hormonal contraceptives on breast cancer risk, were identified with computer-aided literature searches, review articles, and discussions among colleagues. The original data were obtained on 53,297 women with breast cancer and 100,239 women without breast cancer participating in 54 studies. The data were analyzed to determine the relative risk of breast cancer associated with hormonal contraceptive use.

Results.—Compared with women who had never used oral contraceptives, those who had ever used contraceptives had a relative risk of 1.07, a statistically significant excess risk. The risk of breast cancer was weakly associated with increasing duration of use, was greatest among women who first used contraceptives before the age of 20, and decreased with an increased time since first and last use. The time since the last use of contraceptives was the strongest independent predictor of breast cancer risk. The relative risk decreased as follows: 1.24 in current users, 1.16 in women who discontinued use 1 to 4 years earlier, and 1.07 in women who discontinued use 5 to 9 years earlier. In women who discontinued use at least 10 years earlier, there was no significantly increased risk of breast cancer (relative risk of 1.01). These findings were not significantly affected by age or parity. Compared with never users, ever users of hormonal contraceptives had significantly less advanced breast cancers.

Conclusions.—A small but significant increased risk of breast cancer exists for women who use combined oral contraceptives during use and for 10 years after discontinuing use. The excess risk is no longer present by 10 years after ceasing contraceptive use. However, the cancers diagnosed in these women are less likely to be advanced than the cancers diagnosed in women who have never used contraceptives.

Oral Contraceptive Use and Risk of Breast Cancer in Middle-aged Women

Rossing MA, Stanford JL, Weiss NS, et al (Fred Hutchinson Cancer Research Ctr, Seattle; Univ of Washington, Seattle)
Am J Epidemiol 144:161–164, 1996   16–11

Introduction.—The women who first used oral contraceptives when they became available in the 1960s are now middle aged, the time of life when breast cancer is most frequent. However, little is known about the effects of oral contraception on breast cancer risk. The potential link between contraceptive use and breast cancer risk in middle age was evaluated in a case-control study.

Methods.—The population-based study included women in Washington State who were 50 to 64 years old in 1988–1990. There were 537 breast cancer cases and 492 disease-free control subjects. The women were interviewed in detail about their use of oral contraceptives, among other variables.

Results.—The 2 groups were similar in the proportion of women who had ever used oral contraceptives, the total duration of oral contraceptive use, the time since last use, or the age at first or last use. Women whose first use of oral contraceptives was within 20 years of their interview had a slightly increased risk of breast cancer; otherwise, risk did not increase with decreasing time since last use. Oral contraceptive use did not affect breast cancer risk among women in different 5-year age strata, and there was no significant effect when various subgroups of women were compared (i.e., those with vs. without a family history of breast cancer, parous vs. nulliparous women, and users vs. nonusers of hormone replacement therapy).

Conclusions.—Among women who were of reproductive age when oral contraceptives first became available, the use of birth control pills does not seem to increase the risk of breast cancer during middle age. This is true even for women who use oral contraceptives relatively later during their reproductive years (i.e., after age 40).

▶ The information from the massive collaborative reanalysis of data from 54 epidemiologic studies (Abstract 16–10), approximately 90% of all the epidemiologic information published on the topic, as well as the data from the case-control study in Washington State (Abstract 16–11) are reassuring about the risk of breast cancer associated with use of oral contraceptives (OC). As observed in the large Cancer and Steroid Hormone Study done in the United States several years ago, OC use, like early first term pregnancy, may slightly increase the risk of breast cancer when a woman is young and the incidence of the disease is low. Early first term pregnancy has also been shown to have a protective effect against the development of breast cancer in women of older age when the disease is most prevalent and thus reduces the lifetime risk of developing this cancer. Data are not yet available that analyze the effect of OC use on lifetime risk of breast cancer or the risk in women older than age 60. However, the data on breast cancer risk and OC use in middle-aged women, when the disease is more common than in younger women, indicate that there is no effect of OC use on risk of this disease.

It is hoped that OCs, like first term pregnancy at an early age, will prove to reduce the lifetime risk of breast cancer. In the meantime, women should be reassured by the results of these studies that use of oral contraceptives does not affect the risk of breast cancer developing 10 years after stopping use as well as after age 50 when the disease becomes more common. It is also reassuring that, like previous studies, neither of these analyses showed that OC use affected the risk of breast cancer among women with a family history of breast cancer.

D.R. Mishell, Jr., M.D.

Smoking and Cycle Control Among Oral Contraceptive Users

Rosenberg MJ, Waugh MS, Stevens CM (Univ of North Carolina, Chapel Hill)
Am J Obstet Gynecol 174:628–632, 1996   16–12

Background.—Associations between tobacco use and anti-estrogenic effects, such as infertility, early menopause, osteoporosis, and menstrual problems, have been established. To determine whether cigarette smoking adversely affects intermenstrual spotting and bleeding in oral contraceptive users, data from 3 large multicenter clinical trials involving 2,956 women using 3 different oral contraceptives were evaluated.

Patients and Methods.—Study enrollees were healthy, sexually active women with no known contraindications to oral contraceptive use. Participants were between 16 and 45 years of age and had had regular menses for at least 3 cycles before study enrollment. The 3 studies were conducted as open-label clinical trials, using a common protocol that included uniform definitions of spotting and bleeding.

Two or more different monophasic oral contraceptive preparations were compared in the 3 trials. One preparation—75 µg of gestodene plus 30 µg of ethinyl estradiol (Minulet)—was common to all 3 trials. Comparison preparations in 2 studies included desogestrel 150 µg, plus 30 mg of ethinyl estradiol (Marvelon) in 1 trial, and 150 µg of desogestrel plus 20 µg of ethinyl estradiol (Mercilon) in another. Norgestimate 250 µg plus 35 µg of ethinyl estradiol (Cilest) was compared in the third trial. In a daily diary, study participants recorded pills taken, bleeding, spotting, side effects, and any medications taken concurrently. Follow-up was conducted for at least 6 months in all 3 studies. Data obtained during the first 6 months were pooled and analyzed.

Results.—Nearly one third of the 2,956 study enrollees smoked cigarettes. Spotting or bleeding occurred much more frequently in the first cycle compared with later cycles in both smokers and nonsmokers. The percentage of patients reporting spotting or bleeding was 59% for smokers and 52% for nonsmokers in the first cycle and 14% vs. 9% in the sixth cycle. The average was 23% for smokers and 19% for nonsmokers for all 6 cycles. The percentage of smokers reporting spotting or bleeding was significantly higher in each cycle compared with that of nonsmokers (Fig 1).

Significant decreases in the percentage of smokers and nonsmokers with spotting or bleeding were noted over time, although after the first cycle, nonsmokers had a slight but steady decrease in spotting or bleeding for each successive cycle. In comparison, decreases were noted in smokers during the first 2 cycles, after which spotting and bleeding remained essentially constant for cycles 3 through 6. Compared with nonsmokers, the relative risk of spotting or bleeding increased with a greater number of cycles, and, for each cycle, with increasing levels of tobacco use among smokers. Outcomes were not significantly affected by age, alcohol use, height, weight, and study site. For women with any smoking, the relative risk increased for every cycle, with significant differences noted in 5 of 6 cycles. The relative risk for any smoking ranged from 1.30 in the first cycle to 1.86 in the sixth cycle, representing a 30% increased risk for the first cycle and an 86% increased risk in the sixth, compared with nonsmokers. A significant association was found between increasing levels of smoking and increased risk of spotting or bleeding at each cycle.

The most pronounced differences were observed during the last cycles. The highest relative risk was at the final cycle for the highest level of smoking: compared with nonsmokers, women smoking more than 16 cigarettes per day had an almost threefold increase in spotting or bleeding risk.

Conclusions.—An adverse relationship between cigarette smoking and cycle control has been identified in oral contraceptive users, which may be a result of increasing estrogen catabolism. Women who experience spotting or bleeding are considerably more likely to discontinue oral contraceptive use than those not having these problems, thereby increasing the chances of unintended pregnancy.

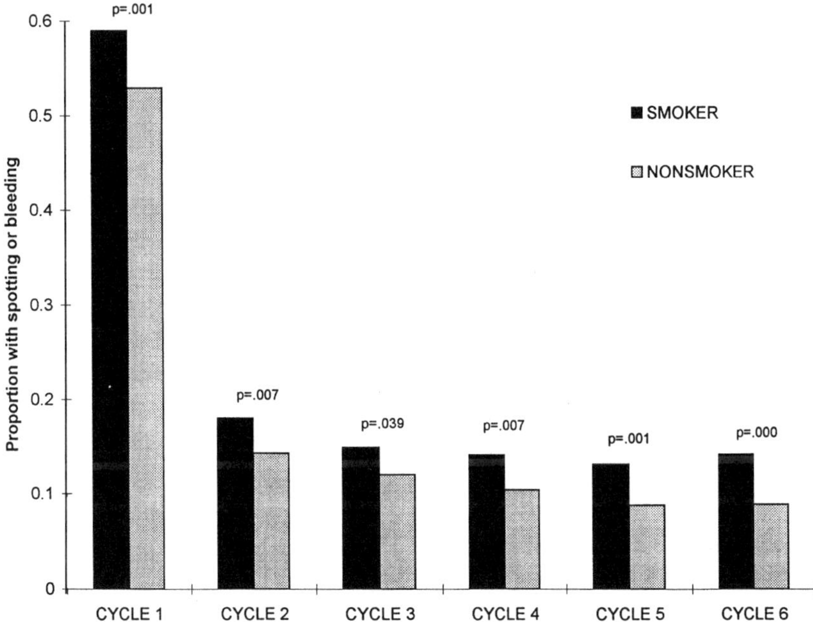

FIGURE 1.—Proportion of oral contraceptive users with spotting or bleeding, by smoking status. (Courtesy of Rosenberg MJ, Waugh MS, Stevens CM: Smoking and cycle control among oral contraceptive users. *Am J Obstet Gynecol* 174:628–632, 1996.)

► Cigarette smoking is known to adversely influence the effects of endogenous estrogen and is associated with an increased risk of menstrual abnormalities, earlier age of menopause, infertility, and osteoporosis, compared with that in nonsmoking women. This study indicates that cigarette smoking also adversely affects the ability of exogenous estrogen to maintain endometrial integrity during the time that oral contraceptives are being ingested. The resultant increased risk of breakthrough bleeding and spotting is bothersome to the contraceptive user and may cause her to stop taking the oral contraceptives, with an increased risk of an unwanted pregnancy.

A recent report suggested that cigarette smokers use an oral contraceptive formulation with only 20 μg of estrogen because there were fewer adverse effects on some parameters of the coagulation profile, compared with products with 30 or 35 μg of estrogen. However, no epidemiologic data indicate that cigarette smokers have an increased risk of venous thromboembolism compared with nonsmokers—or that the minor differences in the coagulation profile occurring with the 2 doses of estrogen in the formulation are associated with an increased risk of thromboembolism. The results of the study in this abstract appear to indicate that cigarette smokers should preferentially use formulations with 30–35 μg of ethinyl estradiol instead of 20 μg to help maintain endometrial integrity and reduce the incidence of breakthrough bleeding.

D.R. Mishell, Jr., M.D.

Pregnancy and Lifestyle Study: The Long-term Use of the Contraceptive Pill and the Risk of Age-related Miscarriage

Ford JH, MacCormac L (Queen Elizabeth Hosp, Woodville, Australia)
Hum Reprod 10:1397–1402, 1995   16–13

Introduction.—Although oral contraceptives have received adverse publicity in the lay media, there are some considerable noncontraceptive health benefits related to the suppression of ovulation. These include reductions in iron-deficiency anemia, menstrual disorders, endometrial cancer, benign breast disease, ovarian cysts, ovarian cancer, and endometrial cancer. Women aged 30 years and older have been shown to have an increased incidence of spontaneous abortions. The ovarian follicular dynamics after long-term use of oral contraceptives have not been determined. The risk of age-related miscarriage with the long-term use of oral contraceptives was investigated.

Methods.—A total of 585 couples planning a pregnancy within the next year completed questionnaires. The women submitted monthly urine samples on the 28th day of each cycle in which conception was attempted. These couples had 1 of 3 outcomes: live birth of an apparently normal child, spontaneous abortion, or 9 months of infertility.

Results.—Most women had used oral contraceptives for 6 months or longer. Only 39 women had never used oral contraceptive pills. The years of pill usage compared with rates of miscarriage were 0–2, 22.2%; 3–4, 17.3%; 5–6, 19.6%; 7–8, 16.7%; and 9 or more, 11.4%. The miscarriage rate was inversely proportional to years of pill use, suggesting that pill use may offer protection against miscarriage. The reduction in miscarriage was only significant in women older than age 30 years. The rate of miscarriage decreased with the number of years of pill use. For all women, the mean rate of miscarriage decreased from 23% with 0–2 years of pill use to 11.3% with 9 or more years of pill use. For women aged 30 years and older, the mean miscarriage rate decreased from 28% with 0–2 years of pill use to 7% for women who used the pill 9 or more cumulative years. Pill use for a longer period did not affect the rate of miscarriage in women aged 25–29 years. However, it greatly reduced the rate in women aged 30–34 years and women 35 years or older.

Conclusions.—The age-related miscarriage rates were 13.4% in women aged 25–29 years, 17.3% in those 30–34 years, and 28.3% in those 35–39 years. A dramatic reduction in miscarriage was observed in women aged 30 years or older who had taken oral contraceptives for 9 or more years. There was about a 50% reduction in the miscarriage rate in women aged 30–34 and 35–39 years at the time of conception. These reductions in miscarriage rates might result from a preservation effect on follicles in long-term users of oral contraceptives.

▶ Several noncontraceptive health benefits have been associated with use of oral contraceptives. The 2 most important previously reported benefits of oral contraceptive use are a reduction in the risk for both ovarian and endometrial cancer developing. The degree of reduction of these cancers is directly related to the duration of oral contraceptive use. The results of this study indicate that there is probably another major benefit of long-term use of oral contraceptives, that of reducing the rate of spontaneous abortion if women conceive after age 30 and have used oral contraceptives for 9 years or longer. Today, many women are delaying the onset of childbearing until after age 30 or more. The rate of spontaneous abortion normally increases from a rate of 13% in women who are pregnant at age 25–29 to 17% at age 30–35, and to 28% at age 35 to 39. Long-term use of oral contraceptives reduced the risk of spontaneous abortion by about 50% in the latter 2 age groups. The authors hypothesized that the reduction in risk of abortion was due to preservation of follicles, which thus lowered the risk of having a trisomic conception. Whether or not this is the mechanism whereby long-term oral contraceptive use reduces the abortion rate of pregnancy in older women, women should be informed of the results of this study if they choose to become pregnant after age 30.

D.R. Mishell, Jr., M.D.

The Risk of Pregnancy After Tubal Sterilization: Findings From the U.S. Collaborative Review of Sterilization
Peterson HB, for the U.S. Collaborative Review of Sterilization Working Group (Natl Center for Chronic Disease Prevention and Health Promotion, Atlanta Ga)
Am J Obstet Gynecol 174:1161–1170, 1996   16–14

Background.—Tubal sterilization is now the most prevalent form of contraception among married and formerly married women in the United States. However, the long-term efficacy of this method has not been documented in any large, prospective studies. Data were obtained from the U.S. Collaborative Review of Sterilization—a large, prospective, multicenter study conducted by the Centers for Disease Control and Prevention—to investigate the long-term efficacy of tubal sterilization.

Methods.—A total of 10,863 women were enrolled in the study from 1978 through 1986. Characteristics of the surgery and complications were recorded during and after sterilization. In addition, the women were contacted by phone about 1 month after the surgery and annually thereafter for follow-up. One hundred seventy-eight women were excluded from the final analysis for various reasons.

Findings.—Follow-up data were available for 89.2% of the participants at 1 year after sterilization, 81% at 3 years, 73% at 5 years, and 57.7% at 8 to 14 years. Pregnancy classified as true sterilization failures occurred in 143 women. Pregnancy was ectopic in 32.9%. Another 14.7% of pregnancies ended in spontaneous abortion, and 18.2% were terminated. The remaining 28.7% of the women were delivered of infants. The cumulative 10-year probability of pregnancy was greatest after clip sterilization, at 36.5 in 1,000 procedures, and lowest after unipolar coagulation and postpartum partial salpingectomy, each at 7.5 in 1,000 procedures. Women sterilized at a young age by bipolar coagulation or clip application had the greatest cumulative risk of pregnancy, at 54.3 and 52.1 in 1,000, respectively.

Conclusion.—Although tubal sterilization is very effective, the risk of failure is greater than has been appreciated. Pregnancy can occur more than 1 to 2 years after the procedure. The risk of pregnancy varies by method of tubal occlusion and patient age.

▶ Female sterilization by surgical removal of a portion of the oviduct or mechanically occluding a portion of the lumen by clips, bands, or electrocoagulation was previously believed to be the most effective form of pregnancy prevention. This belief was based upon studies that reported that failure rates during the first year of use of any type of reversible contraception were higher than the first-year failure rate of female sterilization. The results of this long-term study indicate that pregnancies continue to occur for many years after the sterilization procedure. For women 18 to 27 years of age, 2.8% became pregnant 5 to 10 years after bipolar coagulation of the oviduct. There are several reversible methods of contraception with failure rates similar to those of tubal sterilization. Cumulative 5-year failure rates with Norplant are 1.1 per 100 women; with the Copper T380 intrauterine device (IUD), 1.2 per 100 women; and with female sterilization, 1.3 per 100 women. Furthermore, among women who become pregnant after female sterilization about one third have ectopic pregnancies compared with one fourth with Norplant and 5% with the Copper T380 IUD. Because the Copper T380 IUD has an effective life span of 10 years with a failure rate comparable to female sterilization and a lower ectopic pregnancy rate, as well as being less expensive and more convenient to use, it should be considered as an alternative to tubal sterilization.

D.R. Mishell, Jr., M.D.

The Yuzpe Regimen of Emergency Contraception: How Long After the Morning After?
Trussell J, Ellertson C, Rodríguez G (Princeton Univ, NJ)
Obstet Gynecol 88:150–154, 1996   16–15

Background.—The most common form of emergency contraception consists of an altered dose of regular combined oral contraceptives. This method—called the Yuzpe method—involves taking 1 dosage within 72 hours after unprotected intercourse and a second dosage 12 hours later. This study evaluated whether failure of the Yuzpe method is related to the length of time elapsed between intercourse and treatment.

Methods and Findings.—A literature search found 9 published studies that included the number of women treated and outcomes by time elapsed since unprotected intercourse. Failure rates did not differ significantly when treatment was begun on the first, second, or third day after unpro-

TABLE 1.—Interval Between Unprotected Intercourse and Treatment With Emergency Contraceptive Pills

	First day		Day of treatment after unprotected intercourse Second day		Third day	
Reference	No.	Preg.	No.	Preg.	No.	Preg.
Yuzpe & Lancee[1]* (1977)	428	0	138	0	42	1
Tully[11]† (1983)	242	6	159	4	98	1
Luerti et al[12]‡ (1986)	161	0	156	7	119	1
Friedman & Rowley[13]§ (1987)	260	9	132	6	74	0
Percival-Smith & Abercrombie[14]‖ (1987)	266	6	376	7	225	5
Bagshaw et al[15]* (1988)	331	3	425	6	214	3
Kane & Sparrow[8]¶ (1989)	401	9	338	5	156	7
Zuliani et al[16]*# (1990)	220	4	118	3	69	2
Ho & Kwan[9]* (1993)	217	3	130	6	0	0
Total	2,526	40	1,972	44	997	20

Abbreviations: No. Number of women treated; *Preg.*, number of pregnancies; *LFU*, lost to follow-up.

*Nos. exclude women LFU.

†Nos. include 116 women LFU; "patients who were so motivated as to travel a great distance (30–80 miles) to obtain postcoital contraception would have been similarly motivated to contact us had the method failed"; "had any of our lost to follow-up patients become pregnant we would have heard, if not from them then from colleagues in Family Planning Clinics, or GPs or gynecologists."

‡Nos. include 81 women LFU; "presumably they would have contacted our center in case of pregnancy."

§Nos. include 20 women LFU and 12 women treated with an emergency intrauterine device insertion (none of whom became pregnant).

‖Nos. include 93 women LFU; "it is likely that they would have returned to the clinic for further care" if they had become pregnant.

¶Nos. include 8% of women LFU.

#Nos. and Pregs. not found in original publication but supplied by Guglielmo Zuliani (personal communication, July 10, 1995).

(Courtesy of Trussell J, Ellertson C, Rodríguez G: The Yuzpe regimen of emergency contraception: How long after the morning after? *Obstet Gynecol* 88:150–154, 1996, reprinted with permission from The American College of Obstetricians and Gynecologists.)

tected intercourse. Because of the large sample size, a power of 76% was ensured to reject the null hypothesis of equal failure rates when the odds of failure on the third day were twice those on the first and second days (Table 1).

Conclusions.—The Yuzpe regimen is equally effective at preventing pregnancy whether treatment is begun on the first, second, or third day after unprotected intercourse. Protocols that deny treatment after 72 hours may be unnecessarily restrictive, especially if the alternative of emergent placement of a copper intrauterine device is not possible. Also, insistence on taking the first dosage as soon as possible may be inappropriate when taking the second dosage 12 hours later is difficult.

▶ Although emergency, or postcoital, contraception is not widely used in the United States, the most popular technique is to take 4 tablets of a combination of ethinyl estradiol and levonorgestrel in 2 divided dosages 12 hours apart. Several studies have demonstrated that if only a single act of unprotected intercourse occurs at midcycle, ingestion of 4 of these oral contraceptive tablets will prevent approximately 75% of the pregnancies that would have occurred without ingestion of these agents. The results of this analysis indicate that the incidence of pregnancy occurring when the tablets are initially ingested 1, 2, or 3 days after the unprotected coitus are similar and range from 1.6% to 2.2%. Thus, if women do not have immediate access to this type of oral contraceptive formulation, the same level of protection will occur if they ingest the first tablets within the first 24 hours or 1 or 2 days later.

D.R. Mishell, Jr., M.D.

17 Abortion

Thyroid Autoantibodies in Euthyroid Non-pregnant Women With Recurrent Spontaneous Abortions
Bussen S, Steck T (Univ of Würzburg, Germany)
Hum Reprod 10:2938–2940, 1995   17–1

Introduction.—Autoimmune dysfunction has been implicated in the etiology of recurrent spontaneous abortion (RSA). Thyroid autoantibodies have been associated with an increased risk of RSA, and it has been suggested that the association may be causal. However, this association has not been thoroughly investigated. As a step in this investigation, the incidence of thyroid autoantibodies was determined in euthyroid nonpregnant women with a history of RSA and in euthyroid nonpregnant women without such a history.

Methods.—Sera were obtained from 22 nonpregnant women with at least 3 consecutive pregnancy losses and 2 control groups: 22 nulligravidas and 22 multigravidas, all with no endocrine dysfunction and no history of pregnancy loss. The samples were analyzed for the presence of thyroid peroxidase antibodies and thyreoglobulin antibodies.

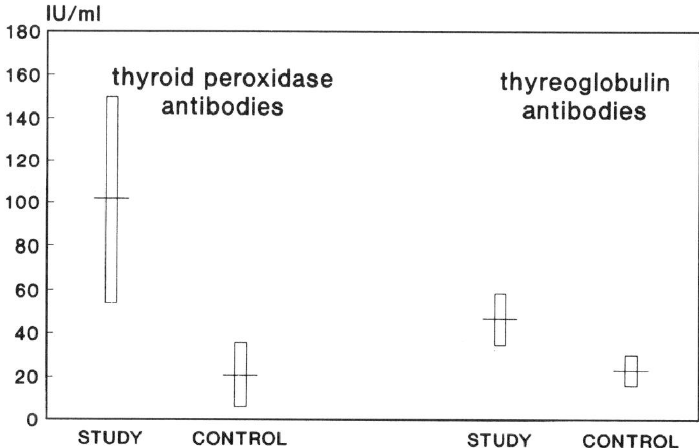

FIGURE 1.—Thyroid peroxidase and thyreoglobulin antibody concentrations in the study and control groups (mean ± SE). (Courtesy of Bussen S, Steck T: Thyroid autoantibodies in euthyroid non-pregnant women with recurrent spontaneous abortions. *Hum Reprod* 10:2938–2940, 1995, by permission of Oxford University Press.)

"

Results.—Positive titers for thyroid peroxidase, thyreoglobulin, or both were found in 36% of the women with a history of RSA, but only 9% of the nulligravida controls and 5% of the multigravida controls, which was a statistically significant difference (Fig 1). Antibodies to thyroid peroxidase were detected in 5 women with RSA and 1 woman in each control group. Thyreoglobulin antibodies were detected in 4 women with RSA, 1 nulligravida, and none of the multigravidas.

Conclusions.—Euthyroid women with a history of RSA have a significantly increased incidence of thyroid antibodies, compared with euthyroid women without a history of RSA. Thyroid antibodies may serve as a marker for RSA related to autoimmune dysfunction. Screening for thyroid antibodies should be included in the evaluation of women with RSA.

▶ Several published studies indicate that there is a much higher incidence of antithyroid antibodies among a group of women with RSA than in a control group. In this study, approximately one third of women with RSA had antithyroid antibodies in their circulation. It appears that these antithyroid antibodies are a risk marker for recurrent abortion but not necessarily a cause of the abortion. All the women were euthyroid, with normal thyroid function tests. Measurements of these antibodies should be performed as part of the diagnostic evaluation of women with recurrent abortion. However, when thyroid antibodies are present, as yet no therapy has been shown to improve pregnancy outcome.

D.R. Mishell, Jr., M.D.

Antiphospholipid Antibodies and β_2-Glycoprotein-I in 500 Women With Recurrent Miscarriage: Results of a Comprehensive Screening Approach

Rai TS, Regan L, Clifford K, et al (St Mary's Hosp, London; Central Middlesex Hosp, London; Univ College Hosp, London)
Hum Reprod 10:2001–2005, 1995   17–2

Background.—Antiphospholipid antibodies (APAs)—the lupus anticoagulant (LA) and/or anticardiolipin antibodies (ACA)—are associated with recurrent miscarriage. However, there is marked interlaboratory variation in the detection of APA. The prevalence of APA in women with 3 or more consecutive pregnancy losses was determined using standardized laboratory protocols.

Methods and Findings.—Five hundred consecutive women, aged 19–45 years, underwent screening for the presence of LA and/or ACA. All had a history of recurrent miscarriage (median, 4; range, 3–16). On the initial sample, 26.4% of the women were LA- or ACA-positive. Of these 132 women, 14.6% were LA-positive; 9%, IgG ACA–positive; and 6.2%, IgM ACA–positive. The first 300 women screened for LA underwent activated partial thromboplastin time (APTT), kaolin clotting time (KCT), and dilute Russell's viper venom time (dRVVT) testing. The dRVVT identified

LA in 6.7% of these women, and the APTT and KCT detected it in 1%. Ninety-six percent of the women with an initial positive dRVVT test ratio had a second test done on a sample obtained 8 weeks or more after the initial sample. In 65.7%, the dRVVT was positive again. Thus, 9.6% of the total group had a persistently positive LA. Nine percent of the overall group had positive IgG ACA findings and 6.2% positive IgM ACA findings on initial testing. Eight or more weeks later, only 36.6% of these women were IgG ACA–positive and 36.0% were IgM ACA–positive. Thus, 3.3% of the women were persistently IgG ACA–positive, and 2.2% were persistently IgM ACA–positive. Positive LA findings were uncorrelated with positive IgG or IgM ACA findings. Two thirds of the APA-positive women had had only early miscarriages. None of the 250 women with negative ACA findings initially had a subsequent positive ACA finding.

Conclusions.—The dRVVT with a platelet neutralization procedure identified LA significantly more often than did the APTT or the KCT in women with recurrent miscarriage. Before primary antiphospholipid syndrome can be diagnosed, APA must have been shown on at least 2 occasions.

▶ The results of this very large series of women with recurrent abortion help to further clarify the association between 2 APAs, LA and ACA, and recurrent abortion. The finding that a positive antibody test may be transient indicates that the test should be repeated after an interval of more than 2 months to determine whether the antibody is permanently present. The finding that the dRVVT was more sensitive than the KCT or the APTT to detect LA indicates that the dRVVT is the best test to be used in women with recurrent abortion to determine whether LA is present. About 15% of women with recurrent abortion of undetermined etiology will have 1 of these antibodies present. If antibodies are present, the abortion occurs more frequently in the first trimester than the second. Whether therapy with prednisone, heparin, or aspirin or a combination of these agents yields a greater incidence of viable pregnancies than does placebo in women with these antibodies remains to be determined, but treatment with heparin and aspirin is now the recommended therapeutic regimen for women with recurrent abortion who have either of these antibodies present.

D.R. Mishell, Jr., M.D.

Antibodies to Oxidized Low-density Lipoprotein and to Cardiolipin in Nonpregnant and Pregnant Women With Habitual Abortion
Tulppala M, Ailus K, Palosuo T, et al (Univ Central Hosp of Helsinki; Natl Public Health Inst, Helsinki)
Fertil Steril 64:947–950, 1995
17–3

Objective.—Because titers of circulating antibody against oxidized low-density lipoprotein (LDL) are elevated in preeclamptic women, a study was planned to identify these antibodies in nonpregnant women and in expectant women with a history of habitual abortion.

Study Population.—Forty-two women who had had 3 to 7 consecutive miscarriages, occurring at a median gestational age of 8 weeks, formed the study group. Half of them had never delivered a child. All these women conceived during a median follow-up of 7 months. Twelve of the 39 initially viable pregnancies ended in miscarriage, whereas 27 led to the birth of a healthy child. Twenty-three healthy nonpregnant women and 22 pregnant women with no past abortions also were studied.

Methods.—A solid-phase enzyme-linked immunosorbent assay was used to measure immunoglobulin G antibodies to malondialdehyde-modified LDL. Anticardiolipin antibodies also were estimated.

Results.—Both groups of pregnant women had relatively low median titers of antibody to oxidized LDL. Nine of the habitual aborters with initially viable pregnancies (23%) had increased antibody titers during pregnancy, whether or not the pregnancy continued or ended in miscarriage. The same proportion of habitual aborters had detectable anticardiolipin antibody when pregnant, but increased titers were more frequent in those who miscarried in their current pregnancies. Three of the 27 ongoing pregnancies were complicated by preeclampsia, and fetal growth retardation was noted in 5 instances.

Conclusion.—These findings do not support a role for antibody against oxidized LDL in determining the outcome of a current pregnancy in habitually aborting women.

High Prospective Fetal Loss Rate in Untreated Pregnancies of Women With Recurrent Miscarriage and Antiphospholipid Antibodies

Rai RS, Clifford K, Regan L (St Mary's Hosp, London)
Hum Reprod 10:3301–3304, 1995   17–4

Introduction.—Antiphospholipid antibodies (APA), lupus anticoagulant, and anticardiolipin antibodies have been linked to the primary antiphospholipid syndrome, which consists of recurrent miscarriage, thrombosis, and thrombocytopenia. Very high miscarriage rates have been reported in retrospective studies of women with APA, but these studies have failed to establish a temporal relationship between APA and pregnancy loss. The untreated pregnancy outcomes of APA-positive women with a history of recurrent miscarriage were prospectively studied.

Methods.—The study included 20 pregnant women with persistently positive tests for APA and a history of 3 or more consecutive pregnancy losses. All women declined treatment—low-dose aspirin, alone or with heparin—for their subsequent pregnancy. None of the women had systemic lupus erythematosus or a history of thromboembolic disease. The pregnancy outcomes were compared with those of 100 consecutive women who had a history of recurrent miscarriage but no apparent underlying cause for their pregnancy losses.

Results.—The miscarriage rate was 90% in the women with APA, compared with 34% in the control group. All but a few of the miscarriages in both groups occurred during the first trimester. Fetal heart activity was twice as likely to be observed before fetal death in the APA group (86% vs. 43%).

Conclusions.—Women with APA and a history of recurrent miscarriage who are not treated during subsequent pregnancies have a high prospective fetal loss rate. Most pregnancy losses in women with APA occur during the first trimester, suggesting the need to study the effects of APA on embryonic implantation and placentation. The optimal treatment for women with APA and a history of recurrent miscarriage remains to be determined in prospective, randomized trials.

► Approximately 15% of women with recurrent spontaneous abortion have been found to have either lupus anticoagulant or anticardiolipin antibodies. The mechanism whereby the presence of these antibodies causes, or is associated with, early pregnancy loss has not been determined. The findings that nearly all abortions occurred in the first trimester and that fetal heart activity was observed in approximately 85% of the women with APA who aborted suggest that there is probably a problem with early implantation and development instead of infarction of placental vessels, as previously thought. Therapy with heparin and aspirin is now being used most frequently to treat this problem, because therapy with corticosteroid and aspirin, which was used previously, was associated with both maternal and fetal complications. Clinicians should be aware that there have been no prospective, randomized clinical trials demonstrating that any treatment of the APA syndrome is superior to no treatment for reducing pregnancy loss.

D.R. Mishell, Jr., M.D.

Second-trimester Pregnancy Loss Is Associated With Activated Protein C Resistance

Rai R, Regan L, Hadley E, et al (St Mary's Hosp, London)
Br J Haematol 92:489–490, 1996   17–5

Background.—Circulating antiphospholipid antibodies—lupus anticoagulant or anticardiolipin antibodies or both—have been noted in 12% of women with second-trimester pregnancy loss, suggesting a thrombotic etiology for second-trimester miscarriage. Most other second-trimester miscarriages are not explained by this finding, however. One important cause of familial thrombophilia and venous thrombosis is inadequate anticoagulant response to activated protein C. In individuals with a history of thrombosis, the prevalence of activated protein resistance (APCR) is reportedly 40%. Given the possible thrombotic etiology of second-trimester miscarriage and the high prevalence of APCR, a study was performed to determine whether an association between APCR and second-trimester pregnancy loss could be identified.

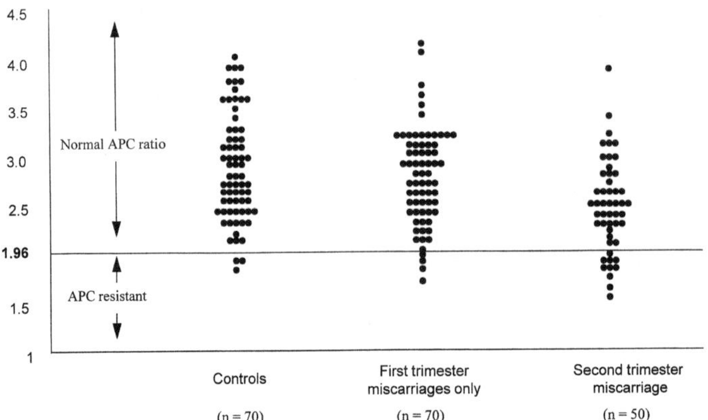

FIGURE 1.—Distribution of activated protein ratios in the 3 study groups. (Courtesy of Rai R, Regan L, Hadley E, et al: Second-trimester pregnancy loss is associated with activated protein C resistance. *Br J Haematol* 92:489–490, 1996. Published by Blackwell Science Ltd.)

Patients and Methods.—Screening for APCR was performed in 120 women evaluated at a specialist recurrent miscarriage clinic. All patients had a history of recurrent miscarriage, including first-trimester pregnancy loss in 70 patients and at least 1 second-trimester miscarriage in the other 50 patients. Seventy women without a history of miscarriage served as controls. None of the women had a history of thrombosis. All women tested negative for lupus anticoagulant and IgG and IgM anticardiolipin, and all had a normal coagulation screen. The prevalence of APCR was compared in the 3 groups.

Results.—Women who had experienced second-trimester miscarriages had a significantly higher prevalence of APCR, noted in 20% of these patients, compared with 5.7% of those who had had first-trimester miscarriages and 4.3% of the controls (Fig 1). This finding suggests that APCR may play an important role in second-trimester pregnancy loss.

Conclusions.—The prevalence of APCR was comparable between women with recurrent first-trimester miscarriages (4 of 70) and controls (3 of 70), a finding consistent with the previously reported incidence of APCR in the general population. Women with second-trimester miscarriages had a significantly higher prevalence of APCR in comparison (10 of 50), suggesting that all women with a history of second-trimester pregnancy loss should undergo APCR screening, and possibly screening for other thrombophilic abnormalities.

▶ Activated protein C cleaves and inactivates 2 of the factors that enhance thrombosis, factor Va and factor VIIIa. A genetic mutation, called factor V Leiden, produces resistance to activated protein C, with resulting increased activity of the thrombophilic factors Va and VIIIa. Individuals with APCR thus have an increased risk of having venous thromboembolism. Because this genetic mutation is relatively common, occurring in 3% to 5% of individuals from Europe or their descendants, it is estimated that approximately 40% of all individuals who have venous thromboembolic disorders have APCR.

The etiology of recurrent spontaneous abortion can be diagnosed in at least one third of women with this problem. This study indicates that the thrombophilic effects of APCR may cause as many as 20% of pregnancy losses in the second trimester among women with a history of recurrent pregnancy loss. Therefore, a test to detect APCR should be undertaken in all women with recurrent pregnancy loss, particularly if it occurs in the second trimester. If the disorder is found to be present, treatment with heparin and low-dose aspirin should be initiated as soon as a subsequent pregnancy is diagnosed in an attempt to prevent thrombosis in the placental vessels.

D.R. Mishell, Jr., M.D.

The Effect of Serum Follicular Phase Luteinizing Hormone Concentrations in Habitual Abortion: Correlation With Results of Paternal Leukocyte Immunization

Carp HJA, Hass Y, Dolicky M, et al (Sheba Med Ctr, Tel Hashomer, Israel; Sackler School of Medicine, Tel Aviv, Israel)
Hum Reprod 10:1702–1705, 1995

17–6

Introduction.—Recurrent miscarriage has been recently linked to aberrant immunologic responses to fetal antigens and increased luteinizing hormone concentrations. In a large series of women who habitually abort, the incidence of increased luteinizing hormone concentrations was determined. Outcomes of further pregnancies were compared in women who habitually abort who have either normal luteinizing concentrations or increased circulating luteinizing concentrations. Elevated circulating luteinizing concentrations were assessed to determine whether they affect the efficacy of immunization with paternal leukocytes.

Methods.—The study included 153 women, aged 20–44 years, who had 3 to 8 miscarriages. On days 5–7 of the cycle, serum luteinizing hormone and follicle-stimulating hormone concentrations were assessed. To determine the presence of antipaternal cytotoxic antibodies, a cytotoxic crossmatch was conducted on all patients, and those testing positive for antipaternal cytotoxic antibodies were excluded. Those who tested negative received immunizations at 3- to 4-week intervals, or some elected to forgo immunization.

Results.—Of the 153 women, 97 (62.2%) had luteinizing hormone concentrations of less than 10 mIU/mL, and 56 (35.9%) had luteinizing hormone concentrations that were greater than 10 mIU/mL. During the study, 103 of 153 couples conceived, and of the 103 pregnancies, 65 (63.1%) resulted in a birth of a live infant. There was no statistical significance between women with low or high luteinizing hormone concentrations, even though the pregnancy outcome was slightly better for women with low concentrations. Higher live birth rates (75.8%) were seen with women immunized with paternal leukocytes than with those who were not immunized (43.6%).

Conclusion.—Although increased luteinizing hormone concentrations are not the major cause of recurrent abortion, they may be associated with habitual abortion in a small population. In some habitual aborters, paternal leukocyte immunization increases the chance of a subsequent live birth.

▶ Controversy exists regarding the 2 parameters analyzed in this study of a large group of women with recurrent abortion. Some investigators have found that women with elevated follicular-phase luteinizing hormone (LH) levels have a greater risk of spontaneous abortion than do women with levels less than 10 mIU/mL, whereas others have not demonstrated that such an association exists. In this study, the live birth rate was 67% in women with low LH levels and 56% in those with high LH levels, but the differences were not statistically significant. Paternal white blood cell immunization has not been found to significantly increase live birth rates compared with controls in most randomized clinical trials. However, a recent meta-analysis of the data from all randomized trials indicated that there might be a slight significant benefit from paternal white blood cell immunization. In this study, paternal white cell infusion was associated with a markedly improved live birth rate (75%), compared with women who elected not to receive the infusion (44%), but this trial was not randomized and the live birth rate in the nonimmunized women was lower than that reported in the control group of other investigators. In conclusion, the data reported in this study do not clarify the confusion regarding the exact relation between elevated LH levels and etiology, and immunization of paternal white blood cells for the therapy of recurrent abortion. Each of these parameters may have a role in the etiology and treatment of recurrent abortion, but more data are needed to determine their precise relation.

D.R. Mishell, Jr., M.D.

A Comparison of Meta-analytic Results Using Literature vs Individual Patient Data: Paternal Cell Immunization for Recurrent Miscarriage
Jeng GT, Scott JR, Burmeister LF (Univ of Iowa, Iowa City; Univ of Utah, Salt Lake City)
JAMA 274:830–836, 1995
17–7

Introduction.—Meta-analysis can be used to validate treatment results by synthesizing the results from multiple studies of a specific topic. However, meta-analytic conclusions can be conflicting when different meta-analytic methods are used. The differences between meta-analysis using individual patient data and meta-analysis of the literature were evaluated using original data from studies on immunotherapy with injections of the paternal white blood cells in women with recurrent miscarriages.

Methods.—Only data from randomized, controlled trials of paternal leukocyte immunization for the management of unexplained recurrent miscarriage were used. Meta-analyses were performed with either data from the literature (MAL) or with individual patient data (MAP). The

Trials	No. of Patients	RR (95% CI)
4 Published	202	1.29 (1.03-1.60)
4 Published (Updated)	239	1.17 (0.97-1.37)
4 Unpublished	140	1.01 (0.74-1.28)
4 Published	202	1.38 (0.89-1.87)
4 Published (Updated)	239	1.18 (0.98-1.42)
4 Unpublished	140	1.01 (0.74-1.28)

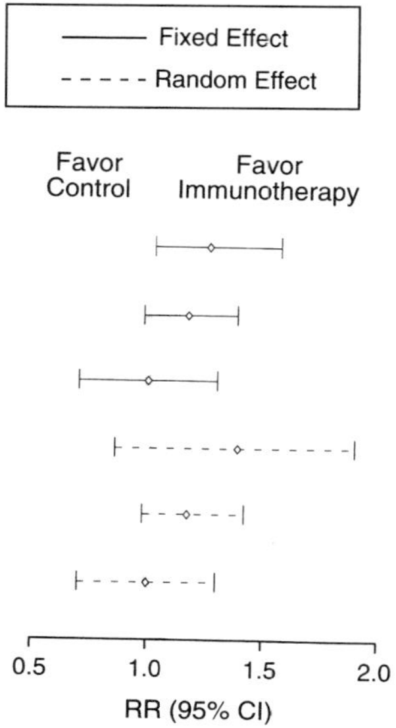

FIGURE 1.—Publication bias: comparisons of published trials (original and updated) and unpublished trials. Number of trials, number of patients, relative live-birth ratios (*RRs*), and 95% confidence intervals (*CIs*) are displayed. (Courtesy of Jeng GT, Scott JR, Burmeister LF: A comparison of meta-analytic results using literature vs individual patient data: Paternal cell immunization for recurrent miscarriage. *JAMA* 274:830–836, Copyright 1995, American Medical Association.)

trends in overall treatment effect with the addition of new trial results were identified with cumulative meta-analysis of sequentially added trial data. Publication bias and the effect of adjustment of prognostic variables were investigated.

Results.—Data were available from 239 patients from 4 published studies and 140 patients from 4 unpublished trials. With MAL, there was a statistically significant effect of immunotherapy using the fixed-effects model but not with the random-effects model. With MAP, there was no statistically significant effect of immunotherapy with either the fixed-effects or the random-effects model. There was a greater benefit of immunotherapy in the published than in the unpublished trials, and a decreased treatment effect was observed as data from succeeding trials were added to the analysis (Fig 1). Patients in the treatment group were older and had more previous miscarriages than did the control group; adjustment for these prognostic factors increased the treatment effect for the MAP.

Conclusions.—Meta-analysis of studies of immunotherapy in the management of recurrent miscarriage yielded significantly different results, depending on the meta-analytic methods, with a consistently greater estimate of a treatment benefit with MAL than MAP. Publication bias and the effect of adjustment of prognostic variables also had a significant effect on the findings. Therefore, the effect of immunotherapy for the management of recurrent miscarriage is still inconclusive.

▶ Only one of several randomized trials of paternal white blood cell infusion for women with recurrent spontaneous abortion of undetermined etiology has shown a significant benefit for such therapy. Because most trials consist of small numbers of women, the technique of meta-analysis has been used to determine whether immunotherapy may have a beneficial effect. However, the results of this methodology using individual patient data sheets from both published and unpublished randomized trials fail to demonstrate that there is a significantly increased live-birth rate with immunotherapy with paternal leukocyte infusion. Such therapy is costly and may be associated with severe adverse long-term effects on the health of the recipients. As benefit has not been proved to exist, such therapy should be considered experimental and should only be performed without cost to the patient as part of an approved investigative clinical trial.

D.R. Mishell, Jr., M.D.

Serum CA 125 and First Trimester Abortion
Scarpellini F, Mastrone M, Sbracia M, et al (Univ of Rome 'La Sapienza')
Int J Gynecol Obstet 49:259–264, 1995
17–8

Introduction.—Present methods for diagnosing fetal demise and miscarriage are limited to clinical findings and ultrasonography. The value of using serum CA 125 with serum β-human chorionic gonadotropin (hCG) in predicting pregnancy outcome was assessed.

Methods.—The CA 125 serum levels were compared with β-hCG levels in 100 women with singleton pregnancies with a gestational age ranging from 6 to 11 weeks. Transvaginal and transabdominal ultrasound examinations were performed to assess the presence of a gestational sac and a viable embryo in utero. One week later, ultrasound was repeated to determine ongoing pregnancies and threatened abortions. Patients were assigned to 1 of 2 groups. Group 1 had 52 women with nonthreatened pregnancies, and group 2 had 48 women with threatened abortions.

Results.—Nineteen women (39.6%) in group 2 aborted and no women in group 1 aborted. The mean serum CA 125 values of women in group 2 were constantly higher compared with values of women in group 1. In 15 of the 19 abortions (78.9%), the CA 125 serum values and β-hCG values were significantly higher compared with those in women with viable pregnancies. The use of the 2 markers together showed a sensitivity of 78.9%, a specificity of 96.5%, a positive predictive value (PPV) of 93.7%, a negative predictive value (NPV) of 87.5%, and an odds ratio of 105. For β-hCG alone, the sensitivity was 57.9%, the specificity was 86.2%, the PPV was 73.3%, the NPV was 75.7%, and the odds ratio was 8.59. For CA 125 alone, the sensitivity was 78.9%, the specificity was 75.8%, the PPV was 68.1%, the NPV was 84.6%, and the odds ratio was 11.7. There was a close correlation between CA 125 values and the ultrasonographic extent of trophodecidual hematoma.

Conclusion.—Evaluation of serum β-hCG and CA 125 helps discriminate better between threatened pregnancies with a poor outcome and those with a favorable outcome. Compared with each one alone, the use of CA 125 and β-hCG together provides a remarkable improvement in specificity and positive and negative predictivity.

▶ The presence of bleeding in the first trimester of a pregnancy is relatively common but causes great concern to the pregnant woman. The results of this study indicate that if a woman has a threatened abortion, the finding of an elevated CA 125 level is associated with a poor prognosis for the pregnancy. When combined with a low level of hCG, under 45,000 mIU/mL, if the CA 125 was above 120 mIU/mL, 15 of the 16 women with threatened abortion in this study did abort the pregnancy. If the CA 125 was less than 95 mIU/mL, all women with threatened abortion did not abort and had a viable pregnancy. Clinicians should consider measuring both β-hCG and CA 125 in women with threatened abortion who have evidence of a viable pregnancy that is visualized sonographically to provide a better prognosis of the outcome of their pregnancies.

D.R. Mishell, Jr., M.D.

The Role of a Single Progesterone Measurement in the Diagnosis of Early Pregnancy Failure and the Prognosis of Fetal Viability

Al-Sebai MAH, Kingsland CR, Diver M, et al (Royal Liverpool Univ, England; Alder Hey Hosp, Liverpool, England)
Br J Obstet Gynaecol 102:364–369, 1995   17–9

Introduction.—Hormonal assessment may be as informative as ultrasound scanning in diagnosing miscarriage, because progesterone production may be defective for days or weeks before miscarriage occurs. In the diagnosis of early pregnancy failure and the prognosis of fetal viability, the value of a single estimation of maternal serum progesterone levels at the time of vaginal bleeding, with or without abdominal pain, was investigated.

Methods.—Four hundred eighty-nine consecutive women in the first 18 weeks of pregnancy were compared with 131 women with singleton intrauterine pregnancies having lower abdominal pain. Of these, 358 women had an intrauterine pregnancy with vaginal bleeding with or without abdominal pain, or they had a tubal pregnancy with lower abdominal pain with or without vaginal bleeding. For estimation of progesterone, a sample of blood was taken.

Results.—In the comparison group of 131 women who had an uncomplicated pregnancy at least until 28 weeks, the mean progesterone level was 86.4 nmol/L. In the threatened-continuing pregnancies, vaginal bleeding with or without abdominal pain was found in 148 women whose pregnancy continued until at least 28 weeks, and their mean progesterone level was 77 nmol/L. In the noncontinuing pregnancy group, 175 women had missed abortions, empty sacs, incomplete abortions, or complete abortions. Their mean progesterone level was 14.5 nmol/L. In the tubal pregnancy group, 35 women had a mean progesterone level of 11.9 nmol/L.

Conclusions.—Significantly lower progesterone levels were found in the tubal pregnancy and the intrauterine noncontinuing groups when compared with the comparison group and the threatened-continuing pregnancies. The cutoff level for serum progesterone was 45 nmol/L to differentiate between viable pregnancies that continued to 28 weeks' gestation and miscarriages or tubal pregnancies. A single measurement of progesterone may be used to diagnose early pregnancy failure and to give an immediate prognosis of fetal viability.

▶ Three techniques have been used to provide information regarding the prognosis of women with threatened abortion. Transvaginal sonography is useful at 8 weeks of gestation or later. Serial human chorionic gonadotropin measurements are of value prior to 7 weeks of gestation. A single progesterone assay, as was found in this study, appears to be useful throughout the first trimester and early second trimester of pregnancy. Clinicians can use 1 or more of these modalities to assist them in offering women with threatened abortion a reliable assessment of the likelihood of having the pregnancy terminate or continue to fetal viability.

D.R. Mishell, Jr., M.D.

Ultrasonographic Characteristics of First-trimester Gestations in Recurrent Spontaneous Aborters
Cunningham DS, Bledsoe LD, Tichenor JR, et al (Natl Naval Med Ctr, Bethesda, Md)
J Reprod Med 40:565–570, 1995   17–10

Background.—Currently, there are no completely reliable methods for distinguishing a normal from an abnormal gestation in recurrent spontaneous aborters (RSAs). Serial ultrasound findings during the first trimester of pregnancy in women with a history of primary recurrent spontaneous abortion were compiled for the first time to determine the dynamics of early normal and abnormal gestations.

Methods.—Forty women were enrolled in the study. Four groups were represented in equal numbers: RSAs and primiparas with successful and unsuccessful gestations. Transvaginal sonograms were acquired every week from 5 to 12 weeks' gestational age.

Findings.—Embryonic heart motion was identified in 40% to 50% of the successful pregnancies in the fifth week of gestation and in the rest by week 6. Heart motion was identified in no more than half the pregnancies that subsequently failed. All failed pregnancies were detected by the eighth week of gestation, including those with previously documented viability. In failed pregnancies, the gestational sac size and crown-rump length were smaller than expected. The sac size difference was apparent as early as week 5, and the crown-rump length difference was apparent by week 7.

Conclusions.—When performed at the right time, ultrasound assessment can serve as an effective prognosticator of a pregnancy. Vaginal ultrasound examination at 8 weeks' estimated gestational age is justified in RSAs to provide realistic feedback to anxious couples.

▶ Normal embryonic development occurs in early gestation much more frequently when spontaneous abortion occurs in RSAs than when it occurs in the general population. In the general population, the abortion is usually due to a chromosomal or genetic disorder in the embryo, whereas in RSAs, the embryo is more frequently normal and abortion occurs because of an abnormality in the maternal environment. Thus, it is not surprising that although the rate of abortion is only 2% to 7% after finding embryonic heart activity in early gestation in the general population, the rate of abortion after finding normal fetal heart activity in early pregnancy in RSAs is 30%. Therefore, the finding of heart rate activity prior to 7 weeks' gestation does not provide as good a prognosis in RSAs as in the general population. However, if heart rate activity is present at 8 weeks' gestation in women both with and without recurrent abortion, the prognosis for a viable infant is quite good and the women can be so informed.

D.R. Mishell, Jr., M.D.

Misoprostol in the Management of Spontaneous Abortion

Chung TKH, Cheung LP, Leung TY, et al (Chinese Univ of Hong Kong; Prince of Wales Hosp, Hong Kong)
Br J Obstet Gynaecol 102:832–835, 1995   17–11

Introduction.—Traditionally, patients with spontaneous abortions have undergone surgical evacuation of the uterus. However, incomplete spontaneous abortion could also be managed with uterotonic agents, including misoprostol, an orally active prostaglandin analogue. The efficacy of misoprostol in patients with spontaneous abortion was investigated to assess its therapeutic role for these patients.

Methods.—Over a 5-month period, 252 women with spontaneous abortions were observed. Those with no evidence on transvaginal ultrasound of significant amounts of conception products were discharged and evaluated 1 to 2 weeks later; evaluation included the performance of a urinary pregnancy test. Women with significant amounts of gestation products were given 400 μg of oral misoprostol every 4 hours for a maximum of 3 doses. They were reassessed clinically and with transvaginal ultrasound the next morning, and those who still retained significant products of gestation underwent surgical evacuation of the uterus.

Results.—The spontaneous abortions occurred at a mean gestation of 9 weeks. Of the 252 women in the study, 141 had ultrasonic evidence of significant retained products of gestation. Of these 141 patients who were given misoprostol, 62% did not require subsequent surgical evacuation of the uterus. There were no significant differences in the infection rate in the groups, with infection occurring in 3% of those treated with misoprostol alone, in 4% of the women who underwent curettage after misoprostol treatment, and in 3% of those discharged without any treatment. Among the women treated with misoprostol, 3 had prolonged bleeding for more than 4 weeks, 11 had irregular bleeding for at least 3 months, and 1 had a molar pregnancy. There were few and minor side effects of misoprostol, including nausea and vomiting, diarrhea, headaches, dizziness, transient pyrexia, and transient hypotension.

Conclusions.—For 78% of the study population, including more than 60% of those treated with misoprostol, curettage was not needed and complications were not increased unacceptably. The avoidance of curettage represents a substantial benefit and cost saving. These findings justify further study of the use of misoprostol as the primary treatment in the management of spontaneous abortion.

▶ In this study of a large group of women with spontaneous incomplete abortion in early pregnancy, use of oral misoprostol effected the emptying of the uterine cavity and avoided the use of a curettage in two thirds of the women. Since as many as 3 doses of misoprostol were given every 4 hours, most women needed to stay in the hospital for at least 12 hours, and some had either prolonged or heavy bleeding after the medical treatment. Most women in the United States with an incomplete abortion are presently treated in an emergency room facility by curettage with local anesthesia; therefore, this medical treatment does not appear to be cost-effective. Nevertheless, with different dosages of misoprostol and use of vaginal administration, it may become cost-effective to use this agent in certain circumstances. More studies of the use of misoprostol for treating spontaneous abortion are warranted.

D.R. Mishell, Jr., M.D.

A Randomized Trial Comparing Misoprostol Three and Seven Days After Methotrexate for Early Abortion

Creinin MD, Vittinghoff E, Galbraith S, et al (Univ of California, San Francisco)
Am J Obstet Gynecol 173:1578–1584, 1995   17–12

Background.—Intramuscular methotrexate followed by misoprostol administered vaginally can induce abortion at 8 weeks' gestation or less. Only 60% of women will have their abortion on the day they receive misoprostol, whether for the first or second time. This proportion might increase if more time were allowed for methotrexate to destabilize the trophoblastic attachment. The benefits of giving misoprostol vaginally 3 vs. 7 days after intramuscular methotrexate were examined in a randomized, controlled trial.

Methods.—Eighty-seven women desiring abortion at 56 days' gestation or less received intramuscular methotrexate, 50 mg/m². They were then randomly assigned to received misoprostol intravaginally 3 days (group 1) or 7 days (group 2) later. Misoprostol was given in four 200-µg tablets, and this dose was repeated 4 days later if necessary. Patients were instructed to avoid high-folate foods for 2 weeks or until the abortion occurred.

Results.—Abortion without a surgical procedure occurred in 83% of women in group 1 (95% confidence interval 69% to 92%) and 98% of women in group 2 (95% confidence interval 87% to 100%). In group 1, 50% of patients had an abortion after the first dose of misoprostol. The rest received a second dose of misoprostol: 35% passed the pregnancy that day and 39% after a delay. In all, 65% of women in group 1 had a complete abortion on the same day as they received the first or second dose of misoprostol. Sixty percent of women in group 2 passed the pregnancy after the initial dose of misoprostol, and 68% aborted on the same day as the first or second dose.

For women in whom abortion was delayed, the mean delay was 24 days after methotrexate injection in group 1 and 28 days in group 2. Vaginal bleeding lasted 9 days in group 1 and 8 days in group 2; spotting lasted 5 days in group 1 and 8 days in group 2; and total bleeding and spotting lasted 14 days in group 1 and 17 days in group 2. None of the women needed curettage because of hemorrhage, and none needed transfusion. The 3 significant predictors of treatment success, on univariate analysis, were study group, odds ratio, 8.2; gravidity of less than 4, odds ratio, 5.7; and parity of less than 2, odds ratio, 4.4. Side effects were infrequent, but included nausea, vomiting, diarrhea, headache, and dizziness after methotrexate and nausea, vomiting, and diarrhea after misoprostol.

Conclusions.—Giving misoprostol intravaginally 7 rather than 3 days after intramuscular methotrexate for early-gestation abortion makes no difference in the immediate success rate. However, the longer wait is significantly more effective in inducing complete abortion. This approach provides a useful alternative to surgical abortion or to medical abortion with antiprogestins and prostaglandin.

▶ The progesterone antagonist RU 486 is not currently available in the United States and will not be available for several years, if ever. Therefore, if women wish to electively terminate an early gestation medically instead of by surgical evacuation, the use of a combination of methotrexate and misoprostol has been found to be effective.

When misoprostol was given 7 days instead of 3 days after methotrexate, the complete abortion rate increased from 83% to 98%. This finding indicates that the 7-day regimen is probably more effective. One drawback of this method is that only about two thirds of the women aborted shortly after misoprostol was given. The other one third of women who aborted needed to wait nearly an additional month to abort. Another problem is that most of the women had uterine bleeding for several weeks, whether they aborted early or late. Despite these disadvantages, the avoidance of a surgical procedure and the ability to be treated in an office setting are reasons why some women may wish to choose this way to electively terminate early gestation.

D.R. Mishell, Jr., M.D.

Methotrexate and Misoprostol for Early Abortion: A Multicenter Trial. I. Safety and Efficacy
Creinin MD, Vittinghoff E, Keder L, et al (Univ of Pittsburgh, Pa; Univ of California, San Francisco; Women's Health Care Services, Wichita, Kansas)
Contraception 53:321–327, 1996   17–13

Background.—Several studies have shown that IM injection of methotrexate 50 mg/m^2 followed by misoprostol insertion induces abortion in the first 56 days of gestation. However, the safety and efficacy of this procedure have yet to be assessed at multiple sites using a single protocol.

Methods.—The current multicenter study included 300 pregnant women seeking elective abortion. Seven days after the IM injection of methotrexate, 50 mg/m^2, the patients returned for vaginally administered

TABLE 3.—Cumulative Abortion Rate (N = 300)

	Abortion Rate	Incomplete Abortion*
Before misoprostol	2 (0.7%)	
After first dose of misoprostol†	158 (52.7%)	4 (2.5%)
After second dose of misoprostol†	203 (67.7%)	8 (3.9%)
By follow-up on day 14	209 (69.7%)	8 (3.8%)
By day 21	232 (77.3%)	11 (4.7%)
By day 28	263 (87.7%)	13 (4.9%)
By day 35	275 (91.7%)	13 (4.7%)
By day 80	277 (92.3%)	14 (5.1%)

*Includes 1 patient with a surgical aspiration for hemorrhage (day 9).
†Within 24 hours of misoprostol administration.
(Reprinted by permission of the publisher from Creinin MD, Vittinghoff E, Keder L, et al: Methotrexate and misoprostol for early abortion: A multicenter trial. I. Safety and efficacy. *Contraception* 53:321–327, 1996. Copyright 1996 by Elsevier Science Inc.)

misoprostol, 800 µg. Four 200-g tablets were placed into the vagina through a speculum. As the speculum was removed, the tablets were pushed into the posterior fornix with a large cotton swab. Patients were permitted to get up immediately after misoprostol was administered. A vaginal ultrasound examination was performed 1 and 5 days later. A surgical abortion was done when cardiac activity was still present after the second ultrasonography. Patients returned 4 weeks later for a follow-up assessment.

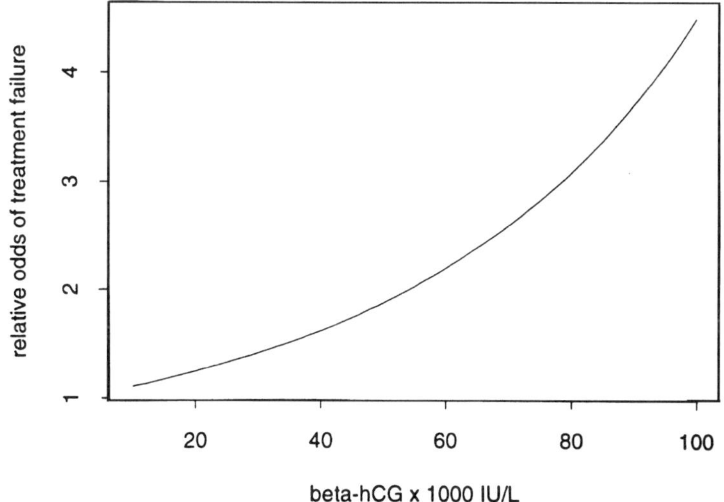

FIGURE 1.—Odds of treatment failure based on serum β-human chorionic gonadotropin (β-hCG) on the day of methotrexate injection. (Reprinted by permission of the publisher from Creinin MD, Vittinghoff E, Keder L, et al: Methotrexate and misoprostol for early abortion: A multicenter trial. I. Safety and efficacy. *Contraception* 53:321–327, 1996. Copyright 1996 by Elsevier Science Inc.)

Findings.—Overall, abortion occurred with no need for surgery in 87.7% of the women. The complete abortion rate was 90.6% in women with gestations of less than 49 days and 81.6% in women with gestations of 50–56 days. In 65% of women, abortion occurred within 24 hours of the initial or repeat misoprostol dose. In the remaining 22.7% of women who aborted, abortion was delayed by a mean of 23.6 days. The success rate after the first misoprostol dose was greater between days 43 and 56 compared to before day 43 (Table 3). In almost all the women, bleeding and/or cramping began within 3.3 hours after the first misoprostol dose. Patients in whom the procedure was immediately successful had vaginal bleeding lasting a mean of 10 days and spotting for a mean of 4 days. In women with delayed abortion, vaginal bleeding lasted a mean of 7 days and spotting a mean of 4 days. None of the women needed a transfusion. In a univariate analysis, gravidity of less than 3, lower gestational age, and lower serum β-human chorionic gonadotropin on the day of methotrexate injection significantly predicted treatment success (Fig 1).

Conclusions.—Methotrexate followed by misoprostol is an effective and safe alternative to surgical abortion and the use of antiprogestins and prostaglandin for medical abortion. The adverse effects of methotrexate and misoprostol administration were minimal.

▶ This large multicenter study confirms the fact that the sequential use of a single IM injection of methotrexate followed by vaginally administered misoprostol is an effective method of electively terminating a pregnancy of less than 7 weeks gestational age from onset of the last menses, with a success rate of about 90%. Problems with this medical therapy are the fact that only two thirds of the women aborted within 24 hours of the last misoprostol dose. Most of the remaining one third of women who do abort do not do so until 2–3 weeks later. In addition, the women who do abort bleed an average of about 2 weeks and in some instances for as long as 6–8 weeks. Finally, about one third of the women experience nausea, vomiting, or diarrhea. Koppersmith et al.[1] reported that about two thirds of women in early pregnancy treated with vaginal misoprostol alone, without methotrexate, had a successful abortion within 48 hours without the gastrointestinal side effects of methotrexate. These investigators did not extend their study beyond that time period but performed vaginal evacuation of the uterine cavity if abortion had failed to occur within 12 hours after receiving the last study medication. Until an antiprogestin is available for use in the United States, if a woman wishes to terminate her pregnancy medically, perhaps vaginal misoprostol alone without methotrexate should still be given. For the one third of women who fail to abort, uterine evacuation can be performed to avoid the prolonged duration of uterine bleeding and need for careful evaluation, as well as avoiding the side effects of methotrexate.

D.R. Mishell, Jr., M.D.

Methotrexate and Misoprostol to Terminate Early Pregnancy

Hausknecht RU (Mount Sinai School of Medicine, New York)
N Engl J Med 333:537–540, 1995   17–14

Introduction.—Medical termination of pregnancy has been available in China and Europe for more than 5 years. Political and social resistance in the United States has delayed testing until recently. The combination of methotrexate and misoprostol for the medical induction of abortion was studied.

Methods.—Of 209 women seeking termination of pregnancy, 178 fulfilled study criteria, which included intrauterine pregnancy of 63 days' duration or less. A complete medical examination that included medical history and a vaginal ultrasound examination was performed. Patients were given an intramuscular injection of methotrexate at a dose of 50 mg/m^2 of body surface area. They returned 5–7 days later for intravaginal insertion of 800 µg of misoprostol. Alternate patients received four 200-µg vaginal suppositories that were held in place by a tampon in the vagina. Patients receiving tablets were asked to leave the tampon in place for 12 hours or until active bleeding started. Seven days after receiving misoprostol, patients returned for a bimanual pelvic examination and vaginal ultrasound examination. Vacuum aspiration was performed or a second dose of misoprostol was given if abortion did not occur.

Results.—Of 178 women, 171 (96%) had successful abortion after the first or second administration of misoprostol. The first dose of misoprostol was unsuccessful in 25 women (14%), and a second dose resulted in 18 complete abortions. Seven patients required suction curettage. No patients had pain or vaginal bleeding in fewer than 2 hours after vaginal insertion of misoprostol. Abortions occurred within 24 hours in 88% of women. No patients required blood transfusions or suction curettage for heavy bleeding. The duration of bleeding after abortion was varied, but all women ceased irregular bleeding after the first spontaneous menstrual period. Two women experienced mild stomatitis attributable to methotrexate that resolved in 48 hours without treatment. Side effects of misoprostol included brief periods of diarrhea in 9 patients, nausea greater than that experienced during pregnancy in 6 patients, and temperature elevation of 38.8°C (102°F) several hours after tablet insertion in 1 patient. Women reported they overwhelmingly preferred medical termination to surgical termination of pregnancy.

Conclusion.—Termination of early pregnancy using methotrexate and intravaginal misoprostol is safe and effective. It gives greater privacy to women and potentially allows medical abortion to become a part of the everyday practice of medicine.

▶ The results of this study indicate that 2 drugs currently available in the United States can be used to successfully terminate early intrauterine gestations. The population treated was unique, as two thirds of the study group had pregnancies with a gestational age of fewer than 6 weeks. Most women requesting pregnancy termination have pregnancies of more than 6 weeks' gestational age when they initially contact a medical facility. No information was given about the gestational age in the pregnancies of the 7 women who required suction curettage, but the failure rate was probably greater among women with pregnancies that were more than 6 weeks' gestational age than those that were less than 6 weeks' gestational age. More information is needed regarding the true success rate of this technique with gestations ranging between 6 and 9 weeks. The author also failed to provide information regarding the number of women who required vacuum aspiration 7 days after the misoprostol was given. If some women required this procedure, they should be considered failures of medical therapy. Because more information is needed regarding the effectiveness of this treatment regimen and the incidence of toxicity, clinicians should not currently offer it to patients unless performed under a research protocol.

D.R. Mishell, Jr., M.D.

Combined Methotrexate and Misoprostol for Early Induced Abortion
Schaff EA, Eisinger SH, Franks P, et al (Univ of Rochester, NY)
Arch Fam Med 4:774–779, 1995   17–15

Background.—In much of the United States, surgical abortion is not readily available, and a safe medical method of abortion that is more than 90% effective would greatly increase access to abortion. The folic acid antagonist methotrexate has been combined with misoprostol for this purpose. The latter agent has been safely used for abortion in Britain and France.

Study Design.—A prospective trial of combined methotrexate and intravaginal misoprostol was carried out in 100 consecutive pregnant women aged 18 years and older who were seen before 8 weeks' gestation and were in good general health. Methotrexate was injected intramuscularly in a dose of 50 mg/m², followed in 3 days by an 800-µg misoprostol suppository. Patients were told to insert the suppository deeply and to rest on their back for at least 30 minutes. Acetaminophen with codeine was used at 4-hour intervals as needed for cramping, and ibuprofen was a backup.

Results.—All but 2 of the 100 women had a complete abortion. Two women required surgery, 1 because a sizing error resulted in continued gestation, and 1 with heavy vaginal bleeding. Four other women had vaginal bleeding but did not require surgery. In about one fourth of women, either bleeding was delayed or the β-human chorionic gonadotropin (β-hCG) level failed to decrease by at least half within a week. An initial β-hCG level less than 10,000 IU/L predicted a delayed response (Table 2). The average time needed for the β-hCG to decline below 10 IU/L was 33 days. When questioned, the women stated convincingly that they would choose this procedure over surgical abortion, even if the response had been delayed.

TABLE 2.—Outcome Variables by Initial β-Human Chorionic Gonadotropin (hCG)

| | Initial β-hCG Value | | |
Variable	<10,000 IU/L (n = 30)	≥10,000 IU/L (n = 70)	P
	No. (%) of Subjects		
Rise in hCG on day 7	6 (20)	4 (6)	<.03
Misoprostol doses			
1	23 (77)	58 (83) ⎤	
>1	7 (23)	12 (17) ⎦	.47
Response to misoprostol			
Immediate	16 (53)	57 (81) ⎤	
Delayed	14 (47)	13 (19) ⎦	.004
Surgical intervention	0	2 (3)	...
	Mean (SD)		
% Decrease in β-hCG			
level, day 7	51.7 (66.5)	76.9 (36.5)	.02
No. of days of bleeding	9.7 (4.2)	12.0 (6.3)	.07
No. of days of heavy			
bleeding	2.3 (1.3)	2.8 (2.1)	.20
No. of days of cramping	4.4 (2.9)	4.9 (4.3)	.51
No. of days until hCG			
level <10 IU/L	25.6 (11.0)	36.8 (16.9)	.001
Overall satisfaction score			
(1=low, 5=high)	4.8 (0.4)	4.6 (0.8)	.24

(Courtesy of Schaff EA, Eisinger SH, Franks P, et al: Combined methotrexate and misoprostol for early induced abortion. *Arch Fam Med* 4:774–779, 1995. Copyright 1995, American Medical Association.)

Conclusion.—The combination of methotrexate and intravaginal misoprostol is a highly effective means of inducing abortion in the first 8 weeks of gestation.

▶ There are now several published studies that indicate that the combination of methotrexate followed a few days later by the prostaglandin analogue misoprostol is an effective method to terminate a normal early intrauterine gestation. The major problem with this method is that for a substantial proportion of women, 27% in this study, uterine bleeding does not begin until about 10 days or more after the medication is administered. In addition, the overall mean duration of bleeding was more than 10 days. The method of preparing the misoprostol in suppository instead of tablet form is innovative and may enhance the success of this medical method of performing elective pregnancy termination in the first 8 weeks of gestation.

D.R. Mishell, Jr., M.D.

18 Ectopic Pregnancy

Fertility After Ectopic Pregnancy: First Results of a Population-based Cohort Study in France
Job-Spira N, Bouyer J, Pouly JL, et al (Hôpital de Bicêtre, Clamart, France; CHU Hôtel-Dieu, Clamart, France; Hôpital Antoine Béclère, Clamart, France)
Hum Reprod 11:99–104, 1996   18–1

Purpose.—Whereas the rate of ectopic pregnancy (EP) has been increasing, there has been significant progress in early diagnosis and conservative management of EP. Presumably, these advances should improve preservation of the fallopian tube and thus reduce infertility and recurrence rates. However, there are no conclusive data on these outcomes. The reproduc-

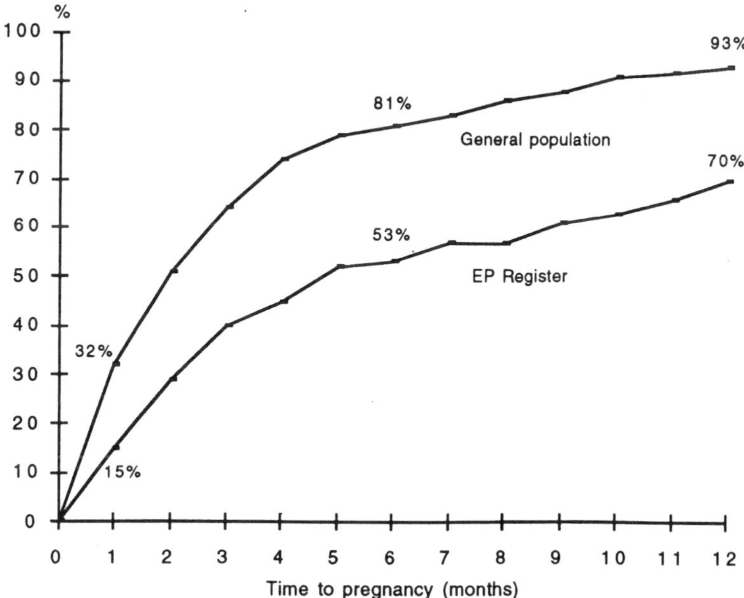

FIGURE 1.—One-year cumulative frequency of first subsequent intrauterine pregnancy in EP Register and general population. (From de Mouzon et al: A prospective study of the relation between smoking and fertility. *Int J Epidemiol* 17:378–384, 1988. Courtesy of Job-Spira N, Bouyer J, Pouly JL, et al: Fertility after ectopic pregnancy: First results of a population-based cohort study in France. *Hum Reprod* 11:99–104, 1996, by permission of Oxford University Press.)

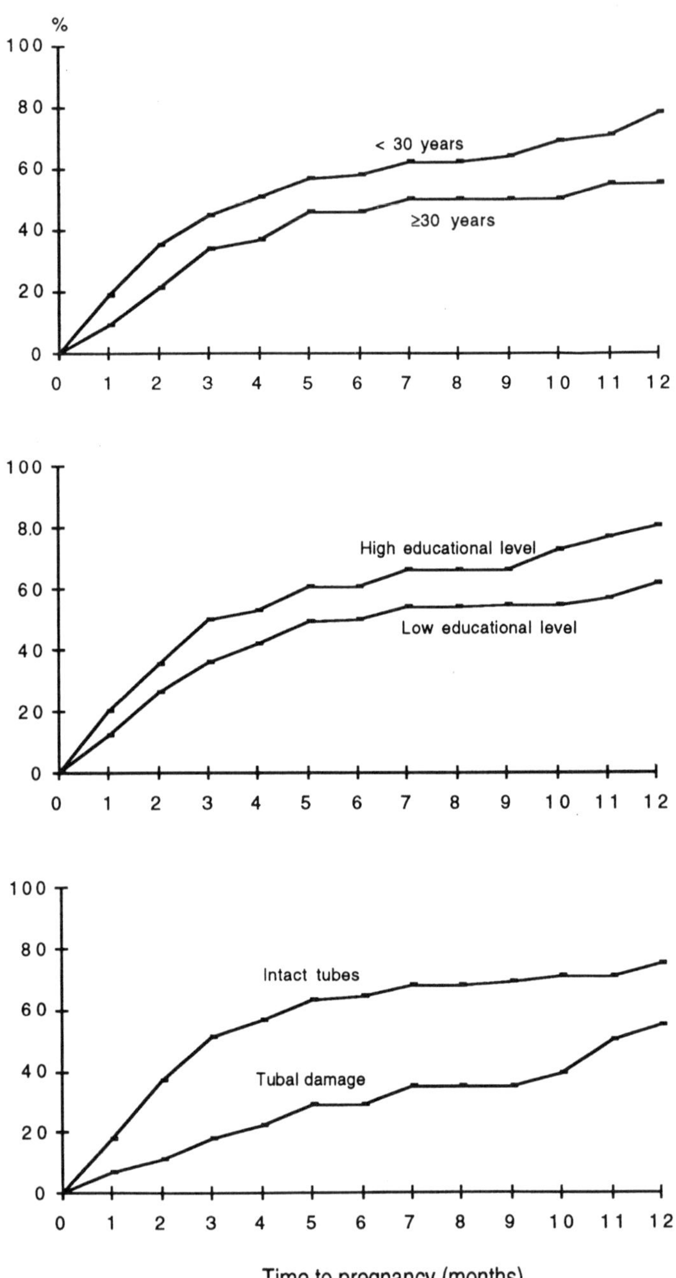

FIGURE 2.—One-year cumulative frequency of first subsequent intrauterine pregnancy according to age, educational level, and prior tubal status. (Courtesy of Job-Spira N, Bouyer J, Pouly JL, et al: Fertility after ectopic pregnancy: First results of a population-based cohort study in France. *Hum Reprod* 11:99–104, 1996, by permission of Oxford University Press.)

tive outcomes of EP managed by modern techniques were evaluated using data from a population-based registry.

Methods.—The registry included 395 women of reproductive age living in 1 area of France who were treated for EP between 1992 and 1994. All women were prospectively followed up until they were 45 years of age to determine their reproductive outcomes. Fifty women were excluded from follow-up because they underwent sterilization or bilateral salpingectomy, and another 30 were lost to follow-up. The final analysis included 155 women with at least 6 months' follow-up. All wished to become pregnant again, and most started trying during the first year after treatment of EP. The main outcome measures were the time to pregnancy (TTP) of the first intrauterine pregnancy (IUP) after EP and the risk of recurrent EP.

Results.—Mean age at EP was 30 years. Seven percent of the women had had a previous EP, 28% had a history of infertility, and 35% had a history of tubal damage. Sixty-nine percent of the women had been pregnant before. The EP was managed conservatively in 70% of women and by salpingectomy in 30%. Sixty percent of the women were successful in their attempts to conceive again. Of 92 intrauterine pregnancies, 47% produced a live birth and 23% ended in miscarriage. There were 10 cases of recurrent EP.

Among women who became pregnant, mean TTP was approximately 5 months. Seventy percent of women achieved an intrauterine pregnancy within 1 year, 53% within 6 months, and 15% within 1 month (Fig 1). The likelihood of achieving pregnancy that ended in a live birth within 1 year was 46%, whereas the probability of recurrent EP was 16%. Women with recurrent EP had a mean TTP of 11 months. The chances of achieving IUP were significantly greater for younger and better-educated women and worse for women with previous tubal damage (Fig 2). Several factors that were significantly related to IUP on univariate analysis—including marital status, vaginal douching, history of appendectomy, history of infertility, and radical vs. conservative treatment of EP—were not significant after adjustment for other factors. The risk of EP was greatest for women with a history of miscarriage or previous tubal damage.

Conclusions.—Of women who try to get pregnant again after EP, 70% will succeed in the first year. The chances of fertility after EP are affected more by the patient's characteristics than by the characteristics and management of the EP. The rate of recurrent EP was approximately 10% in this study, but this will probably increase with longer follow-up. Conservative management does not increase the risk of recurrent EP.

▶ The information from this study is useful because of its completeness of follow-up, excellent type of statistical analysis, and diverse population studied. Therefore, the results should be used when counseling women with an EP about their future reproductive potential. Overall, women with a single EP should have approximately a 70% chance of having an IUP within 1 year and only a 10% chance of having another EP. However, approximately one fourth of the IUPs will end in a spontaneous abortion. A history of a previous spontaneous abortion or the presence of gross tubal pathology at the time of the EP markedly increase the risk of a subsequent EP. Age younger than 30 years and the presence of grossly normal oviducts and the lack of a prior spontaneous abortion will increase the chance of having an IUP. Unlike other studies, it was determined that when adjusting for these risk factors, the type of surgical procedure performed for the EP—salpingectomy or salpingostomy—did not affect the subsequent rate of IUP. Women with an EP who become pregnant again should be monitored by sonography early in pregnancy because of the high incidence of another EP as well as spontaneous abortion.

D.R. Mishell, Jr., M.D.

Conservative Versus Radical Surgery for Tubal Pregnancy: A Review
Clausen I (Kolding Hosp, Denmark)
Acta Obstet Gynecol Scand 75:8–12, 1996   18–2

Introduction.—Currently, many gynecologists prefer conservative to radical surgical treatment for tubal pregnancy, believing that this approach offers the best chance of preserving fertility. However, this theory has not been proved. Therefore, fertility and recurrence of tubal pregnancy were compared in patients treated with either conservative or radical surgery.

Methods.—The literature was searched to identify studies comparing fertility prognosis and recurrence rates of tubal pregnancy among patients undergoing conservative or radical surgical treatment. The studies were organized by design: retrospective noncomparing studies, retrospective comparing studies, prospective selected treatment series, and prospective randomized comparing investigations. The 40 publications included, which were published during the last 40 years, all had clear treatment methods, reported the number of patients, and had data on subsequent pregnancies among women who wanted to become pregnant as well as recurrence rates with 95% confidence limits.

Results.—In the retrospective noncomparing studies, pregnancy rates were 46% in the conservative treatment group and 44% in the radical treatment group, a nonsignificant difference. No significant differences were found in subsequent pregnancy rates between the 2 treatment groups in 14 of 15 retrospective comparing studies or the prospective selected treatment series studies. There were no prospective randomized studies. In the retrospective noncomparing studies, the repeat ectopic pregnancy rate varied considerably in both conservative and radically treated patient groups, with an average rate of 10% after conservative surgery and 15% after radical surgery. The prospective treatment series studies reported an average repeat ectopic pregnancy rate of 13% (Fig 6). No significant differences in recurrence rate were found in the treatment groups in the retrospective comparing studies.

Conclusions.—Current research indicates no differences in prognosis for fertility or in recurrence of tubal pregnancies among patients treated

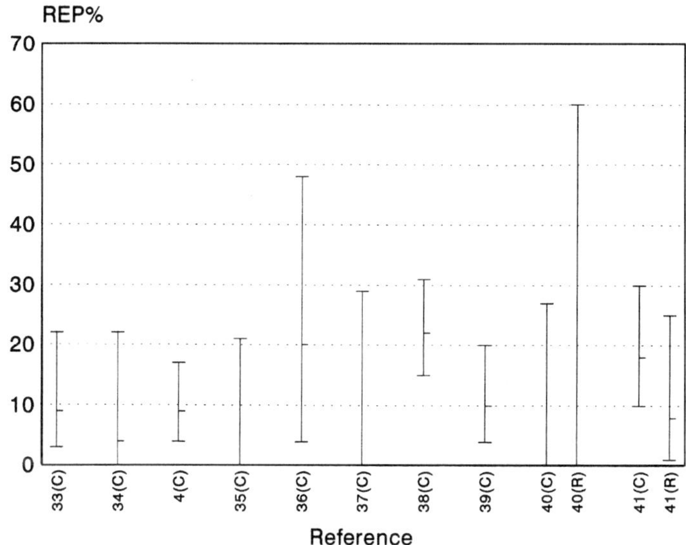

FIGURE 6.—Prospective selected treatment series. Repeat ectopic pregnancy rates (*REP%*) after conservative (C) or radical (R) tubal surgery with 95% confidence limits. (Courtesy of Clausen I: Conservative versus radical surgery for tubal pregnancy: A review. *Acta Obstet Gynecol Scand* 75:8–12, 1996. Munksgaard International Publishers Ltd., Copenhagen, Denmark.)

for tubal pregnancy with either conservative or radical surgery. However, definitive clarification must await prospective, randomized studies.

▶ Since about 1980, the standard treatment for unruptured tubal pregnancy has been salpingostomy instead of salpingectomy. Subsequent intrauterine pregnancy rates have been reported to be higher after conservative than radical tubal surgery, with no significant differences in subsequent ectopic pregnancy rates. As this extensive review reveals, there are marked differences in subsequent intrauterine pregnancy rates after either salpingostomy or salpingectomy, but repeat ectopic pregnancy rates are similar after the 2 procedures, usually in the range of 10% to 20%.

To date, no randomized clinical trials have been undertaken to compare the results of the 2 operative therapies, and it is unlikely that such a trial will be performed in the future. Therefore, because salpingostomy is not a difficult procedure and may improve subsequent viable pregnancy rates, this procedure should be performed if a woman has an unruptured tubal gestation and desires future fertility. Because of the problem of persistent ectopic pregnancy after salpingostomy, monitoring of human chorionic gonadotropin levels postoperatively is mandatory.

D.R. Mishell, Jr., M.D.

Ectopic Pregnancy: Nonsurgical, Outpatient Evaluation and Single-dose Methotrexate Treatment

Gross Z, Rodriguez JJ, Stalnaker BL (Univ of Florida, Pensacola)
J Reprod Med 40:371–374, 1995   18–3

Objective.—Single-dose systemic methotrexate (MTX) has been shown to be safe and effective for the outpatient treatment of unruptured ectopic pregnancy. However, community hospital–based practitioners—who lack the benefits of highly skilled sonographers and specialized laboratories—have been hesitant to use this approach. The use of single-dose MTX treatment extended to the community hospital setting was examined.

Methods.—All women who were seen in the hospital emergency department or outpatient clinics with suspected ectopic pregnancy were studied. All underwent a careful history and physical examination, quantitative human chorionic gonadotropin (hCG) test, endovaginal ultrasonography, and dilation and curettage. Those who met the criteria for ectopic pregnancy and for MTX treatment were offered outpatient treatment with single-dose IM MTX.

Results.—Seventeen patients met the criteria and were managed as outpatients. Treatment failed in 1 patient: she required right salpingectomy for ruptured ectopic pregnancy, after which she experienced no further complications. In the 16 responders, the mean pretreatment hCG level was 3,321 mIU/mL. Single-dose MTX was followed by adequate hCG titer declines, with a continuous decline after day 6. The patients took a mean of 26 days to reach an hCG value of less than 15 mIU/mL. All patients lacked chorionic villi in their uterine curettage specimens, including 10 who had hCG concentrations of greater than 2,000 mIU/mL. In 1 patient, increasing abdominal pain and vaginal bleeding developed 6 days after treatment. She had a repeat transvaginal scan, but no further treatment was required.

Conclusions.—In the community hospital setting, single-dose MTX is a safe and effective treatment approach for selected patients with unruptured ectopic pregnancy. A stepwise diagnostic approach is recommended. In this institution, physicians have stopped performing dilation and curettage for patients who have hCG titers of 2,000 mIU/mL or greater and an empty uterus seen on transvaginal ultrasonography.

▶ The treatment of small (less than 3 cm) unruptured tubal ectopic pregnancies with a single IM injection of MTX is becoming an acceptable practice in both community and academic hospitals. Various protocols are used to provide exclusion as well as inclusion criteria, and different diagnostic evaluations as well as treatment protocols are utilized. If the hCG level is above 2,000 mIU/mL and an intrauterine pregnancy is not visualized sonographically, an ectopic pregnancy should be present. With a lower hCG level, if a steady increase does not occur during the next few days, either a nonviable intrauterine gestation or an ectopic gestation is present. If no choronic villi are present in the uterine cavity, then it is unnecessary to perform a laparoscopy to establish that an ectopic pregnancy is present. The patient can be treated with MTX if she so desires. As shown in this paper, the possibility of tubal rupture after treatment exists, so close monitoring is essential until hCG levels become undetectable.

D.R. Mishell, Jr., M.D.

Treatment of Ectopic Pregnancy by Local Injection of Hypertonic Glucose: A Randomized Trial Comparing Administration Guided by Transvaginal Ultrasound or Laparoscopy

Gjelland K, Hordnes K, Tjugum J, et al (Haukeland Univ, Bergen, Norway)
Acta Obstet Gynecol Scand 74:629–634, 1995   18–4

Objective.—Two forms of hyperosmolar glucose treatment—injections guided by transvaginal ultrasonography and by laparoscopy—were compared in 80 women with an ectopic pregnancy of 4 cm or less as seen by transvaginal ultrasound and a human chorionic gonadotropin (hCG) level no greater than 3,000 IU/L.

Patients.—The patients had an average age of 29 years and had had nearly 3 pregnancies on average. Eight participants had had ectopic pregnancies previously, 3 of them more than once. Nearly 80% of patients had corpus luteum cysts on the side of the ectopic gestation.

Management.—In 39 cases, 20–30 mL of 50% glucose solution was instilled into the affected tube under transvaginal ultrasound guidance. The injection was made using an 18-gauge needle that was inserted through an introducer mounted on the ultrasound probe. Fentanyl or alfentanil was given intravenously if necessary. The remaining 41 patients were anesthetized and received injections under laparoscopic guidance.

Results.—Eighty percent of patients given sonographically guided injections had a successful outcome. Eight patients received a second injection because of an increasing hCG level, but 5 of them had to be operated on. Twenty-one patients in the laparoscopy group were treated successfully. The difference in efficacy was statistically significant. The average interval from saline injection to the elimination of hCG was 24 days in the sonography group and 18 days in patients who had the laparoscopically guided procedure. The median hospital time for all successfully treated patients was 3 days. One patient in each group had severe intra-abdominal bleeding. The treated tube was found to be open in all but 3 of 28 patients who agreed to hysterosalpingography.

Conclusion.—Tubal injection of hyperosmolar glucose under transvaginal ultrasound guidance is a simple and effective means of treating ectopic pregnancy. The treated tube remains patent in a substantial majority of patients.

▶ Systemic methotrexate is the most widely used nonsurgical treatment of small, unruptured tubal pregnancies. However, some individuals with expertise in the technique of sonographically guided transvaginal needle placement have injected various substances including methotrexate, hypertonic glucose, and potassium chloride into the gestational sac, with about a 75% rate of successful resolution of the ectopic pregnancy. The high rate of posttreatment tubal patency (90%) in the affected tubes indicates that this procedure warrants further investigation.

D.R. Mishell, Jr., M.D.

19 Sexuality and Premenstrual Syndrome

The Effect of a Carbohydrate-rich Beverage on Mood, Appetite, and Cognitive Function in Women With Premenstrual Syndrome
Sayegh R, Schiff I, Wurtman J, et al (Harvard Med School, Boston; Massachusetts Inst of Technology, Cambridge)
Obstet Gynecol 86:520–528, 1995

19–1

Background.—The cause of premenstrual syndrome (PMS) remains uncertain, but some of the symptoms—dysphoria and the increased consumption of carbohydrate-rich foods—have been ascribed to deficient serotoninergic neurotransmission in the brain. Increased dietary carbohydrate increases the serum tryptophan, and premenstrual dysphoria is decreased by administering dexfenfluramine, which releases cerebral serotonin and blocks its reuptake.

Objective.—The effectiveness of a carbohydrate-rich beverage was examined in a double-blind, placebo-controlled crossover study that enrolled 24 women who met National Institute of Mental Health criteria for PMS. At least 5 relevant symptoms had been present for a year or longer, had interfered with daily activities in the premenstrual period, and had remitted at the onset of menstruation.

Methods.—Three dietary interventions were tested in women whose symptoms became 30% more severe in the postovulatory phase of 2 menstrual cycles. The experimental beverage (A) contained simple and complex carbohydrates (dextrose and maltodextrin) known to increase the serum ratio of tryptophan to large neutral amino acids. The other beverages resembled A in caloric content but contained mixtures of protein and carbohydrate (B) or carbohydrate alone (C) that did not alter the relative tryptophan level. All drinks supplied nearly 200 calories. They were administered over a 3-month period after a 1-month run-in period during which all research subjects drank beverage B. Mood and appetite were assessed using a computerized phone system, and a battery of cognitive tests was administered.

"

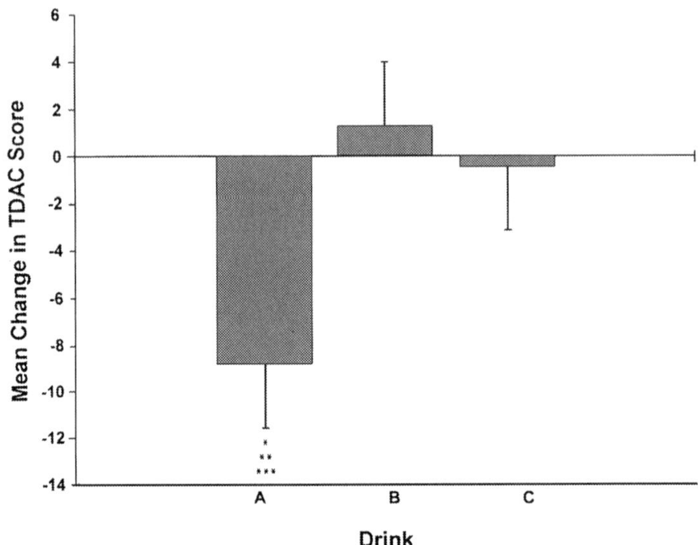

FIGURE 1.—Changes in total mood score (summed tension, anger, depression, and confusion) (*TDAC*) at T180. To adjust for large intersubject variability between cycles in predrink mood, statistical adjustments were made using the T0 score as the covariate. *$P < 0.04$ treatment effect of drink A; **$P < 0.02$ compared with drink B; ***$P < 0.04$ compared with drink C. (Courtesy of Sayegh R, Schiff I, Wurtman J, et al: The effect of a carbohydrate-rich beverage on mood, appetite, and cognitive function in women with premenstrual syndrome. *Obstet Gynecol* 86:520–528, 1995. Reprinted with permission from The American College of Obstetricians and Gynecologists.)

Results.—Drink A was most effective in improving mood 3 hours after ingestion (Fig 1). Earlier mood scores did not differ significantly. Drink A suppressed the craving for sweet and starchy carbohydrates. It also improved scores on a measure of recognition memory, but none of the drinks influenced performance on tests of verbal retrieval or serial addition.

Conclusion.—A carbohydrate beverage designed to elevate the serum tryptophan level relieves dysphoric mood and enhances memory function in women with moderate-to-severe PMS.

▶ It has been postulated that some of the adverse symptoms of PMS, particularly dysphoria and craving for carbohydrate-rich foods, are due to deficiencies in serotonin-mediated neurotransmission in the brain. It has been previously shown in several studies that the administration of fluoxetine, a serotonin receptor blocker that increases brain serotonin levels, significantly improves the symptoms of PMS, compared with placebo.

Studies in the rat have shown that if the diet is changed so that serum tryptophan levels are increased, there is also an increase in serotonin synthesis and brain serotonin levels. In this study, ingestion of a beverage that selectively increased tryptophan levels, in comparison to other amino acids, significantly relieved some of the symptoms of PMS. If such a beverage became commercially available, it could be used by clinicians to treat women with PMS, as it has fewer side effects and risks than do the pharmacologic agents such as fluoxetine currently being used.

D.R. Mishell, Jr., M.D.

Efficacy of Progesterone Vaginal Suppositories in Alleviation of Nervous Symptoms in Patients With Premenstrual Syndrome
Baker ER, Best RG, Manfredi RL, et al (Univ of South Carolina, Columbia; Pennsylvania State Univ, Hershey)
J Assist Reprod Genet 12:205–209, 1995   19–2

Background.—The symptom complex known as premenstrual syndrome (PMS) includes emotional, behavioral, and physical manifestations associated with the luteal phase of the menstrual cycle. Although an underlying endocrine abnormality would appear to be the cause of PMS, no clear evidence supports this hypothesis. To evaluate the efficacy of progesterone (P) in reducing symptoms of PMS, a double-blind, placebo-controlled study was conducted. The rationale for the trial was the potential role of metabolites of P as anxiolytic agents.

Methods.—Participants were recruited within a 12-month period from a PMS clinic. Seventeen of 25 women who met entry criteria completed the 7-month protocol. All were healthy and regularly menstruating and did not use hormonal contraception. Psychiatric testing and interviews determined that none of the women had a major emotional or mental disorder. The protocol started with a 1-month evaluation period followed by a month of placebo. In the third and fourth months, the first group received P and the second group placebo. The fifth month was a washout period with placebo for both groups. In the final 2 months, the first group received placebo and the second group was treated with P. Active treatment consisted of 200-mg vaginal P suppositories, administered twice daily. Study participants were evaluated with a battery of psychological tests and serum hormonal assays.

Results.—The results of hormonal assays confirmed that control and treatment groups were similar. Study and control cycles showed no overall significant difference in ratings of subjective symptoms, based on the outcomes of 7 standard psychological tests. Significant improvement occurred, however, during P cycles in the subcategory of questions relating to guilt and self-image on the schedule for affective disorders and schizophrenia change form.

Conclusions.—There have been a few scattered reports of a beneficial effect of P among women with PMS. In this group of patients with a diagnosis of moderate-to-severe PMS, twice-daily treatment with 200-mg P suppositories alleviated some symptoms relating to tension, mood swings, irritability, anxiety, and lack of control. Whereas overall symptoms showed no significant improvement, certain subsets of women with PMS may benefit from the anxiolytic effects of P.

▶ The results of this study are in agreement with those of many other studies indicating that P does not relieve the overall symptoms of PMS any better than does placebo. The results of this study, however differ from those of other reports as it was found that P was significantly better than placebo for reducing nervous symptoms, such as tension, mood swings, irritability, and anxiety, and improvement was seen with questions relating to guilt and self-imaging. Progesterone and certain of its metabolites are anxiolytic. If the woman's main premenstrual symptoms are nervousness and anxiety, she may note significant improvement with the use of a high dose of P suppositories, 200 mg twice a day. No information was provided regarding the side effects of this high dose of P, but fatigue and sleepiness may occur with its use.

D.R. Mishell, Jr., M.D.

Treatment of Premenstrual Syndrome by Spironolactone: A Double-blind, Placebo-controlled Study

Wang M, Hammarbäck S, Lindhe B-Å, et al (Umeå Univ, Sweden; Uppsala Academy Hosp, Sweden)
Acta Obstet Gynecol Scand 74:803–808, 1995   19–3

Background.—Spironolactone (aldosterone receptor antagonist) is known to antagonize the anesthetic and sedative effects of steroid anesthetics. Encouraging results have been reported in previous studies investigating the use of spironolactone in women with menstrual cycle–linked mood change, known as premenstrual syndrome (PMS). The therapeutic effect of spironolactone on women with PMS was investigated in this double-blind, placebo-controlled, crossover study.

Patients and Methods.—Thirty-five women aged 25–45 years in the study had established cyclic mood changes. Patients were observed during 2 pretreatment cycles and then were randomly assigned to begin treatment with either 100 mg of spironolactone (given orally) or placebo. Tablets were taken on a daily basis during 14 premenstrual days for 3 months, after which patients crossed over to another tablet for an additional 3 months. Symptoms occurring during menstrual cycles were recorded each day using a previously validated visual analogue scale. Specifically, patients were asked to self-rate 4 negative parameters (anxiety and tension, irritability, fatigue, and depression) and 4 positive parameters (cheerfulness, well-being, friendliness, and energy level) of psychological mood as well as 4 somatic subjective symptoms (headache, feeling of swelling, sweet craving, and breast tenderness).

Results.—Compared with pretreatment symptom scores, lower negative and higher positive symptom scores were noted with both spironolactone and placebo treatment cycles, whereas summarized somatic symptom scores were significantly lower only in the spironolactone treatment cycles. No significant differences in negative and positive mood changes were noted before and after crossover in women assigned to begin treatment with spironolactone, with patients continuing to feel better during placebo therapy. Significant improvement in feeling of swelling and breast tender-

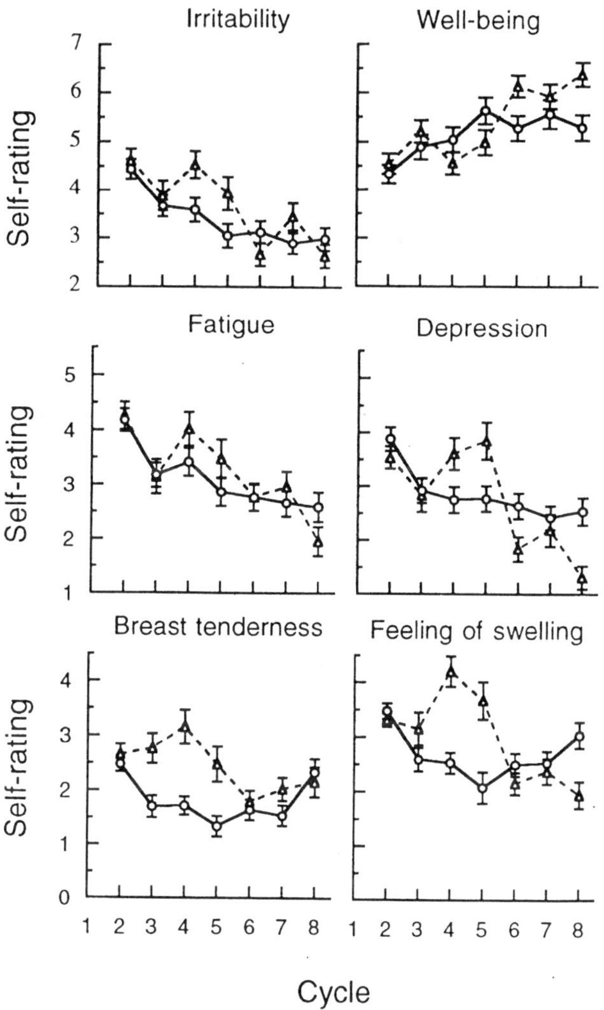

FIGURE 1.—Mean self-rating of the spironolactone first (*circles*) and placebo first (*triangles*) groups for Fatigue, Well-being, Depression, Irritability, Breast tenderness, and Feeling of swelling in the last 8 days of premenstrual phase of cycle 3–8 and mean scores for 2 pretreatment cycles indicated as cycle 2. (Courtesy of Wang M, Hammarbäck S, Lindhe B-Å, et al: Treatment of premenstrual syndrome by spironolactone: A double-blind, placebo-controlled study. *Acta Obstet Gynecol Scand* 74:803–808, Copyright 1995 Munksgaard International Publishers Ltd., Copenhagen, Denmark.)

ness also was noted in these patients. In patients who began treatment with placebo, significant decreases in fatigue, depression, and irritability, and increases in feelings of well-being, were noted after crossover to spironolactone. With the exception of headache, all other somatic symptoms also were improved after crossover to active drug therapy (Fig 1). Among patients who began treatment with spironolactone, improved symptom scores were noted in 83% of negative parameters (vs. 57% in the placebo group), 83% of positive parameters (vs. 50% in the placebo group), and

50% of somatic symptoms (vs. 50% in the placebo group). Placebo effects diminished during treatment in patients who began treatment with placebo, whereas no waning of effects was noted in the spironolactone-first treated group. This suggests a lasting effect of the active drug treatment, because the time effect was only found in patients who began treatment with spironolactone.

Conclusions.—Treatment with spironolactone leads to significant improvements in irritability, depression, feeling of swelling, breast tenderness, and food craving in patients with PMS. This agent therefore appears to be effective in this particular patient population.

▶ Several studies now indicate that spironolactone is more beneficial than placebo in reducing many of the adverse symptoms associated with PMS. The mechanism whereby spironolactone causes this beneficial effect is not known, but it involves actions other than its mild diuretic effect. Because minimal adverse symptoms are associated with the ingestion of 100 mg of spironolactone daily, clinicians may wish to use this agent for the initial therapy for PMS.

D.R. Mishell, Jr., M.D.

20 Surgical Gynecology

Drainage Following Radical Hysterectomy and Pelvic Lymphadenectomy: Dogma or Need?
de B Lopes A, Hall JR, Monaghan JM (Queen Elizabeth Hosp, Gateshead, England)
Obstet Gynecol 86:960–963, 1995   20–1

Background.—Varying proportions of patients have lymphocysts after undergoing extensive dissection of the retroperitoneal lymph nodes. Symptoms may develop when a cyst enlarges or becomes infected. Drainage typically is recommended after radical hysterectomy and pelvic node dissection, but the need for drainage has been questioned because presently the pelvic peritoneum frequently is left open.

Objective.—To determine the clinical value of drainage, a prospective, randomized study was performed in 100 women having a Piver type II radical hysterectomy and comprehensive en bloc dissection of the pelvic lymph nodes.

Methods.—The external iliac, internal iliac, and obturator nodes were dissected bilaterally. The edge of the vaginal cuff was oversewn, leaving the vaginal vault open. The pelvis was not reperitonized. Fifty-one patients were randomly assigned to have suction drains placed in each iliac fossa along the site of node dissection. Patients received antibiotics prophylactically at the time of anesthetic induction. Abdominal ultrasonography was done 8 weeks postoperatively.

Results.—The average total drainage volume was 929 mL. Drains were removed 4 days postoperatively, on average. Patients not having drainage more often reported the loss of serosanguinous vaginal fluid on the first day. Febrile morbidity developed in 3 patients who had drainage and 4 patients who did not. No difference in overall postoperative morbidity was found. Lymphocysts were found on ultrasound study in 16% of patients having drainage and 17% of those who did not have drainage. They were evident clinically in 6% of each group.

Conclusion.—As long as the vaginal cuff and pelvic peritoneum are left open, in patients having radical hysterectomy with retroperitoneal node dissection, suction drainage does not significantly lower the risk of a pelvic lymphocyst developing.

▶ As noted by the authors, this is an initial prospective, randomized study of the use of retroperitoneal drainage in cases of radical hysterectomy. The patients had the vaginal cuff and the pelvic peritoneum left open, with no difference in results regarding the occurrence of lymphocysts or postoperative morbidity. These results are impressive.

I was taught to close the retroperitoneum and use suction catheters. It may well not have affected the results of this study, but I wish the authors had closed the peritoneum in the suction catheter group, because I think they did not really compare the techniques that should be compared. I think this question still needs to be answered: does closing the peritoneum and using suction catheters provide as superior a result as just leaving the peritoneum open? Fortunately, the occurrences of lymphocysts is rare in either case.

A.L. Herbst, M.D.

Loop Electrosurgical Excision Procedure for Squamous Intraepithelial Lesions of the Cervix: Advantages and Potential Pitfalls
Ferenczy A, Choukroun D, Arseneau J (McGill Univ, Montreal; Royal Victoria Hosp, Montreal)
Obstet Gynecol 87:332–337, 1996
20–2

Background.—Loop electrosurgical excision has been proposed as an alternative to cold-knife and CO_2 laser conization for outpatient treatment of cervical cancer precursor lesions. Loop electrosurgical excision has some important advantages, including relative simplicity, low complication rates, and potential cost-effectiveness. As the procedure becomes more popular, however, there have been problems with removal of excessive tissue and overtreatment. A large series of patients undergoing loop electrosurgical excision was studied to identify the advantages and potential dangers of this procedure.

Patients.—The study included 1,189 consecutive patients undergoing loop electrosurgical excision after colposcopy referral after an abnormal Papanicolaou smear during a 4-year period. All procedures, done while the patient received local anesthesia, used colposcopic guidance. Seventy-seven percent of patients were managed in a single session using the "see and treat" approach. The remaining 23% underwent endocervical curettage and cervical biopsies before loop electrosurgical excision. Follow-up information was available for 90% of patients.

Findings.—The follow-up loop electrosurgical excision specimen showed adenocarcinoma in 15 patients and microinvasive squamous cell carcinoma in 6. The evaluation of treatment results included 883 patients, the rest being excluded because of lack of follow-up, a negative loop electrosurgical excision procedure, or lesions other than squamous intraepithelial lesions (SILs). In 14% of patients, the excised specimen did not include any lesional tissue. Ninety-two percent of evaluable patients were free of disease at 6 months' or longer follow-up after a single procedure and 95% after 2 loop electrosurgical excision procedures. Of 309 patients with high-grade SILs, 93% were successfully treated with loop electrosurgical excision. The complication rate was 7%, with most complications consisting of intraoperative and postoperative bleeding. When the loop electrosurgical excision procedure gave a negative result, the referral cytologic diagnosis, colposcopy, or histologic findings were found to be false positive in retrospect. In some cases, smaller specimens of diseased tissue were removed by biopsy before loop electrosurgical excision.

Conclusions.—The increasingly popular loop electrosurgical excision procedure for cervical cancer precursors is associated with some danger of overtreatment. This danger can be reduced by using the traditional diagnostic triage procedure for lesions in which the cytologic and colposcopic findings are not definitive. When the cytologic and colposcopic findings in a persistent lesion are unequivocal, the "see and treat" method is appropriate.

▶ This is a large study from the Canadian group with extensive experience with loop electrosurgical excision procedure. The success rates for treating intraepithelial lesions was reported to be high (more than 90%), and the authors did achieve these results in an outpatient setting with local anesthesia. They also note the advantage of this approach for potential cost savings. Importantly, they limited the size of the loop to 2 × 1 cm and in most cases 2 × 0.8 cm, which prevents removal of excessive cervical tissue.

There are, however, some negatives and areas of concern. The original study comprised 1,189 patients, but 306 were excluded (almost 30%) because of loss to follow-up (119) and negative cone specimens (166) as well as a few with non-SIL pathology. In addition, 25 patients required 2 loop electrosurgical excision procedures, whereas 15 others needed a third procedure. I was particularly concerned about the authors using "see and treat" for atypical squamous cells of undetermined significance. This seems like overkill to me, unless one is dealing with an unreliable patient or with a high-risk patient (one with HIV, for example). The authors note that younger patients were more likely to have negative specimens, some probably due to thermal injury from the loop electrosurgical excision procedure.

The "see and treat" approach obviously has cost-effective appeal. However, as I have written elsewhere, I suspect this procedure is overly used in the United States. It certainly is an appropriate approach for an individual who has had children and who is being evaluated for a high-grade smear consistent with cervical intraepithelial neoplasia, grade 3. It also seems to work well for those from underserved areas who are unlikely to return for follow-up or if the patient herself is unreliable.

A.L. Herbst, M.D.

21 Diagnostic Gynecology

A Decision Analysis of Practice Patterns Used in Evaluating and Treating Abnormal Pap Smears
Roland PY, Naumann RW, Alvarez RD, et al (Univ of Alabama, Birmingham)
Gynecol Oncol 59:75–80, 1995
21–1

Background.—The large-loop excision of the transformation zone (LLETZ) procedure has been shown to be highly effective in treating cervical dysplasia. Several reports have recommended using LLETZ as a single combined diagnostic and therapeutic procedure in patients with cervical dysplasia. The potential for excessive treatment and health care costs of different evaluation and treatment strategies for patients with abnormal Papanicolaou (Pap) smears were compared.

Methods.—Four algorithms were constructed for the management of patients with abnormal Pap smears (Fig 1). With algorithm 1, traditional colposcopic evaluation was followed by cryotherapy for mild dysplasia and LLETZ for moderate-to-severe dysplasia. With algorithm 2, colposcopy was performed, and mild dysplasia was managed with observation, moderate dysplasia with cryotherapy, and severe dysplasia with LLETZ. With algorithm 3, low-grade squamous intraepithelial lesions (LGSILs) were managed with colposcopy, and high-grade squamous intraepithelial lesions (HGSILs) were managed with immediate LLETZ. With algorithm 4, immediate LLETZ was performed on all patients with LGSILs or HGSILs on Pap smears. Within an 18-month period, all new patients with LGSIL or HGSIL Pap smears underwent colposcopic evaluation. Biopsy specimen–proved dysplasia was managed with observation if mild and with LLETZ if moderate or severe. The cervical biopsy specimens and/or LLETZ histology findings in the study population were used to determine the potential for excessive treatment with algorithms using immediate LLETZ without colposcopy. Algorithm costs were calculated using nationwide 50th percentile reimbursement costs for medical procedures and pathology.

Results.—In the study population, 47.6% had LGSIL and 52.4% had HGSIL on the referral Pap smear. Cervical biopsy specimen or LLETZ histology results indicated no dysplasia in 46.7%, mild dysplasia in

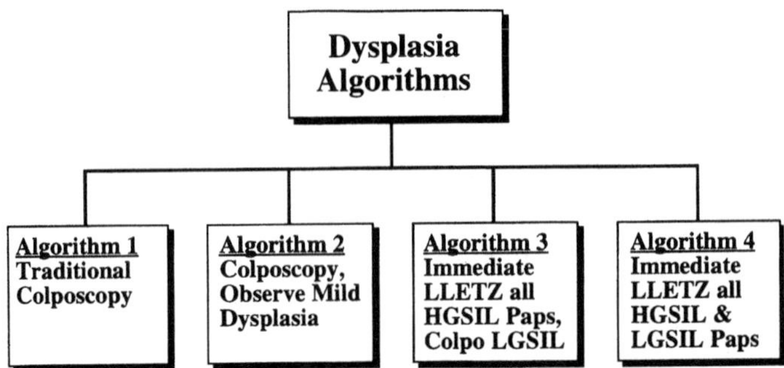

FIGURE 1.—Treatment algorithm summary. *Abbreviations: LLETZ,* large-loop excision of the transformation zone; *LGSIL,* low-grade squamous intraepithelial lesions; *HGSIL,* high-grade intraepithelial lesions. (Courtesy of Roland PY, Naumann RW, Alvarez RD, et al: *Gynecol Oncol* 59:75–80, 1995.)

17.1%, moderate dysplasia in 17.6%, severe dysplasia in 13.4%, and invasion in 0.5% of the patients. Of those with HGSIL Pap smears, 38.2% had no dysplasia and 15.2% had only mild dysplasia. Immediate LLETZ of all patients with LGSIL and HGSIL Pap smears (algorithm 4) would have resulted in the overtreatment of as many as 46.7% of the patients, and immediate LLETZ of all patients with HGSIL Pap smears (algorithm 3) would have resulted in the overtreatment of 38.2% of the patients. Excessive treatment would have been reduced to 18% with algorithm 1 and 2.8% with algorithm 2. The average costs per patient would be $1,019 with algorithm 1, $947 with algorithm 2 (Fig 2), $787 with algorithm 3, and $838 with algorithm 4. Analysis of the incidence of patients with different abnormal Pap smear findings requiring treatment indicated that immediate LLETZ was most cost-effective with HGSIL Pap smears, and traditional colposcopy with cryotherapy of mild dysplasia was most cost-effective with LGSIL Pap smears.

Conclusions.—Continued use of colposcopic examination is recommended to minimize the potential for excessive treatment. The management strategy that best minimizes excessive treatment and is most cost-

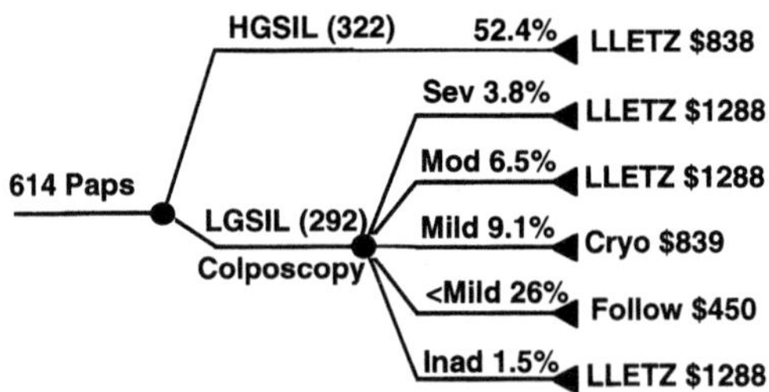

FIGURE 2.—Data tree for traditional colposcopy (algorithm 2). Each *branch* of the data tree is labeled with a diagnosis and resultant action. *Percentages* represent the proportion of the study population that would compose each branch of the data tree. The termination of each branch (*triangle*) lists its total cost. *Abbreviations: Sev,* severe dysplasia; *Mod,* moderate dysplasia; *Inad,* inadequate colposcopy: *LLETZ,* large-loop excision of the transformation zone; *LGSIL,* low-grade squamous intraepithelial lesions; *HGSIL,* high-grade squamous intraepithelial lesions. (Courtesy of Roland PY, Naumann RW, Alvarez RD, et al: *Gynecol Oncol* 59:75–80, 1995.)

effective includes colposcopy, followed by observation of mild dysplasia, cryotherapy of moderate dysplasia, and LLETZ of severe dysplasia. However, immediate LLETZ therapy may be used in patients with HGSIL/severe dysplasia, with colposcopy used in other patients.

▶ This article analyzes quite nicely the cost-effectiveness of a number of different triage options for an abnormal Pap smear. I have reproduced Figure 1 (the protocol) and Figure 2 (the data for colposcopy followed by observation for mild dysplasia; cryotherapy for moderate dysplasia; and LLETZ for severe dysplasia). As is clearly demonstrated, the "see and treat" approach for all lesions of cervical intraepithelial neoplasia (CIN) is expensive and unnecessary and, I suspect, may also be accompanied by potential long-term reproductive problems, particularly when applied to younger nulliparous patients.

The authors emphasize that colposcopy still has an important role in the management of CIN, particularly as it allows one to use less expensive therapeutic approaches for many of the dysplastic lesions (see Fig 2). I would reemphasize that the authors follow cases of mild dysplasia; use cryotherapy for cases of moderate dysplasia; and excise with LLETZ those with severe dysplasia. These are reasonable choices, especially for the purposes of this analysis. However, cases of persistent mild dysplasia probably deserve treatment. Certainly even severe dysplasia can be handled in the office, in many instances, by locally destructive methods, and an LLETZ is not always necessary.

For the reader, I would like to quote most of the final sentence of the article: "the use of immediate LLETZ of all patients with an abnormal Pap smear proves to be excessive in terms of both expense and treatment." One exception is the multiparous patient with a Pap smear consistent with CIN III, in which case immediate LLETZ is an appropriate option.

A.L. Herbst, M.D.

Papanicolaou Smears in Human Immunodeficiency Virus–Seropositive Women During Follow-up

Heard I, Bergeron C, Jeannel D, et al (Hôpital Broussais, Paris; Hôpital Cochin, Paris; Laboratoire Cerba, Pontoise, Cergy-Pointoise, Italy; et al)
Obstet Gynecol 86:749–753, 1995   21–2

Background.—The odds ratio of cervical squamous intraepithelial lesions (SILs) in HIV-seropositive women is estimated to be 4.9. Authorities continue to disagree about the outcomes of cervical abnormalities and cervical intraepithelial neoplasia in HIV-positive women. The 18-month gynecologic follow-up of 60 women with HIV infection was reported.

Methods.—The research subjects were 27 women with initially normal Papanicolaou (Pap) smears and 33 with abnormal Pap smears. The prospective follow-up included smears performed every 6 months for 18 months.

Findings.—At the final follow-up, the cumulative incidence of SIL was 9% in the women with normal smears at entry. Among those with SIL at study entry, the rate of cervical lesions was 95% in untreated women and 61% in those undergoing surgery. Persistence or progression of cervical lesions occurred in 92% of women with low-grade SIL. There were no cases of invasive cancer during the 18-month study.

Conclusions.—The rate of persistent SIL in HIV-infected women is high. Furthermore, conventional treatment in such women is relatively inefficient. The natural history of SIL in women with HIV infection is unlike that in immunocompetent women.

▶ There is a growing literature on the management of the Pap smear in HIV-seropositive women. This is a small study, but it is useful because all the patients had a smear every 6 months with 18 months of follow-up. Even those with an initial normal smear had a 9% subsequent cumulative incidence of a positive smear. However, the most impressive results were for the 33 patients with an initial positive smear, and in this group, 95% of those who were untreated had progression or persistent disease. An alarming 61% of those who were treated failed to have the disease eradicated. These disquieting results are similar to others previously reported. I believe HIV-positive women do require aggressive and careful follow-up and treatment, particularly those with low CD4+ counts.

A.L. Herbst, M.D.

Determinants of High-grade Dysplasia Among Women With Mild Dyskaryosis on Cervical Smear

Parazzini F, Sideri M, Resteli S, et al (Istituto di Ricerche Farmacologiche "Mario Negri," Milan, Italy; Univ of Milan, Italy; Istituto Europeo di Oncologia, Milan, Italy)
Obstet Gynecol 86:754–757, 1995

21–3

Background.—Authorities debate the need for routinely referring women with mild dyskaryosis on a single smear test for colposcopy and biopsy. The epidemiologic characteristics of women with such findings but with cervical intraepithelial neoplasia (CIN) grade II or III at biopsy were elucidated.

Methods.—Two hundred ninety-one women, aged 17 to 69 years, underwent colposcopy and histologic confirmation by biopsy. All women had had mild dyskaryosis on a single smear test. Women with CIN I or no evidence of CIN were compared with women with CIN II or III at biopsy.

Findings.—At biopsy, CIN I was identified in 10%, CIN II in 15%, and CIN III in 8%. The frequency of CIN II or III tended to decline with increasing levels of education. Women with 11 years of education or more had a multivariate odds ratio of 0.5 for CIN II or III compared with women reporting 11 or fewer years of education. Parous women had an odds ratio of 1.8 for CIN II or III compared with nulliparous women.

Compared with women who had never smoked, current smokers had an odds ratio of 2.3 for CIN II or III. Ex-smokers were also at increased risk, with a 3.8 odds ratio. Compared with women who had only 1 sexual partner, women with 2 to 3 or with 4 or more sexual partners had odds ratios of 1.4 and 2.3, respectively, for CIN II or III.

Conclusions.—Among women with a single smear showing mild dyskaryosis, the prevalence of high-grade lesions is increased in less-educated women who had had 1 or more full-term pregnancies and in women who had smoked cigarettes. In addition, the risk of CIN II or III tended to increase with the number of sexual partners.

▶ This is a small study, but it makes an interesting observation, namely that women with risk factors usually associated with CIN development are at an increased risk for having CIN II or CIN III discovered on colposcopically directed biopsy at the time they are being evaluated for a Pap smear that shows only mild dysplasia (dyskaryosis). None of the subjects in this study had a prior abnormal smear, although for some it was their initial cytologic smear. Reliable patients with an initial smear of mild dysplasia can usually be followed with a repeat smear at 4 to 6 months.[1] However, patients with high-risk factors such as HIV and those who are not reliable deserve immediate triage. This study suggests that perhaps we need to be more vigilant for those who have a smear of mild dysplasia and who also have other risk factors, including multiple sex partners, as well as for those who have smoked.

A.L. Herbst, M.D.

Reference

1. Giles JA, Hudson FA, Crow J, et al: Colposcopic assessment of the accuracy of cervical cytology screening. *BMJ* 296:1099–1102, 1988.

PAPNET-Directed Rescreening of Cervicovaginal Smears: A Study of 101 Cases of Atypical Squamous Cells of Undetermined Significance
Ryan MR, Stastny JF, Remmers R, et al (Washington Univ, St Louis, Mo; Virginia Commonwealth Univ/Med College of Virginia, Richmond; VA Med Ctr, Richmond, Va)
Am J Clin Pathol 105:711–718, 1996   21–4

Background.—Squamous cell intraepithelial lesions (SIL) are ultimately found in many women with cervicovaginal smears read as atypical squamous cells of undetermined significance (ASCUS). It is unknown whether rare cells diagnostic of SIL are present but not detected in these "atypical" smears. The PAPNET Cytological Screening System, developed by Neuromedical Systems, offers a possible safeguard against false negative and underdiagnosed cervicovaginal smears. The value of the PAPNET system in detecting cells diagnostic of SIL in atypical smears was investigated.

Methods.—Six reviewers independently read the PAPNET video images of 101 smears diagnosed as ASCUS. Selected cases were then manually reviewed and reclassified on the basis of consensus opinion, using PAPNET-identified microscopic coordinates.

Findings.—Thirty-five images were reclassified as SIL. Twenty-two were classified as low-grade, and 13 were classified as high-grade. On histologic assessment, 37 of the 101 smears were diagnosed as SIL, 65% of which were reclassified as SIL using PAPNET.

Conclusion.—With PAPNET-directed rescreening, a significant number of SIL cases can be detected among smears interpreted as atypical. Thus, PAPNET can serve as a safeguard against the underdiagnosis of cervicovaginal smears.

▶ The PAPNET system has been approved by the Food and Drug Administration to reduce the false negative rate in cytologic smears. By automatically rescreening slides that have been read as "negative," the system identifies and locates for the cytologist cells that are of concern, and these special images are viewed on a screen for review. This allows for the unique identification of "difficult to find" or "few" abnormal cells that can be missed, even in a careful manual rescreening process. This study by Ryan et al. suggests the potential of another application of this advanced technology, namely to rescreen ASCUS smears to uncover which of these contain low-grade SIL or high-grade SIL and which appear to be "benign." Larger studies are needed but, if verified, this would provide a very useful tool for the clinician who, all too often, is receiving an ASCUS report.

A.L. Herbst, M.D.

Postmenopausal Squamous Atypia: A Spectrum Including "Pseudo-koilocytosis"
Jovanovic AS, McLachlin CM, Shen L, et al (Harvard Med School, Boston)
Mod Pathol 8:408–412, 1995   21–5

Background.—The postmenopausal cervix may exhibit a range of epithelial and cellular changes apart from typical atrophy, including hyperchromatic nuclei, varying nuclear size, and multinucleated cells. The alterations closely resemble koilocytotic atypia. It remains uncertain whether these changes, subsumed under the term postmenopausal squamous atypia (PSA), represent age-related epithelial disturbances or condylomatous low-grade squamous intraepithelial lesions related to human papillomavirus (HPV).

Objective.—Changes of PSA were examined in 30 cervical biopsy specimens from 26 women older than 50 years of age to identify HPV nucleic acids and to learn whether PSA can be distinguished from condyloma. All specimens exhibited cytoplasmic halos and various nuclear alterations, sometimes accompanied by atrophy.

Findings.—Moderate-to-marked nuclear enlargement was a feature of 22 of the 30 biopsy specimens. Multinucleation was apparent in 11 specimens. Thirteen specimens exhibited chronic inflammation, but mitotic figures were present in only 1 case. Differences in nuclear size and staining were, in general, less marked than in HPV-related lesions. Nuclear chromatin was evenly distributed, in contrast to the extreme density or granularity seen in koilocytotic atypia. The nuclei usually were in the center of a uniform halo, whereas more irregular halos were seen in koilocytotic atypia. Nucleic acids of HPV were not identified in any case.

Conclusion.—When considering a diagnosis of low-grade squamous intraepithelial disease in a menopausal or postmenopausal woman, PSA should be ruled out.

▶ I have included this morphologic HPV study from Dr. Crum's laboratory at Harvard Medical School because it documents quite well that some cells that look somewhat like koilocytes are, in fact, not infected with HPV and should not be included in the category of low-grade squamous intraepithelial lesions (LGSIL). The article demonstrates some of the microscopic differences between the PSA described by the authors, which they term "pseudo-koilocytosis," and HPV-associated LGSIL. It is worth emphasizing that some of these lesions occurred in atrophic cervical epithelium, a fact to remember when mild squamous atypia is noted in perimenopausal and postmenopausal hypoestrogenic women. A short trial of vaginal estrogen cream could reverse these findings and provide a more accurate reading of a Pap smear. However, this is a histologic study, and of 30 cervical biopsy specimens with pseudokoilocytosis, none demonstrated HPV by the sensitive polymerase chain reaction technique. In contrast, 74% of LGSIL and high-grade squamous intraepithelial lesion biopsy specimens so studied were HPV-positive.

All of this adds to our knowledge that diagnosis of koilocytosis requires stringent morphologic criteria. The fact that stringent criteria are not always followed leads to the overuse of the diagnosis of LGSIL, which is one of the weaknesses of the Bethesda terminology.

A.L. Herbst, M.D.

22 Gynecologic Oncology

Population-based Study of Tamoxifen Therapy and Subsequent Ovarian, Endometrial, and Breast Cancers
Cook LS, Weiss NS, Schwartz SM, et al (Univ of Washington, Seattle)
J Natl Cancer Inst 87:1359–1364, 1995   22–1

Objective.—Tamoxifen has effectively reduced the risk of new primary contralateral breast cancers, prompting interest in using the drug for primary prevention of breast cancer. A population-based, case-control study was planned to determine the risk of second primary cancers of the ovary, endometrium, and other breast developing in women receiving tamoxifen for breast cancer.

Study Population.—Cases included 234 women who had a second primary cancer in the contralateral breast; 39 with a second primary ovarian cancer; and 42 with endometrial cancer. Control women were matched with cases for age, stage of primary breast cancer, and year of diagnosis. There were approximately 2 controls for each case patient.

Findings.—Tamoxifen had been used by 18% of women with a second primary ovarian cancer and 20% of their controls. The respective figures for endometrial cancer cases and controls were 26% and 31%, and for contralateral breast cases and controls, 10% and 18%. In all groups, tamoxifen had been used for fewer than 2 years on average. The risk of contralateral breast cancer was actually decreased in tamoxifen-treated women, especially those treated for longer than 1 year and those who were postmenopausal at the time breast cancer was first diagnosed.

Conclusion.—Relatively short-term tamoxifen therapy did not increase the risk of second primary cancers in these breast cancer patients, but the results may not be extrapolated to women who receive the drug for longer periods.

▶ I have included this negative study regarding tamoxifen and neoplasia because it is important that gynecologists be current on this issue in our role as health providers to women.

As has been noted in many studies, tamoxifen has a potential neoplastic effect on the uterus and also has an estrogenic component that, among other actions, helps to prevent osteoporosis.

This study shows no tamoxifen association with endometrial or ovarian carcinoma for those patients who took the drug for *fewer than 2 years*. As noted by the authors, short-term use may be relatively safe, but longer-term use may well be another issue. My guess is that the frequency of complications, such as endometrial carcinoma, in patients receiving tamoxifen is comparatively low but that abnormal bleeding and hyperplasia will occur more frequently than in those not taking tamoxifen. All of this will require gynecologic investigation.

A.L. Herbst, M.D.

Ovarian Cysts in Premenopausal and Postmenopausal Tamoxifen-treated Women With Breast Cancer
Shushan A, Peretz T, Uziely B, et al (Sharett Inst of Oncology, Jerusalem; Hebrew Univ, Jerusalem)
Am J Obstet Gynecol 174:141–144, 1996   22–2

Objective.—Because tamoxifen produces estrogen-like effects on the vaginal epithelium and hypertrophic endometrial changes in postmenopausal women, the effects of prolonged treatment were studied in 95 consecutive premenopausal and postmenopausal women with breast cancer. Three fourths of patients had stage II or stage III cancer.

Methods.—Patients were given tamoxifen in a daily dose of 20 mg as adjunctive treatment for breast cancer. Vaginal ultrasonography was done using a 5-MHz probe, followed by endometrial biopsy. The ultrasound study was repeated each year. If an ovarian cyst was found, the serum level of CA 125 was estimated.

Results.—Tamoxifen was given for 2 years on average. Ovarian cysts were found in 11 women (11.5%). The incidence was 6% in postmenopausal women and 37.5% in premenopausal patients. The mean times patients received tamoxifen were 19 months for postmenopausal women and 28 months for premenopausal women. Two premenopausal women had complex ovarian cysts. In 8 of 11 cases, the cyst ceased enlarging after tamoxifen treatment had been stopped for 2 months. All women with cysts had normal serum CA 125 levels. All 3 cysts that were removed proved to be benign.

Discussion.—A literature review yielded 17 reports of premenopausal women who were treated with tamoxifen for ovarian cysts. Ovarian cysts are not unusual in premenopausal or postmenopausal women given tamoxifen as adjunctive treatment for breast cancer. Most cysts disappear when tamoxifen is withdrawn.

▶ It has been well established that abnormalities of the endometrium occur with increasing frequency in patients treated with taxmoxifen. This article from Israel indicates that ovarian cysts, albeit of small size, are common as well. Specifically, 11% of the 95 women studied had cysts detected by vaginal ultrasound, and 5 of the 11 women were postmenopausal.

Two points are worth emphasizing. First, all of the cysts were less than 50 mm or 5 cm in diameter. Second, the cysts regressed when the tamoxifen was stopped. Because tamoxifen is being increasingly used in patients with breast cancer as well as being evaluated as a possible preventive strategy against breast cancer, all gynecologists should be aware of these findings and recognize that these cysts do not appear to be any threat to the patient's health.

A.L. Herbst, M.D.

Complications of Pelvic Radiation Therapy for Gynecologic Malignancies in Elderly Women

McGonigle KF, Lavey RS, Juillard G, et al (Univ of California, Los Angeles)
Int J Gynecol Cancer 6:149–155, 1996   22–3

Introduction.—Older women with cancer often receive less aggressive cancer therapy than their younger counterparts. Pelvic irradiation for gynecologic malignancies causes serious complications in up to 10% of women of all ages, and older women are especially likely to receive radiation therapy as the primary treatment for gynecologic cancer. The frequency and severity of complications of pelvic radiation therapy in elderly women were assessed.

Methods.—The retrospective study included 60 women older than 65 years of age who underwent pelvic irradiation for gynecologic malignancies. Thirty-one had endometrial cancer, 26 had cervical cancer, and 3 had proximal vaginal cancer. The grading system of the Gynecologic Oncology Group was used to grade all complications, which were divided into acute and chronic categories. The impact of radiation therapy and patient and disease characteristics on complications was assessed by univariate and multivariate analyses.

Results.—Five percent of patients had acute grade 3 or 4 gastrointestinal (GI) complications. Of 49 patients followed for longer than 3 months, 57% had chronic complications. Mild diarrhea and cystitis were the most frequent chronic complications. More severe examples included small bowel obstruction, life-threatening GI bleeding, and urethrovaginal fistula. The 3-year actuarial rate of chronic GI or genitourinary (GU) complications was 63%; for complications greater than grade 1, the rate was 24%. Of the 14 grades 2 to 4 chronic complications recorded, 12 occurred in the GI tract. There was a 45% 3-year actuarial chronic complication rate in the GI tract, compared with a 17% rate in the GU tract. The chronic GI complications occurred in a median of 8 months and the chronic GU complications in a median of 19 months. Multivariate analysis suggested that patients with 2 or more concomitant medical problems and those receiving a 45-Gy or higher dose of external beam radiation therapy were more likely to have chronic complications.

Conclusion.—Elderly women receiving pelvic irradiation for gynecologic malignancies have high rates of moderate-to-severe GI complications. These complications are particularly likely to occur in women with multiple preexisting medical conditions and in those receiving higher radiation doses. Pelvic irradiation should be used judiciously in elderly women, and treatment strategies that will reduce GI complications should be pursued.

▶ I have included this report on 60 women over 65 years of age to emphasize that our therapies are often much more toxic in this group. It is worrisome that chronic complications occurred in 57% of the patients followed for longer than 3 months and by 3 years reached 63%. It is of particular concern that about one quarter of the patients had grade 2, 3, or 4 GI or GU complications at the 3-year period. Obviously, there will be times patients in this age group will need radiation treatment. However, we should be extremely cautious in administering radiation therapy to this group, particularly when we are considering it in an "adjuvant" setting.

A.L. Herbst, M.D

The Management of a Persistent Adnexal Mass in Pregnancy

Platek DN, Henderson CE, Goldberg GL (Albert Einstein College, Bronx, NY)
Am J Obstet Gynecol 173:1236–1240, 1995   22–4

Background.—Almost 1% of gravid women have an adnexal mass diagnosed on ultrasonography during routine obstetric management. The pathologic features and pregnancy outcomes of women with persistent adnexal masses managed conservatively or surgically were reviewed.

Methods.—Thirty-one patients with persistent adnexal masses in pregnancy between January 1988 and June 1994 were identified at 1 center. These patients had simple or complex masses of 6 cm or greater in diameter that persisted on ultrasonographic assessment. Women with cysts that resolved spontaneously by 16 weeks' gestation and women who received diagnoses after delivery were excluded from the study.

Findings.—Nineteen patients (59%) had surgical intervention, and the rest were managed conservatively. Of those undergoing surgery, 9 patients had functional cysts; 6, mature cystic teratomas; and 4, other benign cysts. Surgery was performed at a mean gestational age of 18.6 weeks. Two complications occurred within 12 hours of surgery: spontaneous abortion in 1 patient and rupture of the membranes in another. Of the 12 patients treated nonoperatively, 7 were managed conservatively and 5 had percutaneous drainage of simple cysts that were symptomatic.

Conclusions.—The incidental finding of an adnexal mass in pregnancy is becoming more common. The operative treatment of this complication should be reconsidered because of the complications associated with abdominal surgery. A randomized clinical trial is needed to determine the best management of an adnexal mass in pregnancy.

▶ An adnexal mass requiring intervention during pregnancy is a rare event, and this nonrandomized study brings up some interesting points. First, the use of ultrasound not only provides earlier detection, but a more accurate assessment of an adnexal mass. I agree with the authors that it is wise to follow a mass larger than 6 cm at least to the 16th week for the likelihood of spontaneous regression. If it does not regress, then depending on size and symptoms, an operative procedure may be advisable. It is worth noting that one spontaneous abortion occurred in a patient in this study operated on at 17 weeks. I prefer, if possible, to restrict operation during pregnancy to the 22–22-week interval. Three patients in this series had transvaginal ovarian cyst aspirations, a controversial procedure. As noted by the authors, this procedure, if used, should be individualized. The authors did it either to avoid dystocia or because of concern for incipient torsion. As an oncologist, I am concerned about aspirating ovarian cysts because I have seen it done on supposedly benign cysts that did turn out to be malignant. I would urge extreme caution in this area and would restrict any consideration of aspiration to unilocular cysts that are clearly identified on ultrasound without any other ultrasound findings, e.g., papillations, solid areas, and septa.

A.L. Herbst, M.D.

Ovarian

Tamoxifen in Patients With Advanced Epithelial Ovarian Cancer

van Der Velden J, Gitsch G, Wain GV, et al (Royal Hosp for Women, Sydney, Australia)
Int J Gynecol Cancer 5:301–305, 1995   22–5

Background.—The outcomes of second-line treatment in patients with persistent or recurrent epithelial ovarian cancer are generally unsatisfactory. In the past decade, tamoxifen has been reported to be an active salvage therapy in such patients. An experience with tamoxifen in patients with persistent or recurrent epithelial ovarian carcinoma was evaluated.

Methods.—Thirty patients were given tamoxifen after platinum-based chemotherapy evoked no response. Twelve patients were given tamoxifen

TABLE 2.—Reported Experience With Tamoxifen for Persistent or Recurrent Epithelial Ovarian Cancer

Study reference no.	No. of patients	Complete response (CR) (*n*)	Partial response (PR) (*n*)	Stable disease (*n*)	CR+PR (%)
3	13	0	1	4	7.7
5	29	1	7	12	27.6
6	23	0	0	19	0.0
7	22	0	0	1	0.0
8	37	1	2	6	8.1
9	53	0	1	5	1.9
10	105	10	8	40	17.1
11	29	2	3	18	17.2
This study	30	2	0	10	6.6
Total	341	16	22	115	11.1

(Courtesy of van Der Velden J, Gritsch G, Wain GV, et al: Tamoxifen in patients with advanced epithelial ovarian cancer. *Int J Gynecol Cancer* 5:301–305, 1995.)

for persistent disease, and 18 were treated for recurrent cancer after a disease-free interval.

Findings.—Complete remissions occurred in 2 patients (6.6%). One remission lasted 41 months and the other lasted 12 months. There were no partial responses to treatment, but disease was stable in 10 patients (33.3%) for a mean duration of 11.5 months. None of the patients had significant toxicity as a result of tamoxifen (Table 2). Seven patients had warm flushes.

Conclusions.—Tamoxifen can induce complete responses in patients with persistent and recurrent ovarian cancer, with minimal adverse effects. Thus, it has a place as second-line treatment for such patients. Tamoxifen therapy should probably be initiated when CA 125 titers increase progressively, before there is gross evidence of recurrent disease.

▶ A number of reports have concerned the possible use of tamoxifen for ovarian cancer, and there has been some enthusiasm for its use with well-differentiated lesions. The mechanism of action of this antiestrogen to affect ovarian carcinoma is not clear. Steroid hormone receptors have been identified in some ovarian epithelial carcinomas, but, unlike in endometrial cancers, the receptors do not appear to affect ovarian carcinoma cell growth.

At any rate, this study from Australia shows 2 of 30 complete responses lasting 12 and 41 months in patients previously treated with *cis*-platinum. The world experience is reproduced in Table 2. The pertinent information is that 16 of 341 patients had a complete response, i.e., less than 5%, a small proportion; even when partial responses are added, the proportion only rises to 11%. I am always skeptical of figures regarding "stable disease," particularly in well-differentiated tumor and, therefore, tend to discount that figure. However, it is worth noting in the present series that 1 of the complete responses occurred in a patient with a grade III tumor. The response rate is low, but this is a great advantage when it occurs, since there is virtually no toxicity.

A.L. Herbst, M.D.

Preoperative CA 125: An Independent Prognostic Factor in Patients With Stage I Epithelial Ovarian Cancer
Nagele F, Petru E, Medl M, et al (Univ Hosp of Vienna; Univ Hosp of Graz, Austria; Gen Hosp Salzburg, Austria; et al)
Obstet Gynecol 86:259–264, 1995   22–6

Background.—The tumor marker CA 125 has proved useful for monitoring the clinical course of ovarian cancer. It has also been correlated with responsiveness to chemotherapy, International Federation of Gynecology and Obstetrics (FIGO) stage of disease, and postoperative residual tumor mass. In patients with advanced disease, CA 125 is useful for predicting survival. The prognostic effects of preoperative CA 125 levels on the survival of patients with FIGO stage I epithelial ovarian cancer were compared with 3 well-established prognostic factors: histologic grade, FIGO substage, and patient age.

Methods.—Traditional variables and CA 125 levels were retrospectively assessed in 201 patients treated at 5 centers from 1984 to 1993. Patients were excluded from the analysis if they had borderline tumors or nonepithelial ovarian carcinomas or if CA 125 levels had not been determined before surgery.

Findings.—Univariate analysis showed that patients whose test results were positive for CA 125 had a significantly reduced overall survival. Survival prognosis was also significantly influenced by substage and histologic grade. When the effects of preoperative CA 125 levels and histologic grade were correlated, all 3 subgroups with CA 125 levels equal to or exceeding 65 units/mL were related to reduced survival probability. In a multivariate analysis, preoperative CA 125 was the strongest prognostic factor for survival. The risk of dying of disease was 6.4 times greater in patients with positive CA 125 findings. Although FIGO substage continued to significantly affect survival, histologic grade and age were not important prognostically.

Conclusions.—The tumor marker CA 125 appears to be the best independent prognosticator in patients with stage I epithelial ovarian cancer. Randomized trials designed to assess the efficacy of additional therapy in early-stage disease should be stratified according to preoperative serum CA 125 levels.

▶ CA 125 has been used in a variety of settings and thus far has proven most valuable in detecting recurrences in patients with ovarian carcinoma. This article provides a useful prognostic observation with preoperative CA 125 in regard to stage I ovarian tumors. Those patients whose preoperative value was 65 IU or more had a decidedly worse prognosis. The authors suggest those with stage I tumors, grades I and II, who fall into the elevated CA 125 category be considered for adjuvant chemotherapy, whereas those with grade III tumor who have a low CA 125 may not need such therapy. As the authors note, randomized trials are appropriate, but these observations offer an additional point to be considered when contemplating adjuvant chemotherapy in stage I tumors. There were 34 stage I tumors with CA 125 of 65 IU or more, and this subset had a 29.6% risk of dying of disease, compared with a 34.9% for those with elevated CA 125 and grade II tumors and 76.9% for those with elevated CA 125 and grade III tumors. Unquestionably, the grade III tumors with elevated CA 125 should receive chemotherapy, but it is not clear how much we can improve survival, particularly in the grade I tumors, which so frequently are chemoresistant—another reason for the suggested randomized trial.

A.L. Herbst, M.D.

A Risk Model for Ovarian Carcinoma Patients Using CA 125: Time to Normalization Renders Second-look Laparotomy Redundant

Frasci G, Conforti S, Zullo F, et al (Univ Federico II, Naples, Italy; Univ of Regio, Calabria, Italy; Natl Tumor Inst of Naples, Italy; et al)
Cancer 77:1122–1130, 1996

22–7

Background.—Second-look laparotomy (SLL) has long been a part of the treatment strategy for patients with epithelial ovarian carcinoma. However, patients with negative SLL findings apparently do not do as well as previously believed. Several other factors seem to influence the prognosis of patients with ovarian carcinoma. Whether SLL can be made redundant by adding CA 125 normalization times to a prognostic model based on pretreatment factors in women with ovarian carcinoma was determined.

Methods.—Fifty-four consecutive patients with ovarian carcinoma undergoing SLL between 1985 and 1990 were studied. All had abnormal CA 125 serum levels at diagnosis. These levels normalized during chemotherapy. Pretreatment variables relevant for prognosis were selected in a Cox model.

Findings.—Independent predictors of survival included size of residual tumor at the start of treatment and Eastern Cooperative Oncology Group performance status. Time to CA 125 serum level normalization also proved to be an independent prognostic indicator. When CA 125 and SLL findings were both included in the model, only CA 125 had independent prognostic relevance. Patients were stratified into 6 subgroups with different outcomes based on performance status, tumor size, and time to CA 125 normalization. The 5-year survival rate was 80% among patients with good prognostic pretreatment variables and patients with an intermediate prognosis at the start of treatment who had CA 125 values that normalized quickly. The 5-year survival rate for the remaining patients was only 16%.

Conclusion.—The survival of patients with advanced ovarian carcinoma can be predicted accurately by combining certain pretreatment variables and CA 125 normalization times in a prognostic model, obviating the need for SLL. Larger prospective trials are now needed to validate this risk model.

CA 125 Kinetics: A Cost-effective Clinical Tool to Evaluate Clinical Trial Outcomes in the 1990s

Buller RE, Vasilev S, DiSaia PJ (Univ of Iowa, Iowa City; City of Hope Natl Med Ctr, Duarte, Calif; Univ of California, Irvine)
Am J Obstet Gynecol 174:1241–1254, 1996

22–8

Background.—Several studies have investigated the treatment of advanced epithelial ovarian cancer with higher doses of chemotherapeutic agents. To optimize treatment protocols, practical methods are needed to evaluate treatment response. Routine assessment laparotomy is expensive.

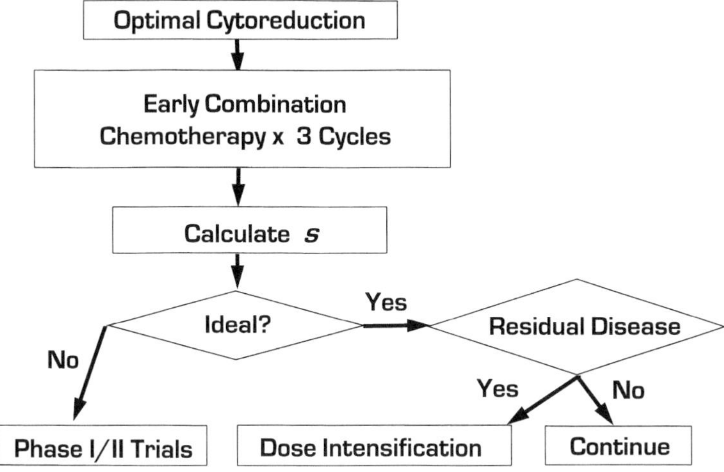

FIGURE 6.—Ovarian cancer treatment algorithm based on slope of the CA 125 exponential regression curve. (Courtesy of Buller RE, Vasilev S, DiSaia PJ: CA 125 kinetics: A cost-effective clinical tool to evaluate clinical trial outcomes in the 1990s. *Am J Obstet Gynecol* 174:1241–1254, 1996.)

Measuring the rate of reduction in serum CA 125 concentrations is a promising method of evaluating treatment response to chemotherapy. The association between the slope of the CA 125 regression curve and conventional prognostic indicators was analyzed in patients with ovarian cancer.

Methods.—A total of 126 patients treated for ovarian cancer were studied. Serum CA 125 concentrations were measured before and after surgery, and a regression curve was constructed using these data. Sixty-five patients had optimal cytoreduction. A reassessment laparotomy was done in 68 patients, with negative findings in 30 patients, of whom 18 had recurrences during the mean follow-up of 1,031 days. The dose intensity was calculated for each chemotherapeutic agent in each patient. The relationships between survival and the regression rate of CA 125, as well as other treatment and prognostic variables, were analyzed with univariate and multivariate analyses.

Results.—The CA 125 concentrations were normalized in 86 patients by the fourth chemotherapy cycle. The CA 125 regression curve correlated best with platinum treatment intensity, treatment equivalence, and overall treatment intensity. Univariate analysis revealed that survival was most strongly predicted by the slope of the CA 125 regression curve, the numbers of treatment cycles before CA 125 normalization, residual disease, and platinum treatment intensity. In multiple regression analysis, the slope of the CA 125 regression curve and the number of treatment cycles before CA 125 normalization were the most significant predictors of survival, with more predictive power than the conventional prognostic indicators, including age, stage, grade, chemotherapy intensity, and residual disease. However, there were no significant predictors of survival in the 28 patients without residual disease. The most important determinants of the slope of the CA 125 regression curve were the intercept of the regression equation, stage, age, and the interval between surgery and chemotherapy initiation.

Conclusions.—The determination of CA 125 kinetics is a useful method for monitoring response to chemotherapy in patients with epithelial ovarian cancer. Its cost-effectiveness further recommends its role in a treatment algorithm (Fig 6). It is recommended that patients with epithelial ovarian cancer undergo optimal cytoreduction, followed by 3 cycles of conventional combination chemotherapy with periodic measurements of serum CA 125 concentrations. The CA 125 regression curve, plotted from these measurements, can then dictate further treatment planning.

▶ I have paired these 2 articles (Abstracts 22–7 and 22–8), which deal with CA 125 kinetics and prognosis in ovarian epithelial carcinoma. Admittedly, CA 125 is not elaborated by 15% to 20% of these tumors. For those tumors that do elaborate CA 125, these studies suggest that the speed of reversion of CA 125 levels from an elevated level to a normal value is a strong indicator of prognosis.

In the Buller article, the slope of the regression curve "s" was a most important factor in predicting survival. In fact, those who were completely cytoreduced and had an ideal regression curve for their CA 125 values were alive and in over 4 years of follow-up, had not yet reached a median survival. In contrast, 33 of 44 patients with slow (less than ideal) slopes to the regression curve had residual disease at SLL, and this group had a survival rate of only 9%. Buller et al. constructed an algorithm that relates the slope of the regression curve to outcome and provides a guideline to therapists for either switching chemotherapy or continuing with the current regimen. This type of approach, I believe, provides us with a useful tool in thinking about therapy in this difficult disease,

The Frasci article evaluated 54 patients who underwent SSL. Those who had rapid normalization of CA 125 values did markedly better than those who did not. Both of these papers offer good evidence that CA 125 can provide important prognostic information and, in many cases, eliminate the need for SLL.

A.L. Herbst, M.D.

Laparoscopic Surgical Staging of Ovarian Cancer
Childers JM, Lang J, Surwit EA, et al (Univ of Arizona, Tucson)
Gynecol Oncol 59:25–33, 1995   22–9

Objective.—Although laparoscopy has been used to identify extraovarian metastases, its value in the surgical staging of ovarian cancer has yet to be determined. The accuracy, advantages, and disadvantages of laparoscopic staging of ovarian cancers were retrospectively studied.

Methods.—In the first group of women, aged 27–80 years, 40 patients had 44 second-look laparoscopic staging procedures for advanced disease after surgical debulking and chemotherapy. In the second group of women, there were 14 women, aged 17–75 years, with presumed early ovarian cancer, 5 of whom were unstaged when their tumors were surgically removed.

Results.—In the second-look group, 24 of the 44 procedures demonstrated persistent cancer. At surgery, 5 patients had microscopic disease only, located in the omentum, para-aortic nodes (2 patients), pelvic peritoneum, and peritoneal washings. All of these patients had recurrences. In 20 of the second-look patients, no metastatic disease was found, but 8 of these patients had recurrences. Six second-look patients had serious complications, and 3 required laparotomy. Eight of the 14 patients undergoing staging for the first time had metastatic disease, including 2 patients with adenocarcinoma; 3 patients with pelvic disease, which was confined to a fallopian tube in 1 patient and confined to the pelvic peritoneum in 2 patients; and 3 patients with metastatic adenocarcinoma of the para-aortic lymph nodes. Two patients had significant complications. Hospital stays ranged from 1 to 3 days.

Conclusion.—Laparoscopic surgical staging of ovarian cancer appears to be effective and accurate. Additional validation studies are recommended.

▶ This group from Tucson has been among those in the forefront in regard to the potential use of laparoscopic surgery in gynecologic oncology. The results presented here appear quite good insofar as the operating time (a major problem for those who are not well experienced in the technique) was short, and the knowledge gained in terms of positive biopsies and/or para-aortic node disease seems appropriate. The hospital stay was short (average, 1.6 days). All the major intraoperative complications were corrected laparoscopically, a feat not likely to be accomplished by many laparoscopic surgeons currently.

As the authors correctly note, we have much to learn in this area. It is possible that laparoscopic evaluation may prove to be as valuable and safe as laparotomy; however, a comparative multi-institutional trial would be needed. I believe we must remember the admonition of the authors, namely that laparoscopic skills are difficult to achieve. Furthermore, to obtain results similar to those reported, at least 2 highly skilled laparoscopists are required. I agree with the conclusion of the authors that it will be a number of years before such a pool of trained surgeons is available. In the meantime, I hope those who are acquiring these skills will be judicious and cautious in the application of these new techniques. All of us have witnessed severe and unnecessary patient complications with ill-advised efforts to utilize this new and potentially excellent approach.

A.L. Herbst, M.D.

Laparotomy to Complete Staging of Presumed Early Ovarian Cancer

Stier EA, Barakat RR, Curtin JP, et al (Mem Sloan-Kettering Cancer Ctr, New York)

Obstet Gynecol 87:737–740, 1996   22–10

Introduction.—Patients with stage I epithelial ovarian cancer have 5-year survival rates of greater than 95%. Most patients with ovarian cancer have advanced disease at diagnosis and have 5-year survival rates of 21%. Because most early ovarian cancers are discovered during procedures for presumed benign disease, the necessary biopsies for identifying occult disease and to properly stage disease are not performed. The findings and complications of laparotomies performed for restaging presumed early ovarian cancer were reported.

Methods.—Forty-five patients with stage IIB or earlier ovarian cancer underwent restaging surgery. The mean patient age was 34 years. The presumed stages from the initial surgery were as follows: 28 stage IA, 3 stage IB, 12 stage IC, 1 stage IIA, and 1 stage IIB. The mean time from initial operation to restaging was 56 days. Before reoperation, no patients had evidence of disease progression and none had received adjuvant therapy.

Results.—The disease stage was reclassified to a higher stage in 7 of 45 patients (16%) after second laparotomy. Two patients with initial stage IA disease were restaged to IB and IC, respectively. Another patient with borderline tumor was restaged from IIB to IIIA. One patient each with invasive epithelial adenocarcinoma was reclassified from: IC poorly differentiated adenocarcinoma to IIIB; stage IC, grade 2 mucinous cystadenocarcinoma to IIIA; and IC granulosa cell tumor to IIB. There were no intraoperative complications after restaging. Fifteen patients (33%) experienced postoperative complications. Adjuvant chemotherapy was able to be withheld in 18 patients with invasive cancer for whom restaging confirmed low-risk stage IA/B disease. The course of treatment was changed for 1 patient as a result of restaging. She was given adjuvant chemotherapy.

Conclusion.—The major benefit of restaging surgery is accurate prognostic information. This operation provides little benefit to those patients who require chemotherapy based on initial findings.

▶ This study of 45 patients with ovarian cancer from Memorial Sloan-Kettering Cancer Center addresses a pertinent question, i.e., "Should one re-explore ovarian cancer after initial incomplete staging?" As noted by the authors, some therapists do this laparoscopically, but there are not currently a large number of individuals in the United States who are fully qualified and competent with that approach.

The article concludes that a repeat operation can provide useful prognostic information, such as the lack of need for adjuvant chemotherapy for low-stage, low-grade cases. There is no clear benefit, in terms of cure, for patients with advanced disease, and there have been isolated reports of successful intervention by initial chemotherapy, which is usually given for 3 to 4 cycles followed by a full staging laparotomy. I believe it is difficult to provide firm guidelines in these cases because there is such great potential for individual variation. However, in general, I have preferred the chemotherapy-reoperation approach except in cases of grade 1 or borderline tumors. Then the question of reoperation would be primarily to remove disease not previously resected. If there is uncertainty, laparoscopic evaluation first would be an important initial consideration.

A.L. Herbst, M.D.

Preliminary Analysis of the Behavior of Stage I Ovarian Serous Tumors of Low Malignant Potential: A Gynecologic Oncology Group Study
Barnhill DR, Kurman RJ, Brady MF, et al (Walter Reed Army Med Ctr, Washington, DC; Johns Hopkins Med Insts, Baltimore, Md; Roswell Park Cancer Inst, Buffalo, NY; et al)
J Clin Oncol 13:2752–2756, 1995   22–11

Objectives.—A consensus on the management of ovarian epithelial tumors of low malignant potential (LMP) has yet to be reached. To investigate further, the Gynecologic Oncology Group conducted a long-term prospective study to evaluate the biological behavior of ovarian LMP tumors, the effectiveness of melphalan chemotherapy in patients with clinically detectable residual disease after surgical staging and those whose tumors progressed or recurred after surgical therapy, and the response rate to cisplatin in those who failed to respond to melphalan therapy.

Management.—Between 1983 and 1992, 146 patients with stage I serous LMP tumors underwent removal of the affected ovary (or ovaries) and a complete staging operation. None of the patients had endosalpingiosis. The median age was 43.7 years. Twenty-one patients had a unilateral salpingo-oophorectomy with retention of the uterus and a normal-appearing contralateral ovary; 123 had total bilateral abdominal hysterectomy and bilateral salpingo-oophorectomy. The tumor was ruptured in 10% of patients, the peritoneal cytology was positive in 12%, and external surface excrescences were present in 15%. In 7 patients who initially had an ovarian cystectomy and were then surgically explored, none had residual tumor in the ovary in which the cystectomy had been performed or in the contralateral normal-appearing ovary. None of the patients received adjuvant chemotherapy or radiation therapy.

Outcome.—All patients survived without recurrence during a median follow-up of 42.4 months (range, 1.8–108 months).

Conclusion.—Ovarian serous LMP tumors limited to the ovaries rarely, if ever, recur. These findings support a conservative surgical approach for the treatment of ovarian LMP tumors. After careful surgical exploration and thorough pathologic sampling with negative findings, unilateral salpingo-oophorectomy or possibly ovarian cystectomy is adequate therapy for women of reproductive age.

▶ This collaborative study from the Gynecologic Oncology Group reemphasizes a number of important points regarding borderline mucinous ovarian tumors. I was happy to note that no patient in the stage I study group received adjuvant chemotherapy and 21 patients had unilateral adnexectomy as their treatment, with preservation of the contralateral normal-appearing ovary in four of these patients who eventually became pregnant. I agree with the authors' conclusion that limited resection after meticulous exploration is sufficient and appropriate treatment for these patients.

A.L. Herbst, M.D.

Clear Cell Carcinoma of the Ovary: A Distinct Histologic Type With Poor Prognosis and Resistance to Platinum-based Chemotherapy in Stage III Disease

Goff BA, Sainz de la Cuesta R, Muntz HG, et al (Harvard Med School, Boston; Univ of Washington, Seattle)
Gynecol Oncol 60:412–417, 1996

22–12

Purpose.—Clear cell carcinoma is recognized as a distinct type of epithelial ovarian cancer. Although some studies suggest that the survival rate is similar for patients with clear cell vs. serous ovarian adenocarcinomas, others report that survival is shorter for patients with clear cell disease. Studies of cisplatin-based chemotherapy for epithelial ovarian cancers have included few patients with clear cell disease. The response to treatment and the prognostic factors for response in patients with clear cell ovarian cancer were assessed.

Methods.—The study compared 24 patients with stage III clear cell ovarian cancer treated during a 10-year period with 34 women with stage III papillary serous tumors treated during a 2-year period. Treatment consisted of cytoreductive surgery followed by conventional platinum-based chemotherapy. Median follow-up in survivors was 44 years.

Results.—Endometriosis was found in the surgical specimen in 37.5% of women with clear cell disease vs. 3% of those with papillary serous carcinoma. The rate of thromboembolic events was 42% vs. 18%, respectively. Progressive disease occurred in 70% of patients with clear cell carcinoma, including clinical progression during chemotherapy in 52% of patients. Progressive disease was found at second-look surgery in 4 patients, and a complete response occurred in only 2. By comparison, 29% of patients with papillary serous disease had progression during chemotherapy.

Median survival was 12 months for the patients with clear cell carcinoma vs. 22 months for those with papillary serous disease. On univariate analysis, age younger than 50 years was a negative prognostic factor for women with clear cell carcinoma. Endometriosis, thromboembolic events, and optimal cytoreductive surgery were not significant predictors of survival.

Conclusions.—The clinical characteristics and prognosis of patients with clear cell carcinoma of the ovary are different from those of patients with papillary serous tumors. Platinum-based chemotherapy does not produce a good response rate in patients with clear cell disease, most of whom show disease progression during therapy. In treatment trials, patients with clear cell histology should be differentiated from other patients with epithelial ovarian carcinomas and should be targeted for studies of alternative treatment approaches.

▶ This small series of 24 patients with stage III clear cell carcinoma of the ovary concludes that ovarian tumors with this histology not only have a poor prognosis, but also seem resistant to platinum-based chemotherapy. Perhaps somewhat surprisingly, these patients fared worse than a comparable group of patients with a papillary serous histology. The median lengths of survival were 12 months vs. 22 months, respectively. Even for those who were optimally debulked, the papillary serous group did better. In fact, a number of the patients with clear cell carcinoma actually had progression of disease while receiving platinum-based chemotherapy. All of this is quite discouraging and, as the authors suggest, we need a more effective alternative form of treatment for this highly lethal variety of ovarian carcinoma.

A.L. Herbst, M.D.

Primary Peritoneal Serous Papillary Carcinoma: A Study of 25 Cases and Comparison With Stage III-IV Ovarian Papillary Serous Carcinoma

Ben-Baruch G, Sivan E, Moran O, et al (Tel-Aviv Univ, Israel)
Gynecol Oncol 60:393–396, 1996   22–13

Objective.—Primary peritoneal serous papillary carcinoma (PPSC) occurs in women without ovarian disease or with only minimal involvement of the ovarian surface. It is unknown whether patients with PPSC are significantly different in their epidemiologic characteristics from those with papillary serous ovarian carcinoma (PSOC). There is disagreement about the relative prognoses of these 2 conditions and about the ability to perform optimal surgical debulking in PPSC. The clinical findings and treatment results of patients with PPSC and PSOC were compared.

Methods.—The study included 22 patients with PPSC and 63 patients with PSOC. The patients were seen at 1 department during an 11-year period. All underwent primary surgery designed to achieve optimal cytoreduction, followed by platinum-based combination chemotherapy. The clinical characteristics and treatment outcomes were compared between the 2 groups.

Results.—Mean age was approximately 60 years in each group. Between groups there were no significant differences in menopausal status, parity, ascites fluid volume, proportion of patients with stage IV disease, or proportion of patients undergoing optimal debulking. Median disease-free interval was 15 months for the patients with PPSC and 18 months for those with PSOC. Median survival was 21 and 26 months and 5-year survival was 18% and 24%, respectively. When the residual tumor measured 2 cm or more, median survival was 20.5 months in the patients with

PPSC and 24 months in those with PSOC. For patients with smaller residual tumors, median survival was 46 and 41 months, respectively. The survival advantage associated with smaller residual tumor was significant only for patients with PSOC.

Conclusions.—The clinical findings and treatment outcomes are similar for women with PPSC and PSOC. Treatment for PPSC seems to be the same as that for stage II to IV PSOC, the best approach being optimal debulking plus platinum-based chemotherapy. The presence of a pathophysiologic association between PPSC and PSOC remains to be determined.

▶ I have paired this article with the Goff et al. article (Abstract 22–12) on ovarian clear cell carcinoma because all of these types of malignancies are rare and, unfortunately, they share a poor prognosis. In this study, primary peritoneal serous tumors did slightly worse than the papillary serous ovarian cancers discussed by Goff et al. The median disease-free survivals were 15 and 18 months, which certainly are not very good. Not surprisingly, survival improved when residual disease postoperatively was less than 2 cm. Cisplatin, Adriamycin, and cyclophosphamide were frequently used together as a chemotherapy regimen; this is 1 regimen that our group has certainly favored for this group of tumors, although we certainly do not have proof that it is superior to any other regimen. Unlike the patients with clear cell adenocarcinoma in the Goff series, the patients in this report did, fortunately, seem to benefit from platinum-based chemotherapy.

A.L. Herbst, M.D.

Platinum-based Chemotherapy for Advanced-stage Serous Ovarian Carcinoma of Low Malignant Potential

Barakat RR, Benjamin I, Lewis JL Jr, et al (Mem Sloan-Kettering Cancer Ctr, New York; Univ of Pennsylvania, Philadelphia)

Gynecol Oncol 59:390–393, 1995

22–14

Objective.—A platinum-based chemotherapy regimen was evaluated in 21 women having advanced-stage (stage III or IV) papillary serous carcinoma considered to be of low malignant potential. Treatment was administered after cytoreductive surgery.

Patients.—The average age at diagnosis was 41 years; 71% of the women were premenopausal. Most patients reported abdominal or pelvic pain or pressure at the outset. Most underwent total abdominal hysterectomy with bilateral salpingo-oophorectomy and debulking of the tumor. Eight of 20 evaluable patients had gross residual disease measuring 2 cm or less in diameter. Twelve patients had only microscopic disease after surgery.

Treatment.—Three to 10 cycles of combination chemotherapy were given, the average number being 5. All patients received cisplatin in doses of 50–100 mg/m^2 and cyclophosphamide in doses of 500–750 mg/m^2. In addition, 10 patients received doxorubicin in a usual dose of 50 mg/m^2.

Outcome.—Ten of 16 patients (62.5%) were free of disease at second-look surgery, performed after chemotherapy was completed. Three patients (19%) had progressive disease. Three of the 7 patients with gross residual disease after initial surgery responded at least partially. All 10 patients with negative laparotomy findings remained free of disease at last follow-up. Five of the 6 patients with residual disease received further treatment. During an average follow-up exceeding 5 years, only 1 patient died of disease. Two of 3 patients had a partial response documented at third-look laparotomy, and the third patient remained stable.

Recommendations.—Presently these patients are offered IV cisplatin and paclitaxel. Those with gross residual disease after initial surgery are offered a second-look operation. If persistent disease is present, further chemotherapy including intraperitoneal treatment may be helpful. Patients with only microscopic residual disease probably will not benefit from a second-look operation.

▶ I have included this retrospective study of stage III and IV borderline ovarian carcinomas because I think that it sends an erroneous message. The authors indicate in the discussion that they now offer cisplatinum and paclitaxel (Taxol) chemotherapy to all patients with stage III and IV borderline ovarian carcinomas even though they counsel the patients that there is no evidence for survival advantage with this treatment. I believe that this is poor advice for these patients.

As noted by the authors, the literature suggests that about one fourth (26%) of those with macroscopic borderline tumors have a complete response to chemotherapy as do 68% of those with microscopic disease. They also note that approximately 21% of the patients with stage III to IV disease will die of the disease process. Using these figures, one can calculate a maximum theoretical benefit. This would amount to 26% (those with the macroscopic disease who would get a complete response) of the 21% (those who would die without treatment), which means that approximately 5% of these patients would benefit, assuming that 100% of those were treated. However, we know from evidence in the literature from Senekjian et al.[1] as well as others that those with noninvasive implants tend to do quite well and will likely survive. Furthermore, there is no evidence for a benefit of treatment even to this group with invasive implants. It does appear that those with invasive implants will do badly, although it is not at all clear that chemotherapy can help even this small group of patients.

Because those with noninvasive implants do exceedingly well without any further treatment, I continue to avoid using toxic chemotherapy in this group of patients. I do consider further treatment in those with stage III to IV disease who have invasive implants. In this way, many patients will continue to do well without therapeutic intervention and will not have to experience the toxicity of aggressive chemotherapy.

A.L. Herbst, M.D.

Reference

1. Senekjian EK, Hubby M, Bell D, et al: Clear cell adenocarcinoma (CCA) of the vagina and cervix in association with pregnancy. *Gynecol Oncol* 24:207, 1986.

Does Aggressive Therapy Improve Survival in Suboptimal Stage IIIc/IV Ovarian Cancer?: A Canadian–American Comparative Study

LoCoco S, Covens A, Carney M, et al (Univ of Toronto; Duke Univ, Durham, NC)

Gynecol Oncol 59:194–199, 1995   22–15

Objective.—To detect any differences in the treatment or outcome of patients with inadequately debulked epithelial ovarian cancers, experience at 2 tertiary care cancer centers in the United States and Canada was reviewed.

Study Population.—Sixty-one Canadian and 68 American patients had more than 1 cm of residual stage IIIc or stage IV disease after attempted debulking.

Patients and Treatment.—Patients at the American and Canadian centers did not differ significantly with regard to age, performance status, histology, tumor grade, or stage distribution. Optimal debulking was achieved in 19% of Canadian and 26% of American patients during the period under review (1987–1989). More American patients were operated on by a gynecologic oncologist. The mean extent of residual disease was 7.5 cm in Canada and 4.9 cm in the United States. More American patients underwent bowel surgery, but significant complications and hospital length of stay did not differ significantly. More than 90% of both groups received platinum-based treatment as primary chemotherapy. The number of oncologic laparotomies averaged 2.5 in the United States and 1.7 in Canada.

Outcome.—The median survival was 21 months in Canada and 20 months in the United States. The respective 5-year survival rates were 10% and 11%. Analysis of pooled data from the 2 centers showed that age was the only independent prognostic factor.

Implication.—Pending the development of new treatment strategies or better means of salvaging patients with inadequately debulked advanced-stage ovarian cancer, "more treatment is not necessarily better."

▶ I have included this retrospective operative study because I believe it makes a very good point, namely, that it does not benefit the patient with ovarian carcinoma to undergo radical operation if the result leaves the patient with gross tumor. All of the patients in this study had residual disease greater than 1 cm after operation for stage III disease or had stage IV disease at the time of operation. As can be seen from Table 1 in the original article, more extensive operations were accomplished at the Duke Center in comparison with the center at Toronto. In addition, the patients at Duke also received more chemotherapeutic regimens with increased grade 3 or more hematologic toxicity (38% vs. 18%). Most important, no survival benefit accrued to the group and, in fact, the 5-year survival rates at both centers were virtually identical—11% and 10%.

All this indicates to me that radical operative therapy does not appear to benefit the patients with ovarian carcinoma who cannot be debulked to small volume disease of less than 1 cm. As noted by the authors, we very much need better agents and regimens to improve our results with this disease.

A.L. Herbst, M.D.

Cyclophosphamide and Cisplatin Compared With Paclitaxel and Cisplatin in Patients With Stage III and Stage IV Ovarian Cancer

McGuire WP, Hoskins WJ, Brady MF, et al (Emory Univ, Atlanta, Ga; Mem Sloan-Kettering Cancer Ctr, New York; Roswell Park Cancer Inst, Buffalo, NY; et al)

N Engl J Med 334:1–6, 1996

22–16

Background.—The combination of an alkylating agent and cisplatin has become standard therapy for patients with advanced epithelial ovarian cancer. Although response rates are high, long-term survival is disappointing with this treatment. Paclitaxel has been found to have a high response rate in women with platinum-resistant ovarian cancer and can be safely combined with cisplatin. The efficacy of cisplatin combined with either cyclophosphamide or with paclitaxel in the treatment of advanced ovarian cancer was compared in a prospective, randomized, phase 3 trial.

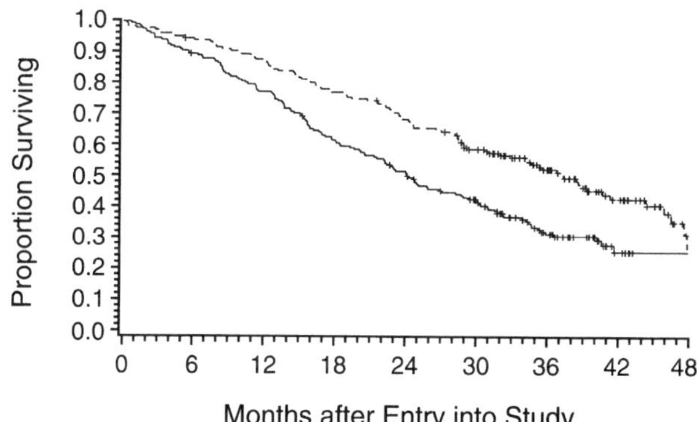

Treatment	No. Alive	No. Dead	Total	Median Survival (mo)
—— Cisplatin + cyclophosphamide	65	137	202	24
---- Cisplatin + paclitaxel	86	98	184	38

FIGURE 2.—Survival according to treatment group. (Reprinted by permission of *The New England Journal of Medicine* from McGuire WP, Hoskins WJ, Brady MF, et al: Cyclophosphamide and cisplatin compared with paclitaxel and cisplatin in patients with stage III and stage IV ovarian cancer. *N Engl J Med* 334:1–6, Copyright 1996, Massachusetts Medical Society.)

Methods.—A total of 410 women with stage III or IV epithelial ovarian cancer and residual disease after surgery were randomly assigned to receive treatment with either cisplatin and cyclophosphamide or cisplatin and paclitaxel every 3 weeks for 6 courses. All adverse effects were graded. Clinical response was evaluated in patients with clinically measurable disease, and overall and progression-free survival was calculated.

Results.—The cisplatin/paclitaxel group had significantly more toxicity. However, the cisplatin/paclitaxel group also had a significantly greater overall response rate (73% vs. 60%), complete response rate (51% vs. 31%), progression-free survival (18 vs. 13 months), and overall survival (38 vs. 24 months, Fig 2).

Conclusions.—The combination of cisplatin and paclitaxel has greater therapeutic efficacy and results in longer survival in patients with advanced epithelial ovarian cancer than the combination of cisplatin and cyclophosphamide.

▶ This is a large and important study by the Gynecologic Oncology Group that establishes the regimen of paclitaxel (Taxol) with cisplatin to be superior to cyclophosphamide and cisplatin in the treatment of advanced ovarian cancer. The reader should note that all patients had residual masses greater than 1 cm after initial operation.

Although the results are impressive and statistically significant, the improvement is still not very great. For example, progression-free survival was only 5 months longer in the paclitaxel group (18 vs. 13 months). More important, the median survival was 14 months longer in the paclitaxel group (38 vs. 24 months, see Figure 2). Follow-up is not long enough to provide data on 5-year survival, but Figure 2 suggests it is of the order of 30% to 35%. Admittedly, this is a poor prognostic group with residual disease before treatment, but we clearly have a long way to go in terms of effective therapy for this disease.

The authors also provide in the discussion some very important observations and warnings. For example, they note that some practitioners have substituted carboplatinum for cisplatin even though there are no data to prove that this regimen is as effective. In fact, the latter combination is in a phase 1 trial. Furthermore, they observed that some therapists have switched from 24-hour to 3-hour paclitaxel infusions because second- and third-line trials have shown equivalent efficacy for 3-hour paclitaxel alone, with less toxicity. However, in vitro data suggest that duration of exposure to paclitaxel is the primary determinant of effectiveness. We are all under great pressure to reduce costs, but it is clearly not appropriate or fair to patients to substitute less expensive regimens for which good data are lacking. I prefer cisplatin and paclitaxel given as a 24-hour infusion.

A.L. Herbst, M.D.

Assessment of Dose-intensive Therapy in Suboptimally Debulked Ovarian Cancer: A Gynecologic Oncology Group Study

McGuire WP, Hoskins WJ, Brady MF, et al (Emory Univ, Atlanta, Ga; Univ of the Health Sciences, Bethesda, Md; Mem Sloan-Kettering Cancer Ctr, New York; et al)

J Clin Oncol 13:1589–1599, 1995   22–17

Background.—A prospective trial of dose intensity and its effect in ovarian cancer using the current standard 2-drug therapy has not been reported. Women with advanced ovarian cancer were studied to evaluate the effect of chemotherapy dose intensity on survival and progression-free survival.

Methods.—Four hundred eighty-five patients with epithelial ovarian cancer and residual masses greater than 1 cm after surgery (stage III presentation) or stage IV presentation were randomly assigned to receive either standard therapy or intense therapy. Standard therapy consisted of IV cyclophosphamide, 500 mg/m², and IV cisplatin, 50 mg/m², every 3 weeks for 8 courses. Intense therapy consisted of cyclophosphamide, 1,000 mg/m², and cisplatin, 100 mg/m², every 3 weeks for 4 courses. Patients were not allowed to have any deviations in doses, but deviations were allowed in timing of subsequent doses. Before the next course could be administered, patients were required to have a white blood cell count greater than or equal to 3×10^9/L and a platelet count greater than or equal to 100×10^9/L.

Results.—Of the 485 patients, 458 met all eligibility criteria and were assessed for survival and progression-free survival. The intense-therapy group received the same total dose of the 2 drugs as did the standard therapy group, but the dose intensity was 1.97 times greater. Both groups of patients had similar clinical and pathologic response rates, response duration, and survival. The intense-therapy group had significantly progressively more severe hematologic, gastrointestinal, and renal toxicities and more febrile episodes and septic events than did the standard-therapy group. Seventeen percent of patients in the intense-therapy group and 7% of patients in the standard-therapy group were removed from the study because of toxicity.

Conclusions.—In these patients with bulky ovarian epithelial cancers, modest increases in chemotherapy dose intensity (without increasing the total dose) did not improve survival or progression-free survival. The increased-intensity treatment did, however, cause more severe toxicity.

▶ The struggle to provide an improved regimen for treating ovarian carcinoma continues. This well-done Gynecologic Oncology Group study looked at cisplatin and cyclophosphamide, and the patients were randomized and stratified by institution and clinical measurability of disease. The analysis results looked at the usual parameters of response, second-look operation, survival, etc. It is of interest that the total dose of each drug was identical in both arms of the study, the only difference being that in 1 arm, the dosage was given over 8 cycles, whereas in the other arm, double the dose was given in 4 cycles. The high-dose arm resulted only in more toxicity but did not improve overall survival or progression-free survival. It is unfortunately well established that increasing the dose cannot be relied on to yield a better result for the patient.

A.L. Herbst, M.D.

Surgical Management of Malignant Ovarian Germ-cell Tumors: 10 Years' Experience of 129 Patients

Peccatori F, Bonazzi C, Chiari S, et al (Univ of Milan, Monza, Italy)
Obstet Gynecol 86:367–372, 1995   22–18

Background.—Malignant ovarian germ-cell tumors are relatively uncommon, constituting approximately 10% of all ovarian tumors. Because of their rarity, the optimal surgical procedures for the management of malignant ovarian germ-cell tumors have not yet been established. To help define the role of various surgical procedures in different clinical situations, the surgical management of a large number of patients with malignant ovarian germ-cell tumors treated at a single institution was retrospectively evaluated.

Patients and Findings.—One hundred twenty-nine patients who had undergone surgery within a 10-year period were evaluated. The mean age at diagnosis of ovarian germ-cell tumor was 21 years. Dysgerminoma was noted in 57 patients, nondysgerminoma in 39 patients, and pure immature teratoma in 33 patients. On the basis of International Federation of Gynecology and Obstetrics criteria, 79 women had stage I disease, and 5 were first referred at recurrence, 11 at stage II, 35 at stage III, and 4 at stage IV.

Twenty-nine patients underwent primary surgery at the study institution, whereas the remaining 100 women were referred after surgery. Fertility-sparing surgery was done in 108 patients. Among the 44 patients with advanced conditions, tumors were reduced to less than 2 cm in diameter in 13 women. In the other 31 patients, residual tumors greater than 2 cm in diameter were noted before chemotherapy. Surgical or radiologic restaging was performed in 85 of the 100 referred patients, with an increase in staging noted in 16 patients. Eighty-four patients were treated with chemotherapy after surgery. Of the 65 women who were evaluated for response, 58 achieved a complete response, and 4 a partial response, and 3 did not respond to first-line treatment. A second laparotomy was done in 3 patients with immature teratoma for a growing mass. Mature teratoma or grade I immature teratoma was noted in all patients on histologic evaluation, and no further chemotherapy was administered. Thirty-one of 84 patients underwent second-look surgery, with positive findings observed in 4 women. The overall survival for all patients was 96%. Six patients, including 3 with dysgerminoma and 3 with endodermal sinus tumor, died of their disease. The mean follow-up from first surgery was 55 months, and no patient was lost to follow-up.

Conclusions.—Fertility-sparing surgery does not have an effect on the recurrence rate or survival, and therefore it is recommended for all ovarian germ-cell tumors. Extensive tumor-reductive surgery should be performed in patients with immature teratoma only and is not suggested for other histologic types. In certain patients, restaging can be effective, although chemotherapy treatment, when required, appears to be more important. Second-look surgery is only minimally useful.

▶ It is encouraging to note that fertility-sparing surgery has become part of the management of ovarian germ-cell tumors. I wish the authors would have included this concept, which they document so well in the title of this article. It is impressive that of the 129 cases, fertility-sparing procedures were initially performed in 108 (84%), including stages III and IV as well as those that were recurrent. Of course, all this is possible because of the effectiveness of chemotherapy in the eradication of these diseases. The predominant agents used were platinum and bleomycin, to which either vinblastine or etoposide was added. The results are impressive, with only 6 patients so far dead, with a mean follow-up of 55 months. As noted by the authors, the use of a second-look operation is controversial. It may have a place in patients who appear to have growing tumor after chemotherapy, particularly in cases of teratoma. I also agree with the authors that wedge biopsy of a contralateral normal-appearing ovary is not warranted, and I would apply this guideline to cases of dysgerminoma as well. The use of imaging procedures, such as ultrasound, to follow the pelvis and CT to evaluate the retroperitoneal nodes allows for a rational follow-up of these patients, with chemotherapy available and usually effective should a recurrence develop.

A.L. Herbst, M.D.

Cisplatin-based Chemotherapy in Dysgerminoma of the Ovary: Thirteen-year Experience at the Institut Gustave Roussy

Culine S, Lhomme C, Kattan J, et al (Institut Gustave Roussy, Villejuif, France; Centre Leon Berard, Lyon, France)
Gynecol Oncol 58:344–348, 1995

22–19

Objective.—Cisplatin-based chemotherapy was administered to 12 patients with pure dysgerminoma of the ovary after initial operative treatment. The drugs variably administered with cisplatin included actinomycin D, cyclophosphamide, vinblastine, bleomycin, and etoposide. Five of the 12 patients had no gross residual disease after the initial surgery. None of the patients received adjuvant radiotherapy.

Results.—All 6 patients who received chemotherapy as primary postoperative treatment were free of disease when followed up 18 months to 15 years later. Treatment failed in 3 of 6 patients who received chemotherapy as a part of salvage treatment for recurrent disease. One of these patients was a primary failure, 1 later relapsed, and 1 died of sepsis without evidence of treatment-related neutropenia. The other patients achieved complete clinical remission and remained free of disease 50–95 months after the start of chemotherapy. No clinical evidence of pulmonary or neurologic toxicity was found in the 9 patients who survived without disease.

Conclusion.—These results endorse the use of cisplatin-based chemotherapy in patients with pure ovarian dysgerminoma.

▶ The effectiveness of chemotherapy in the treatment of germ cell tumors is well established. This small series from the well-known Institut Gustave Roussy in France confirms its potential efficacy. Unfortunately, the group is small (12 patients), and 5 different protocols were used. Probably the most frequent combination in current use in the United States is bleomycin, etoposide, and cisplatin.

I would use such therapy after primary operation in patients with stage IC or higher dysgerminoma. I would probably withhold such treatment in stage IA unless the tumor were quite large (greater than 10–12 cm), in which case a fertility-preserving procedure is appropriate. But the role of adjuvant chemotherapy with its accompanying toxicity is at least a debatable point. It was "successfully" used by the authors in 1 case in this series.

A.L. Herbst, M.D.

The Efficacy of Cranial Irradiation in Ovarian Cancer Metastatic to the Brain: Analysis of 32 Cases

Corn BW, Greven KM, Randall ME, et al (Thomas Jefferson Univ, Philadelphia; Bowman Gray School of Medicine, Winston-Salem, NC; Univ of Miami, Fla; et al)
Obstet Gynecol 86:955–959, 1995
22–20

Introduction.—Ovarian cancers other than germ-cell tumors rarely metastasize to the brain. Recent studies indicate that carboplatin may be the preferred treatment and also that focal irradiation may help palliate metastases of ovarian cancer at various sites.

Series.—A review of tumor registries at 5 university cancer centers yielded 4,027 cases of ovarian cancer seen in the years 1965 to 1994. Thirty-two women had cerebral metastases, and all of them received fractionated irradiation to the whole brain in a median total dose of 30 Gy. In addition, 5 patients received systemic chemotherapy and 26 patients received corticosteroid therapy, usually with dexamethasone.

Results.—The most common features seen initially were headache and a seizure. The overall median survival time after the detection of brain metastasis was 4 months. Patients whose Karnofsky performance status was 70 or greater had a median survival of 33 weeks. Twenty-three of the 32 patients responded symptomatically to treatment, and in 16 cases palliation persisted to the time of death. The median time of palliation in those who responded was 6 months. A high performance status and the absence of active extracranial lesions predicted symptomatic improvement. The only treatment-related complications were sepsis (in a patient given chemotherapy) and a steroid-induced gastric ulcer.

Conclusion.—Whole-brain irradiation is a reliable means of palliating women who have cerebral metastases of ovarian cancer; in some cases, it may lengthen survival.

▶ This article deals with the exceedingly rare complication of brain metastases in ovarian cancer. I have included it, however, because of the effective palliative results. It is worth noting that most patients do not survive more than a few months, but palliation was effectively achieved in 23 of the 32 patients and 16 of these were benefited until they died of the disease. The authors emphasize that those with a good performance status did the best.

It appears to me that this is a useful mode of management for the rare occurrence of ovarian carcinoma brain metastases, particularly if the patient has a reasonable performance status. This offers us a useful way to deal with the dangerous complication of this disease.

A.L. Herbst, M.D.

Endometrioid Adenocarcinoma of the Ovary and Its Relationship to Endometriosis

McMeekin DS, Burger RA, Manetta A, et al (UCI Med Ctr, Orange, Calif; Long Beach Mem Med Ctr, Calif)
Gynecol Oncol 59:81–86, 1995

22–21

Background.—The clinical presentation of patients with endometriosis-related tumors has not been well documented. In addition, the biological behavior of these tumors is poorly understood. A 13-year historical cohort determined whether endometriosis-associated tumors were different from typical endometrioid adenocarcinomas in clinicopathologic variables and disease outcome.

Methods.—All women with endometrioid adenocarcinoma of the ovary diagnosed between 1979 and 1991 were included in the review. Pathology reports were analyzed to determine whether coexisting endometriosis was present. Cancers adjacent to endometriosis on the same ovary or arising within endometriosis were classified as endometriosis-associated endometrioid adenocarcinoma (EAEA). All others were considered typical endometrioid adenocarcinoma (TEA).

Findings.—Sixty-nine percent of the 91 patients with endometrioid adenocarcinoma of the ovary had TEA and 31% had EAEA. Patients with TEA and with EAEA differed significantly in age at diagnosis, with more patients with TEA being older than 55 years; nulliparity, with more patients with EAEA being nulliparous; stage, with stages I and II being more common among patients with EAEA; and disease status at the completion of primary surgery, with a greater proportion of patients with EAEA undergoing complete tumor resection. Eleven percent of patients with TEA and 25% with EAEA had synchronous atypical endometrial hyperplasia of uterine carcinoma. The estimated 5-year disease-free interval was significantly longer in patients with EAEA than in those with TEA. However, the 5-year survival difference was nonsignificant. Disease stage was the only independent prognostic factor that predicted both disease-free interval and survival.

Conclusions.—Endometrioid adenocarcinoma of the ovary associated with endometriosis may have a more favorable biological behavior than TEA. Women with EAEA are significantly younger, have an earlier disease stage when seen initially, and have a longer disease-free survival than do patients with TEA.

▶ This article nicely compares the behavior of EAEA of the ovary with the TEAs of the ovary, which exist without evidence of endometriosis. This series of 91 patients had 30 cases of tumors associated with endometriosis, a comparatively unusual event. As noted by the authors, malignant transformation of endometriosis is believed to be rare. The findings indicate that endometriosis-associated tumor occurred in younger patients who tended to be more frequently nulliparous and had a better prognosis, in part due to the fact that most were diagnosed at a low stage. In addition, synchronous endometrial carcinomas tended to occur in the EAEA group. It is of interest that in all 12 of these cases, the synchronous endometrial tumor was well differentiated and confined to the inner third of the myometrium. Endometriosis with endometrioid adenocarcinomas of the ovary does not occur often, but these patients do appear to have a survival advantage in comparison to those with tumors that occur without evidence of endometriosis.

A.L. Herbst, M.D.

Uterine

Screening by Ultrasonography for Endometrial Carcinoma in Postmenopausal Breast Cancer Patients Under Adjuvant Tamoxifen

Cecchini S, Ciatto S, Bonardi R, et al (Natl Cancer Inst, Genoa, Italy; Careggi Hosp, Florence, Italy)
Gynecol Oncol 60:409–411, 1996   22–22

Background.—There is concern that women taking long-term tamoxifen as an adjuvant or preventive treatment may be at increased risk of endometrial carcinoma. Vaginal sonography has been suggested as a surveillance test for endometrial changes in this patient population. The ability of sonography to detect endometrial changes in women receiving long-term tamoxifen therapy and to select patients needing further investigation was studied.

Methods.—The analysis included 737 asymptomatic, postmenopausal breast cancer patients who were receiving adjuvant tamoxifen therapy.

The average duration of tamoxifen therapy was 50 months. All patients underwent endometrial ultrasonography with a 3.5-MHz abdominal or a 6-MHz vaginal convex transducer. An endometrial thickness of 6 mm or more was defined as abnormal. When this finding was present, outpatient endometrial biopsy was recommended.

Results.—Twenty-eight percent of patients had abnormal endometrial thickness, which was significantly associated with patient age and duration of tamoxifen treatment. Biopsy was refused by 25 of these 209 patients; another 76 were followed up with sonography because of cervical stenosis. Endometrial carcinoma was detected in only 1 of the 108 patients who underwent biopsy, and this result was consistent with age-specific incidence rates. Another patient was confirmed as having endometrial hyperplasia, and all the rest were found to have endometrial atrophy. Endometrial carcinoma did not develop in any additional patients, and no additional endometrial changes have been observed at sonographic follow-up.

Conclusions.—In a study of women receiving adjuvant tamoxifen therapy, no increased prevalence of endometrial disease is apparent to date. Sonography shows an apparent increase in endometrial thickness in some patients, which may result from tamoxifen-induced changes in the endometrial stroma and myometrium. The authors plan annual endometrial sonographic follow-up in the study cohort.

▶ I have included this ultrasound study of postmenopausal patients receiving tamoxifen for breast cancer because it is a timely topic of great concern both to the patient and to her gynecologist. Of interest is the fact that the patients had been given tamoxifen for more than 4 years and approximately 30% of the 737 patients studied had endometrial stripes of 6 mm or more. Ultimately, biopsies were obtained from 108 patients with thick endometrial stripes and these yielded only 1 case of endometrial carcinoma. Most of the patients had no pathology. This is certainly a reassuring study, and I prefer not to routinely biopsy patients who are taking tamoxifen. However, I do office endometrial sampling if the patient bleeds.

A.L. Herbst, M.D.

Secretory Endometrial Adenocarcinoma in a Patient on Tamoxifen for Breast Cancer: A Report of a Case
Folk JJ, Mazur MT, Eddy GL, et al (State Univ of New York, Syracuse; Crouse Irving Mem Hosp, Syracuse, NY)
Gynecol Oncol 58:133–135, 1995
22–23

Background.—Tamoxifen, a nonsteroidal compound with weak estrogenic activity, is used as palliative breast cancer therapy, as prophylaxis for women at high risk for breast cancer and for the remaining breast after mastectomy, and as a treatment for advanced, node-positive disease. Several reports of endometrial carcinoma associated with tamoxifen therapy have been published within the past 10 years. In a new case report, well-differentiated secretory endometrial adenocarcinoma occurring in a postmenopausal woman given low-dose tamoxifen was evaluated. This is thought to be the first report of secretory carcinoma of the endometrium related to the use of tamoxifen.

> *Case Report.*—Woman, 68, was evaluated for an episode of vaginal bleeding 5 years after undergoing a right mastectomy for breast carcinoma. The patient had been taking 10 mg of oral tamoxifen twice daily since breast surgery. A benign endometrial polyp and complex endometrial hyperplasia were noted on hysteroscopy and uterine dilation and curettage. Multiple tissue fragments with complex atypical hyperplasia and secretory changes were observed in the uterine curettings, as were separate fragments of a benign polyp. Closely spaced glands separated by a thin stromal layer were characteristic of the hyperplasia. Extensive subnuclear and supranuclear vacuolization, producing a secretory change comparable to that found in normal early-secretory-phase endometrium, was observed in the glandular epithelium. Because of the distinct crowding of the glands, the pattern was considered atypical. Examination of the polyp showed large, irregular glands with minimal mitotic activity in a dense, fibrotic stroma. These findings were consistent with tamoxifen-associated polyps.
>
> Laparoscopic-assisted vaginal hysterectomy with bilateral salpingo-oophorectomy was performed 4 weeks after hysteroscopy and uterine curettage. A 3- × 1.8- × 1.5-cm polypoid lesion with surrounding granular tissue was obtained, and histopathologic analysis showed a grade I secretory adenocarcinoma, according to criteria of the International Federation of Gynecology and Obstetrics, originating from the atypical complex secretory hyperplasia. A residual benign polyp with secretory glands was also found in the tissue pieces. A cribriform and papillary patterns, together with considerable subnuclear and supranuclear vacuoles, were noted in the adenocarcinoma. Uniform nuclei, with small nucleoli and a low mitotic rate, were also observed. The myometrium was superficially invaded by the carcinoma, to a depth of 0.2 cm.

Conclusions.—The pathogenesis of the secretory change observed in this adenocarcinoma remains unknown, and it is possible that this change was not associated with tamoxifen use. Focal secretory changes affecting the glands in tamoxifen-associated polyps and in complex atypical hyperplasia occurring after treatment with tamoxifen have, however, previously been observed. Whatever the reason for the secretory change observed in this patient, this report adds to other descriptions of the histologic patterns occurring in tamoxifen-related endometrial carcinoma.

▶ I have included this case report because there has been increasing attention regarding tamoxifen utilized for breast cancer and subsequent uterine neoplasia. In spite of all of the concern, carcinoma really appears to be quite rare. I thought it interesting that secretory carcinoma developed in a patient while taking this medication, particularly as secretory carcinoma is such a rare variant of that disease. In any event, as gynecologists, we should be alert to our patients who are being treated with this drug secondary to breast carcinoma. I generally do not do endometrial sampling unless the patient is symptomatic.

A.L. Herbst, M.D.

Assessment of Myometrial Infiltration and Preoperative Staging by Transvaginal Ultrasound in Patients With Endometrial Carcinoma

Weber G, Merz E, Bahlmann F, et al (Univ of Mainz, Germany)
Ultrasound Obstet Gynecol 6:362–367, 1995   22–24

Introduction.—Carcinoma of the endometrium is the most common gynecologic malignancy. Both the depth of tumor invasion in the myometrium and the degree of differentiation have been shown to have important prognostic value in patients with endometrial carcinoma, and precise preoperative assessment of these 2 factors is crucial in treatment planning. The value of transvaginal sonography for preoperative staging and evaluation of myometrial invasion was studied prospectively in patients with endometrial carcinomas.

Methods.—The preoperative sonographic findings and postoperative histologic data were compared in 80 patients with an endometrial carcinoma. Transvaginal sonography was performed in the sagittal and transverse planes to assess endometrial thickness and structure, endometrial demarcation, evidence of intrauterine fluid, and the degree of cervical and adnexal tumor infiltration.

Results.—All 80 patients had increases in endometrial thickness of more than 1.5 cm in premenopausal patients and more than 0.5 cm in postmenopausal patients, irregular demarcation of the boundary of the endometrium, and heterogeneous endometrial structure. Sonography revealed infiltration of up to 50% of the myometrium in 60% of the patients and of more than 50% of the myometrium in 34%. Accordance was found between the sonographic findings and the postoperative histologic data in 85% of the patients for the depth of tumor infiltration in the myometrium and in 87.5% of the patients for tumor staging.

Conclusions.—Transvaginal sonography is an inexpensive and noninvasive method of obtaining valuable diagnostic information in patients with endometrial carcinoma; it has considerable clinical utility in planning appropriate surgical treatment. Optimal prognostic data would be obtained by performing simultaneous imaging of the endometrium in all 3 planes.

▶ This is an interesting study of transvaginal ultrasound's ability to predict the spread and thus the stage of endometrial carcinoma in the uterus. The ultrasound was effective to detect the presence of carcinoma by evaluating endometrial thickness with values greater than 1.5 cm in premenopausal patients and greater than 0.5 cm in postmenopausal patients, indicating carcinoma. To evaluate myometrial invasion, the investigators chose a penetration of one half. The sonographic findings correlated with the postoperative histologic findings in 87.5% of the cases (70 of 80). Eight of the other cases were understaged (3 because of missed cervical involvement) by sonography and in 2 others, cervical involvement indicated by ultrasound was not confirmed histologically.

It would appear this is a potentially useful technique in helping to plan intraoperative therapy. However, it appears to result in errors, particularly with regard to cervical involvement. I have not yet incorporated preoperative routine vaginal ultrasonography into the evaluation of patients with endometrial carcinoma, but I will be looking for further and larger studies because the technique does seem promising.

A.L. Herbst, M.D.

Staging Laparotomy for Endometrial Carcinoma: Assessment of Retroperitoneal Lymph Nodes
Chuang L, Burke TW, Tornos C, et al (Univ of Texas, Houston)
Gynecol Oncol 58:189–193, 1995   22–25

Background.—In the 1988 International Federation of Gynecology and Obstetrics staging scheme for uterine corpus cancer, stage IIIC is defined as tumor spread to retroperitoneal lymph nodes. However, this scheme does not include recommendations on how to detect lymph node metastasis.

Methods.—The techniques of lymph node assessment in 295 patients at risk were reviewed. Patients had clinical stage I disease and preoperative biopsy specimens demonstrating grade 2 or 3 adenocarcinoma or papillary serous, clear-cell, or mixed carcinoma. The retroperitoneal space was divided arbitrarily into 10 lymphatic zones: left and right para-aortic, common iliac, external iliac, hypogastric, and obturator.

Findings.—Eighty-two percent of the patients had some type of node sampling involving an average of 3 zones. Of 244 patients sampled, 33 (13.5%) had nodal metastases. Involvement was gross in 20 patients and microscopic in 13. Fifty-one patients had no node sampling, 193 had some nodes biopsied, and 51 had node sampling with a minimum of 1 para-aortic plus at least 1 right and left pelvic specimen. Retroperitoneal recurrences thought to originate from lymph node sites in patients whose nodes tested negative were identified. In the first group, findings were positive in 8%; in the second, 5%; and in the third, 0%. Twenty-four percent of the patients with biopsy specimen–proved metastases had lymphatic-site failures.

Conclusions.—Failure to systematically sample pelvic and para-aortic nodes is associated with a risk of undetected extrauterine metastasis. An accurate estimate of whether nodes truly test negative may be achieved through a selective approach to sampling that includes biopsy specimens from para-aortic and bilateral pelvic lymphatic zones.

▶ The authors evaluated the pelvic and peritoneal nodes in patients with endometrial carcinoma who underwent a staging procedure. There remains some uncertainty about which patients need such an approach. The authors chose those with serous or clear-cell histology and any grade II or grade III tumor or a grade I tumor greater than 50% of the myometrium invaded. In their series, 13.5% (33 of 244 cases) had positive nodes. I prefer to restrict the node dissection to those with grade III tumors and any degree of myometrial invasion and grade I or II tumors with more than one third of the myometrium invaded in medically appropriate candidates.

However, the authors have made an important point, namely, that metastases are found in clinically nonsuspicious nodes. Furthermore, lymph node sampling should include representative sites of the pelvic and the para-aortic nodes. However, a complete node dissection, which certainly can be difficult, if not hazardous, in the somewhat obese patient, probably is not necessary and does not add much useful information.

A.L. Herbst, M.D.

Pathologic Models to Predict Outcome for Women With Endometrial Adenocarcinoma: The Importance of the Distinction Between Surgical Stage and Clinical Stage—A Gynecologic Oncology Group Study
Zaino RJ, Kurman RJ, Diana KL, et al (Pennsylvania State Univ, Hershey; Johns Hopkins Med Insts, Baltimore, Md; Roswell Park Cancer Inst, Buffalo, NY; et al)
Cancer 77:1115–1121, 1996   22–26

Introduction.—Models of prognostic factors created from multivariate analysis can be used to predict the probability of recurrence or death from tumor in patients with cancer. Models were created from univariate and multivariate analyses to predict the risk of death from tumor based on the clinical stage and surgical stage for women with endometrial carcinoma.

Methods.—Patients with clinical stage I and occult stage II endometrial adenocarcinoma underwent clinicopathologic evaluation as part of a Gynecologic Oncology Group investigation. The International Federation of Gynecology and Obstetrics staging criteria of 1971 were used. The primary therapy for all patients was total abdominal hysterectomy, bilateral salpingo-oophorectomy, selective pelvic and para-aortic lymphadenectomy, and peritoneal cytologic sampling. Postoperative therapy was individualized by the treating physician. All pathologic slides were reviewed by a subcommittee of 6 pathologists. Cell types were classified and recorded. Tumors were evaluated for cell type and architectural grade. Of 819 patients evaluated, 597 had surgical stage I or occult stage II disease. These patients were followed until death or for a minimum of 5 years.

TABLE 2.—Clinical Stage I and II Tumors: The Proportional Hazards Modeling of Relative Survival Time

Variable	Regression coefficient	Relative risk	Significance test* (*P* value)
Endometrioid			—†
Grade 1	—	1.0	
Grade 2	0.47	1.6	12.7 (0.0004)
Grade 3	0.94	2.6	
Clear cell			10.5 (0.001)
Grade 1	2.00	7.1	
Grade 2	1.33	3.8	2.7 (0.1)
Grade 3	0.71	2.0	
Serous			6.7 (0.01)
Grade 1	1.06	2.9	
Grade 2	1.47	4.4	2.7 (0.1)
Grade 3	1.89	6.6	
Endometrioid with			
squamous differentiation			0.3 (0.6)
Grade 1	−0.25	0.8	
Grade 2	−0.04	1.0	0.5 (0.5)
Grade 3	0.17	1.2	
Villoglandular			2.2 (0.1)
Grade 1	−0.94	0.4	
Grade 2	0.28	1.3	3.2 (0.08)
Grade 3	1.50	4.5	
Myometrial invasion			
Endometrium only	—	1.0	
Superficial	0.19	1.2	
Middle	0.46	1.6	23.9 (0.0001)
Deep	1.08	3.0	
Positive washings	1.09	3.0	35.5 (0.0001)
Age	0.17	—	
Age	−0.000985	—	24.9 (0.0001)
45 (arbitrary reference)	—	1.0	
55	0.715	2.0	
65	1.233	3.4	
75	1.554	4.7	
Vascular space involvement	0.41	1.5	4.6 (0.03)

Note: P value for grading is for overall grade within cell type.

*Wald chi-square test.

†Typical endometrial is reference for all cell types.

(Courtesy of Zaino RJ, Kurman RJ, Diana KL, et al: Pathologic models to predict outcome for women with endometrial adenocarcinoma: The importance of the distinction between surgical stage and clinical stage—A Gynecologic Oncology Group study. *Cancer* 77:1115–1121, Copyright © 1996. Reprinted by permission of Wiley-Liss, Inc., a division of John Wiley & Sons, Inc.)

Results.—Univariate analysis showed significant differences for patients with stage I and occult stage II disease in the probability of death from tumor based on cell type, architecture grade, depth of invasion, vascular space involvement, and presence of positive perineal cytology. Multivariate analysis revealed that many, but not all, of the risk factors were independent variables for stage I and occult stage II disease. The significant factors were the architectural grade of endometrioid adenocarcinoma, depth of myometrial invasion, serous and clear cell types, and age at diagnosis. The relative contribution of individual factors to probability of death (relative risk) can be calculated using the first model (Table 2). The predicted survival time can be assessed for varying relative risks using the

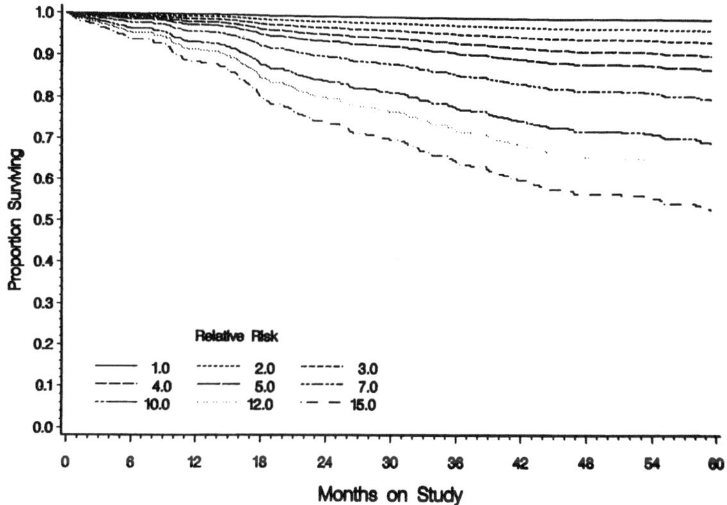

FIGURE 1.—Predicted survival time by initial tumor relative risk in clinical stage I and II patients. (Courtesy of Zaino RJ, Kurman RJ, Diana KL, et al: Pathologic models to predict outcome for women with endometrial adenocarcinoma: The importance of the distinction between surgical stage and clinical stage—A Gynecologic Oncology Group study. *Cancer* 77:1115–1121, Copyright © 1996. Reprinted by permission of Wiley-Liss, Inc., a division of John Wiley & Sons, Inc.)

second model (Fig 1). Using these models, a simple calculation can determine the relative risk of death for an individual patient from the data for each independent prognostic variable. For any given relative risk, the survival curve for surgical stage I and II disease was better, compared with that of clinical stage I and II disease.

Conclusion.—Age, depth of myometrial invasion, and, to a lesser extent, histologic grade and cell type are independent prognostic variables for stage I and II endometrial adenocarcinoma. Models that designate the relative risk associated with each independent prognostic variable were created. This data can be used to determine prognosis and the need for postoperative adjuvant therapy.

▶ This is an interesting and useful study from the Gynecologic Oncology Group concerning the behavior of endometrial carcinoma. The authors have evaluated both clinical and surgical stages. Table 2 and Figure 1, which relate to clinical staging and outcome, have been reproduced.

Not surprisingly, the age of the patient and the depth of invasion were the most powerful predictors of survival, as well as histologic grade and cell type. The analysis is based on 819 patients and provides a useful guideline for predicting survival. For example, given a patient with stage I, grade 3 serous carcinoma with middle one third myometrial invasion, there would be a value of 10.56. From Table 1, i.e., grade 3 serous (6.6) × middle one third myometrial invasion (1.6) = 10.56. Taking this value to Figure 1 corresponds to a 5-year survival rate of 65%. Using the data compiled by Zaino et al., one could then predict survival, and this will provide therapists with a useful mechanism for deciding whether adjuvant therapy may be necessary. The major problem with the article is that the graphs that are reproduced for both clinical and surgical staging are extremely small and difficult to interpret. It would be helpful if they could be produced in the future in a larger size.

A.L. Herbst, M.D.

Adjuvant Radiation Therapy is Not Necessary in the Management of Endometrial Carcinoma Stage I, Low-risk Cases

Poulsen HK, Jacobsen M, Bertelsen K, et al (Odense Univ, Denmark)
Int J Gynecol Cancer 6:38–43, 1996   22–27

Introduction.—Although endometrial carcinoma is traditionally managed by a combination of surgery and radiation therapy, there is considerable variation in the treatment approach. In particular, there is ongoing debate regarding the mode, timing, and effects of adjuvant radiation therapy. In 1986, the Danish Endometrial Cancer Group agreed to national guidelines by which only those high-risk patients with stage I endometrial carcinoma would receive adjuvant radiation therapy. The long-term results of patients treated by this protocol were reviewed.

Methods.—The analysis included 1,214 women with newly diagnosed endometrial carcinoma treated from 1986 to 1988. They accounted for all such patients with a diagnosis of endometrial carcinoma in Denmark during this time. Treatment consisted of total abdominal hysterectomy and bilateral salpingo-oophorectomy, without preoperative radiation therapy. Eighty-six percent of the women had no macroscopic residual tumor and/or microscopic tumor tissue in the resection margins. Those with grade 1 or 2 tumors and 50% or less myometrial invasion were classified as P-stage I low-risk, and those with grade 1 or 2 tumors and more than 50% myometrial invasion and those with grade 3 tumors were classified as P-stage I high-risk. Patients in the P-I low-risk classification received no postoperative radiation therapy, whereas those in the P-I stage high-risk group—as well as those in the P-II, and P-III (group 1) categories—received external radiation therapy. Follow-up ranged from 68 to 92 months.

TABLE 6.—Recurrences at 68–92 Months Follow-up in Endometrial Carcinomas
(P-Stages, I, II, and III, Group 1)

P-stage	n (%)
P-stage I, low-risk	45 / 641 (7)
P-stage I, high-risk	36 / 235 (15)
P-stage II	30 / 105 (29)
P-stage III, Group I	27 / 58 (47)
Total	138 / 1039 (13)

(Courtesy of Poulsen HK, Jacobsen M, Bertelsen K, et al: Adjuvant radiation therapy is not necessary in the management of endometrial carcinoma stage I, low-risk cases. *Int J Gynecol Cancer* 6:38–43, 1996.)

TABLE 7.—Death From Endometrial Carcinoma (P-Stages I, II, and III, Group 1) at 68–92 Months Follow-up

P-stage	n (%)
P-stage I, low-risk	28 / 641 (4)
P-stage I, high-risk	25 / 235 (11)
P-stage II	23 / 105 (22)
P-stage III, Group 1	26 / 58 (45)
Total	102 / 1039 (10)

(Courtesy of Poulsen HK, Jacobsen M, Bertelsen K, et al: Adjuvant radiation therapy is not necessary in the management of endometrial carcinoma stage I, low-risk cases. *Int J Gynecol Cancer* 6:38–43, 1996.)

Results.—The patient classifications were P-I low-risk, 641 patients; P-I high-risk, 235 patients; P-II, 105 patients; and P-III (group 1), 58 patients. Recurrence rates at follow-up were 7% in the P-I low-risk group, 15% in the P-I high-risk group, 29% in the P-II group, and 47% in the P-III (group 1) group (Table 6). With salvage therapy, 15 of 17 P-I low-risk patients with vaginal recurrences were still alive at a median follow-up of 64 months. The crude survival rate for P-stage I low-risk patients was 90% (Table 7).

Conclusions.—The use of adjuvant radiation therapy in patients with stage I endometrial carcinoma can be limited to high-risk cases. For P-stage I low-risk patients, total abdominal hysterectomy and bilateral salpingo-oophorectomy appears to be adequate treatment. A low recurrence rate and good survival can be achieved with no need for preoperative or postoperative radiation therapy.

▶ This is a useful article describing a prospective Danish study of 1,039 cases of endometrial carcinoma. I shall confine my comments to the stage I results even though some cases of stage II and III were included.

The low-risk patients were categorized as those with grades I or II tumors that invaded 50% or less of the myometrium and no further therapy was given after operation. The high-risk stage I group consisted of those with grade 3 or grades 1 and 2 with greater than 50% myometrial invasion for whom whole pelvic irradiation to 4,500 cGy was given. Unfortunately, the serous and clear cell tumors were not excluded, so some were counted in the low-risk group, which is not consistent with many studies that would consider these as high-risk types.

However, the results for the low-risk group in particular are impressive. With no further therapy, only 45 of 641 (7%) had recurrence and of these only 4 died (see Tables 6 and 7). It is clear there is a definable group of patients with endometrial carcinoma who do not need postoperative radiation therapy. In fact 15% of 17 vaginal recurrences in the low-risk group were effectively treated by subsequent radiation. As noted by the authors, adjuvant radiation for this low-risk group runs the risk of increased complications with little potential benefit.

A.L. Herbst, M.D.

Radiation Therapy as Exclusive Treatment for Medically Inoperable Patients With Stage I and II Endometrioid Carcinoma of the Endometrium

Fishman DA, Roberts KB, Chambers JT, et al (Yale Univ, New Haven, Conn)
Gynecol Oncol 61:189–196, 1996   22–28

Introduction.—Primary surgery and individualized radiation therapy is the most widely accepted treatment approach for women with stages I and II endometrial cancer. About 10% to 20% of patients with endometrial cancer have medical conditions that render them medically inoperable. These patients usually have multiple medical problems, have excessive perioperative risk, and frequently die from intercurrent disease. Fifty-four patients with stage I or II endometrial cancer who were considered medically inoperable and received primary radiation were retrospectively compared with 108 well-matched controls who received surgery with or without adjuvant radiation therapy.

Methods.—All patients with operable disease underwent an abdominal procedure. Radiation treatments were appropriate to stage and similar whether patients were considered operable or inoperable. Survival rates were determined for both treatment groups.

Results.—All medically inoperable patients had received at least 2 serious medical diagnoses. Most patients who were considered inoperable had cardiac or hypertensive disease. The median ages of patients with inoperable and operable disease were 76 and 70 years, respectively. Patients with inoperable disease were heavier than those who could undergo surgery. Obesity was not a cause for inoperability in this cohort. Patients with inoperable stage I disease had a mean disease-free interval (DFI) and overall survival of 36 and 37 months, respectively. The actuarial 5-year cancer-specific survival rate was 80% and the overall survival rate was 30% for this cohort. Patients with operable stage I disease had a mean DFI of 74.5 months and an overall survival of 75 months. The corresponding 5-year cancer-specific and overall survival rates for this patient group were 98% and 88%, respectively. For stage II disease, patients who were inoperable had a median DFI and median survival of 50 months each. The actuarial 5-year cancer-specific survival and overall survival for these patients were 85% and 24%, respectively. By comparison, patients with operable stage II disease had a median DFI and survival of 70 months, an actuarial 5-year cancer specific rate of 85%, and a 5-year overall survival rate of 100%.

The differences in median DFI and overall survival were significantly better for patients in the operable group, compared with those in the inoperable group for both stage I and stage II disease. Significantly more patients with inoperable stage I disease were likely to die of intercurrent disease, compared with patients with operable disease (28 of 32 vs. 3 of 15). Intercurrent deaths were not significantly higher for patients with inoperable stage II disease, compared with those with operable stage II disease (7 of 10 vs. 1 of 3). When cancer-related deaths were evaluated, patients with inoperable stage I disease had a mean survival of 62.3 months, and those with stage II disease had a mean survival of 72 months. These figures are similar to those for patients with operable disease. The primary radiation toxicity was diarrhea that was medically managed. Patients with inoperable disease were significantly more likely to experience diarrhea when compared with patients with operable disease.

Conclusion.—Patients with inoperable stage I or stage II endometrial cancer benefit from exclusive radiation therapy. It is well-tolerated and has results that approach those of patients with operable disease.

▶ This study spans the years 1975–1992 and examines radiation as the sole therapy for medically inoperable patients with stages I and II endometrial carcinoma. The results are impressive and, perhaps, to some surprising. The numbers are small insofar as only 54 patients were studied. However, given the 17-year duration of the study, it is likely that those treated more recently were treated in a more efficient manner than those who had their initial therapy in the 1970s. Interestingly, death from intercurrent disease was the main problem, and those who did not die of intercurrent disease had survivals that were close to that of patients who could have had an operation. The median survival for operable patients with stage I disease was 62.3 months and for stage II disease it was 72 months. The very excellent results in this study confirm the benefit of radiation therapy in patients who cannot undergo an operation.

A.L. Herbst, M.D.

Postoperative Radiation Therapy for Surgically Staged Endometrial Cancer: Impact of Time Factors (Overall Treatment Time and Surgery-to-Radiation Interval) on Outcome
Ahmad NR, Lanciano RM, Corn BW, et al (Fox Chase Cancer Ctr, Philadelphia)
Int J Radiat Oncol Biol Phys 33:837–842, 1995   22–29

Introduction.—There are few data on the impact of time factors on the outcome of postoperative radiotherapy in patients with endometrial cancer. The importance of these factors was explored using data from a cohort of patients with endometrial cancer treated in a consistent manner over a period of 22 years.

Methods.—A total of 195 patients with surgically staged endometrial cancer received postoperative radiation therapy between 1971 and 1993. All patients were treated with total abdominal hysterectomy, and 38% also underwent pelvic or para-aortic lymph node sampling or both. All patients underwent postoperative whole pelvic radiation therapy, and 69% also were given a vaginal cuff boost with either low-dose rate or high-dose rate brachytherapy. The impact of various tumor and treatment factors (including the surgery-to-radiation interval, overall radiation treatment time, and external beam treatment time) on local control and on disease-specific survival was analyzed.

Results.—The cohort had an overall actuarial 5-year local control rate of 85%. Multivariate analysis showed that tumor grade, pathologic stage, external radiation dose, and surgical lymph node evaluation were significant independent prognostic indicators and that a surgery-to-radiation interval of more than 6 weeks was a marginally significant predictor of reduced local control. The overall actuarial 5-year disease-specific survival rate was 86%. In multivariate analysis, the following significant independent predictors of disease-specific survival were identified: depth of myometrial invasion, tumor grade, pathologic stage, and a surgery-to-radiation interval of more than 6 weeks.

Conclusions.—Although the overall radiation treatment time and external beam treatment time did not significantly affect either local control or disease-specific survival, an interval between surgery and radiation therapy exceeding 6 weeks was a significant independent predictor of reduced disease-specific survival and was a marginally significant predictor of reduced local control in patients with endometrial carcinoma. Therefore, radiation therapy should be administered as soon as possible after surgery and within 6 weeks.

▶ This is a nonrandomized study of 195 patients with endometrial carcinoma who received postoperative radiation at 1 treatment center. The types of radiation were mixed; that is, external beam alone or with a vaginal boost. The major observation from multivariate analysis was that disease-specific survival was significantly enhanced if radiation treatment was started within 6 weeks of operation. The common practice is to begin such treatment within 4 to 6 weeks postoperatively, and the study corroborates that this is indeed good practice.

A.L. Herbst, M.D.

Endometrial Carcinoma: Relative Effectiveness of Adjuvant Irradiation vs Therapy Reserved for Relapse

Ackerman I, Malone S, Thomas G, et al (Univ of Toronto; Univ of Ottawa, Canada; Sunnybrook Regional Cancer Centre, North York, Canada)
Gynecol Oncol 60:177–183, 1996
22–30

Introduction.—For many years, endometrial carcinoma has been managed by surgery with adjuvant radiation therapy (RT). However, no studies have examined the use of adjuvant therapy in patients at high risk of recurrence compared with observation and radical therapy reserved for patients with pelvic relapse only. Patterns of relapse after treatment for endometrial carcinoma were studied, along with factors associated with effective salvage and the possibility of reserving adjuvant RT for patients with relapse.

Patients.—The investigators reviewed the records of 304 patients with endometrial cancer treated during a 4-year period. Of this group, 54 had recurrent endometrial carcinoma. Thirty-two patients had received primary therapy with surgery alone and 22 with surgery plus RT. The patients with recurrent cancer were assigned to 1 of 2 groups, based on the extent of their disease at initial presentation. Fifteen were considered low risk, having grade 1 or 2 endometrial carcinoma with limited myometrial invasion or grade 3 tumors confined to the endometrium. The 39 patients with grade 3 tumors with any myometrial invasion or tumors of any grade with more than 50% myometrial invasion were considered high risk.

Findings.—Long-term survival was achieved in 40% of patients. Seventy-two percent of patients who did not receive adjuvant pelvic RT as their primary therapy had isolated pelvic recurrence, whereas 77% of those who did receive adjuvant RT initially had distant relapse. Treatment failure occurred in the pelvis alone in 54% of patients, with 46% having some distant failure. Sixteen of 28 patients with isolated pelvic relapse had vaginal mucosal involvement only, the other 12 having involvement of the parametrium, pelvic sidewall, or both.

All survivors were followed up for at least 5 years. Radical RT was used in 21 of the 28 patients with isolated pelvic relapse, and pelvic disease was controlled until death or last follow-up in 14. Pelvic control was maintained in 79% of patients with mucosal involvement only, compared with 43% of those with extramucosal involvement. There were no instances of major treatment-related toxicity. On univariate analysis, tumor size, RT dose, and disease-free interval were not significantly related to either pelvic control or survival. The anatomic extent of the pelvic recurrence showed a nonsignificant trend toward a relationship with pelvic control.

Conclusions.—Many patients with endometrial carcinoma and recurrent disease confined to the pelvis can achieve long-term disease-free

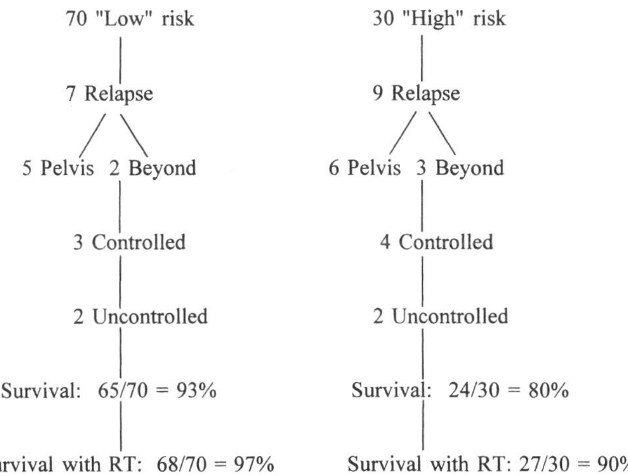

FIGURE 2.—Algorithm of expected outcome of adjuvant pelvic radiotherapy. (Courtesy of Ackerman I, Malone S, Thomas G, et al: Endometrial carcinoma—relative effectiveness of adjuvant irradiation vs therapy reserved for relapse. *Gynecol Oncol* 60:177–183, 1996.)

survival with pelvic control. The findings suggest the need to reexamine the role of routine adjuvant pelvic RT. In this situation, RT may have only a small overall benefit in terms of pelvic control and survival (Fig 2).

▶ This study looks at an interesting point: namely, the role of salvage RT for patients who have had a primary pelvic recurrence of endometrial carcinoma. The authors divide primary endometrial carcinoma into high and low risk by commonly used criteria: low risk, grades 1 or 2 less than 50% myometrial invasion; and high risk, grade 3 with any degree of myometrial invasion or any grade with more than 50% myometrial invasions. For those who divide the myometrium into thirds, many would want outer third myometrial invasion in grade 1 especially to be considered "high risk."

Not surprisingly, those who initially did not have adjuvant RT tended to fail in the pelvis, whereas those who received such treatment tended to fail distally. It is impressive that in 14 of 21 patients pelvic control was achieved after radiation for pelvic recurrence and the calculated actuarial survival was 38%.

Although the numbers in this study are small, the authors note that those with grade 3 disease and deep myometrial invasion are the most likely group to benefit from adjuvant RT. Furthermore, the authors make the point that those with pelvic recurrence, not previously radiated, can be cured with pelvic irradiation.

The authors constructed an interesting algorithm for expected outcomes with adjuvant pelvic irradiation (see Figure 2). In this example 100 patients were evaluated, with 70 having low-risk disease and 30 high-risk disease, which are numbers generally expected. Clearly, the low-risk group has no benefit with pelvic irradiation. Only 7 would be expected to relapse and 3 of these can be helped with follow-up radiation therapy to achieve 93% survival. For the high-risk group, a 100% adjuvant RT gives a 90% survival rate. Without adjuvant therapy in this group and follow-up radiation for pelvic recurrence, an 80% rate is theoretically achieved. Thus, for the high-risk group there is a 10% theoretical advantage for 100% adjuvant radiation. All of this indicates that future therapeutic trials should be strict in the criteria used to warrant adjuvant RT for endometrial carcinoma.

A.L. Herbst, M.D.

Chemotherapy Plus Sequential Hormonal Therapy for Advanced and Recurrent Endometrial Carcinoma: A Phase II Study
Pinelli DM, Fiorica JV, Roberts WS, et al (Univ of South Florida, Tampa)
Gynecol Oncol 60:462–467, 1996   22–31

Objective.—Although surgery and radiotherapy has a high cure rate in patients with endometrial cancer, many patients with advanced disease or metastases will require systemic therapy. Many chemotherapeutic agents have been used in this situation, most recently carboplatin. Because endometrial adenocarcinomas are sensitive to hormones, the combination of an oral progestin and a platinum-based chemotherapeutic agent might be a reasonable approach to the treatment of advanced or recurrent disease. The combination of sequential cyclic hormone therapy and carboplatin chemotherapy was studied for use in outpatient management of advanced or recurrent endometrial cancer.

Methods.—The phase II trial included 18 patients with confirmed endometrial carcinoma extending outside of the pelvis or with recurrent disease. All received 300 mg/m² of carboplatin every 4 weeks for 6 courses or until disease progression occurred. They also received hormonal therapy with megestrol acetate, 80 mg twice daily, alternating with tamoxifen citrate, 20 mg twice daily, every 3 weeks. The objective clinical response, progression-free interval, and survival were assessed.

Results.—There were 13 evaluable patients. Complete response rate was 31%, partial response rate 46%, and progression rate 15%; 1 patient was left with stable disease. Objective responses occurred in 86% of patients with stable disease. Complete responders had a median progression-free interval of 14 months, with 2 patients alive and with no evidence of disease at 41 and 59 months. Grade 2 or 3 hematologic toxicity occurred in 54% of patients but always resolved within 2 weeks. In 1 patient, the carboplatin dose had to be reduced to 200 mg/m². Median survival was 11 months overall and 33 months for complete responders.

Conclusions.—In this study of treatment for advanced or recurrent endometrial cancer, the combination of carboplatin chemotherapy with sequential hormonal therapy with megestrol acetate and tamoxifen had promising results. The treatment is well tolerated, has minimal toxicity, and can be given on an outpatient basis. Receptor positivity is significantly related to patient response and survival.

▶ This is a useful report of what I believe is a potentially attractive approach to the treatment of endometrial carcinoma. The authors combined hormone therapy (tamoxifen and megestrol acetate alternating) with carboplatin. Of 13 evaluable patients, 4 had a complete response with the median progression-free interval of 14 months. Although this may seem a modest result, it is quite good considering that 4 patients had also received chemotherapy previously and 1 of these had a complete response to the combined protocol. The authors noted a correlation of response with endometrial carcinoma receptor status, which does differ from the results of the initial report of this approach by Ayoub et al.[1]

As noted by the authors, the Gynecologic Oncology Group is evaluating tamoxifen and megestrol acetate to treat endometrial carcinoma. Hopefully, the next large national cooperative study will combine hormone therapy with a maximum effective multiagent chemotherapy protocol to try to improve our results for recurrent endometrial carcinoma.

A.L. Herbst, M.D.

Reference

1. Ayoub J, Audet-La Point P, Metrot Y: Efficacy of sequential cyclical hormonal therapy in endometrial cancer and its correlation with steroid hormone receptor status. *Gynecol Oncol* 31:327-337, 1988.

Postsurgical Surveillance of Patients With FIGO Stage I/II Endometrial Adenocarcinoma

Berchuck A, Anspach C, Evans AC, et al (Duke Univ, Durham, NC)
Gynecol Oncol 59:20–24, 1995   22–32

Introduction.—Although most patients with endometrial adenocarcinoma have disease confined to the uterus and have a low recurrence rate, they typically undergo intensive postsurgical surveillance for 3–5 years. However, the value of this surveillance is unclear because recurrent disease is associated with a poor prognosis. The value of postsurgical surveillance was determined by investigating its influence on survival.

Methods.—The records of 354 patients treated surgically for International Federation of Gynecology and Obstetrics stage I/II endometrial adenocarcinoma between 1978 and 1987 were reviewed. Data were collected on clinicopathologic features, treatment modalities, outcome, and disease status at last follow-up. Among patients with recurrent disease, the presence of signs or symptoms or evidence on a Papanicolaou (Pap) smear or chest radiograph was noted.

Results.—Of the 354 patients, initial surgical treatment included total abdominal hysterectomy, adnexectomy, and pelvic peritoneal cytology in 45% and the previously mentioned procedures plus selective pelvic and aortic lymphadenectomy in 55%. Recurrent disease developed in 44 patients (12%) and had no significant association with the extent of the initial surgical treatment. When the recurrence was diagnosed, 61% had symptoms, 68% had suspicious physical findings, and 84% had either symptoms and/or physical findings. Evidence of recurrence was found on the Pap smear in 25% and on chest radiographs in 20%. Eight of the 44 patients (18%) with recurrent disease are still alive without disease after salvage therapy. Among the survivors are 50% of the patients with isolated vaginal recurrent disease and only 6% of the patients with other patterns of recurrent disease. Of the 8 survivors, 3 had symptoms of recurrence, 6 had physical examination signs, 3 had a positive Pap smear, and none had a positive chest radiograph.

Conclusions.—Survival is not significantly influenced by postsurgical surveillance in patients with recurrence of early-stage endometrial cancer. A cost-benefit analysis indicates that the typical postsurgical surveillance program costs approximately $700,000 to salvage 8 of 44 patients with recurrent disease. However, this analysis does not account for the psychological benefit of reassurance for most patients without recurrence. Biannual visits for 5 years without Pap smears or chest radiographs may be a more cost-effective postsurgical surveillance strategy for these patients.

▶ As we enter the time of cost containment and cost-benefit analyses, we will be seeing many more articles evaluating current practices and their effectiveness as well as cost. All this makes the current article quite timely.

The analysis shows that recurrence of stages I or II endometrial carcinoma is infrequently discovered by either Pap smear (25%) or chest radiographs (20%). As the authors correctly note, second-line treatment (except for pelvic irradiation in previously nonirradiated patients) tends not to be effective. Therefore, in many instances, "early" detection will not translate into prolonged survival. Nonetheless, an annual chest radiograph and Pap smear are comparatively inexpensive, and the former can be easily accomplished at the time of annual mammography for these patients. The authors note the potential "reassurance value" of a negative test, and I continue to obtain these in patients being followed for endometrial carcinoma.

A.L. Herbst, M.D.

Phase II Trial of Hydroxyurea, Dacarbazine (DTIC), and Etoposide (VP-16) in Mixed Mesodermal Tumors of the Uterus: A Gynecologic Oncology Group Study
Currie JL, Blessing JA, McGehee R, et al (Johns Hopkins Hosp, Baltimore, Md; Roswell Park Cancer Inst, Buffalo, NY; Univ of Mississippi, Jackson; et al)
Gynecol Oncol 61:94–96, 1996   22–33

Introduction.—The treatment approach for early-stage mixed mesodermal tumors (MMT) of the uterus is total hysterectomy, bilateral salpingo-oophorectomy, and lymph node sampling, often followed by adjunctive radiotherapy. Chemotherapy is usually unsuccessful in the presence of advanced or recurrent disease. Reported are results of a groupwide phase II study of the Gynecologic Oncology Group (GOG) of 33 untreated patients with advanced or recurrent uterine MMT treated with the combination of hydroxyurea, dacarbazine (DTIC), and etoposide (VP-16)

Methods.—All patients had failed local therapeutic measures and were considered incurable with surgery or radiation. The therapeutic regimen was administered for 4 days and was repeated every 4 weeks for 12 courses, unless toxicity was a problem. The fourth day of the initial course was omitted if patients had had prior radiation therapy or were over 75 years of age. The women received hydroxyurea, 2 g, in divided doses on the first day; DTIC, 700 mg/m², and VP-16, 100 mg/m², on day 2; and VP-16, 100 mg/m² IV, on days 3 and 4. Stable disease was considered to be no progression of disease for 2 months.

Results.—The median patient age was 66 years. Twenty-six of 33 evaluable patients had had a previous hysterectomy. Of 32 patients who could be evaluated for treatment response, GOG performance status was as follows: 11 grade 0, 14 grade 1, and 7 grade 2. Eleven of these 32 patients had undergone adjuvant radiation therapy. There was an overall response rate of 15.7% with 2 complete responses and 3 partial responses. The median duration of response was 6.3 months. Patients with complete responses underwent a median of 9.5 courses of therapy, and those with partial responses underwent a median of 6 cycles of therapy. Seventeen patients (53.1%) had stable disease for a median of 6 cycles. Ten patients (31.2%) had increasing disease with a median of 2 courses of treatment. Toxicity was considered acceptable. Five patients had grade 3 toxicity and 11 experienced grade 1 or 2 toxicity.

Conclusion.—The drug regimen of hydroxyurea, DTIC, and VP-16 had modest activity and acceptable toxicity in patients with advanced or recurrent MMT. Two patients had a complete response, 3 had a partial response, and 17 had stable disease.

Combination Chemotherapy With Hydroxyurea, Dacarbazine (DTIC), and Etoposide in the Treatment of Uterine Leiomyosarcoma: A Gynecologic Oncology Group Study

Currie JL, Blessing JA, Muss HB, et al (Johns Hopkins Hosp, Baltimore, Md; Roswell Park Cancer Inst, Buffalo, NY; Wake Forest Univ, Winston-Salem, NC; et al)
Gynecol Oncol 61:27–30, 1996   22–34

Introduction.—The virulent nature of the rare leiomyosarcomas of the uterus requires aggressive surgical treatment for early-stage disease. Radiation therapy has been unsuccessful when disease is recurrent or advanced at diagnosis. Thirty-nine patients with advanced or recurrent leiomyosarcoma underwent treatment with hydroxyurea, dacarbazine (DTIC), and etoposide (VP-16) as part of a group-wide phase II study of the Gynecologic Oncology Group (GOG).

Methods.—All patients were considered incurable with surgery or radiation. Treatment consisted of 2 g of hydroxyurea, 700 mg of DTIC per m^2, and 300 mg of VP-16 per m^2 in divided doses every 4 weeks for 12 weeks, unless toxicity was a problem. Stable disease was considered to be no disease progression for 2 months.

Results.—The median patient age was 55.6 years. Thirty-eight patients were evaluable for response and toxicity. The GOG performance grade for these patients was as follows: 20 grade 0, 15 grade 1, and 3 grade 2. Eleven patients had already received adjunctive radiation therapy. The overall response rate was 18.5%; there were 2 complete responses and 5 partial responses. Six responders had disease outside the pelvis. The median response duration was 12.1 months. Twenty patients (52.6%) had stable disease for a median of 5 courses. Eleven patients (28.9%) with increasing disease received a median of 1 treatment course. The median survival was 15.0 months. Adverse treatment effects were considered modest. The platelet count decrease was grade 3 in 1 patient and grade 1 in 4 patients. The white blood cell count toxicity included 1 grade 4, 10 grade 3, and 17 grade 1 or 2.

Conclusion.—Compared with doxorubicin-based regimens, the activity of hydroxyurea, DTIC, and VP-16 is not inferior and may be less toxic. The moderate activity of this regimen may be used to treat recurrent or advanced leiomyosarcoma.

▶ I have paired these articles (Abstracts 22–33 and 22–34) because they give some recent data from the GOG on the chemotherapy of sarcomas of the uterus, a difficult therapeutic problem. The regimen in both studies was the same: 2 g hydroxyurea, 500 mg/day every 6 hours; DTIC, 700 mg/m^2 on day 2 started 6 hours after hydroxyurea; and VP-16 at 300 mg/m^2 (100 mg each on days 2, 3, and 4). This regimen was repeated every 4 weeks. The results were, at best, fair, with 2 complete and 5 partial responses out of 39 patients with leiomyosarcoma and 2 complete and 3 partial responses for the 33 patients with MMT. We still need a more effective regimen; currently, a number of agents including Taxol and ifosfamide are being tested.

A.L. Herbst, M.D.

Fallopian Tube

Primary Fallopian Tube Adenocarcinoma: Clinical Complete Response After Salvage Treatment With High-dose Paclitaxel
Tresukosol D, Kudelka AP, Edwards CL, et al (Chulalongkorn Univ, Bangkok, Thailand; Univ of Texas, Houston)
Gynecol Oncol 58:258–261, 1995   22–35

Background.—Primary fallopian tube cancer is an uncommon, highly aggressive tumor, and its optimal management has yet to be established. A patient with primary fallopian tube cancer who underwent salvage treatment with paclitaxel for late recurrence of pelvic disease after adjuvant chemotherapy for early-stage disease was studied. This is the first report describing the activity of paclitaxel—a drug that has proved effective against platinum-resistant ovarian cancer—in fallopian tube cancer.

Case Report.—Woman, 62, was referred for salvage treatment because of a platinum-resistant fallopian tube adenocarcinoma. Although secondary cytoreductive surgery was attempted, the outcome was less than favorable. The bulky residual disease did not respond to platinum-based therapy, and disease progression to the retroperitoneum became apparent. Obstructed venous return, ureteral obstruction, and renal infection were noted, the latter of which required a third laparotomy and a nephrectomy. Platinum reinduction again proved to be ineffective, and salvage treatment with high-dose paclitaxel, a drug with proven activity against platinum-resistant epithelial ovarian cancer, was initiated. The patient achieved a complete response after 2 cycles of paclitaxel, given intravenously at a dose of 200 mg/m^2 over 24 hours. Three additional cycles were administered, and colony-stimulating factor was also given prophylactically. In this patient, cumulative fatigue and significant mental depression precluded continuation of paclitaxel therapy. The association between paclitaxel and mental depression is presently unclear, although the depression gradually resolved after discontinuing treatment. The patient has remained in complete remission 16 months after terminating paclitaxel, with an 18-month remission duration. During paclitaxel treatment, dose reductions were not required, and no evidence of grade 3 or 4 myelosuppression was observed.

Conclusions.—Paclitaxel has proved to have activity against fallopian tube carcinoma and is recommended for patients with recurrent platinum-resistant disease. Patients undergoing paclitaxel treatment need to be carefully monitored, however, because the drug is associated with significant, although tolerable, toxic effects.

▶ This case of platinum-resistant fallopian tube carcinoma demonstrates that patients with this unusual disease can have a complete response to paclitaxel (Taxol). In this case, a high dose was used (200 mg/m^2) over 24 hours, and granulocyte colony-stimulating factor was also given. Thus far, the complete remission has lasted 1½ years, certainly a worthwhile and impressive response.

A.L. Herbst, M.D.

Cervical

Adenocarcinoma *In Situ* of the Uterine Cervix: Management and Outcome
Widrich T, Kennedy AW, Myers TM, et al (Cleveland Clinic Found, Ohio)
Gynecol Oncol 61:304–308, 1996   22–36

Introduction.—The issue of hysterectomy vs. cervical conization for adenocarcinoma in situ of the uterine cervix is particularly important because most women with this lesion are of reproductive age. A retrospective review of the management and outcome of 46 women with cervical adenocarcinoma in situ was conducted to determine the results of conization versus hysterectomy, as well as results achieved by different conization approaches.

Methods.—Patients' histologic slides of biopsy specimens, endocervical curettings, conization specimens, and hysterectomy specimens were reviewed by 2 pathologists to confirm the diagnosis of adenocarcinoma in situ. Results of cold knife conization and standard large loop excision of the transformation zone (LLETZ) methods were reviewed.

Results.—The mean patient age was 38.4 years. There were 9 diagnoses from 1980 to 1987 and 37 from 1988 to 1994. Eight patients had had a previously abnormal Papanicolaou smear within 2–8 years of diagnosis of adenocarcinoma in situ. There were 25, 18, and 3 cold knife conizations,

LLETZ, and laser conizations, respectively. There were 45 patients with evaluable resection margins. Of these, 18 (40%) were involved with adenocarcinoma in situ, and the remaining 27 were not involved. Eight of 24 patients (33%) who underwent cold knife conization had margins involved with adenoma in situ, compared with 9 of 18 patients (50%) who underwent LLETZ. Of 46 patients, 7 in the cold knife cone group and 4 in the LLETZ group underwent immediate hysterectomy, and 2 in the cold knife group and 4 in the LLETZ group underwent reconization. Recurrent adenocarcinoma developed in 1 of 18 patients (6%) managed with initial cold knife conization; 4 of 14 patients (29%) with LLETZ; and 1 of 3 patients (33%) who underwent laser conization. Invasive adenocarcinoma developed in 1 patient with a positive margin after initial LLETZ and a negative margin after reconization. Of 24 patients with negative margins who underwent conization rather than hysterectomy, 2 (8.3%) had recurrent adenocarcinoma in situ at 10 and 27 months, respectively, after initial conization.

Conclusion.—Adenocarcinoma in situ is being seen with increasing frequency, particularly in younger women. The LLETZ approach yielded inferior results and a higher rate of recurrence, compared with cold knife conization. Patients with initial conization margins uninvolved by adenocarcinoma in situ can be managed adequately with conization alone if they agree to close follow-up examinations.

Can Cervical Adenocarcinoma *In Situ* Be Safely Managed by Conization Alone?
Muntz HG (Virginia Mason Med Center, Seattle)
Gynecol Oncol 61:301–303, 1996   22–37

Introduction.—The use of cervical conization in the conservative management of cervical adenocarcinoma in situ remains controversial. Residual cervical adenocarcinoma has been detected in subsequent hysterectomy specimens in which the carcinoma was supposedly completely excised by cone biopsy. The question of conservative management of women with this disease is addressed.

Accepting the Risk.—Some women are willing to accept the low risk of preinvasive neoplasia to preserve their reproductive ability. The practice of managing adenocarcinoma in situ with conization alone must be considered only in carefully selected women whose initial conization is of adequate size, with uninvolved margins and normal endocervical curettage. The patients must agree to close follow-up. Defining the adequacy of conization is difficult in clinical practice. Investigations report differing guidelines for adequate conization. Negative margins can never be justified with cervical adenocarcinoma in situ. The risk of persistent disease is about 60%. This figure is based on the evaluation of post cone hysterectomy specimens. Clinicians must carefully manage women who have undergone a small conization or the more superficial large loop electrosurgical excision procedure (LEEP). Women who undergo conservative treatment must be counseled carefully because of the small number of patients managed conservatively, the short follow-up in published series, and concern about whether cervical cytology can reliably diagnose recurrent adenocarcinoma in situ before progression to invasive cancer. Follow-up intervals of reported series average only 3 years.

Conclusion.—It will take a large, prospective investigation to determine just how safe conservative management is for patients with cervical adenocarcinoma in situ. The number of patients is too small and the length of follow-up is too short in current published reports to define safe management of these women. Meanwhile, physicians are encouraged to perform a good initial scalpel conization and avoid shallow or fragmented LEEP conizations in the presence of suspected cervical glandular dysplasia.

▶ I have paired the article by Widrich (Abstract 22–36) and the accompanying editorial (Abstract 22–37) because they deal with an important and timely topic, i.e., the fertility-sparing therapy of adenocarcinoma in situ of the cervix. Only 46 patients were studied, but good results were obtained, particularly with cold knife conization. Large loop excision of the transformation zone was used, but it was accompanied by a higher frequency of negative margins and a greater recurrence rate in comparison with cold knife conization. The authors state that this may be because of a smaller volume of tissue removed by LLETZ.

Although there is concern for subsequent development of adenocarcinoma, I believe that cold knife conization is usually appropriate therapy and the reliable patient may be followed, particularly if the cone margins are negative. As noted by Muntz in his editorial, there is a risk of residual in situ disease, even if the cone margin is negative, and the rate is at least 8%, perhaps a bit higher if high rates noted in some small series are included. Nonetheless, it does appear that the preferred therapy is cold knife conization, and shallow or fragmented LEEP specimens should be avoided. Careful follow-up—particularly with endocervical brush instruments for improved endocervical cytology samples—should help.

A.L. Herbst, M.D.

Mature Results of a Phase II Trial of Concomitant Cisplatin/Pelvic Radiotherapy for Locally Advanced Squamous Cell Carcinoma of the Cervix

Fields AL, Anderson PS, Goldberg GL, et al (Albert Einstein College of Medicine, Bronx, NY)
Gynecol Oncol 61:416–422, 1996   22–38

Introduction.—Concomitant chemoradiation has been under investigation for over a decade in an attempt to improve response rates, pelvic control, and possible survival in patients with cervical carcinoma. Reported are the mature results of a 5-year follow-up of a prospective phase

II trial of concomitant cisplatin and pelvic radiotherapy in 59 patients with locally advanced squamous cell carcinoma of the cervix.

Methods.—All patients had untreated, histologically confirmed invasive squamous cell carcinoma of the cervix confined to the pelvis. Patients underwent external-beam radiation therapy at 1.8 to 2 Gy/day, 5 fractions per week, for 4–5 weeks. Intracavity cesium insertions were administered concomitantly. Intravenous cisplatin, 20 mg/m², was administered daily for 5 days at 21-day intervals. Patients were followed at appropriate intervals for treatment response and toxicity.

Results.—Fifty-five patients were evaluable for treatment response. Of these, 16 were stage IB/IIA, 11 were stage IIB, 24 were stage III, and 4 were stage IVA. Two patients (3.6%) had progressive disease during treatment. Thirty-three patients underwent either fine-needle aspiration or laparotomy lymph node evaluation. Of these, 15 (45.5%) had confirmed pelvic node metastases. Toxicity was severe but was considered manageable. Patients received a median of four cisplatin treatments, with an interruption in planned dose in 7 patients. All planned radiation therapy was administered to all patients. Eighteen patients required treatment delays. Seventeen percent (3 of 18) of patients requiring treatment delays were dead of disease, compared to 38% (14 of 37) of patients who had no lapses in treatment time. The total pelvic failure rate was 28% (13 of 46). Five of 46 patients (11%) failed in the pelvis alone. Eleven of 48 patients with complete response experienced recurrence. There were 46 patients who were evaluable at 5 years. The overall survival rate was 73% for stage IB/IIA, 60% for stage IIB, 67% for stage III, and 25% for stage IV. All patients with partial response or progressive disease died at a median of 10 months of disease. The 60-month disease-free survival rate was 73% for stage IB/IIA, 50% for stage IIB, 67% for stage III, and 25% for stage IV.

Conclusion.—Findings suggest that concomitant cisplatin/pelvic radiotherapy is safe and tolerable for locally advanced cervical carcinoma. The lack of statistical significance in this investigation is probably a reflection of the small number of patients. Despite this and the fact that there was no control group, the response rate was impressive enough to warrant further investigation.

► This is a follow-up study of an initial effort published in 1989 using chemoradiation to treat advanced squamous cell carcinoma of the cervix. The authors have used short-duration chemotherapy for 20–30 minutes, administering 20 mg/m² daily for 5 days every 21 days during external-beam radiation therapy after the daily external-beam radiation doses were given and after the brachytherapy doses were removed. Most patients received 4 cycles, and, as expected, some patients could not tolerate more than 2–3 cycles of chemotherapy.

Nonetheless, the results are very encouraging. Of 55 patients, a complete response was noted in 87%. Of course, the 5-year survival rate is the important statistic and these results are quite good, i.e., stage IB/IIA, 73%; stage IIB, 60%; a most impressive 67% for stage III; and 25% (1 of 4) for stage IV. These are excellent results and, I believe, worthy of further evaluation with a trial of a larger number of patients.

A.L. Herbst, M.D.

Sarcoma Botryoides of the Cervix Treated With Limited Surgery and Chemotherapy to Preserve Fertility
Lin J, Lam SK, Cheung TH (Prince of Wales Hosp, Shatin, Hong Kong)
Gynecol Oncol 58:270–273, 1995   22–39

Background.—Sarcoma botryoides in the uterine cervix is rare. It usually occurs in adolescents and is treated by surgery and adjuvant chemotherapy. It may be possible to limit surgery to local excision in patients with stage I disease, in which the tumor is confined to the cervix.

Case Report.—Woman, 20, sought medical attention for vaginal bleeding. The diagnosis of benign cervical polyps was made, and resection was performed. Six months later, vaginal bleeding recurred, and a repeat polypectomy was performed. Careful histologic examination showed pleomorphic spindle-shaped tumor cells, some showing skeletal muscle differentiation with striation. Rhabdomyosarcoma was diagnosed. On ultrasound assessment, a bulky but well-defined cervix was identified. Because there were no signs of metastases, the disease was staged as group IA. Hysteroscopy and cone biopsy, with a 5-cm base and 2-cm length, were performed. Tumor cells were found to have infiltrated about 1 cm into the cervical stroma. The superior resection margin was involved, and the lateral resection margins were close. No further resection was planned. Instead, chemotherapy consisting of vincristine, actinomycin, and cyclophosphamide was begun. Six months after chemotherapy was completed, a repeat cone biopsy showed no evidence of further tumor. At 36 months after diagnosis, the patient continued to be free from disease, with a normal menstrual cycle.

Conclusions.—In this patient with stage IA sarcoma botryoides of the cervix, treatment was limited to cervicectomy followed by adjuvant chemotherapy to preserve reproductive function. After 3 years, the patient remained well, suggesting that such therapy may be sufficient for early-stage disease.

▶ These extremely rare tumors usually occur in the vagina of young patients under the age of 8 years. There have been a few case reports of the tumor being in the cervix, and as emphasized in this case, chemotherapy has an important place in the management of this disease. It is also of interest that the prognosis of the cervical tumors may be better than that for their vaginal counterparts.

A.L. Herbst, M.D.

Stage I Squamous Cell Cervical Carcinoma in Pregnancy: Planned Delay in Therapy Awaiting Fetal Maturity

Sorosky JI, Squatrito R, Ndubisi BU, et al (Univ of Iowa, Iowa City; Univ of Florida, Jacksonville; Milton S Hershey Med Ctr, Hershey Pa)
Gynecol Oncol 59:207–210, 1995

22–40

Introduction.—Cervical cancer is the most common malignant condition to develop in pregnant women. Women with stage I disease have a 5-year survival expectancy similar to nonpregnant women, but it is not clear whether delaying treatment until the fetus matures will influence their survival.

Series.—Seven patients who were pregnant when diagnosed as having stage IB cervical carcinoma chose to delay treatment in order to optimize the fetal outcome; they were followed up prospectively through pregnancy. One other woman conceived in the cycle after cancer was diagnosed; her diagnosis-to-treatment interval was 282 days. The patients made their decision despite being advised to have surgery within several weeks of diagnosis. Seven women had elective cesarean section combined with radical hysterectomy in the third trimester after fetal pulmonary maturity was confirmed. One patient was operated on when the membranes ruptured at 35 weeks' gestation.

Results.—All tumors were less than 2.5 cm in size. The mean interval from diagnosis to elective treatment was nearly 16 weeks. In no case did disease progress clinically. Serial MRI confirmed the presence of stable disease in 1 patient and suggested an increasing tumor volume in another; the latter finding was not confirmed pathologically. All patients were free of disease after an average follow-up of just over 3 years. One neonate had spontaneous pneumothorax.

Conclusion.—In this small series, delaying treatment of stage I cervical cancer until the fetal lungs mature has not adversely affected the outcome.

▶ This article makes an important point, namely, that the treatment of stage I cervical cancer during pregnancy is no emergency, and waiting for fetal viability does not appear to compromise the curability of the patients. All of the patients in this small series had cervical carcinomas less than 2.5 cm in diameter. Although the mean follow-up was only 33 months, no patient has had a recurrence and there was no clinical progression of the disease noted during any of the pregnancies. It is of interest that 1 patient delayed treatment for almost the entire pregnancy, because she evidently conceived in the cycle following the diagnosis of cervical carcinoma.

The results of this series are similar to those reported by my colleagues[1] in cases of diethlystilbestrol-associated clear-cell adenocarcinoma, in which a delay of treatment up to 21 weeks did not appear to have any adverse effect. All of these data are reassuring to physicians and patients who wish to delay treatment of early invasive cervical carcinoma to allow fetal viability.

A.L. Herbst, M.D.

Reference

1. Senekjian EK, Hubby M, Bell D, et al: Clear cell adenocarcinoma (CCA) of the vagina and cervix in association with pregnancy. *Gynecol Oncol* 24: 207, 1986.

The Adverse Effect of Treatment Prolongation in Cervical Carcinoma

Petereit DG, Sarkaria JN, Chappell R, et al (Univ of Wisconsin, Madison)
Int J Radiat Oncol Biol Phys 32:1301–1307, 1995   22–41

Objective.—In head/neck cancer, treatment delay may result in a loss of local control, possibly because of the proliferation of surviving tumor clones during protracted radiotherapy. The relation of total treatment time to pelvic control and survival was studied in women given radiotherapy for squamous cell carcinoma of the uterine cervix.

Methods.—A total of 209 women with stage IB to IIIB cervical cancer were treated with a combination of external-beam radiotherapy and low-dose-rate intracavitary irradiation. They received a whole-pelvis dose of at least 51 Gy at 1.7 Gy per fraction via 2–4 fields, followed by intracavitary therapy if technically feasible. The median doses to points E and A were 60 and 80 Gy, respectively, and the median treatment time was 55 days. Patients were followed up for a median of 7½ years.

Results.—The most common cause of delay was logistical, involving the interval between external and intracavitary treatment when combined with holidays. Radiation complications and poor tumor shrinkage were the next most common reasons. The overall 5-year survival was 60%, and the pelvis was controlled in 80% of patients. The 5-year pelvic control rate was 87% when treatment time was fewer than 55 days and 72% when it was longer. Survival also was adversely affected with longer treatment times (65% vs. 54%). No such effects were apparent in women with stage IIB disease. The 5-year survival declined by 0.6%, and pelvic control by 0.7%, for each added day of treatment beyond 55 days. Treatment time could not be related to the risk of late complications.

Implications.—Prolonged radiotherapy for cervical cancer is associated with decreased 5-year local control and survival rates. In addition to avoiding treatment breaks, fractionation regimens that minimize treatment time might be helpful.

Carcinoma of the Uterine Cervix. I. Impact of Prolongation of Overall Treatment Time and Timing of Brachytherapy on Outcome of Radiation Therapy

Perez CA, Grigsby PW, Castro-Vita H, et al (Washington Univ, St Louis, Mo)
Int J Radiat Oncol Biol Phys 32:1275–1288, 1995   22–42

Objective.—The treatment records of 1,224 women with histologically proved stage IB to stage III cervical carcinoma, managed exclusively by definitive radiotherapy, were reviewed to confirm previous reports of poorer outcomes when treatment is prolonged.

Methods.—External-beam radiotherapy was combined with 2 intra-cavitary insertions to deliver doses of 70–90 Gy to point A. High-energy photon therapy was administered. The overall treatment time was 7 weeks or fewer in 81% of patients with stage IB disease and 74% of those with stage IIA disease. Longer treatment times were more frequent for patients with more advanced disease. Patients were followed up for a minimum of 3 years; survivors were seen for a median of 12 years.

Findings.—Cause-specific survival (CSS) of patients with stage IB was significantly greater when treatment time was 9 weeks or fewer. In those with stage IIA tumors, the 10-year CSS was 73% when the treatment time was 7 weeks or fewer and 43% at best when it was longer. No significant association was evident for patients with stage III disease except those who received 85 Gy or more to point A, who did better when the treatment time did not exceed 9 weeks. Some correlations were observed between the overall treatment time and the risk of pelvic failure.

Conclusion.—It appears best to minimize radiotherapy time for patients with cervical carcinoma and to avoid unnecessary interruptions and delays.

▶ I have paired these 2 articles (Abstracts 22–41 and 22–42) because they emphasize the important point that prolongation of radiation treatment time leads to a decrease in therapeutic success.

In the Petereit et al. study, the dividing line was 55 days, and the authors estimate a survival decrease of 0.6% a day for each day of prolongation, whereas for pelvic control it was 0.7% per day. These results apply to all tumor stages, a very remarkable observation.

The Perez et al. study chose 49 days for its cutoff and noted the best values for that group, followed by those treated for 7.1 to 9 weeks, and the worst for those who were treated for more than 9 weeks. One might assume that local toxicity during treatment was a major contribution to these delays, but the authors note that holiday and weekends were the major contributing factor. With radiation treatment equipment being so expensive and the tremendous pressures on all of us for cost containment, perhaps we should consider using these facilities 7 days per week. Obviously this would shorten treatment time and would also necessitate some dosage adjustments for toxicity, but the notion might not be as far-fetched as it may initially seem.

A.L. Herbst, M.D.

Adenocarcinoma as an Independent Risk Factor for Disease Recurrence in Patients With Stage IB Cervical Carcinoma

Eifel PJ, Burke TW, Morris M, et al (Univ of Texas, Houston)
Gynecol Oncol 59:38–44, 1995

22–43

Background.—The many studies of the effect of histology on prognosis among patients with International Federation of Gynecology and Obstetrics stage IB adenocarcinoma (AC) and with squamous cell carcinoma (SCC) of the cervix have yielded inconsistent results. Previous studies have been limited by methodologic problems, such as small patient numbers. The influence of histologic type on outcome in 1,767 radiation-treated patients with stage IB AC and SCC of the cervix was investigated.

Methods and Findings.—The patients were treated between 1960 and 1989. Two hundred twenty-nine had AC and 1,538 had SCC. The overall 5-year survival rate for patients with SCC was 81%, and for those with AC it was 72%. The maximum cervical diameter of less than 4 cm was documented more often in patients with AC than in those with SCC (53% vs. 47%). Among the 903 patients with tumors measuring 4 cm or greater, 73% with SCC and 59% with AC survived for 5 years or longer. The rate of pelvic disease recurrence did not differ between groups, but the rate of distant metastases was greater for patients with AC (Table 3). Prognosis was strongly associated with tumor size and lymphangiogram findings but not age or tumor morphology in patients with tumors of 4 cm or greater. There was a nonsignificant trend toward better survival in 165 patients undergoing adjuvant hysterectomy. In a multivariate analysis, the association between histology and survival was highly significant and independent. Patients with AC of 4 cm or greater in diameter had a 1.9 times higher estimated risk of death than did patients with SCC.

Conclusions.—The prognosis of patients with AC of the cervix does appear to be worse than that of patients with similar stage and diameter SCC. This difference mainly reflects a greater rate of distant metastases in patients with AC.

TABLE 3.—Risk of Pelvic or Distant Relapse at 5 Years

Size	Histology	No. of patients	Pelvic*		Distant†		Any site	
					Actuarial risk of relapse			
<4 cm	SCC	706	2.6%		7.4%		9.6%	
	AC	113	6.3%	*P* < 0.01	15.2%	*P* = 0.01	16.9%	*P* = 0.03
≥4 cm	SCC	797	13.1%		21.2%		26.4%	
	AC	106	16.7%	*P* = 0.16	36.8%	*P* < 0.01	43.6%	*P* < 0.01

*Progressive or recurrent pelvic disease detected at any time after initial treatment.
†Extrapelvic recurrence detected at any time after initial treatment.
Abbreviations: SCC, squamous cell carcinoma; *AC,* adenocarcinoma.
(Courtesy of Eifel PJ, Burke TW, Morris M, et al: Adenocarcincoma as an independent risk factor for disease recurrence in patients with stage IB cervical carcinoma. *Gynecol Oncol* 59:38–44, 1995.)

▶ It is debated in the literature whether ACs of the cervix have a worse prognosis then their SCC counterparts. This extensive analysis from the M.D. Anderson Cancer Center of stage IB cases provides excellent evidence that the ACs do worse, even correcting for the important variable of tumor size. Table 3 has been reproduced because it demonstrates quite nicely that the ACs do worse for comparable stage and size. Although the rates of pelvic recurrence in tumors 4 cm or larger do not reach statistical significance, all the other categories do. The SCC tumors also had a survival advantage, 81% vs. 72%. For those tumors 4 cm or greater, the 5-year survival rates were 73% vs. 59%.

We still do not have the answer for the ideal treatment of these tumors. Assuming no evidence of extrauterine spread, I prefer to treat ACs of the cervix that are apparent stage IB with preliminary brachytherapy and a radical hysterectomy for those lesions that are less than 4 cm in diameter. For larger lesions, I prefer pelvic radiation therapy and implant, followed by an extrafascial hysterectomy. I cannot quote data to "prove" that this is correct, but I also know of no data to indicate that there is currently a superior alternative approach.

A.L. Herbst, M.D.

Prognostic Factors in Patients With Cervix Cancer Treated by Radiation Therapy: Results of a Multiple Regression Analysis

Fyles AW, Pintilie M, Kirkbride P, et al (Princess Margaret Hosp, Toronto; Univ of Toronto)
Radiother Oncol 35:107–117, 1995

22–44

Background.—Tumor characteristics such as stage according to the International Federation of Gynecology and Obstetrics, size, depth of invasion, and nodal involvement have been found to predict prognosis in patients with cervical cancer. Certain host-related factors also appear to be important. A number of clinical and treatment variables were studied to determine their predictive value for disease-free survival (DFS) and pelvic control.

Methods and Findings.—Data on 965 patients treated by radiation therapy between 1976 and 1981 were analyzed retrospectively. The best prognosticator was stage, followed by radiation dose and duration of treatment. When the analysis was limited to patients given radical doses of 75 Gy or more, dose became nonsignificant. Other variables adversely affecting DFS and local control were young age at diagnosis, nonsquamous histology, and need for transfusion during therapy (Fig 5). Para-aortic nodal involvement observed on lymphogram was correlated with reduced DFS, but pelvic lymph node involvement alone was not. In patients with stage I and IIA disease, the most powerful predictor of survival was tumor size. The extent of pelvic sidewall involvement was significant in patients with stage III disease. Histologic grade, documented for only 712 patients, also appeared to be a predictive factor.

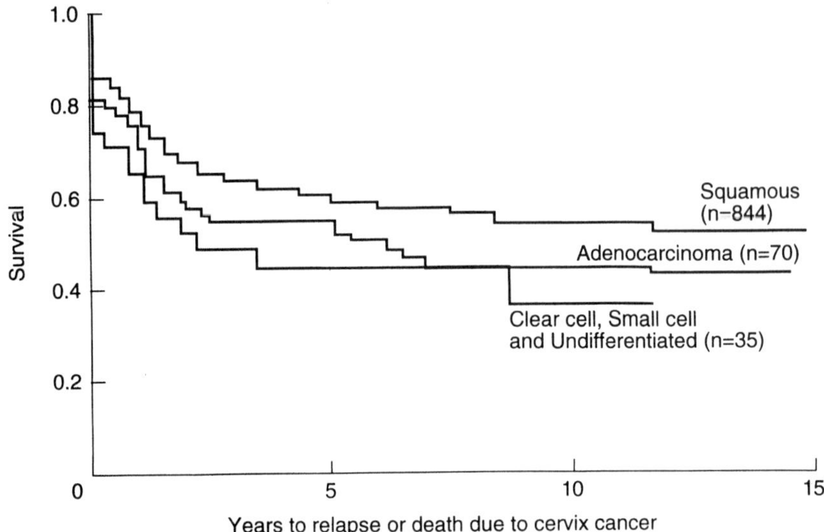

FIGURE 5.—Disease-free survival according to pathologic subtype. (Reprinted from Fyles AW, Pintilie M, Kirkbride P, et al: Prognostic factors in patients with cervix cancer treated by radiation therapy: Results of a multiple regression analysis. *Radiother Oncol* 35:107–117, 1995, with kind permission of Elsevier Science–NL, Sara Burgerhartstraat 25, 1055 KV.)

Conclusions.—Revising current staging systems to include tumor size or bulk in stages I to III and to redefine stage IIIA should be considered. Investigators also need to control for other prognostic variables, such as age, anemia or requirement for transfusion, and duration of radiation therapy, when designing clinical trials.

▶ This very large series from the well-known unit at Princess Margaret Hospital in Canada confirms what has been indicated in other smaller studies regarding the treatment of cervical carcinoma. Not surprisingly, para-aortic node involvement worsened the prognosis, but perhaps surprisingly, pelvic node involvement did not seem to lower the disease-free survival interval. However, these data are based on the interpretation of lymphangiograms, not histologic verification.

I think that it is extremely important to note that, in stages I and IIA, increasing the dose of radiation above 7,500 centigray (cGy) has no beneficial effect. There was an improved survival in higher stages for doses up to 8,500 cGy, but the authors noted that there may have been a selection bias in that the more healthy and fit patients were chosen for the higher doses.

Not surprisingly, stage was the most predictive as was tumor size in regard to survival, particularly where it could be reasonably accurately measured in stages I and IIA. Patients who required transfusion did worse in the multivariant analysis presumably because they had large hemorrhagic tumors. Although the initial hemoglobin was also a poor prognostic factor and transfusion was not always effective in reversing this, as noted by the authors, the current concern regarding HIV may mitigate against aggressive transfusion policies in these patients.

Adenocarcinoma did worse than squamous cell carcinomas in this series, but the number of adenocarcinoma cases was small and it is still debatable whether this subset of tumor has a poorer prognosis. I was surprised to note that the clear-cell carcinomas were lumped with the small-cell and undifferentiated tumors. Unquestionably, the latter 2 have a poor prognosis, but from the data my colleagues and I have accumulated for clear-cell carcinomas of the cervix,[1] it would appear that, stage for stage, the survival for clear-cell carcinoma is comparable to or perhaps even better than that for squamous cell carcinoma of the cervix.

A.L. Herbst, M.D.

Reference

1. Herbst AL, Mishell DR, Stenchever MA, et al: *Comprehensive Gynecology*, ed 2. St Louis, Mosby, 1992.

Prognostic Factors for Local and Distant Recurrence in Stage I and II Cervical Carcinoma

Werner-Wasik M, Schmid CH, Bornstein L, et al (New England Med Ctr Hosps, Boston; Tufts Univ, Boston)
Int J Radiat Oncol Biol Phys 32:1309–1317, 1995   22–45

Objective.—The influence of tumor-related variables such as tumor size and parametrial involvement on the outcome of treatment was investigated in 125 women having International Federation of Gynecology and Obstetrics stage I or stage II carcinoma of the uterine cervix who were scheduled for curative radiotherapy. The patients had a median age of 55 years and were followed for at least 2 years, and for a median of 40 months after treatment. Twelve patients also underwent extrafascial hysterectomy, and 8 received chemotherapy.

Recurrence.—Twenty-three patients had local failure, and there were 16 distant failures. Tumor stage did not significantly predict recurrences overall, but initial failure at a distant site was likelier with increasing stage. Recurrence became more likely as tumor size increased. Involvement of pelvic or para-aortic nodes was a significant prognostic factor, associated with a relative risk of 2.4. The extent of parametrial involvement also was a factor in recurrence. Neither high tumor grade nor adenocarcinoma increased the risk of failure.

Survival.—Thirty patients (24%) died of cervical cancer and 10 others of intercurrent disease with no evidence of recurrent cancer. Ten women had 11 second primary cancers outside the radiation portals. Sixty-eight percent of women were living without disease at 5 years. The chance of this declined with advancing tumor stage and with the presence of bulky disease.

Complications.—Forty-six treatment-related complications occurred in 37 patients. Most of them involved the bowel or genitourinary system. Severe complications were much more frequent in patients having pelvic surgery, and this was the only factor that correlated significantly with the overall risk of complications. Bulky disease was significantly associated with an increased risk of serious complications.

Conclusion.—These findings warrant considering the bulk of cervical tumor and the extent of parametrial disease when staging cervical carcinoma.

▶ The recurrent theme in this article is that in stages I and II cervical carcinoma, tumor size and not surprisingly extent of parametrial involvement (stage II) are strong predictors of behavior. The former correlated with local recurrence and the latter with distant metastases. The authors make another interesting point, which is that the rate of brachytherapy in excess of 60 cGy/hr increases the risk of grade 4 radiation complications. For comparison, most therapy centers give approximately 40–55 cGy/hr, which does provide some margin of safety.

A.L. Herbst, M.D.

Second Primary Cancer After Treatment for Cervical Cancer: An International Cancer Registries Study

Kleinerman RA, Boice JD Jr, Storm HH, et al (Natl Cancer Inst, Bethesda, Md; Danish Cancer Society, Copenhagen; Univ Hosp, Uppsala, Sweden; et al)

Cancer 76:442–452, 1995   22–46

Background.—The pattern of second cancers after cervical cancer treatment provides meaningful data on the risk of radiation-related malignancies. A considerable number of patients with cervical cancer experience long-term survival after treatment with radiotherapy and can therefore be studied for late treatment-related effects. The pattern of risk of second cancers over time after treatment of cervical cancer was thus investigated in a large number of patients who had long-term follow-up.

Patients and Findings.—Incident second cancers in 86,193 patients with cervical cancer were investigated. Cancers were reported to 13 population-based cancer registries in 5 countries. Of these patients, 49,828 women were treated with radiotherapy. There were 7,543 second cancers observed, compared with 6,015 cancers expected according to population rates (observed/expected = 1.2). Lung cancer was responsible for approximately 50% of the excess cancers. Among patients undergoing radiation therapy, 3,750 were alive 30 or more years after treatment. A twofold risk of cancers of heavily irradiated organs was observed in these patients, with most excess cancers observed in the rectum, vagina, vulva, ovary, and bladder. Patterns of risk over time supported a radiation etiology for these cancers. Significant increases in nonchronic lymphocytic leukemia and bone and kidney cancers were also associated with radiation therapy. A significant risk of second cancers was found in patients managed surgically and was likely associated with cigarette smoking and shared risk factors with cervical cancer.

Conclusions.—Large numbers of patients undergoing curative treatment for cervical cancer experience long-term survival; many receive a diagnosis of second cancers very late in life. An increased risk of second cancers was associated with radiation therapy and can persist for 30 or more years after treatment of organs receiving more than 1 Gy. Because the risk of new primary cancers remains high after primary diagnosis of cervical cancer, these patients should be routinely followed up for life.

▶ This article reminds us that, in a certain group of patients, second primary malignancy will develop after treatment for cancer of the cervix, and the heightened risks of many of the pelvic cancers is related to late effects of radiation—specifically for those cancers more than 30 years after treatment. Vaginal, vulvar, ovarian, and bladder cancers were elevated in the radiated group. As expected, due to shared cofactors, vaginal and vulvar carcinomas were also elevated in the nonradiated group. The data regarding the uterus were confounded by an uncertain rate of subsequent hysterectomy, and subsequent oophorectomy may have altered the ovarian results. Nonetheless, the data from this collaborative study from 13 population-based registries in 5 countries are convincing that radiation for cervical carcinoma is associated with approximately a doubling of risk of secondary cancers by 30 years after the relevant exposure.

A.L. Herbst, M.D.

Resection of Bulky Positive Lymph Nodes in Patients With Cervical Carcinoma

Hacker NF, Wain GV, Nicklin JL (Royal Hosp for Women, Paddington, Australia)
Int J Gynecol Cancer 5:250–256, 1995   22–47

Background.—Although external-beam therapy can sterilize small lymph node metastases in patients with cervical carcinoma, it is not likely to be successful against bulky nodal disease. At 1 facility, all bulky, positive lymph nodes are therefore identified and resected before radiation therapy is begun. The morbidity and outcomes of patients undergoing resection of bulky positive lymph nodes for stages IB, II, and III cervical cancer were evaluated.

Patients and Findings.—Thirty-four patients undergoing resection of bulky positive lymph nodes within a 5-year period were evaluated. These nodes were detected at radical hysterectomy in 23 patients and by pelvic and abdominal CT before radiation therapy for more advanced cervical cancer in 11 patients. Pelvic external-beam radiation was initiated in 33 patients after nodal resection. Twenty-eight patients also received pelvic and para-aortic radiation, and 23 received 4 cycles of cisplatin chemotherapy. The median number of resected positive nodes was 4 (range, 1–44). All macroscopic nodal metastases were resected in each patient. Positive nodes were limited to the pelvic region in 17 patients. In another 9 patients, these nodes involved the iliac group, and in 8 patients they involved the para-aortic area. Five patients experienced significant acute morbidity, including a lacerated external iliac vein, necrotizing fasciitis, postoperative cytomegalovirus hepatitis, and 2 instances of infected lymphocysts. Six patients also experienced serious long-term morbidity, including radiation enteritis, leading to small-bowel obstruction in 5, and ischemic bowel in the distribution of the superior mesenteric artery in 1. All patients were observed for a mean of 36 months, at which time 23 patients were alive. Of these, 20 patients were disease-free. Among patients undergoing radical hysterectomy, the actuarial 5-year survival was 80% in those with pelvic and common iliac lymph node involvement and 48% for those with positive para-aortic nodes. In patients with completely resected bulky pelvic and common iliac nodes, survival was similar to that observed for patients with micrometastases.

Conclusions.—In patients with cervical cancer, efforts should be directed toward identifying those with bulky positive lymph node metastases; these nodes should be resected before initiating radiation therapy.

▶ I have always been skeptical about resecting tumor-containing nodes in cervical carcinoma because the outcome has generally been considered to be poor. However, this report from Australia on 34 patients offers a provocative approach. The authors resected gross nodule metastases and, depending on node location, pelvic or pelvic and para-aortic radiation was used (50.4 Gy with a 4-field technique at 180 centigray/day). *Cis*-platinum was also used in 23 of the patients. The group was small and the mean follow-up only 36 months. Nonetheless, for the stages IB–IIA patients who had a radical hysterectomy with positive node removal, the 5-year survival was calculated to be 80%. This certainly is an impressive number. I would be somewhat cautious in my optimism regarding these results but do believe they are sufficiently good to warrant further clinical evaluation.

A.L. Herbst, M.D.

Vulvar

Pelvic Exenteration for Primary and Recurrent Vulvar Cancer

Miller B, Morris M, Levenback C, et al (Univ of Texas, Houston)
Gynecol Oncol 58:202–205, 1995

22–48

Introduction.—Treatment plans for carcinoma of the vulva include preoperative radiation therapy, chemotherapy, radiation therapy, interstitial radiation therapy, and surgery, which in some cases is the only curative therapy. To evaluate treatment outcomes and define indications, data on women with vulvar cancer who had pelvic exenteration were reviewed.

Methods.—Charts of 21 women (median age, 57 years) with pelvic exenteration for vulvar malignancy were reviewed. Eight women had advanced primary tumors, with a mean tumor diameter of 5 cm, and 13 had recurrent disease, with a mean tumor diameter of 4 cm. In 12 women, a posterior exenteration was performed, 6 had anterior exenteration, and 3 had total exenteration. Those with primary tumors had radical vulvectomy and inguinal lymphadenectomy.

Results.—The most frequent postoperative complication was infection, which occurred in 15 women, followed by pulmonary problems in 4 women and cardiac problems in 3 women. No deaths were related to treatment. Further surgery was necessary for 5 women to correct late postoperative sequelae. After treatment of primary tumor, 4 of 8 women had a recurrence: 1 was local, 2 were in the inguinal area, and 1 was local and in the pelvis. A second recurrence developed in 9 of 13 women treated for recurrent tumors, with the second recurrences in the pelvis. For patients treated for primary disease, the 5-year survival rate was 70%, and for those treated for recurrent disease, the 5-year survival rate was 38%. The median time to recurrence was 12 months, with a range of 3 to 196 months.

Conclusion.—For selected patients with advanced vulvar malignancy, pelvic exenteration is indicated. Before exenteration, the presence of nodal metastasis should be excluded.

▶ Exenteration is not usually used for vulvar carcinoma, especially for primary treatment. I prefer to use preoperative radiation for large vulvar tumors encroaching on the urethra or anus followed by a partial radical vulvectomy to excise the affected area. However, radiation vulvitis can be an annoying sequela. The authors certainly obtained good results in their selected cases, and the 38% 5-year survival rate for those who had exenteration for recurrent disease shows the operation does have a place in certain special cases.

A.L. Herbst, M.D.

23 Human Papillomavirus

Prospects for a Vaccine Against Human Papillomavirus
Hines JF, Ghim S-J, Schlegel R, et al (Brooke Army Med Ctr, San Antonio, Tex; Georgetown Univ, Washington, DC)
Obstet Gynecol 86:860–866, 1995   23–1

Background.—Recent research has increased understanding of the biology of human papillomaviruses (HPVs). Immunologically active forms of HPV pseudocapsids can now be prepared in quantity and accurately in vitro. Mounting evidence also suggests that cervical cancer also stimulates cell-mediated immune responses. The data supporting the use of recombinant viral capsid proteins as a prophylactic subunit vaccine against HPV infection were reviewed.

Methods and Findings.—The MEDLINE database and reference lists were searched to identify English-language studies of strategies for prophylactic and treatment vaccination against HPV infection. The several reports found included descriptions of systems producing recombinant HPV major capsid proteins as antigens for biochemical, molecular, and immunologic studies and assessments of cell-mediated immune responses to HPV-induced, tumor-related peptides. Recombinant HPV major capsid proteins, which self-assemble into virus-like particles, are produced in quantity. These proteins mimic the conformation of native virions, react with neutralizing antibodies, and are type-specific. The cytotoxic T-lymphocyte responses resulting from HPV early viral peptides retard tumor progression and protect against tumor development after challenge in animal models (Figs 1 and 3).

Conclusions.—Recombinant papillomavirus virus-like particles are very antigenic, protective in animal models, and lack potentially carcinogenic viral DNA. Thus, they are ideal candidates for a prophylactic vaccine against HPV infection. Human papillomavirus tumor peptide immunization may be beneficial in preventing tumors as well as in tumor regression and rejection. Vaccines against HPV infection may help decrease the incidence of cervical dysplasia and carcinoma worldwide, especially in developing countries.

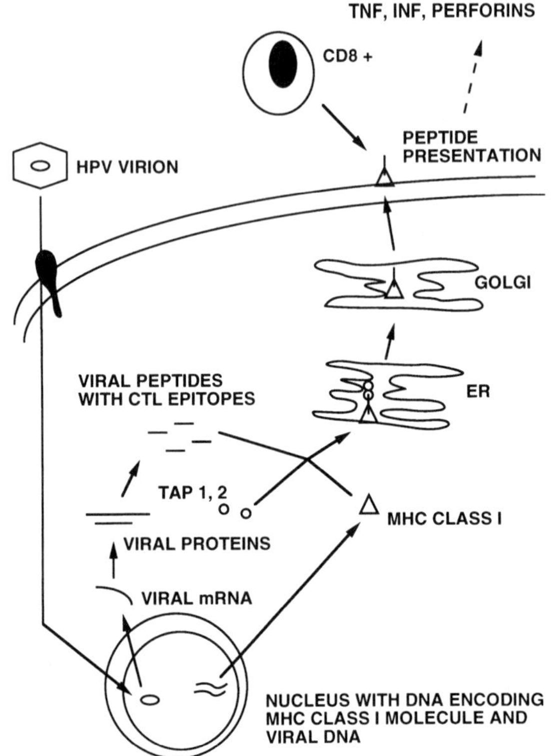

FIGURE 1.—Mechanism of peptide presentation and initiation of cell-mediated cytolysis. Human papillomavirus (*HPV*) virions infect target cells and viral DNA is delivered to the host nucleus. Viral messenger RNAs (*mRNA*) are transcribed and new viral proteins are synthesized on free ribosomes in the cytosol. Some of the newly synthesized viral proteins are degraded into peptide fragments that contain cytotoxic T-lymphocyte (*CTL*) epitopes. These peptides are presented to the endoplasmic reticulum (*ER*) by transport-associated proteins 1 and 2 (TAP 1, 2). Viral peptide fragments complex in the cleft of major histocompatibility complex (*MHC*) class I molecules. The major histocompatibility complex class I-peptide complex traffics through the endoplasmic reticulum and the Golgi apparatus. Finally, the viral peptide is presented at the cell surface and interaction with cytotoxic T lymphocytes (CD8+) causes the release of the cytokines tumor necrosis factor (*TNF*), perforin, and interferon (*IFN*). This promotes subsequent cell-mediated target cell destruction. (Courtesy of Hines JF, Ghim S-J, Schlegel R, et al: Prospects for a vaccine against human papillomavirus. *Obstet Gynecol* 86:860–866, 1995. Reprinted with permission from The American College of Obstetricians and Gynecologists.)

▶ I have included this theoretical discussion of the potential of HPV vaccination because it provides the reader with an excellent overview of the cellular mechanisms of HPV infection and also indicates how, in the future, a vaccine may be developed. This would be a major therapeutic advance against these widely prevalent and often chronic infections.

A few points are worth emphasizing. First, cell-mediated immunity is the primary host response to eradicate HPV infection, and Figure 1 shows the molecular mechanism involved. The CD8+ lymphocyte is the cytotoxic "T" cell, which releases cytokines in response to HPV viral peptide on the surface of the infected cells. This leads to cell mediated destruction of the target infected cell.

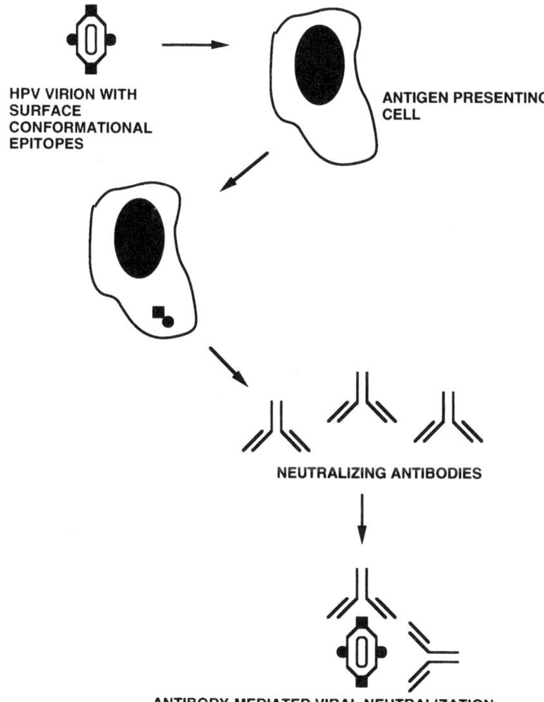

FIGURE 3.—Antibody-mediated viral neutralization. Neutralizing, conformational epitopes are expressed on the surface of human papillomavirus (*HPV*) virions. The epitopes (antigens) are recognized by lymphocytes and specific neutralizing antibodies are generated. These neutralizing antibodies bind specifically to surface epitopes and inhibit viral infection. (Courtesy of Hines JF, Ghim S-J, Schlegel R, et al: Prospects for a vaccine against human papillomavirus. *Obstet Gynecol* 86:860–866, 1995. Reprinted with permission from The American College of Obstetricians and Gynecologists.)

The article also considers the theoretical role of reinfused cytotoxic T cells stimulated by HPV oncoprotein peptides as potential future immunotherapy against cervical cancer. However, I think the most intriguing possibility is the potential role of vaccination in the prophylaxis of HPV infection. The model is illustrated in Figure 3. There are in vitro and animal models to indicate that neutralizing antibodies produced by injection papillomavirus subunits (neutralizing conformation epitopes) that reside on the surface of the viron can lead to the production of neutralizing antibodies by B cells. As noted by the authors, immunologically active virus-like particles used to produce vaccines are antigenic and protective in animal models. Yet, these are not oncogenic since they lack viral DNA. All of this may be very theoretical but certainly provides hopeful basis for the future development of HPV vaccine in humans.

A.L. Herbst, M.D.

Viral Testing for Genital Human Papillomavirus Infections: Recent Progress and Clinical Potentials

Ferenczy A (McGill Univ, Montreal)
Int J Gynecol Cancer 5:321–328, 1995   23–2

Background.—Human papillomavirus (HPV) DNA testing may play a role in the routine screening for cervical neoplasia, diagnostic triage of patients with inconclusive cervical cytologic smears, and quality control of cytologic and pathologic practices. Recent progress in and the clinical potential of viral testing for genital HPV infections were reviewed.

Human Papillomavirus DNA Testing.—Clinically, viral testing can be done to detect a subset of patients with minor-grade abnormalities on their cytologic smears who have a high oncogenic risk of HPV and to provide quality control of cytologic and histologic diagnoses. Several factors influence HPV positivity, regardless of the test used. These factors include age, phase of the menstrual cycle, exogenous hormone, and immunocompetence. Young patients, patients in the luteal phase of their cycle, oral contraceptive users, pregnant women, and immunosuppressed patients have greater detection rates. In such patients, viral replication is increased, resulting in a greater viral load and a greater likelihood of HPV DNA detection.

Screening With HPV Testing.—Viral testing has the potential to decrease the rates of false negative and false positive smears. Routine cytology may be combined with HPV DNA testing to reduce false negative smears. Studies of patients with precolposcopic cytology suggesting atypical squamous cells of undetermined significance or low-grade squamous intraepithelial lesions have shown that the sensitivity of the HPV mix viral tests using 14 or 9 probes ranged from 70% to 85%. When HPV DNA testing and cytology were used, the detection rates of histologically high-grade cervical intraepithelial neoplasia increased from 93% to 100%. The specificity of viral testing can be improved by limiting testing to women older than age 35 years, when the peak of persistent, high oncogenic risk virus-positive high-grade lesions occurs.

Conclusions.—The use of HPV DNA testing will contribute to more cost-effective screening programs, especially when older women are targeted. The results of ongoing large-scale prospective studies of women in routine practices are needed before the use of HPV testing can become widespread.

▶ This is an informative review article by Dr. Ferenczy, who has been an active investigator into cervical intraepithelial neoplasia and HPV. The entire review is worth reading for those who wish to stay current with changes in this area and the future potential of HPV testing. Areas covered are screening with HPV testing; using HPV as a supplement to triage low-grade abnormal smears; and the potential of HPV testing to be utilized for cytologic laboratory quality assurance.

As I have written elsewhere, I do not use HPV typing, at the moment, in my clinical practice, but there are accumulating data that it may well be useful in the future to the gynecologist, particularly in regard to the decision of how to manage low-grade lesions including the pesky diagnosis of atypical squamous cells of undetermined significance (ASCUS).[1]

A few points are worth emphasizing. First, in spite of the mountains of data (some conflicting) about the management of the abnormal Pap smear as well as the appropriate frequency of routine screening, we do not have definitive information regarding the most cost-effective approach. This is an area usefully considered in this review. Second, I am not convinced that HPV typing is useful for screening. The HPV positivity is influenced by a number of factors, including patient age, phase of the menstrual cycle, use of exogenous hormones, pregnancy, and immunocompetence. Furthermore, as is suggested by Dr. Ferenczy, the test when performed, is most specific for those over the age of 35 years, and a single positive test for those in their 20s is of dubious value. I am intrigued with a personal communication reported in the article by another HPV researcher, Dr. A. Lorincz, that cervical intraepithelial neoplasia risk returns to control levels after 4 years of HPV positivity and those who remain cytologically normal. There obviously are a number of facts yet to be learned in this area before we can make generalizations about routine clinical use. In addition, it is important to realize that data for the use of HPV testing and screening trials are not available. Most of the published information deals with studies of individuals who have cytologically positive smears.

The decision for the use of HPV testing for quality control is not so clear, and as I have noted elsewhere, computer-assisted evaluation of normal smears with neural nets offers a useful technology to reduce the number of false negative smears that we now encounter. There is the potential to use a "cocktail" of HPV types to decide whether to colposcope those with a low-grade abnormal smear, such as ASCUS, referred to previously. This is a central issue, and an ongoing National Cancer Institute trial and its results will be of great interest. If it is a highly specific test, the question will then be one of cost-effectiveness. That, too, is a subject of debate, since some have preliminarily found that HPV testing may not be a cost-effective approach.[2]

A.L. Herbst, M.D.

References

1. Cox JT, Lorincz AT, Schiffman MH, et al: Human papillomavirus testing by hybrid capture is useful in triaging women with a cytologic diagnosis of atypical squamous cells of undetermined significance. *Am J Obstet Gynecol* 172:946–954, 1995.
2. Goff BA, Muntz HG, Bell DA, et al: Human papillomavirus typing in patients with Papanicolaou smears showing squamous atypia. *Gynecol Oncol* 48:384–338, 1993.

Persistent Genital Human Papillomavirus Infection as a Risk Factor for Persistent Cervical Dysplasia

Ho GYF, Burk RD, Klein S, et al (Albert Einstein College, Bronx, NY)
J Natl Cancer Inst 87:1365–1371, 1995   23–3

Background.—Cervical dysplasia is classified into 3 grades. It is thought to have the potential for successive progression through these stages to invasive squamous carcinoma of the cervix. However, all cases of cervical dysplasia do not progress; in fact, many mild lesions spontaneously regress. Factors determining persistence vs. regression of cervical dysplasia were investigated.

Methods.—Over the course of 15 months, 70 patients with histologically confirmed grade 2 cervical intraepithelial neoplasia were evaluated first at 6-week and then at 3-month intervals. Evaluation consisted of Papanicolaou smear, colposcopy, and exfoliation of cervicovaginal cells for detection of human papillomavirus (HPV) DNA. The DNA was typed by both polymerase chain reaction (PCR) and Southern blot hybridization techniques. "Low viral loads" were detectable only with the more sensitive PCR technique. The data were grouped in pairs of 2 successive visits. Only lesions detected at each of 2 successive visits were considered to indicate persistent cervical dysplasia. Persistent dysplasia was then correlated with various risk factors using a statistical model for time-dependent data. Lifestyle variables were assessed at baseline with a structured questionnaire.

Results.—Lifestyle variables such as age, ethnicity, sexual behavior, smoking, education, and use of oral contraceptives did not correlate with persistent cervical dysplasia. Continual HPV infection in paired data sets and a persistent high viral load were both associated with persistence of cervical dysplasia. The highest risk for persistent cervical dysplasia was found among those women with type-specific persistent infection (determined by PCR) in successive visits, particularly if viral load was high. Those with a low level of type-specific persistent infection or non–type-specific persistent infection showed a lesser risk. Women with continual genital HPV as detected by Southern blot analysis at 2 successive visits showed a fourfold higher risk of persistent cervical dysplasia than did women without HPV. The association of persistent HPV infection with persistent cervical dysplasia at a succeeding, rather than at the same, time interval was weaker. Persistent infection with HPV and persistence of cervical dysplasia may therefore be synchronous.

Discussion.—Aspects of genital HPV infection such as DNA positivity, viral type, and level of viral load may vary over time, affecting the natural history of cervical dysplasia. A lesion may become chronic rather than regress if persistent HPV infection is type specific and harbors a high viral load. Of women with mild or moderate lesions of cervical dysplasia, those likely to experience spontaneous regression may perhaps be distinguished from those whose lesions will persist or progress (and who need immediate medical attention) by repeated testing for genital HPV infection. Factors that govern the natural pathway of cervical dysplasia should be identified.

New Epidemiology of Human Papillomavirus Infection and Cervical Neoplasia
Schiffman MH (Natl Cancer Inst, Bethesda, Md)
J Natl Cancer Inst 87:1345–1347, 1995   23–4

Stages of Cervical Carcinogenesis.—The first stage of cervical carcinogenesis is initiated when an oncogenic type of human papillomavirus (HPV) is transmitted to the cervical epithelium. Most initial infections do not lead to a diagnosed cytologic abnormality. When cervical intraepithelial neoplasia (CIN) is diagnosed, the lesion is usually low grade (CIN I, including koilocytotic atypia). The HPV infection and early cytologic changes following it typically regress spontaneously within months to years, presumably because of a host response primarily mediated by the cellular arm of the immune system. A small minority of affected patients experience eventual progression to CIN III lesions; risk of progression increases with increased duration of lower-grade lesions.

Report by Ho et al.—The study by Ho et al. focuses on the determinants of persistence and progression vs. regression of CIN. Prospective evaluation of 100 women with lesions originally diagnosed as CIN II was conducted. Clinicians and epidemiologists would like to dichotomize disease in the CIN II category as either low grade (mild, often transient cytologic effect of HPV) or high grade (precursor to cancer requiring immediate treatment). One third of the patients studied by Ho et al. showed regression to normalcy, demonstrating the biological and/or diagnostic heterogenicity of the CIN II classification. These data, along with the fact that some CIN II lesions contain types of HPV not known to be independently associated with cancer, indicate that many CIN II lesions pose low risk. A conceptual "high-grade" category might then include CIN III lesions and those CIN II lesions deemed severe (perhaps those marked by aneuploidy). Ho et al. also demonstrated that HPV infection measured at the molecular level was mirrored by persistence of CIN.

Discussion.—The details of transience and persistence of HPV infections are still largely unknown. Some cases of CIN III appear to develop via another causal pathway. Of the first cytologic abnormalities diagnosed after infection with HPV, 5% to 10% are CIN II or CIN III as opposed to CIN I, indicating that disease in some women may not progress through the CIN I or CIN II stages. This route to CIN III appears to be a relatively minor alternative path of development. Human papillomavirus infection appears to mirror the current state of CIN more strongly than its future state. Measurements of HPV were best able to predict CIN at the same, rather than the subsequent, interval.

▶ The study by Ho et al. (Abstract 23–3) is an important, but complicated analysis of HPV infection in patients with documented CIN II (moderate dysplasia). The HPV-DNA was measured by the sensitive polymerase chain reaction (PCR) and Southern blot hybridization techniques, the latter being less sensitive, but if positive would indicate a higher viral load. The study lasted 18 months with Papanicolaou, colposcopy, and HPV measurements made every 3 months.

I have included the accompanying Schiffman editorial because it gives a useful insight into the interpretation of the Ho data as well as a summary of the current thinking regarding the development of cervical neoplasia.

As noted by Schiffman, CIN is thought to be initiated in most cases by persistent HPV infection. Several important points are worth emphasizing. These infections usually regress over a period of months or years. In addition, most initial HPV infections, even those with oncogenic HPV types, do not lead to diagnostic morphologic abnormalities. With persistent HPV infection, some degree of neoplasia usually develops, and in most instances these are probably low grade. Even most of these changes will spontaneously regress whereas a few likely will progress to CIN III, a high-grade lesion with a strong potential for further progression to invasive carcinoma, if left untreated. To round out this picture, Schiffman also noted that about 10% or fewer of cervical neoplasias are HPV-negative, a definite minority, but still representative of an important alternate route for neoplastic development. It also appears that a few persistent HPV infections may have CIN II or CIN III as the initial morphologic expression, and unpublished data by Schiffman and colleagues suggest that this may appear in 5% to 10% of incident cases they have studied.

To return to the article by Ho et al., it carries a number of important messages. As previously noted, the presence of a high viral load is indicative of neoplasia. However, the presence of a high viral load does *not* predict accurately the findings at a subsequent visit. In other words, a high viral load at one visit does not strongly predict future behavior. Most importantly, this article, which intensely studies CIN (moderate dysplasia), indicates that this diagnosis consists of a mixture of lesions with varying potentials to progress or regress. In fact, in this study, approximately *one third* of the cases of moderate dysplasia spontaneously regressed. As noted correctly by Schiffman, the important issue is to find a way to predict which lesions are virulent and will progress as opposed to those that will regress. I think this is of particular importance to the clinician who gets a report of high-grade squamous intraepithelial lesions, which, of course will include some cases of moderate dysplasia that will spontaneously regress.

A.L. Herbst, M.D.

Human Papillomavirus in False Negative Archival Cervical Smears: Implications for Screening for Cervical Cancer
Walboomers JMM, de Roda Husman A-M, Snijders PJF, et al (Free Univ, Amsterdam; Gooi-Noord Hosp, Blaricum, The Netherlands)
J Clin Pathol 48:728–732, 1995   23–5

Introduction.—Cytologic screening for cervical cancer has low sensitivity (50% to 85%). Because of their unreliability, Papanicolaou (Pap) smears are repeated relatively frequently. Recent studies have shown a strong association between cervical cancer and the presence of oncogenic human papillomavirus (HPV) types. The presence of HPV in false negative archival cervical smears was investigated.

Methods.—Twenty-seven false negative archival cervical smears from 18 women who had a diagnosis of cervical cancer within 6 years of the smears were mixed with 89 Pap smears from 50 women seeking treatment for a variety of gynecologic complaints. The DNA was isolated from these smears and from cervical biopsy specimens from the 18 patients with cervical cancer and were analyzed and typed for HPV with polymerase chain reaction (PCR) techniques.

Results.—Of the 27 false negative archival cervical smears from women with cervical cancer, 24 were positive for HPV, 2 were HPV-negative, and 1 had inadequate DNA for PCR. There were high-risk HPV types in 23 smears. The 9 patients with 2 smears had the same HPV type detected in both smears. In the control group, a high-risk HPV type was detected in 5 of the 28 patients with 1 cervical smear (including 2 patients with cervical intraepithelial demographic and lifestyle variables). The association of these variables with persistent dysplasia was analyzed.

Results.—Of 350 paired colposcopic examinations, 186 demonstrated persistent dysplasia. High HPV loads were detected at 106 visits (52.5%), of which 60 (56.6%) had type-specific persistent infection, and all but 4 had a high-risk HPV type. Human papillomavirus, as detected by PCR, was persistent in 75.9% observations, of which 82.3% showed type-specific persistent infection. Age, ethnicity, education, age at first coitus, duration of oral contraceptive use, number of male sexual partners, and smoking status were not associated with persistent dysplasia. Only persistent HPV infection and viral load were associated with persistent dysplasia, with patients with a type-specific persistent HPV infection and a continual high viral load at the highest risk for persistent dysplasia. The risk of persistent dysplasia was increased fourfold in patients with genital HPV infection detected with Southern blot analysis at consecutive visits; the association between continued PCR-detected HPV infection and persistent dysplasia was less strong.

Conclusions.—Repeated HPV testing in women with mild and moderate cervical dysplasia may distinguish between those with lesions likely to regress spontaneously and those with lesions likely to persist or progress.

▶ I have included this retrospective study of false negative smears because it adds to the understanding that HPV is involved in many of the precursor lesions of cervical carcinoma years before the diagnosis is made. Of the 18 patients studied by the authors, only 2 did not show HPV by PCR, and these cases had inadequate smears for cytologic interpretation.

False negative Pap smears are a worrisome problem for all of us. As I have noted elsewhere, current National Cancer Institute trials will evaluate whether HPV testing can help us properly triage our patients, particularly those with a reading of atypical squamous cells of undetermined significance.

Computer technology is also being applied in this area through having negative Pap smears rescreened with computer assistance. One such device displays the cells of potential concern on a screen for visual inspection (PAPNET, Neuromedical Systems, Suffern, New York). Utilizing this technology, the risk of false negative smears can be markedly reduced. In my role as a medical consultant, I have come to believe that this is an effective approach.

A.L. Herbst, M.D.

Histologic and Biomolecular Aspects of Papillomatosis of the Vulvar Vestibule in Relation to Human Papillomavirus

de Deus JM, Focchi J, Stávale JN, et al (Escola Paulista de Medicina, São Paulo, Brazil)
Obstet Gynecol 86:758–763, 1995

23–6

Background.—Papillomatosis of the vulvar vestibule is often observed during colposcopic assessment of young patients with no history of sexual promiscuity or any history of sexual activity at all. Gynecologists and pathologists have frequently diagnosed vulvar condyloma in such patients, subjecting them to repeated, even damaging treatments. The histologic and biomolecular aspects of papillomatosis of the vulvar vestibule were studied and compared with normal vulvar epithelium and condyloma acuminatum.

Methods.—Twenty-five women with papillomatosis of the vulvar vestibule seen initially with no abnormal clinical, cytologic, or colposcopic changes in the cervix or vagina were studied. Molecular hybridization and histology of biopsy material taken from the inner surface of the labia minora were performed. Findings were compared with those from 24 women with condyloma acuminatum of the vulvar vestibule and from 10 women with normal vulvar epithelium and no cervicovaginal changes. All patients were age 35 years or younger. None was pregnant.

Findings.—By molecular hybridization, papillomatosis of the vulvar vestibule was rarely positive for human papillomavirus (HPV). Positivity was found by dot blot hybridization in 4% and by polymerase chain reaction in 6.7%. These percentages were comparable to those in the group with normal vulvar epithelium. However, the corresponding proportions for the group with condyloma acuminatum of the vestibule were 50% and 100%, which were significantly higher. The biomolecular assessment of vestibular papillomatosis demonstrated that focal koilocytosis was unassociated with HPV infection.

Conclusions.—Papillomatosis of the vulvar vestibule should be considered a paraphysiologic formation of the vulvar epithelium. It is not associated with HPV. In the absence of more explicit clinical-histologic evidence, vulvar HPV infection should not be diagnosed. There is no need for biopsies or treatment in such patients.

▶ As noted by the authors, prior publications have shown that papillomatosis of the vulva is a normal event that occurs in the vulvar vestibule. It is not related to disease or to HPV infection. This article provides some nice illustrations of the papillomatosis condition, which appears as regular rough granulations of the vulva with each papilla being discrete. Application of acetic acid does not produce white epithelium, and these authors have demonstrated that these papillae are HPV-negative. They do not require biopsy, which is the main point of the article. The authors also note that some reports suggesting the presence of koilocytes in papillomatosis probably represent normal cells that have the appearance of a perinuclear halo or perinuclear vacuolization. However, these cells have nuclear atypia and are thus not koilocytes. I would reemphasize that this is a normal condition and does not require biopsy or treatment.

A.L. Herbst, M.D.

24 Gestational Trophoblastic Disease

High-dose Chemotherapy With Autologous Bone Marrow Transplantation for Refractory Metastatic Gestational Trophoblastic Disease
Giacalone PL, Benos P, Donnadio D, et al (Hopital Arnaud de Villeneuve, Montpellier, France; Hopital Lapeyronie, Montpellier, France)
Gynecol Oncol 58:383–385, 1995
24–1

Introduction.—A relatively few patients with trophoblastic disease fail to respond to standard chemotherapy and require second- or third-line treatment. There is as yet no consensus on the most effective regimen of multiagent chemotherapy for these patients.

Case Report.—Woman, 28, underwent curettage of hydatiform mole at 9 weeks' gestation and a second procedure 3 months later, after which the level of plasmatic human chorionic gonadotropin (hCG) declined. After 5 months, the level again increased, and pelvic ultrasonography demonstrated a 1-cm mass in the myometrium as well as anechogenic cysts in the ovaries. Three courses of chemotherapy failed to reduce the plasmatic hCG level below 350 IU/L, although the ultrasound scan became negative. A few months later, a 6-cm nodular mass appeared within the myometrium, and hysterectomy revealed a choriocarcinoma that invaded the full thickness of the uterine wall. The level of β-hCG increased to 4,750 IU/L but declined to 350 IU/L after further chemotherapy with dactinomycin and etoposide. Subsequently autologous marrow transplantation was performed in conjunction with high-dose cyclophosphamide, etoposide, and melphalan therapy. The marrow was markedly suppressed, and the patient required treatment for streptococcal septicemia. The plasma hCG was negative 6 weeks after marrow transplantation, and the patient continued in clinical and biological remission 3 years after treatment.

Conclusion.—Autologous marrow transplantation permits high-dose chemotherapy to be given in this setting while limiting the time of bone marrow suppression.

▶ As noted elsewhere, the preliminary results of high-dose chemotherapy with autologous bone marrow transplantation have been disappointing in ovarian tumors, the primary gynecologic disease in which advanced therapy has been tried.

This case report describing 1 patient with no evidence of disease 3 years after multiagent high-dose chemotherapy with autologous bone marrow transplantation is somewhat encouraging and suggests we should at least consider this modality in these young patients with chemotherapy-refractory disease.

A.L. Herbst, M.D.

25 Breast Diseases

Reanalysis and Results After 12 Years of Follow-up in a Randomized Clinical Trial Comparing Total Mastectomy With Lumpectomy With or Without Irradiation in the Treatment of Breast Cancer
Fisher B, Anderson S, Redmond CK, et al (Pittsburgh, Pa)
N Engl J Med 333:1456–1461, 1995   25–1

Introduction.—Previously published reports of Protocol B-06 of the National Surgical Adjuvant Breast and Bowel Project (NSABP) concluded that lumpectomy followed by breast irradiation was an effective treatment for breast cancer. Since those reports, it was discovered that a researcher at 1 study hospital, St. Luc Hospital in Montreal, had falsified information on patients enrolled in the protocol. This discovery prompted separate audits of St. Luc Hospital and other institutions participating in the study. The results of both audits were investigated, along with an update of the study findings an average of 12 years after randomization.

Methods.—Patients with breast cancer with negative or positive axillary nodes and with tumors measuring no larger than 4 cm in diameter were enrolled into Protocol B-06 from 1976 to 1984. They were then randomly assigned to receive treatment with total mastectomy, lumpectomy followed by breast irradiation, or lumpectomy without irradiation. The current report covers analyses of 3 patient cohorts, including an intention-to-treat analysis of all 2,105 randomly assigned patients. Also analyzed were 1,851 eligible patients with known nodal status who agreed to follow-up and their assigned therapy. This cohort excluded the 6 patients from St. Luc Hospital for whom biopsy dates had been falsified. A third cohort, totaling 1,529 patients, included all patients in the second cohort minus the rest of the patients from St. Luc Hospital.

Results.—In all 3 cohorts, there were no significant survival differences between patients undergoing total mastectomy, lumpectomy alone, or lumpectomy plus breast irradiation (Fig 1). The treatment results were similar for overall survival, disease-free survival, and survival free of distant disease (Figs 2 and 3). Twelve-year cumulative incidence of recurrent tumor in the same breast was 35% for patients undergoing lumpectomy alone vs. 10% in those treated with lumpectomy and breast irradiation (Fig 4). These figures were 32% for lumpectomy vs. 12% for lumpec-

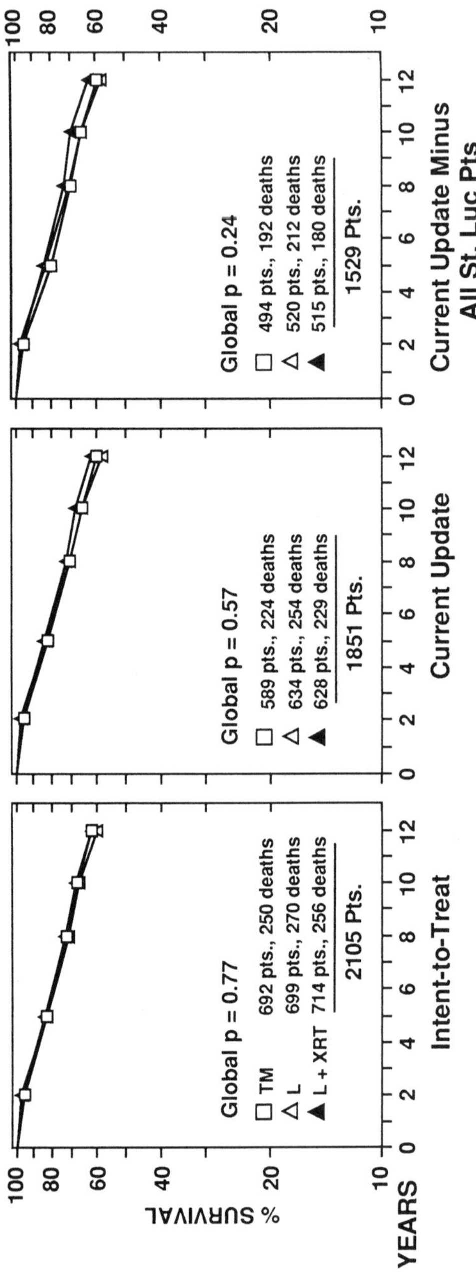

FIGURE 1.—Life-table analysis showing overall survival among patients in the 3 cohorts who were treated by total mastectomy (*square*), or lumpectomy (*open triangle*), or lumpectomy and breast irradiation (*filled triangle*). The number of deaths includes those occurring after 12 years. (Reprinted by permission of *The New England Journal of Medicine* from Fisher B, Anderson S, Redmond CK, et al: Reanalysis and results after 12 years of follow-up in a randomized clinical trial comparing total mastectomy with lumpectomy with or without irradiation in the treatment of breast cancer. *N Engl J Med* 333:1456–1461, Copyright 1995, Massachusetts Medical Society.)

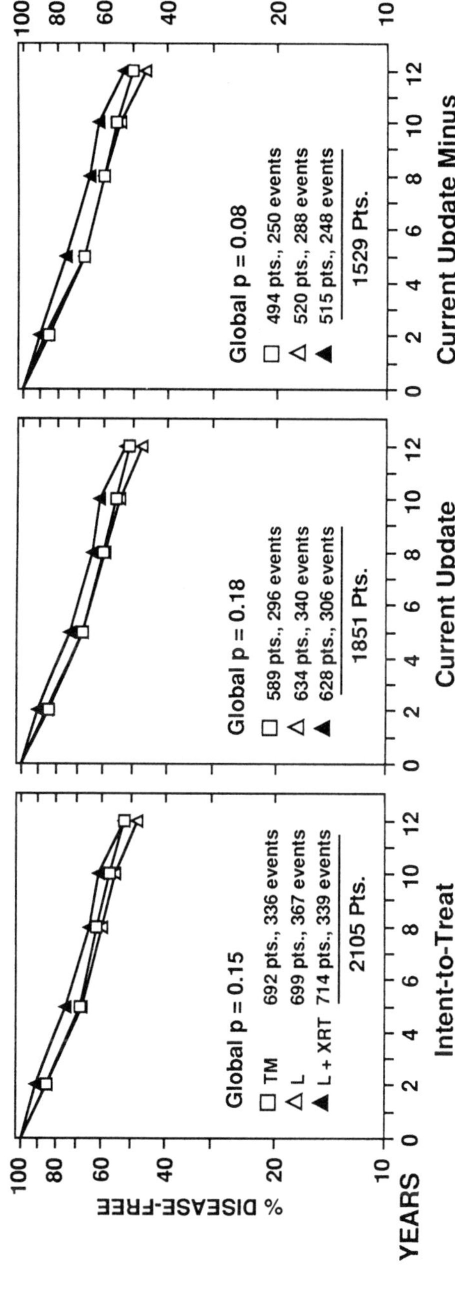

FIGURE 2.—Life-table analysis showing disease-free survival among patients in the 3 cohorts who were treated by total mastectomy (*squares*), lumpectomy (*open triangles*), or lumpectomy and breast irradiation (*filled triangles*). The number of events includes those that occurred after the 12-year follow-up. (Reprinted by permission of *The New England Journal of Medicine* from Fisher B, Anderson S, Redmond CK, et al: Reanalysis and results after 12 years of follow-up in a randomized clinical trial comparing total mastectomy with lumpectomy with or without irradiation in the treatment of breast cancer. *N Engl J Med* 333:1456–1461, Copyright, 1995, Massachusetts Medical Society.)

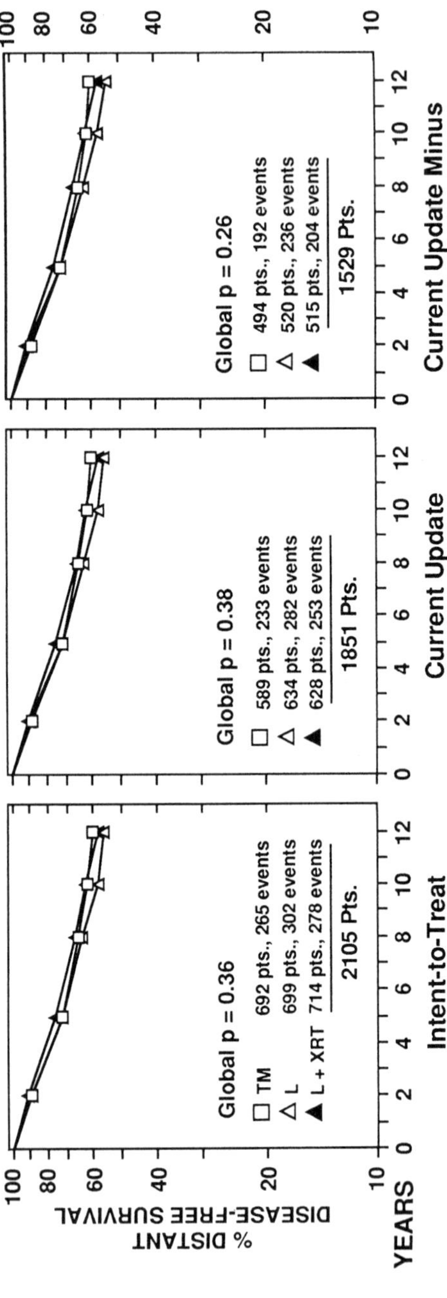

FIGURE 3.—Life-table analysis showing distant-disease-free survival among patients in the 3 cohorts who were treated by total mastectomy (*squares*), lumpectomy (*open triangles*), or lumpectomy and breast irradiation (*filled triangles*). The number of events includes those that occurred after the 12-year follow-up. (Reprinted by permission of *The New England Journal of Medicine* from Fisher B, Anderson S, Redmond CK, et al: Reanalysis and results after 12 years of follow-up in a randomized clinical trial comparing total mastectomy with lumpectomy with or without irradiation in the treatment of breast cancer. *N Engl J Med* 333:1456–1461, Copyright 1995, Massachusetts Medical Society.)

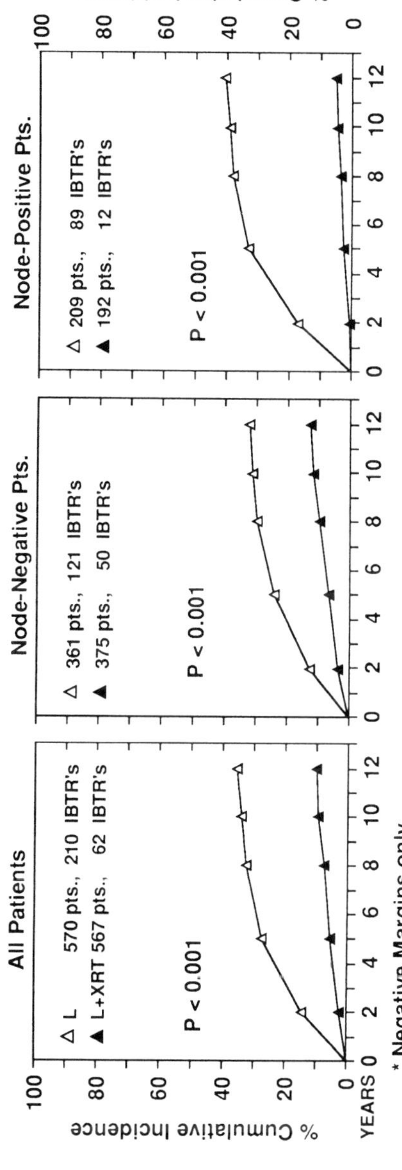

FIGURE 4.—Cumulative incidence of ipsilateral breast tumor recurrence (IBTR) after lumpectomy (*open triangles*) or lumpectomy and breast irradiation in 1,137 patients in the current-update cohort (cohort B) who had either negative or positive results from testing of nodes and tumor-negative specimen margins: The *P* values were calculated from average annual rates of recurrence in the ipsilateral breast. The number of recurrences includes those that occurred after the 12-year follow-up. Negative margins only. (Reprinted by permission of *The New England Journal of Medicine* from Fisher B, Anderson S, Redmond CK, et al: Reanalysis and results after 12 years of follow-up in a randomized clinical trial comparing total mastectomy with lumpectomy with or without irradiation in the treatment of breast cancer. *N Engl J Med* 333:1456–1461, Copyright 1995, Massachusetts Medical Society.)

tomy and breast irradiation in patients with node-negative cancer, and 5% vs. 41% in patients with node-positive cancer who also received chemotherapy.

Conclusions.—Despite the well-reported falsifications of data in Protocol B-06, the results appear to be the same as previously reported: Lumpectomy and irradiation is a suitable treatment for women with stage I or II breast cancer. The careful design of the study prevented the actions of a single person from altering its findings and conclusions.

▶ The results of the NSABP Protocol B-06 were called into question after irregularities in the eligibility criteria of some cases from a single center out of the 89 institutions participating in the protocol were made public. This reanalysis of all the data, after audit by NSABP and National Cancer Institute, with extension of the length of follow-up to 12 years, confirms the original conclusions.[1, 2] Breast-conserving therapy was as effective (except for unacceptable levels of local recurrence in the lumpectomy without irradiation group—see Figure 4) as the traditional modified radical mastectomy for stage I and II breast cancer. As confirmed by the following Supplementary Papers and the NIH Consensus Conference,[3] breast-conserving therapy is the preferred treatment for stage I and II breast cancer. Dr. Fisher and his NSABP group are to be congratulated for this painstaking review and unequivocal validation of his original publication,[1] which has fundamentally changed the treatment of breast cancer for most women in the United States.

W.H. Hindle, M.D.

References

1. Fisher B, Bauer M, Margolese R, et al: Five-year results of a randomized clinical trial comparing total mastectomy and segmental mastectomy with or without radiation in the treatment of breast cancer. *N Engl J Med* 312:665–673, 1985.
2. Fisher B, Redmond C, Poisson R, et al: Eight-year results of a randomized clinical trial comparing total mastectomy and lumpectomy with or without irradiation in the treatment of breast cancer. *N Engl J Med* 320:822–828, 1989.
3. NIH Consensus Conference: Treatment of early-stage breast cancer. *JAMA* 265:391–395, 1991.

Supplementary Papers

Jacobson JA, Danforth DN, Cowan KH, et al: Ten-year results of a comparison of conservation with mastectomy in the treatment of stage I and II breast cancer. *N Engl J Med* 332:907–911, 1995.

▶ This is an update of the National Cancer Institute's randomized clinical trial covering 237 patients comparing traditional total mastectomy with breast-conserving therapy (lumpectomy, axillary node dissection, and radiotherapy) for stages I and II breast cancer. The disease-free survival, overall survival, and local-regional recurrences are similar to the results of other randomized clinical trials, including the NSABP B-06.

W.H. Hindle, M.D.

Recht A, Houlihan MJ: Conservative surgery without radiotherapy in the treatment of patients with early-stage invasive breast cancer: A review. *Ann Surg* 222:9–18, 1995.

▶ This thoughtful review article seeks to answer the question of whether there is a subset of women with stages I and II breast cancer who can adequately be treated by surgery alone, i.e., omitting the currently accepted radiation therapy as a component of breast-conserving therapy. Local recurrences are the problem. What is the threat to overall survival when a local recurrence occurs? It may be minimal. Is mastectomy necessary for all local recurrences? There are no published data with follow-up of re-resection (or a "second lumpectomy") of locally recurrent breast cancer. As the initial surgical treatment, does quadrantectomy reduce the rate of local recurrence to the same rate as that of anterior chest wall recurrence after total mastectomy? The authors suggest that carefully designed prospective, randomized, clinical trials with stringent guidelines and completely informed patients should be undertaken.

W.H. Hindle, M.D.

Early Breast Cancer Trialists' Collaborative Group: Effects of radiotherapy and surgery in early breast cancer: An overview of the randomized trials. *N Engl J Med* 333:1444–1445, 1995.

▶ This overview analysis of 36 randomized trials with mortality data for 28,405 women treated for breast cancer revealed that "the addition of radiotherapy to surgery resulted in a rate of local recurrence that was three times lower than the rate with surgery alone, but there was no significant difference in 10-year survival... ." Twenty-year survial data will be of keen clinical interest as will the increased rate of noncancer deaths for women over 60 years of age at randomization who received irradiation as part of their initial cancer therapy. This report is an example of the statistically reliable and clinically meaningful data on breast cancer outcome that should provide objective medical evidence–based recommendations in the not-too-distant future.

W.H. Hindle, M.D.

Breast Cancer in Women 70 Years of Age or Older

Masetti R, Antinori A, Terribile D, et al (Catholic Univ, Rome)
J Am Geriatr Soc 44:390–393, 1996   25–2

Background.—Although age is known to be an important variable affecting breast cancer biology and management, breast cancer in older women is not well researched. The impact of age as a prognostic factor in older women with breast cancer was investigated.

Methods.—One hundred ninety women aged 70 to 89 years were treated between 1967 and 1991. The mean age was 75 years. Another group of patients matched for T and N categories and surgical procedures, with a mean age of 52 years, served as a comparison.

Findings.—The 10-year actuarial breast cancer–specific survival rates in the older and younger groups were 66% and 56%, respectively. The 10-year actuarial disease-free survival rates were 54% and 45%, respectively. In both age groups, tumor size and nodal stage were significant prognostic factors in univariate and multivariate analyses.

Conclusion.—Surgery that allows the best chance for definitive cure with the lowest risk of recurrence is indicated for women with breast cancer, regardless of age. Treatments that do not include at least excisional biopsy can be justified only for patients with high-grade comorbid conditions that contraindicate surgery.

▶ Elderly women (defined as 70 years of age or older in this report) have received scant attention as a specific group of women with breast cancer. As with this study, most analyses of women in this age group reveal that, except for their age and possible comorbid medical conditions, the diagnosis, treatment, and outcome of breast cancer are similar to those of younger women. These authors stress the importance of surgical resection for local control of the cancer. Regardless of her age, every woman with breast cancer should be evaluated as a unique individual. The diagnostic and treatment recommendations should be relevant to her general health, her fully informed consent, and her family considerations.

W.H. Hindle, M.D.

SUPPLEMENTARY PAPER

Solin LJ, Schultz DR, Fowble BL: Ten-year results of the treatment of early-stage breast carcinoma in elderly women using breast-conserving surgery and definitive breast irradiation. *Int J Radiat Oncol Biol Phys* 33:45–51, 1995.

▶ This comparison of the outcomes of 173 women aged over 65 years with those for 385 women aged 50–64, all of whom had breast-conserving therapy for breast cancer at the University of Pennsylvania Cancer Center, documents an expected increased risk of death from intercurrent disease in the over-65 group. However, there was no significant difference in the 10-year survival, relapse-free survival, freedom from distant metastases, and local failure between the 2 age groups. The data in this study contradict the notion that breast cancers in the elderly (over 65) are indolent and have a distinctly different biological behavior than do breast cancers in women under 65. Furthermore, breast-conserving therapy is as "preferred" for women age 50–64 and women over 65 as it is for women under 50.

W.H. Hindle, M.D.

Improved Survival in Young Women With Breast Cancer

Anderson BO, Senie RT, Vetto JT, et al (Mem Sloan-Kettering Cancer Ctr, New York; Oregon Health Sciences Univ, Portland; Cornell Univ, New York)
Ann Surg Oncol 2:407–415, 1995   25–3

Objective.—It has been proposed that younger women with breast cancer have a relatively poor outlook. This may not take recent therapeutic advances into account. For this reason, outcomes were reviewed in 81 women aged 30 years or younger who had definitive surgery for primary breast cancer in the period 1950–1969 and in 146 others operated on in 1970–1989. The respective median follow-up intervals were 14 and 7 years.

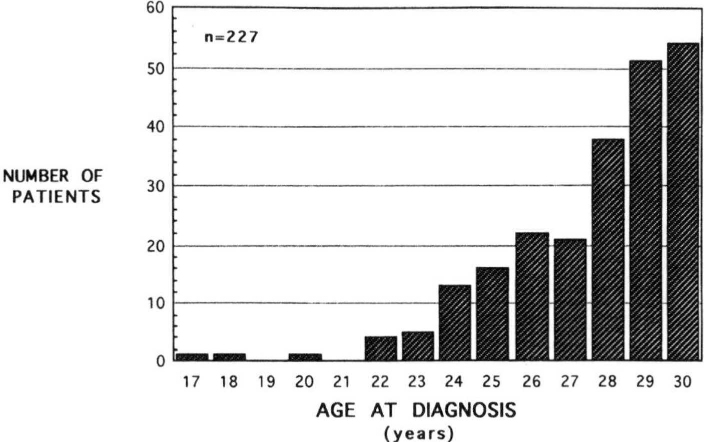

FIGURE 1.—Age at diagnosis for 227 young women (younger than 30 years of age) with primary operable breast cancer. (Courtesy of Anderson BO, Senie RT, Vetto JT, et al: Improved survival in young women with breast cancer. *Ann Surg Oncol* 2:407–415, 1995.)

Observations.—The overall median age at the time breast cancer was diagnosed was 28 years (Fig 1). Ages at diagnosis and at menarche were similar in the 2 groups, as were tumor size, histology, and number of involved lymph nodes. Less extensive resections were done in the later review period, and fewer women received adjuvant radiotherapy than in the earlier years. Actuarial survival was increased in the later group (Fig 3). Local recurrences were more frequent in the later era and adversely affected recurrence-free survival. Although systemic chemotherapy correlated with improved survival, adjuvant measures of all types—including chemotherapy—correlated with decreased overall and recurrence-free survival rates. Nevertheless node-positive patients who received chemotherapy did relatively well (Fig 5).

Conclusion.—Younger women with breast cancer do not necessarily have a poorer outlook, independent of the stage at diagnosis. Given current management, the prognosis for women aged 30 years or younger with early cancers is similar to that of older women having comparable disease.

► These comparative data on the outcome of young women treated for invasive breast cancer at the Memorial Sloan-Kettering Cancer Center are invaluable. The perception had been that young age per se was an adverse prognostic factor of breast cancer outcome. These data demonstrate that such is not the case. In fact, with current methods of treatment, the duration of survival has increased. However, as with women of all ages who elect breast-conserving therapy (BCT), there is an increased rate of local recurrence, but the overall survival rate is unchanged. Thus, BCT is a valid option for younger women with stage I and II invasive breast cancer. Prior to making her choice of mode of therapy and to giving her informed consent,

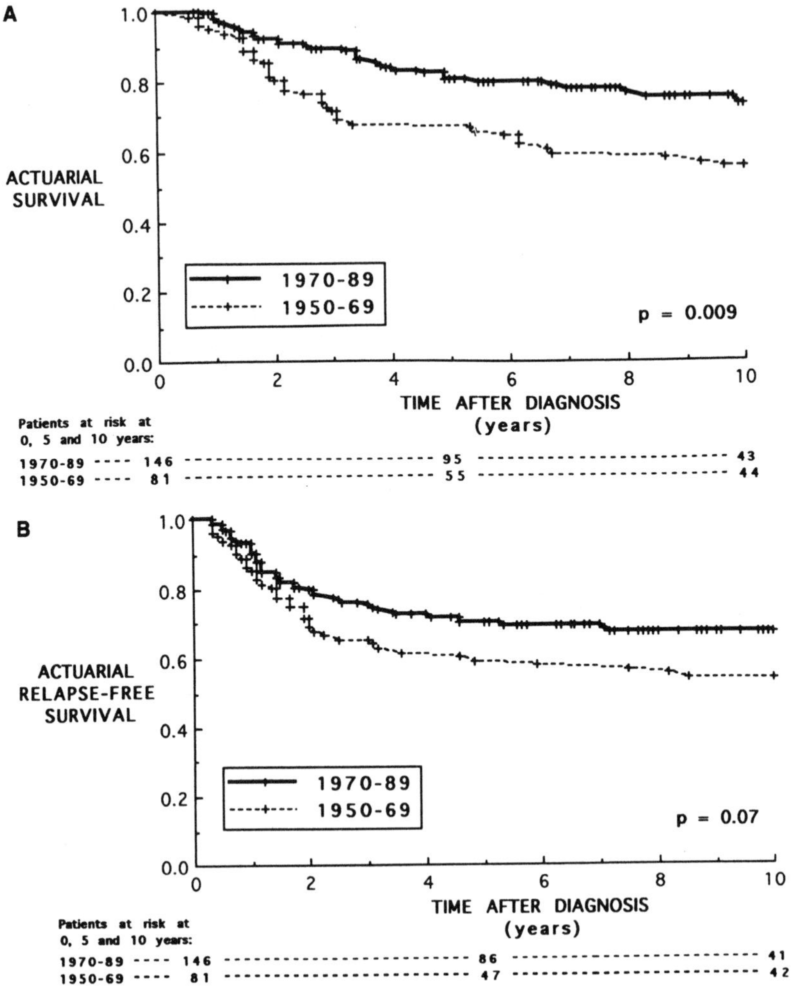

FIGURE 3.—Actuarial survival (**A**) and recurrence-free survival (**B**) after definitive operation for breast cancer in young women (younger than 30 years of age) from 2 consecutive 20-year eras (1950–1969 or 1970–1989). Actuarial survival was increased ($P = 0.009$) for women from the later era. Actuarial recurrence-free survival appeared to be increased for women from the later era, but this trend did not achieve statistical significance ($P = 0.07$) (Courtesy of Anderson BO, Senie RT, Vetto JT, et al: Improved survival in young women with breast cancer. *Ann Surg Oncol* 2:407–415, 1995.)

the patient with invasive breast cancer must be counseled about the increased rate of local recurrence with BCT. The equivalent overall survival by modified radical mastectomy and BCT should be emphasized.

W.H. Hindle, M.D.

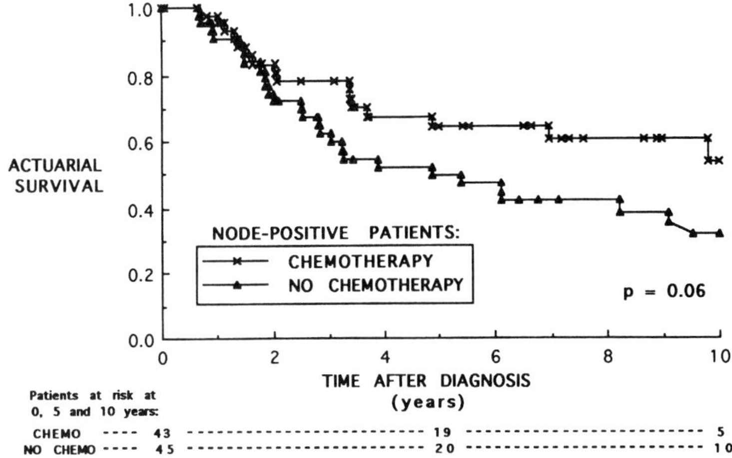

FIGURE 5.—Actuarial survival after definitive operation for node-positive breast cancer in young women (younger than 30 years of age) who did or did not receive chemotherapy. A trend toward increased actuarial survival (*P* = 0.06) was observed for node-positive women who did receive chemotherapy. (Courtesy of Anderson BO, Senie RT, Vetto JT, et al: Improved survival in young women with breast cancer. *Ann Surg Oncol* 2:407–415, 1995.)

Breast Cancer in Young Patients

Sariego J, Zrada S, Byrd M, et al (Hahnemann Univ, Philadelphia)
Am J Surg 170:243–245, 1995

25–4

Objective.—Many consider breast cancer in young women to be an aggressive disease. In an effort to formulate screening and treatment guidelines for young patients, the results of definitive operative treatment were reviewed in 81 women aged 35 years or younger who were treated before mid-1984 at a single medical center. All but 4 women underwent radical or modified mastectomy.

Results.—Infiltrating ductal carcinoma was diagnosed in 93% of patients. Disease was localized to the breast in 36 patients, whereas 36 had disease in ipsilateral axillary nodes and 9 had distant metastases at the time of diagnosis. Sixty-five percent of patients were living 5 years after treatment and 49% at 10 years. Age did not significantly influence survival

TABLE 1.—Survival As a Function of Age

Age (y)	5–Year Survival	10–Year Survival
≤20	50% (1/2)	50% (1/2)
21–25	67% (2/3)	67% (2/3)
26–30	69% (24/35)	54% (19/35)
31–35	63% (26/41)	44% (18/41)

(Reprinted by permission of the publisher from Sariego J, Zrada S, Byrd M, et al: Breast cancer in young patients. *Am J Surg* 170:243–245, Copyright 1995 by Excerpta Medica Inc.)

TABLE 2.—Survival As a Function of Cancer Stage

Cancer Stage	5–Year Survival	10–Year Survival
Localized tumor	89% (32/36)	78% (28/36)
Regional nodal metastases	56% (20/36)	31% (11/36)
Distant metastases	11% (1/9)	11% (1/9)

(Reprinted by permission of the publisher from Sariego J, Zrada S, Byrd M, et al: Breast cancer in young patients. *Am J Surg* 170:243–245, Copyright 1995 by Excerpta Medica Inc.)

(Table 1). Stage of disease was a significant prognostic factor (Table 2). Age at the time of diagnosis did not significantly relate to the extent of disease. After correcting for stage of disease, survival was comparable to that of women older than 35 years of age who were treated in the same period.

Conclusion.—The major prognostic variable for younger women, as for all patients with breast cancer, is the stage of disease.

▶ This report complements that by Anderson et al. (Abstract 25–3). In this review, 2 patients were 20 years old or younger at the time of diagnosis of their invasive breast cancer. In the Anderson report, there were 3 such young women. Although the incidence of breast cancer in this age group is extremely low, it does occur. A dominant breast mass must be definitely diagnosed regardless of a woman's age. Clinical or mammographic impression does not suffice. Otherwise, invasive breast cancers will be missed and the prognosis adversely affected. Although cost-effectiveness economics restrict reimbursement of screening mammography for young women, in clinical practice, the appropriate management of each patient should be individualized and fully discussed. Guidelines and recommendations change with new data and with the pressures of outside (nonmedical) forces, e.g., politics and available funding. However, good medical practice dictates that a palpable dominant breast mass must be definitely diagnosed—at any age.

W.H. Hindle, M.D.

Younger Women With Breast Carcinoma Have a Poorer Prognosis Than Older Women

Chung M, Chang HR, Bland KI, et al (Roger Williams Med Ctr, Providence, RI; Brown Univ, Providence, RI)
Cancer 77:97–103, 1996

25–5

Introduction.—Only 4% of breast cancers occur in women younger than 35 years of age. Reportedly, these women have a worse prognosis than older women, but it is not clear whether this reflects more advanced cancer at the time of diagnosis or an actual difference in tumor biology.

Objective.—Survival was related to age and stage of breast cancer in a series of 3,722 women seen from 1985 to 1992 with invasive breast carcinoma. A majority of patients were 50–80 years of age when the cancer was diagnosed, but 210 (5.6%) were aged 40 years and younger.

Observations.—A relatively high proportion of women aged 40 years and younger had stage II disease. After an average follow-up of 7 years, the 5-year cancer-specific survival rate was lowest (70%) for the youngest women but almost as low (71.5%) for those older than 80 years. Five-year disease-free survival was lowest for the oldest women and next poorest for those aged 40 and below at the time of diagnosis. Except for stage I disease, women aged 40 years and younger had a worse 5-year cancer-specific survival rate than other age groups according to stage. Locoregional disease was adequately treated in the youngest patients, but it was inadequately treated in 40% of the oldest women. Only 3.5% of women aged 80 years and older received adjuvant chemotherapy, and 6% were not treated.

Interpretation.—It appears that young women with breast cancer have a relatively poor outlook, even if treated appropriately. Women aged 40 years and younger are more likely to have more advanced disease at the time of diagnosis, and it may be that they have a biologically more aggressive form of breast cancer.

▶ Historically, it has been a clinical observation that younger women have more aggressive breast cancers, with a resultant poorer prognosis, than older women. Using the criterion of "40 years or younger" as the definition of "younger," this study of data from the Hospital Association of Rhode Island Tumor Registry documents a 69.7% 5-year cancer-specific survival rate for younger women compared with 80.3% for the 41–50 age group. The 5-year disease-free survival rate was 60.79% for the younger than 40 age group and 73.22% for the 41–50 age group. However, the lowest 5-year disease-free survival rate was 39.88% for the oldest (older than 80 years) group.

The authors conclude for the 40-and-younger age group, this difference in survival is not solely a reflection of more advanced disease (at diagnosis) but may reflect differences in tumor biology (i.e., metastasis of smaller cancers).

Such a difference in biological behavior could be a major factor in the lack of statistically significant screening mammography data showing a decreased mortality rate from breast cancer for women less than 50 years of age. However, the goal in clinical practice remains the same: Find nonpalpable breast cancers by screening mammography *before* metastasis has occurred. Furthermore, there are published data that chemotherapy had improved survival for women 30 years of age or younger, although the stage of presentation remained unchanged (Abstract 25–3).

W.H. Hindle, M.D.

Supplementary Papers

Jeffrey KM, Wei JP: Carcinoma of the breast in women 30 years old and younger: A retrospective analysis with review of the literature. *Breast Dis* 9:75–80, 1996.
▶ This report from the Medical College of Georgia adds 17 cases to the published literature. Pertinent articles about women 40 years of age and younger were reviewed for family history, pregnancy and parity, location, oral contraceptive use, histology, presentation, method of diagnosis (including mammography), and treatment. This information for this young age group was summarized. No striking variations were noted compared with older age groups. Although a progressively increasing incidence of breast cancer for this age group is noted, the prognosis with treatment seems less "grave" than historically perceived.

W.H. Hindle, M.D.

Peer PGM, Verbeek ALM, Mravunac M, et al: Prognosis of younger and older patients with early breast cancer. *Br J Cancer* 73:382–385, 1996.
▶ This report from The Netherlands presents similar age-related graphs to the article by Chung. These data are restricted to stage I (T1) breast cancers. In all age groups, cancers 1 cm or less had a longer breast cancer specific survival than larger cancers. Acknowledging an apparent early metastatic potential in the younger age group (younger than 50 years), the authors suggest that screening mammography would have to detect a "substantial proportion" of invasive cancer "before their size exceeds 1 cm" in order to obtain a statistically significant decrease in breast cancer mortality.

W.H. Hindle, M.D.

Current Opinion: Hormone Replacement Therapy After a Diagnosis of Breast Cancer
Sands R, Boshoff C, Jones A, et al (Chelsea and Westminster Hosp, London; Royal London Hosp; Royal Free Hosp, London)
J North Am Menopause Soc 2:73–80, 1995   25–6

Background.—The increased survival among women with breast cancer is not always associated with a good quality of life. Some treatments induce a premature menopause, and traditionally hormone replacement therapy (HRT) for menopausal symptoms in such women is contraindicated. The acute and long-term health problems associated with menopause in women who have had breast cancer and the use of HRT in these women were reviewed.

Arguments Against HRT Use.—Unopposed estrogen treatment has been clearly associated with a risk of endometrial cancer related to treatment dose and duration. Many clinicians' concerns about using HRT in women treated for breast cancer come from epidemiologic, biological, and clinical evidence. Many epidemiologic risk factors for breast cancer are associated with endocrinologic reproductive variables. Laboratory studies of animals have shown that estrogens produce mammary tumors and act as growth factors for established breast cancer cell lines.

The use of HRT apparently does not substantially increase breast cancer risk in the normal population in case-control studies. However, 2 of 4

TABLE 2.—Meta-Analysis of Breast Cancer Incidence Among Hormone Replacement Therapy Users vs. Nonusers

Reference	Effects of ever-use RR (95% CI)	Use more than 15 yr RR (95% CI)	Special risk group ? RR (95% CI)
Armstrong	0.96 (0.98–1.05)	1.04 0.88–1.24)	Nil identified
Dupont and Page	1.08 (0.96–1.2)	No conclusion	Nil identified
Steinberg et al.	1.0	1.3 (1.2–1.6)	Family history 3.4
Grady and Ernster	No increase	1.25	Nil identified

Abbreviations: RR, relative risk: *CI*, confidence interval.
(Courtesy of Sands R, Boshoff C, Jones A, et al: Current opinion: Hormone replacement therapy after a diagnosis of breast cancer. *J North Am Menopause Soc* 2:73–80, 1995.)

meta-analyses demonstrate a duration exposure risk of about 25% to 30% higher than in controls with use for more than 15 years (Table 2). Determining the possible interactions between HRT and individual risk factors for breast cancer is important. Breast cancer risk in women with a family history is apparently unaffected by HRT use.

Data Analysis.—Only 5 studies on the use of HRT in women treated for breast cancer have been published (Table 3). None of these studies found an increased risk of relapse for women receiving HRT. However, these studies reported a total of only 277 women at different disease stages who were followed up for a relatively short length of time and given a variety of HRT formulations and dosages.

Conclusions.—Decisions about HRT use in women who have had breast cancer must include consideration of the risks and benefits. In women with advanced disease and debilitating symptoms from estrogen

TABLE 3.—Hormone Replacement Therapy in Women With a History of Breast Cancer

Study	HRT	Number	Median age	Stage I.S.	1	2	3	4	Follow-up (months)	Outcome
Wile et al.	Varied	25	51	2	13	7	1	2	35	88% NED 12% REL
Disaia	Varied	77	50	6	43	17	5	6	59	92% NED 8% REL
Stoll and Parbhoo	CONJ 0.625 NORG	50	?		—				24	100% NED
Powles et al.	Varied	35	51		12	14	9		43	94% NED 6% REL
Eden et al.	Varied	90	47		—				>72	93% NED 7% REL

Abbreviations: NED, no evidence of disease; *REL*, relapse; *NORG*, norgestrel (0–15 mg).
(Courtesy of Sands R, Boshoff C, Jones A, et al: Current opinion: Hormone replacement therapy after a diagnosis of breast cancer. *J North Am Menopause Soc* 2:73–80, 1995.)

deficiency, for example, the use of estrogen replacement would be largely palliative, and their life expectancy would be relatively short. Prospective studies are needed to assess the effects of HRT in postmenopausal women who have had a diagnosis of breast cancer.

▶ Clinical practice founded on evidence-based medicine requires reappraisal of traditional "authoritative" dogmatic positions. Long-term outcome data on the analysis of estrogen replacement therapy (or HRT with the addition of progesterone) on the incidence and subsequent course of breast cancer are rarely available. All published reports are observational, and prospective, randomized trials are lacking. However, convincing data are available as to the increased risk of cardiovascular disease (and mortality) and osteoporosis (and subsequent associated mortality) for estrogen-deficient women.

Each patient must evaluate her own quality of life and risk tolerance—with and without estrogen replacement therapy. Physicians should serve as educators and sources of current accurate medical data to be rendered to the patient as objectively as possible. We do not have clear-cut definitive answers. This "Current Opinion" is an updated summary of the clinically meaningful published data pertinent to HRT for women who have been successfully treated for breast cancer.

W.H. Hindle, M.D.

A Case-Control Study of Combined Continuous Estrogen–Progestin Replacement Therapy Among Women With a Personal History of Breast Cancer
Eden JA, Bush T, Nand S, et al (Royal Hosp for Women, Paddington, Australia; Univ of Maryland, Baltimore)
J North Am Menopause Soc 2:67–72, 1995   25–7

Background.—Because estrogen has long been implicated as the main hormone in the pathogenesis of breast cancer, estrogen therapy is usually denied to women who have had breast cancer. Premenopausal women who have had early-stage breast cancer and produce their own endogenous estrogen for years are then denied hormone replacement therapy (HRT) at menopause. The risks of cardiovascular events or fractures, which may be reduced by HRT, can be life-threatening. In some women with breast cancer, menopausal symptoms are so severe that their quality of life is diminished without HRT. A nested case-control study of combined continuous estrogen-progestin replacement therapy among women with a history of breast cancer was conducted.

Methods and Findings.—Data on 901 women with surgically confirmed breast cancer seen at 3 centers in Sydney, Australia, were reviewed. The effect of therapy on all-cause mortality and tumor recurrence rate was determined. Ninety women had taken estrogen because of severe menopausal symptoms after diagnosis and treatment of breast cancer. Most

TABLE 2.—Demographics for Estrogen Users and Their Controls

Variable	Estrogen users $n = 90$	Controls $n = 180$
Age at diagnosis (yr)	47 (24–71)	48 (27–96)
Max. tumor diameter (cm)	1.8 (0.40–7.0)	1.5 (0.20–10.0)
Nodes involved	0 (0–18)	0 (0–18)
Tamoxifen usage	12 (13%)	39 (22%)
ER measured	22 (24%)	42 (23%)
Total follow-up (yr)	7 (0.3–30)	6 (0.3–29)
Deaths	0	11 (6%)

Note: Despite matching, estrogen users tended to be younger, to use tamoxifen less often, and to have larger primary tumors than did the controls, although the magnitude of these differences was small. Estrogen users also had significantly longer follow-up than did controls (despite matching for years of diagnosis), but this difference was explained by the observation that there were no deaths among estrogen users and 11 deaths among controls.

Abbreviation: ER, estrogen receptor.

(Courtesy of Eden JA, Bush T, Nand S, et al: *J North Am Menopause Soc* 2:67–72, 1995.)

took combined continuous estrogen-progestin therapy, usually an oral estrogen with a moderate progestin dose. Controls were women from the same database who did not take sex steroids after their disease was diagnosed (Tables 2 and 3). None of the estrogen users died during the mean 7-year follow-up. Ten percent of the nonusers died. Recurrence developed in only 7% of the estrogen users compared with 17% of nonusers. The former had a relative risk of 0.4. The relative risk of recurrence among women taking progestin alone was 0.22.

Conclusions.—The short-term use of combined continuous HRT by women with a history of breast cancer appears to be safe, possibly even reducing the risk of cancer recurrence. Continuous combined HRT may confer significant advantages over the older cyclic treatment regimens.

▶ This epidemiologic short-term study provides adequate numbers to give meaningful confidence intervals for the calculations of relative risk. The results are encouraging (and probably comforting) to clinicians faced with women with symptomatic estrogen deficiency who have been treated for breast cancer. It seems doubtful that estrogen replacement for women with estrogen-deficiency symptoms can be reliably "double-blinded" because, in most cases, it would soon be obvious to the patients and their physicians which women were actually on estrogen replacement therapy and which

TABLE 3.—Demographics for Progestin-Alone Users and Their Controls

Variable	Progestin users n = 30	Controls n = 120
Age at diagnosis (yr)	48 (36–77)	47 (27–96)
Max. tumor diameter (cm)	2.1 (0.5–6.0)	2.0 (0.5–6.0)
Nodes involved	0 (0–10)	0 (0–18)
Total follow-up (yr)	5 (1–25)	4 (1–25)
Deaths	0	10 (8%)

(Courtesy of Eden JA, Bush T, Nand S, et al: *J North Am Menopause Soc* 2:67–72, 1995.)

women were on placebos; nevertheless, well-constructed, long-term, prospective, clinical trials are urgently needed.

These data support the conclusions of the previous paper by Sands et al. (Abstract 25–6).

W.H. Hindle, M.D.

Hormone Replacement Therapy in Breast Cancer Survivors: A Cohort Study

DiSaia PJ, Grosen EA, Kurosaki T, et al (Univ of California, Irvine)
Am J Obstet Gynecol 174:1494–1498, 1996   25–8

Objective.—Traditionally, hormone replacement therapy has not been used in women with a history of breast cancer for fear of activating quiescent disease—putting "fuel on the fire," so to speak. However, this practice deprives thousands of women of the benefits of hormone replacement therapy. A recent analysis found no evidence to support the theoretical increased risk of hormone replacement therapy–induced breast cancer regrowth. A further cohort study was conducted to identify any adverse effects of hormone replacement therapy in breast cancer survivors.

Methods.—The study included 41 women with a history of breast cancer who were receiving hormone replacement therapy. Each patient was matched to 2 breast cancer patients who were not receiving hormone replacement therapy. All patients resided in the area covered by a single cancer registry. The 2 groups were compared for subsequent disease experience—i.e., recurrent breast cancer and multiple primary cancers— and for survival.

Results.—Subsequent disease occurred in 15% of patients receiving hormone replacement therapy and 9% of the comparison patients, a nonsignificant difference. Four-year survival and disease-free survival were comparable in the 2 groups (Tables 3A and 3B).

Conclusion.—Hormone replacement therapy has no apparent adverse effects on disease recurrence rate or survival in women with a history of

TABLE 3A.—Analysis of Survival Time (in Months) in Study and Comparison Breast Cancer Patients

Survival	*HRT patients*	*Comparison patients*
No.	41	82
No. of patients dead from breast cancer	2	6
4 yr survival rate ± SE (mo)	68.9 ± 1.9	46.2 ± 0.6
Comparison of survival curves		NS, *p* < 0.5415
Cox regression		Age: NS
		Stage of disease: NS
		HRT vs comparison: NS

Notes: Outcome: death from breast cancer. In all 8 deaths, cause of death was breast cancer.
Abbreviations: HRT, hormone replacement therapy; *SE,* standard error; *NS,* not significant.
(Courtesy of DiSaia PJ, Grosen EA, Kurosaki T, et al: Hormone replacement therapy in breast cancer survivors: A cohort study. *Am J Obstet Gynecol* 174:1494–1498, 1996.)

TABLE 3B.—Analysis of Disease-Free Time (in Months) in Study and Comparison Breast Cancer Patients

Survival	*Patients*	*Comparison patients*
No.	41	82
No. of patients with subsequent disease	6	7
Mean disease-free time ± SE (mo)	50.6 ± 1.9	45.5 ± 0.9
Comparison of disease-free curves		NS, $p < 0.3212$
Cox regression		Age: NS
		Stage of disease: NS
		HRT vs comparison: NS

Note: Outcome: recurrent disease or multiple primary.
Abbreviations: SE, standard error; *NS,* not significant; *HRT,* hormone replacement therapy.
(Courtesy of DiSaia PJ, Grosen EA, Kurosaki T, et al: Hormone replacement therapy in breast cancer survivors: A cohort study. *Am J Obstet Gynecol* 174:1494–1498, 1996.)

breast cancer. A prospective, randomized trial of this issue is needed. The authors' experience suggests that tamoxifen can be combined with hormone replacement therapy with no apparent loss of biological effect.

▶ Dr. DiSaia continues to pioneer the use of estrogen replacement therapy (ERT) for estrogen-deficient women who have been treated for invasive breast cancer and to urge prospective randomized clinical trials with adequate statistical power. Although long-term observations are critical because of the propensity of breast cancer to recur (to again be clinically manifest) at posttreatment intervals up to 30 or more years, observational evidence continues to accumulate (albeit based on small numbers and the limited time such patients have been followed) showing no adverse effect with the dosage of ERT most commonly prescribed.

It is of keen clinical interest that no adverse interaction was noted in this study when tamoxifen and ERT were given concurrently. As the number of women taking tamoxifen continues to increase, it is imperative to have data on the effect of ERT on the tamoxifen-induced hot flashes; the adverse effect, if any, upon the suppression of breast cancer by tamoxifen when ERT is added; and the results of prescribing ERT after the tamoxifen therapy is completed (currently, after 5 years). Clearly, well-designed multicenter clinical trials are indicated and urgently needed.

W.H. Hindle, M.D.

SUPPLEMENTARY PAPER

La Vecchia C, Negri E, Franceschi S, et al: Hormone replacement treatment and breast cancer risk: A cooperative Italian study. *Br J Cancer* 72:244–248, 1995.
▶ This is a hospital-based case-control study of 2,569 histologically confirmed breast cancer patients and 2,588 controls. However, only 7.5% of the cases and the controls reported ever being on hormone replacement therapy (HRT). None of the multivariate odds ratios (ORs) were more than 2, which limits the trends to epidemiologic significance of "low association," which are not meaningful in clinical practice. The highest OR was for women who had taken HRT for more than 5 years and who had stopped HRT within 10 years. No effect was found for women who had stopped HRT more than 10 years prior to the study. This

"short-term" epidemiologic increased risk is similar to that reported in several studies of the effect of pregnancy and breast cancer risk. The authors conclude: "This study confirms the absence of a strong association between HRT and breast cancer risk, although the risk estimate was above unity for women who had used HRT for 5 years or longer." They also note that "there was no significant interaction between exogenous oestrogen use and age at diagnosis [of breast cancer]... ." Overall, this study adds to the data demonstrating a lack of clinically meaningful increased risk of breast cancer for women who take HRT.

W.H. Hindle, M.D.

Oral Contraceptives and Breast Cancer Risk Among Younger Women

Brinton LA, Daling JR, Liff JM, et al (Natl Cancer Inst, Bethesda, Md; Fred Hutchinson Cancer Research Ctr, Seattle; Emory Univ, Atlanta, Ga; et al)
J Natl Cancer Inst 87:827–835, 1995   25–9

Background.—Several investigators have found an association between oral contraceptive use and breast cancer in younger women. However, chance or bias, including selective screening of contraceptive users, may have contributed to this finding. Oral contraceptives were first available in the United States in the early 1960s. Thus, a population-based case-control study was designed to explore the association between oral contraceptive use and breast cancer in a recent cohort of women younger than age 45 years who had access to oral contraceptives throughout their reproductive life.

Methods and Findings.—Patients with breast cancer were matched to healthy controls in Atlanta, Seattle, and central New Jersey. Oral contraceptive use for 6 months or longer among women younger than 45 years age was correlated with a relative risk (RR) for breast cancer of 1.3 (Table 2). Among patients with breast cancer occurring before 35 years of age, the RR was 2.2 for those using oral contraceptives for 10 or more years. Women who began using oral contraceptives before 18 years of age and

TABLE 2.—Relative Risks (RR) of Breast Cancer by Use of Oral Contraceptives According to Varying Ages of Study Participants

| | Patients | | Control subjects | | | | Adjusted |
Age, y	No.	% users*	No.	% users*	RR†	RR‡	95% CI
All <45	1648	76.4	1505	71.4	1.30	1.27	1.1–1.5
<35	268	76.9	291	66.3	1.64	1.74	1.2–2.6
35–39	488	77.7	474	70.9	1.44	1.36	1.0–1.88
40–44	892	75.6	740	73.6	1.13	1.12	0.9–1.4
45–49§	276	73.6	264	69.7	1.23	1.23	0.8–1.8
50–54§	250	55.2	240	59.2	0.85	0.94	0.6–1.4

*Users of oral contraceptives for 6 months or longer.
†Adjusted for age. Further adjusted for study site in women younger than age 45 years.
‡Adjusted further for race, number of births, and age at first birth.
§All participants were from Atlanta study site. For comparison, adjusted RRs associated with use of oral contraceptives among younger Atlanta participants were 1.77 (95% confidence interval [CI], 0.8–4.0), 1.06 (95% CI, 0.6–2.0), and 1.31 (95% CI, 0.8–2.0), respectively, for the 3 age groups (younger than 35, 35–39, and 40–44 years).
(Courtesy of Brinton LA, Daling JR, Liff JM, et al: *J Natl Cancer Inst* 87:827–835, 1995.)

TABLE 4.—Relative Risks (RR) and 95% Confidence Intervals (CIs) of
Breast Cancer by Combined Measures of Oral Contraceptive Use Patterns: Women
Younger Than Age 45 Years

| | Used 6 mo to <5 y | | Used 5–9 y | | Used ≥ 10 y | |
	No.	RR (95% CI)	No.	RR (95% CI)	No.	RR (95% CI)
No. of years since first use						
<15	136	1.44 (1.1–1.9)	66	1.55 (1.0–2.3)	22	1.27 (0.7–2.4)
15–19	221	1.14 (0.9–1.4)	120	1.45 (1.1–2.0)	93	1.58 (1.1–2.2)
≥20	292	1.29 (1.0–1.6)	190	1.10 (0.8–1.4)	119	1.11 (0.8–1.5)
No. of years since last use						
<5	80	1.66 (1.1–2.4)	87	1.49 (1.0–2.1)	131	1.37 (1.0–1.8)
5–9	66	1.28 (0.9–1.9)	71	1.49 (1.0–2.2)	66	1.13 (0.8–1.7)
≥10	503	1.21 (0.9–1.5)	218	1.14 (0.9–1.5)	37	1.34 (0.8–2.3)
Age at first use, y						
<18	79	1.04 (0.7–1.5)	80	1.55 (1.1–2.2)	75	1.47 (1.0–2.2)
18–21	342	1.32 (1.1–1.6)	224	1.21 (0.9–1.5)	122	1.12 (0.8–1.5)
≥22	228	1.29 (1.0–1.6)	72	1.21 (0.8–1.8)	37	1.68 (0.9–3.0)

*Adjusted for study site, age, race, number of births and age at first birth. All risks relative to women with no use or use
of oral contraceptives for fewer than 6 months (389 patients and 431 controls).
(Courtesy of Brinton LA, Daling JR, Liff JM, et al: *J Natl Cancer Inst* 87:827–835, 1995.)

continued use for more than 10 years had a RR of 3.1. The RRs of women
using oral contraceptives within 5 years of their cancer diagnosis were
greater than the RRs of those who had not (Table 4). This effect was most
pronounced for women younger than age 35 years. Oral contraceptive use
was strongly associated with cancers diagnosed at advanced stages. These
associations were not attributable to selective screening. Women aged 45
years and older had no risks associated with oral contraceptive use.

Conclusions.—Chance or bias most likely does not explain the excess of
early-onset breast cancers reported among long-term or recent oral contraceptive users. The association of oral contraceptives and breast cancer
in young women appears to have a biological basis.

▶ Multiple studies document no overall increase or decrease in the RR of
breast cancer for women who take oral contraceptive therapy (OCT). Relative risk trends have been reported for subsets of women. Duration of more
than 10 years of OCT, beginning OCT at an early age (before 18 years of age),
and OCT use within 5 years of diagnosis for women younger than age 35 are
the subsets identified in this study as having a statistically significant RR of
2.0 or more. These levels of risk are of epidemiologic interest and are
considered a "weak association" but are not clinically meaningful. Such data
should not alter clinical practice or management. Of all the calculations in
this study, only the RR of 3.1 for continued long-term use (longer than 10
years) reaches a clinically relevant level. The authors calculate that the
absolute risk of breast cancer in women younger than 35 years of age would
be increased by 1 case per year per 100,000 women in the general population by the OCT usage patterns in this study. Although this information

should be added to informed consent for OCT, the etiology of breast cancer remains unidentified.

W.H. Hindle, M.D.

Should We Schedule Breast Surgery Based on a Woman's Menstrual Cycle?

Hines OJ, Love SM (Univ of California, Los Angeles)
Breast J 1:173–179, 1995   25–10

Background.—Recent research suggests that the timing of surgery for breast cancer may affect outcomes and survival among premenopausal

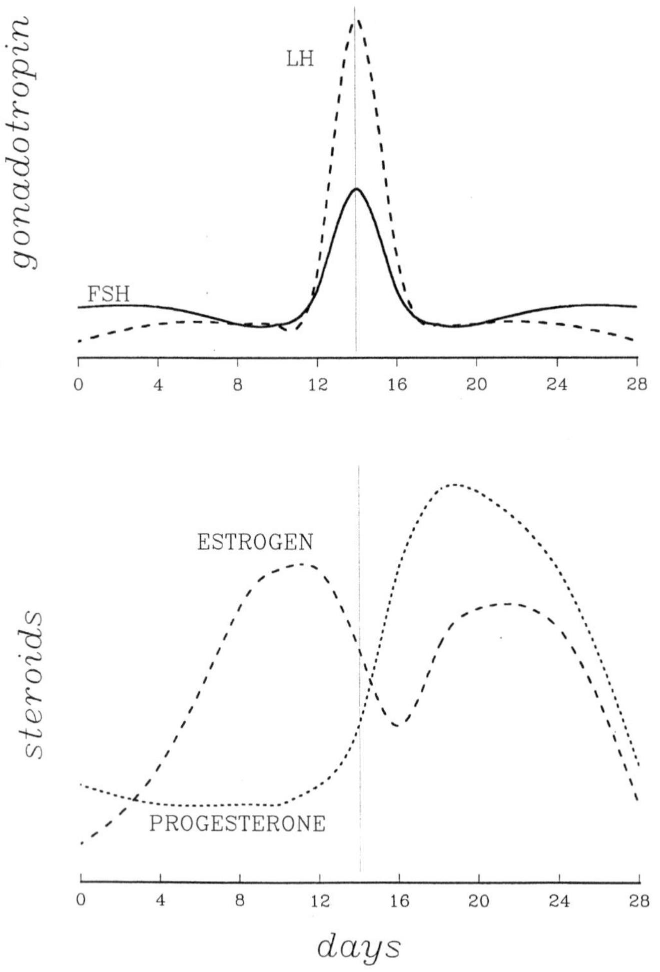

FIGURE 1.—The normal gonadotropin and steroid changes during the menstrual cycle. (Courtesy of Hines OJ, Love SM: Should we schedule breast surgery based on a woman's menstrual cycle? *Breast J* 1:173–179, 1995.)

TABLE 1.—Menstrual Cycle Affects Outcome

Author	No. of pts.	Cycle Days	Disease-free Survival (%)	Overall Survival (%)
Hrushesky	19	0–6, 21–36	58	79
	22	7–20	86*	95*
Veronesi	525	1–14	63.3‡	—
	650	15–36	75.5*‡	—
Seniea†	141	1–14	57‡	—
	142	15–28	71*‡	—
Marques	(63)	1–14	30.2	49.3
		15–28	39.1	71.9*
Badwe†	75	3–12	—	54
	174	0–2, 13–32	—	84*
Saad†	37	1–12	40	40
	59	13–28	72*	79*
Spratt†	20	0–6, 21–36	—	30
	20	7–20	—	71*
Badwe	(210)	[progesterone] > 1.5 ng/ml		
		[progesterone] < 1.5		
Ville	35	1–14	60	83
	54	15–28	78	91

*Statistically significant.
†Ten-year survival statistics.
‡Node-positive patients only.
(Courtesy of Hines OJ, Love SM: Should we schedule breast surgery based on a woman's menstrual cycle? *Breast J* 1:173–179, 1995.)

TABLE 2.—Menstrual Cycle Does Not Affect Outcome

Author	No. of Pts.	Cycle Days	Disease-free Survival (%)	Overall Survival (%)
Corder	58	3–12	59	77
	99	0–2, 13–32	65	78
Gnant	131	3–12	83.0	70.4
	254	0–2, 13–32	80.4	71.6
Kroman	526	3–12	—	80
	1036	0–2, 13–32	—	79
Nathan	40	3–12	—	56
	92	0–2, 13–33	—	58
Sauerbrei	227	1–14	62	74
	235	15–28	64	80
Rageth	104	1–6, 21–36	72	86
	120	7–20	65	81
Garcia-Conde*	117	1–6, 21–34	=	=
	106	7–20	=	=
Powles	44	22–5	45†	41
	37	7–21	54†	49
Powles	43	3–12	—	80
	162	0–2, 13–32	—	85
Low	47	3–12	70	53
	78	0–2, 13–32	74	60
Goldhirsch	84	3–12	62	77
	141	0–2, 13–32	60	79
Ville	54	0–6	79.6	65
	89	21–36	79.7	64
	136	7–20	79.4	68.4
Sainsbury†	64	3–12	—	69
	75	0–2, 13–32	—	50

*No actual data available.
†Ten-year survival.
(Courtesy of Hines OJ, Love SM: Should we schedule breast surgery based on a woman's menstrual cycle? *Breast J* 1:173–179, 1995.)

women. Basic research supports the plausibility of this. The importance of the timing of surgery in the menstrual cycle for early breast cancer was investigated.

Timing of Breast Cancer Surgery.—The predictable hormonal shifts occurring in the menstrual cycle, divided into the follicular and luteal phases (Fig 1), affect the local environment of the breast and breast cancer. Research has clearly demonstrated that surgical manipulation of tumor induces micrometastasis. A substantial amount of evidence now indicates that estrogen may produce an environment more prone to micrometastases as well as an immune system that is less able to manage them. Progesterone may protect against the effects of estrogen, resulting in improved disease-free and overall survival rates during the luteal phase. Although the findings of studies examining this association are conflicting, there appears to be a 30% advantage for patients having surgery during progesterone predominance.

Conclusions.—The debate about the effects of breast surgery timing is far from over (Tables 1 and 2). However, until a methodologically sound, prospective study can be done, there is no harm in scheduling breast cancer surgery for the early luteal phase. Patients undergoing surgery at this time may have significantly better survival rates than those operated on during the follicular phase.

▶ This clinically oriented summary of the literature on this controversial subject should be read by anyone performing or scheduling breast surgery, particularly breast biopsy and cancer surgery. Furthermore, women who are being scheduled for breast surgery of any type should be made aware of these data during the taking of their informed consent for surgery. Although the scientific evidence is not clear or consistent, the possibility exists that the hormonal milieu at different times in the menstrual cycle somehow affects the viability of "dislodged" cancer cells and the occurrence of micrometastasis. The disease-free survival and, in fact, overall survival may be favorably influenced by having breast surgery performed during the early luteal phase of the patient's menstrual cycle. Until evidence-based medical data clarify this perplexing issue, breast surgeons would be well advised to take advantage of this potential benefit for menstruating women and to inform their patients of the compelling circumstances if such timing does not seem possible.

W.H. Hindle, M.D.

BRCA1 Mutations in a Population-based Sample of Young Women With Breast Cancer

Langston AA, Malone KE, Thompson JD, et al (Fred Hutchinson Cancer Research Ctr, Seattle; Univ of Washington, Seattle)
N Engl J Med 334:137–142, 1996   25–11

Background.—It is accepted that inherited mutations in the *BRCA1* gene correlate with a high risk of breast and ovarian cancers in some families. It remains uncertain, however, whether and to what extent these mutations contribute to breast cancer in the general population.

Objective.—The frequency and types of *BRCA1* mutations were examined in 80 women who received a diagnosis of breast cancer before age 35 years, and who were not selected on the basis of family history. The participants were from a large population-based study of early-onset breast cancer.

Methods.—Genomic DNA was analyzed for *BRCA1* mutations by analyzing single-strand conformation polymorphisms and by screening with allele-specific oligonucleotides (Fig 1). Alterations were defined by DNA sequencing.

Findings.—Six of the 80 women studied were found to have germ-line mutations of *BRCA1*. In addition, 4 rare sequence variations of uncertain

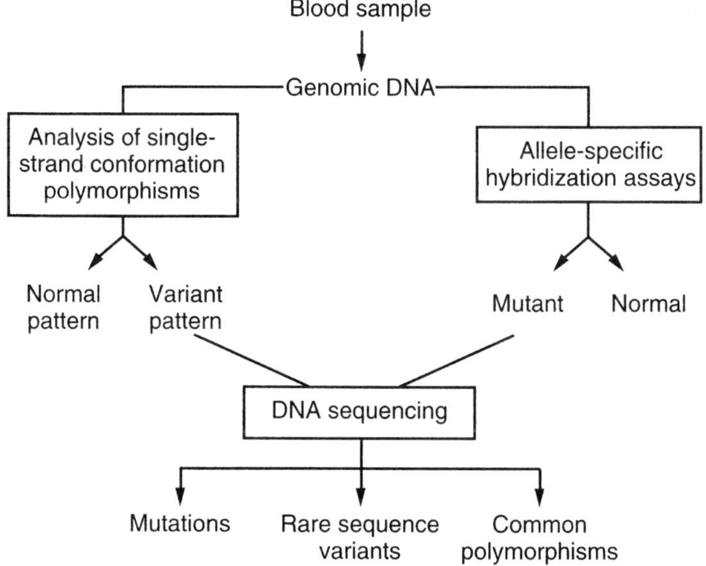

FIGURE 1.—Strategy used to screen for *BRCA1* mutations. The analysis of sequence data permitted each alteration to be assigned to 1 of the following categories: mutations that affect the structure and function of the gene, rare sequence variants of unknown functional consequence, and polymorphisms that are common in the general population, irrespective of breast cancer status. (Reprinted by permission of *The New England Journal of Medicine* from Langston AA, Malone KE, Thompson JD, et al: *BRCA1* mutations in a population-based sample of young women with breast cancer. *N Engl J Med* 334:137–142, 1996.)

functional significance were identified. Two mutations and 3 sequence variations were found among 39 women who reported no family history of breast or ovarian cancers. Of 73 unrelated subjects forming a reference population, none had a *BRCA1* mutation and only 1 had 1 of the sequence variants.

Implication.—Mutations of *BRCA1* may be present in 10% or more of younger women with breast cancer and is not limited to those with a positive family history.

▶ In this study of young women diagnosed with breast cancer before the age of 35 years, 10% were found to have mutations in the *BRCA1* gene on chromosome 17q. This exemplifies the limitations of known genetic testing for susceptibility to invasive breast cancer. By contrast, in another study, 90% of women having mammography or visiting their obstetrician-gynecologists said they would take a test to detect genetic susceptibility to breast cancer.[1]

With the imminent commercial availability of *BRCA1* testing, clinicians will be faced with advising their patients, counseling those women with a family history of breast cancer, and selecting those to whom they recommend *BRCA1* testing. There are no agreed upon guidelines. The giving of current accurate information is the first step in advising your patients. Few will benefit from *BRCA1* testing, and some will suffer anxiety and guilt whether or not they elect to be tested. For whom is *BRCA1* testing medically indicated? There is no consensus. Who should be informed of (or is entitled to know) the results? These are unanswered ethical and moral questions. What is appropriate advice to a woman (or man) found to have *BRCA1* mutations? We do not know.

Thus, *BRCA1* testing presents a series of paradoxical dilemmas. Does the typical clinician have the time (or is it cost-effective medical practice) to undertake the proper advising and counseling of women requesting *BRCA1* testing? Trained and experienced genetic counselors are few; in fact, they are almost rare. The detailed family pedigree should include breast, ovarian, colorectal, and prostate cancer in any of the relatives (male or female). Confirming the diagnosis in each case for each relative is tedious and requires persistence. Perhaps the most urgent medical need is for the development of available genetic counseling services.

W.H. Hindle, M.D.

Reference

1. Chaliki H, Loader S, Levenkron JC, et al: Women's receptivity to testing for a genetic susceptibility to breast cancer. *Am J Public Health;* 85:1133–1135, 1995.

SUPPLEMENTARY PAPERS

Peto J, Easton DF, Matthews FE, et al: Cancer mortality in relatives of women with breast cancer: The OPCS study. *Int J Cancer* 65:275–283, 1996.
▶ This study from the Office of Population Census and Surveys (OPCS) of the United Kingdom studied 3,295 breast cancer patients and 11,678 first-degree

relatives and is based on mortality data rather than incidence data as in the Cancer and Steroid Hormone study. The standardized mortality ratio was calculated for all types of cancer in both males and females. The authors concluded: "These results, together with penetrance estimates from linked families, suggest that approximately one woman in 800 carries *BRCA1*, the susceptibility gene on chromosome 17q, and that this gene causes about 1% all breast cancers." The public should be made aware of this conclusion.

W.H. Hindle, M.D.

McKinley AG, Russell SEH, Spence RAJ, et al: Hereditary breast cancer and linkage analysis to *BRCA1*. *Br J Surg* 82:1086–1088, 1995.
▶ In this report from Belfast, more than 1,000 women diagnosed with breast cancer were contacted by questionnaire, and 164 families with a history of 3 or more members with breast cancer were identified. Full pedigree details were obtained for 123 women. Venous blood samples were obtained from 24 families. In 12 of these families, DNA analysis confirmed that *BRCA1* was related to breast cancer susceptibility. This is consistent with other published data that 50% of hereditary breast cancer families are not linked to *BRCA1*.

W.H. Hindle, M.D.

Johannsson O, Ostermeyer EA, Håkansson S, et al: Founding *BRCA1* mutations in heredity breast and ovarian cancer in southern Sweden. *Am J Hum Genet* 58:441–450, 1996.
▶ Direct sequencing for 9 germ-line mutations (more than 100 have been identified) in *BRCA1* revealed that 73% of the kindreds with *BRCA1* mutations were breast-ovarian cancer families. In addition, prostate, pancreas, skin, and cancer of the lung, malignant melanoma, oligodendroglioma, and carcinosarcoma were identified in *BRCA1* mutation/haplotype carriers. The genetic susceptibility of malignancy is profoundly complex and the precise etiology remains obscure.

W.H. Hindle, M.D.

Breast Cancer: Getting the Diagnosis Right
Henderson MA, Cawson JM, Bilous M (St Vincent's Hosp, Melbourne, Australia; Westmead Hosp, Sydney, Australia)
Med J Aust 163:494–499, 1995   25–12

Purpose.—Breast cancer is a common condition for which early treatment improves survival. It can be very difficult to differentiate benign early breast cancer from benign breast lesions. The available diagnostic tools for breast cancer are imprecise, leading to delayed diagnosis for a small number of patients. The steps in breast cancer diagnosis were reviewed.
Symptoms and Clinical Examination.—Women should be asked about any new lumps or recent changes in the breast; this is the most common presentation of breast cancer. In a few women, pain is the major first symptom (Box 1). Lumps that vary with the menstrual cycle are likely benign. Uncommon and nonspecific symptoms of breast cancer include changes in the size, shape, or color of the breast and nipple discharge.

BOX 1.—Frequency of Presenting Symptoms of Breast Cancer

Lump	67%
Lump plus pain	16%
Pain	6%
Nipple discharge*	7%
Other	2%

Note: Figures are based on 133 patients with breast cancer from the Breast Unit, St Vincent's Hospital, Melbourne, Australia, 1991–1994.

*With or without lump retraction of the nipple.

(Courtesy of Henderson MA, Cawson JM, Bilous M: Breast cancer: Getting the diagnosis right. *Med J Aust* 163:494–499. Copyright 1995. The Medical Journal of Australia—reproduced with permission.

Symptomatic women who have a family history of breast cancer or a personal history of breast neoplasia need especially close attention.

In the clinical breast examination, the patient should be examined first sitting and then lying down. Superficial and deep palpation are performed, and any abnormal findings are charted on a breast diagram. The characteristics of the tumor and surrounding tissue, the site and depth of the lesion, and the examiner's experience will all influence the ability to palpate breast cancers. It can be difficult to distinguish the tumor from normal breast tissue and to tell suspicious lumps from normal physiologic changes. Furthermore, the physical characteristics of breast cancers may vary widely.

Imaging Referrals.—After clinical examination, the patient may be referred for imaging studies, such as mammography or ultrasound If possible, fine-needle aspiration cytology or cyst aspiration should not be performed until radiologic studies have been done. The radiologist should receive a clear description of the patient's signs and symptoms, together with a diagram. Good communication between the clinician and the radiologist and personal involvement of the radiologist provide the best results. The radiologic report should state how likely the lesion is to be malignant and specify other useful diagnostic tests. The clinician should be aware that the sensitivity of mammography varies considerably.

Biopsy.—The various forms of breast biopsy each have their advantages and disadvantages (Box 3). Fine-needle aspiration biopsy is simple, quick, and cost effective. This technique gives the best results when the aspirator and cytopathologist work cooperatively and are experienced in biopsy performance and interpretation. The accuracy of breast cancer diagnosis is greater than 99% with triple assessment: clinical examination combined with radiologic and cytologic assessment. Fine-needle aspiration cytology can also confirm the diagnosis in patients with lesions considered probably benign.

Summary.—In addition to a review of the clinical examination, radiologic studies, and biopsy assessment of breast cancer, the article presents a management overview, including an algorithm for the management of solid breast masses. With careful clinical examination, directed imaging

BOX 3.—Biopsy Methods

Fine needle aspiration cytology

Advantages
- Simple diagnostic test
- Inexpensive
- Avoids open biopsy in some cases and assists planned operations
- Can be performed as an outpatient procedure
- Avoids the need for a frozen tissue section
- Low complication rate

Disadvantages
- Requires skilled personnel
- Risk of delay in diagnosis if unsatisfactory or false negative result
- Cannot differentiate between in-situ and invasive malignancy

Core biopsy

Advantages
- Inexpensive
- Can be performed as an outpatient procedure
- Can distinguish between in-situ and invasive disease
- Avoids open biopsy in some cases and assists planning of surgery
- Relatively low complication rate
- Provides material for routine histological examination

Disadvantages
- More uncomfortable than fine needle aspiration cytology
- Bleeding/bruising more common than with fine needle aspiration
- Like fine needle aspiration there is a possibility of sampling error

Open biopsy

Advantages
- Lesion completely excised
- Provides complete and definitive pathological diagnosis
- Tissue available for hormone receptor and other prognostic factor analysis
- Unlike fine needle aspiration and core biopsy, there should be no sampling error

Disadvantages
- Expensive
- Requires open operation, anaesthetic, hospital admission

(Courtesy of Henderson MA, Cawson JM, Bilous M: Breast cancer: Getting the diagnosis right. *Med J Aust* 163:494–499. Copyright 1995. The Medical Journal of Australia—reproduced with permission.

studies, and fine-needle aspiration cytology, the diagnosis of breast cancer can be made with a high level of accuracy.

▶ Whether or not they are responsible for the diagnosis of breast lesions, all primary health care providers for women should be aware of the diagnostic information in the *Medical Journal of Australia's* "MJA practice essentials" on breast cancer. The writing style is readable, clear, and concise. The information is clinically pertinent and useful in daily practice. Although each physician will have to adapt this information and clinical approach to the local medical practice situation, this article provides a pertinent "how to" guide to breast cancer diagnosis. This is highly recommended reading for all obstetricians and gynecologists.

W.H. Hindle, M.D.

SUPPLEMENTARY PAPERS

Dew JE, Eden JA: Gynaecological complications of women treated with tamoxifen for breast cancer. *Aust NZ Obstet Gynaecol* 35:198, 1995.

▶ Many, if not most, of the 1,500,000 breast cancer survivors in the United States are on tamoxifen therapy and may continue on that hormonal treatment for the remainder of their lives. Furthermore, it is now clear from numerous reports that tamoxifen has an estrogenic effect on the uterus and specifically on the endometrium. Enlargement of the uterus, enlargement of leiomyomata, myohypertrophy, endometrial polyps, and endometrial hyperplastic changes, including atypia and invasive carcinoma, are to be clinically expected, just as are such uterine changes in women on unopposed estrogen therapy. The subendometrial changes of women on tamoxifen, resulting in subendometrial cystic spaces and edema, seem to be unique to that therapy. Some investigators liken these subendometrial changes to adenomyosis, but histologic studies do not seem to support that interpretation. Unlike in women on unopposed estrogen therapy, the endometrial stripe as measured by vaginal probe ultrasound is not a reliable indicator of malignancy. With time, most women on tamoxifen have thickening of the endometrium. Biopsy of thickened endometrial stripes wider than 4–5mm is not applicable, as it is with women on unopposed estrogen therapy. Women on tamoxifen should have regular gynecologic evaluations and immediate investigation of any uterine (vaginal) bleeding. The diagnostic techniques should be the same that the clinician uses for uterine bleeding in women on unopposed estrogen therapy. In addition, as illustrated in 1 of these case reports, tamoxifen therapy can induce ovulation in premenopausal and perimenopausal women and, in fact, has been used successfully in Japan for ovulation induction in women who have failed such induction on clomiphene (which is closely related chemically). Of course, none of these uterine concerns are applicable to a woman who has had a hysterectomy.

W.H. Hindle, M.D.

Robinson DC, Bloss JD, Schiano MA: A retrospective study of tamoxifen and endometrial cancer in breast cancer patients. *Gyn Oncology* 59:186–190, 1995.

▶ In this case-controlled study of 1,017 patients at Wilford Hall Medical Center (Lackland Air Force Base, San Antonio, Texas), of those with adequate records and uteri present, endometrial cancer developed in 4 of 108 women taking tamoxifen compared with 4 of 478 women who were not taking tamoxifen. The calculated odds ratio was 15.2 (confidence interval 2.8–84.4) for the development of endometrial carcinoma in the women taking tamoxifen.

W.H. Hindle, M.D.

Cohen I, Beyth Y, Tepper R, et al: Adenomyosis in postmenopausal breast cancer patients treated with tamoxifen: A new entity? *Gynecol Oncol* 58:86–91, 1995.
▶ This series from Israel covers 14 women on tamoxifen who had hysterectomies for indications unrelated to their tamoxifen therapy. Eight (57%) had adenomyosis. One patient had a large fundal "adenomyotic lump." This is 4 times the rate in this institution of adenomyosis seen in the uteri of women who are not on tamoxifen. This adds to the increased incidence of estrogen-like stimulated findings of endocervical polyps, endometrial carcinoma, endometrial hyperplasia, endometrial polyps, enlarged uteri, enlargement of leiomyomata, and myohypertrophy described in uteri of women on tamoxifen therapy.

W.H. Hindle, M.D.

Gelber RD, Cole BF, Goldhirsch A, et al: Adjuvant chemotherapy plus tamoxifen compared with tamoxifen alone for postmenopausal breast cancer: Meta-analysis of quality-adjusted survival. *Lancet* 347:1066–1071, 1996.
▶ This assessment of data from 9 clinical trials (3,920 patients) concluded: "With 7 years of follow-up, adjuvant chemoendocrine therapy did not provide more quality-adjusted survival time than tamoxifen alone for women aged 50 years or older with node-positive breast cancer."

W.H. Hindle, M.D.

Guthrie TH Jr.: Breast cancer litigation: A retrospective analysis. *Breast J* 1:376–379, 1995.
▶ In this review of the author's 16 cases as an expert witness and 224 other cases from the medical literature, the major allegation was related to diagnosis in 89% of the cases. Ten percent were related to incorrect interpretation of mammograms or biopsies. The typical litigant was 20 years younger than the median age at the time of diagnosis for all breast cancer patients. A common feature of many cases was that on the initial visit the breast examination was thought to be normal and no specific follow-up was recorded.

W.H. Hindle, M.D.

Mitnick JS, Vazquez MF, Kronovet SZ, et al: Malpractice litigation involving patients with carcinoma of the breast. *J Am Coll Surg* 181:315–321, 1995.
▶ This is a detailed review of 118 cases from Westlaw Transmission, a computer database. Gynecologists accounted for 47% of the physicians sued. The typical plaintiff was 44 years old. Most of the women identified a mass in their breast that was "not impressive" or thought to be "fibrocystic disease" by their primary care physician.

W.H. Hindle, M.D.

Crivellari D, for the International (Ludwig) Breast Cancer Study Group: Routine tests during follow-up of patients after primary treatment for operable breast cancer. *Ann Oncol* 6:769–776, 1995.
▶ This report evaluated the routine follow-up blood test of 4,105 breast cancer patients. Analysis of alkaline phosphatase, serum glutamic oxaloacetic transaminase, gamma-GT, bilirubin, serum calcium, and serum creatinine revealed that "alkaline phosphatase was the most effective blood test to distinguish patients with relapse from those without relapse."

W.H. Hindle, M.D.

Association of Directors of Anatomic and Surgical Pathology: Recommendations for reporting of breast carcinoma. *Am J Clin Pathol* 104:614–619, 1995.

▶ Inconsistent, incomplete, and unclear pathology reports have made comparison of data difficult and have confused clinicians. These recommendations and an appended breast cancer checklist are intended to provide uniformity in surgical pathology reporting and a precise, complete, informative report for the clinician. Although compliance with the recommendations is voluntary for pathologists, hopefully clinicians involved with breast cancer diagnosis and therapy will "insist" that these recommendations be followed.

W.H. Hindle, M.D.

Pregnancy Termination in Relation to Risk of Breast Cancer
Newcomb PA, Storer BE, Longnecker MP, et al (Univ of Wisconsin, Madison; University of California at Los Angeles; Univ of Chicago; et al)
JAMA 275:283–287, 1996   25–13

Introduction.—It is accepted that full-term pregnancy—especially at an early age—lowers the risk of breast cancer. It is not clear, however, whether abbreviated pregnancy has a similar effect. Some observations suggest that women whose pregnancy is terminated before the first birth and younger women undergoing abortion are at increased risk.

Objective.—A population-based, case-control study was carried out in 45 Midwestern and New England states to determine whether abortion alters the risk of breast cancer. A total of 6,888 women less than 75 years of age with newly diagnosed breast cancer were compared with 9,529 randomly selected control women younger than 65 years of age.

Results.—Early termination of pregnancy was noted in 27% of the case group and 25.5% of control women. More than 95% of abortions in both groups were spontaneous. The relative risk of breast cancer for women reporting either spontaneous or induced abortion was 1.12. Parity did not influence the association. Induced abortion was associated with a relative risk of 1.23. Age at the time of first abortion was not a factor, and there was no indication that an increasing number of abortions altered the risk of breast cancer.

Conclusion.—The weak positive association noted in this study between abortion and the risk of breast cancer may be a result of reporting bias.

▶ Even with the large numbers of cases giving statistical power to the calculation of relative risk in this analysis, all these relative risk increases have confidence intervals crossing or at 1.00, 1.01, or 1.02. These are, indeed, levels of "weak association" that barely reach statistical significance. Furthermore, as the authors point out, there are multiple confounding variables and potential reporting and other biases. The overall impact of all this is that there is no clinically meaningful correlation between pregnancy termination (spontaneous or induced) and the relative risk of breast cancer.

W.H. Hindle, M.D.

SUPPLEMENTARY PAPER

Tavani A, LaVecchia Franceschi S, et al: Abortion and breast cancer risk. *Int J Cancer* 65: 401–405, 1996.

▶ This multicenter case-controlled study of 2,569 patients with breast cancer, stratified for age at diagnosis, number of children, time of abortion in relation to first birth, and family history of breast cancer, showed no significant relationship between spontaneous or induced abortions (or both together) and the risk of breast cancer.

W.H. Hindle, M.D.

Prospective Assessment of Breastfeeding and Breast Cancer Incidence Among 89,887 Women
Michels KB, Willett WC, Rosner BA, et al (Harvard School of Public Health, Boston; Harvard Med School, Boston)
Lancet 347:431–436, 1996   25–14

Background.—Many researchers have investigated the relationship between breast-feeding and breast cancer risk. However, the results have been conflicting. This association was assessed prospectively in a large group of women.

Methods.—The 89,887 women investigated were participants in the United States Nurses' Health Study. The participants provided breast-feeding histories in 1986. During 6 years of follow-up, 1,459 women received a diagnosis of invasive breast cancer.

Findings.—There was no significant association between the history of breast-feeding and the subsequent development of breast cancer, after adjustment for established breast cancer risk factors. Breast-feeding duration was not inversely associated with breast cancer. Women who had breast-fed for 2 years or more had a relative risk of 1.11. Women who had had only one child and who breast-fed had a lower incidence of breast cancer. Lactation in premenopausal women, who tended to be near menopause because of the cohort age structure, was associated with a relative risk of 1.16. The relative risk among premenopausal women who had lactated for 1 year or longer was 1.10.

Conclusion.—These data do not suggest an overall association between breast-feeding and breast cancer incidence. No general protective effect, as previously reported, was found. However, the risk of breast cancer was lower among women who had had only one child and who had breast-fed.

▶ The statistical power of the United States Nurses' Health Study is impressive (513,015 person-years of follow-up), and the well-designed analysis of the data presented in this report is clinically meaningful, even though, at this time, the follow-up is limited to 6 years. After adjusting for established risk factors for breast cancer, the relative risk was 0.93 with 95% confidence intervals of 0.83–1.03. Further analysis of (1) duration of breast-feeding, (2) giving birth only once, (3) status as a premenopausal woman near menopause, and (4) status as a premenopausal woman who had lactated for more than a year, did not reveal statistically significant variations in the association (relative risk) between breast-feeding and the occurrence of breast cancer.

No overall association between breast-feeding and breast cancer risk (either increased or decreased) was identified. Thus, breast-feeding should be promoted based on its intrinsic value to the mother and her infant. The relative risk of breast cancer is not clinically pertinent to a physician's recommendation or a woman's decision regarding breast-feeding.

Prior reports have been conflicting and have usually acknowledged possible selection and reporting biases. Overall, most recent studies have shown either a low (or even marginal) level of protective effect, or no impact, of breast-feeding upon the relative risk of breast cancer.[1-5]

W.H. Hindle, M.D.

References

1. Newcomb PA, Storer BE, Longnecker MP, et al: Lactation and a reduced risk of premenopausal breast cancer. *N Engl J Med* 330:81–87; 1994.
2. Yang CP, Weiss NS, Band PR, et al: History of lactation and breast cancer risk. *Am J Epidemiol* 138:1050–1056; 1993.
3. United Kingdom National Case-Control Study Group: Breast feeding and risk of breast cancer in young women. *BMJ* 307:17–20; 1993.
4. Layde PM, and the Cancer and Steroid Hormone Study Group: The independent associations of parity, age at first full term pregnancy, and duration of breastfeeding with the risk of breast cancer. *J Clin Epidemiol* 42:963–973; 1989.
5. McTiernan A, Thomas DB: Evidence for a protective effect of lactation on risk of breast cancer in young women. *Am J Epidemiol* 124:353–358; 1986.

SUPPLEMENTARY PAPERS

Katsouyanni K, Lipworth L, Trichopoulou A, et al: A case-control study of lactation and cancer of the breast. *Br J Cancer* 73:814–818, 1996.
▶ This hospital-based study from Athens with 820 breast cancer patients found no association between breast-feeding and breast cancer risk among postmenopausal women and an odds ratio of 0.50 (confidence interval 0.23–1.41) among premenopausal women who had breast-fed for more than 24 months. The authors list other studies that "support the hypothesis that breastfeeding of prolonged duration may reduce the risk of breast cancer among premenopausal women but not among postmenopausal women."

W.H. Hindle, M.D.

Romieu I, Hernández-Avila M, Lazcano E, et al: Breast cancer and lactation history in Mexican women. *Am J Epidemiol* 143:543–552, 1996.
▶ In this case-controlled study from 6 Ministry of Health hospitals in Mexico City, the interviews of 349 women with diagnosed breast cancer were compared with 1,005 National Household Sampling Frame controls. The age adjusted odds ratio was 0.39 (confidence interval 0.25–0.62) for parous women who had ever lactated and 0.47 (confidence interval 0.27–0.83) for women who had breast fed for 12–24 months.

W.H. Hindle, M.D.

Current Management of Ductal Carcinoma In Situ

Barth A, Brenner RJ, Giuliano AE (Saint John's Hosp and Health Ctr, Santa Monica, Calif)
West J Med 163:360–366, 1995   25–15

Introduction.—Ductal carcinoma in situ of the breast is characterized by proliferation of malignant epithelial cells in the ductal system without microscopic evidence of invasion through the basement membrane. This cancer is typically diagnosed through routine screening mammography in women without symptoms of disease. In 1990 13% of all breast cancers in the United States and 20% to 30% of all mammographically detected carcinomas were ductal carcinomas in situ. The natural history and unresolved issues in diagnosis and treatment of this cancer are briefly reviewed.

Diagnosis.—Microcalcifications, typically clustered and either with or without associated soft-tissue abnormality, are the most frequent mammographic findings. The cancer is rarely in the form of a defined mass. Definitive diagnosis is by mammographic-localization breast biopsy, and definitive surgical resection may also be performed on highly suspicious lesions at this time. Diagnosis of ductal carcinoma in situ via histopathologic techniques is not always straightforward. Some pathologists classify this cancer as either comedo, which is characterized by an outer ring of malignant cells and an intraluminal necrosis, or noncomedo. Comedo ductal carcinoma has been associated with more aggressive clinical behavior.

Natural History.—Not all lesions of ductal carcinoma in situ become clinically significant or progress to invasive breast cancer. Local recurrence

TABLE 1.—Local Recurrence and Cause-Specific Death Rates Following Mastectomy for Ductal Carcinoma in Situ

Source	Patients, No.	Follow-up, yr	Local Recurrence, No. (%)	Died of Disease, No. (%)
Farrow, 1970	181	2–20	2	4
Ashikari et al, 1971	110	1–10	2	1
Westbrook and Gallagher, 1975	60	5–25	1	0
Brown et al, 1976	39	1–15	0	0
Carter and Smith, 1977	38	6.2	0	1
Rosner et al, 1980	182	5	—	3
Lagios et al, 1982	53	3.7	2	1
Von Reuden and Wilson, 1984	47	1–22	0	0
Sunshine et al, 1985	68	>10	0	3
Fentiman et al, 1986	76	4.8	1	1
Schuh et al, 1986	51	5.5	0	1
Kinne et al, 1989	101	11.5	1	1
Ciatto et al, 1990	210	5.5	3	1
Fisher et al, 1991	28	7.1	0	1
Silverstein et al, 1995	167	6.5	2	0
Total	1,411		14 (1.0)	18 (1.3)

TABLE 2.—Recurrence After Breast-Conserving Therapy (Excision and Irradiation)

Source	Patients, No.	Follow-up, yr	Recurrences, No. (%)		
			Total	Invasive	Noninvasive
Haffty et al, 1990	60	3.6	4	1	3
Fisher et al, 1991	27	7.1	2	1	1
Solin et al, 1991	259	6.6	28	14	14
Silverstein et al, 1995	133	7.8	16	8	8
Cataliotti et al, 1992	34	7.8	3	3	0
Fisher et al, 1993	399	3.6	28	8	20
Ray et al, 1994	56	5.1	5	1	4
Total	968		86 (8.9)	36 (42)	50 (58)

(Courtesy of Barth A, Brenner RJ, Giuliano AE: Current management of ductal carcinoma in situ. *West J Med* 163:360–366, 1995.)

or progression may be predicted by considering nuclear grade, ploidy, proliferation rate, *her-2/neu* oncogenic overexpression, and absence of *Nm23* gene expression. Most patients receiving excision biopsy without further therapy experience a recurrence in the same quadrant; multifocality (same quadrant) is believed more clinically important than multicentricity (other quadrant). Multicentricity occurs in approximately 29% of cases. Incidence of occult invasion has been suggested to correlate with size of the malignant lesion. Rate of metastasis to axillary lymph nodes seems low.

Treatment.—Formerly, patients with ductal carcinoma were treated primarily with mastectomy, which has a high cure rate. Breast-conserving therapy consisting of excision and irradiation has been evaluated for application in ductal carcinoma in situ (Table 1). Recurrence rates after excision with radiation therapy and after excision alone have been compared (Table 2). Comedo necrosis and margin status may be independent predictors of recurrence. Recurrence after lumpectomy only has also been researched in several nonrandomized studies (Table 3).

TABLE 3.—Recurrence After Wide Local Excision Only

Source	Patients, No.	Follow-up, yr	Recurrences, No. (%)		
			Total	Invasive	Noninvasive
Amesson et al, 1989	38	5	5	2	3
Carpenter et al, 1989	28	3.2	5	1	4
Gallagher et al, 1989	13	8.3	5	3	2
Lagios et al, 1990	79	5.7	10	5	5
Fisher et al, 1991	21	7.1	9	5	4
Silverstein et al, 1992	26	1.5	2	1	1
Schwartz et al, 1992	72	4	11	3	8
Cataliotti et al, 1992	46	7.8	5	5	0
Fisher et al, 1993	391	3.6	64	32	32
Total	714		116 (16)	57 (49)	59 (51)

(Courtesy of Barth A, Brenner RJ, Giuliano AE: Current management of ductal carcinoma in situ. *West J Med* 163:360–366, 1995.)

Conclusions.—Several prospective, randomized trials of breast-conserving treatment for ductal carcinoma in situ are under way. Published results indicate that long-term risk of death is greater for patients undergoing breast-conserving therapy (3% to 5%) than for patients undergoing mastectomy (1% to 2%). Breast-conserving treatments may prove a valid alternative for the majority of patients, however, pending more precise determination of risk stratification.

▶ The appropriate treatment of ductal carcinoma in situ is probably the most controversial and perplexing of all the premalignant and malignant lesions of the breast. The optimum therapy for ductal carcinoma in situ remains an enigma. This conference review from the John Wayne Cancer Institute in Santa Monica, California, summarizes the pertinent medical literature (with 78 listed references) and gives the authors' current recommendations.

Since the utilization of screening mammography, ductal carcinoma in situ and its proper treatment has become a major women's health care issue. The urgent clinical questions seem endless. What is the natural history and biological behavior of ductal carcinoma in situ? What percentage of these lesions undergo malignant transformation and become invasive? What percentage of these lesions spontaneously regress? When does invasion occur? When do metastases occur? Why is there local recurrence? What is the relative risk of invasive cancer in the remaining ipsilateral breast tissue and in the contralateral breast? Though mastectomy as treatment of ductal carcinoma in situ appears to approach 100% ipsilateral "cures," is mastectomy surgical overtreatment? What is the value of radiation therapy in cases of ductal carcinoma in situ?

It is clear that ductal carcinoma in situ is a heterogeneous lesion even when the histologic type appears similar. Furthermore, the precise histologic diagnosis can be variable within a single lesion. Even with strict histologic criteria there can be interobserver variability and lack of pathologic diagnostic consensus.

Clinicians face the near impossible dilemma of explaining all this to their patients. Historically, total mastectomy was almost universally recommended for the treatment of this heterogeneous group of preinvasive lesions. Definitive outcome (survival) data on alternate methods of treatment are not available and, although prospective studies are under way, it will be years before confirmed data are published. Yet, for many women with histologically diagnosed ductal carcinoma in situ, breast-conserving therapy is a valid option, although the precise criteria for selecting appropriate candidates for breast-conserving therapy continues to be debated.

This review is a clear concise summary of current data and gives specific clinical recommendations. Health care providers who order screening mammography or are involved in the resultant diagnoses and treatment of nonpalpable breast lesions are well advised to read (and understand) this review. It will assist you in accurately counseling your patients.

W.H. Hindle, M.D.

Incidence of and Treatment for Ductal Carcinoma In Situ of the Breast

Ernster VL, Barclay J, Kerlikowske K, et al (Univ of California, San Francisco)
JAMA 275:913–918, 1996
25–16

Background.—The widespread use of screening mammography has resulted in a marked increase in the incidence of ductal carcinoma in situ (DCIS) of the breast. Incidence and treatment trends between 1973 and 1992 were investigated. In addition, total numbers of DCIS diagnosed and treated by mastectomy since 1983, when screening mammography started to become popular, were estimated.

Methods and Findings.—Population-based breast cancer incidence and treatment data collected by the National Cancer Institute's Surveillance, Epidemiology, and End Results Program were included in the analysis. In the early 1980s, the incidence of DCIS began to increase markedly. The mean annual rate increases changed from 0.3% between 1973 and 1983 to 12% between 1983 and 1992 among 30- to 39-year-old women, from 0.4% to 17.4% among 40- to 49-year-old women, and from 5.2% to 18.1% among women 50 years of age or older (Figs 1 and 2). In 1992, the total estimated number of cases of DCIS in the United States was 200%

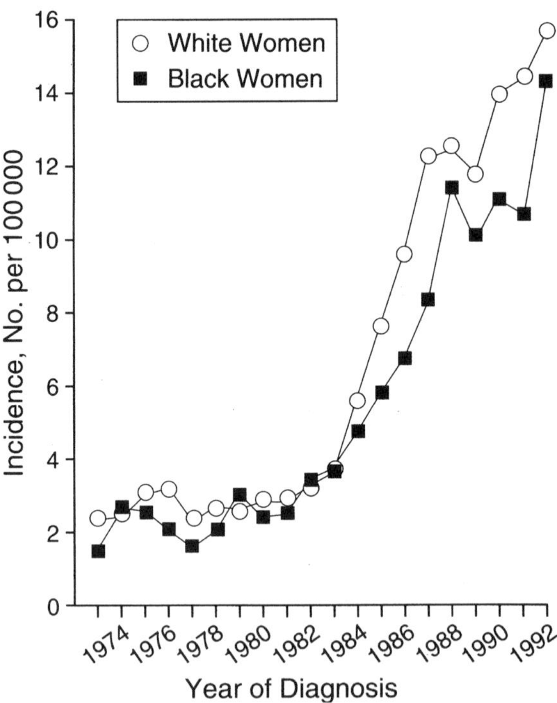

FIGURE 1.—Age-adjusted incidence rates for ductal carcinoma in situ of the breast from 1973 to 1992 for white and black women in the United States. (Courtesy of Ernster VL, Barclay J, Kerlikowske K, et al: Incidence of and treatment for ductal carcinoma in situ of the breast. *JAMA* 275:913–918, Copyright 1996, American Medical Association.)

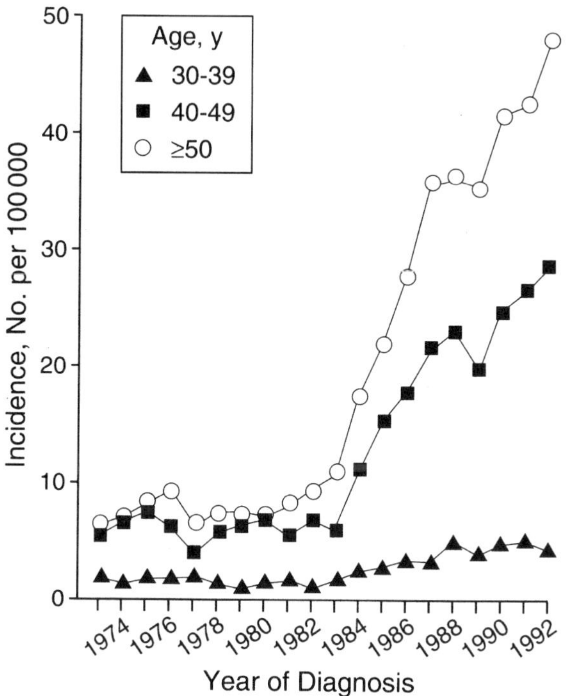

FIGURE 2.—Age-specific incidence rates for ductal carcinoma in situ of the breast from 1973 to 1992 for United States women, all races combined. (Courtesy of Ernster VL, Barclay J, Kerlikowske K, et al: Incidence of and treatment for ductal carcinoma in situ of the breast. *JAMA* 275-913–918, Copyright 1996, American Medical Association.)

TABLE 2.—Percentage of Newly Diagnosed Ductal Carcinoma In Situ Cases Treated by Mastectomy in 1992 by Geographic Area

SEER Site	Percentage Treated by Mastectomy
Connecticut	28.8
San Francisco-Oakland, Calif SMSA	39.1
Metropolitan Detroit, Mich	42.3
Seattle-Puget Sound, Wash	46.3
Utah	49.8
Hawaii	50.1
Iowa	52.4
Metropolitan Atlanta, Ga	54.6
New Mexico	57.7
All areas	43.8

Note: Geographic areas are as designated by the National Cancer Institute's Surveillance, Epidemiology, and End Results Program.
Abbreviation: SMSA, standard metropolitan statistical area.
(Courtesy of Ernster VL, Barclay J, Kerlikowske K, et al: Incidence of and treatment for ductal carcinoma in situ of the breast. *JAMA* 275:913–918, Copyright 1996, American Medical Association.)

TABLE 3.—Age-Specific Estimated Numbers of Newly Diagnosed Ductal Carcinoma In Situ (DCIS) Cases and Estimated Number of Mastectomies Performed for DCIS in the United States, 1992

Age, y	Estimated No. of DCIS Cases*	Treated by Mastectomy, %	No. of Mastectomies for DCIS*
<30	83	49.7	41
30–39	1030	47.1	485
40–49	4920	45.6	2243
50–59	5234	46.1	2413
60–69	5971	42.4	2531
≥70	6130	41.3	2529
Total	23 368		10 242

*Extrapolated from the National Cancer Institute's Surveillance, Epidemiology, and End Results (SEER) Program data by applying age-specific DCIS incidence rates from the SEER areas to the female population count in each age group in the United States in 1992.

(Courtesy of Ernster VL, Barclay J, Kerlikowske K, et al: Incidence of and treatment for ductal carcinoma in situ of the breast. *JAMA* 275:913–918, Copyright 1996, American Medical Association.)

greater than expected, based on 1983 rates and trends between 1973 and 1983. The proportion of DCIS cases treated by mastectomy decreased markedly between 1983 and 1992, and those treated by lumpectomy increased. In 1992, lumpectomy and radiation were performed in 23.3% of the patients, lumpectomy alone in 30.2%, and no surgery in 2.6%. Treatment patterns varied greatly by geographic region. In New Mexico, 57.7% of patients with DCIS underwent mastectomy, whereas only 28.8% in Connecticut had this procedure (Table 2). Although the proportion of patients treated by mastectomy decreased, the rise in DCIS incidence rates resulted in an increase in the absolute number of patients treated by mastectomy until 1990. In 1992, an estimated 10,242 patients with DCIS were treated by mastectomy (Table 3).

Conclusion.—The incidence rates of breast DCIS have markedly increased since 1983 in association with the widespread introduction of mammographic screening. Although detecting invasive breast cancer early is known to be beneficial, the value of such detection of DCIS is unknown. The proportion of patients with DCIS undergoing mastectomy may be inappropriately high, especially in some regions of the United States.

▶ Using national data, this report documents the impact of the widespread utilization of screening mammography upon the incidence of DCIS and the regional and age group variations in the treatment of DCIS by mastectomy. These data verify the concerns expressed and complement the information in the article by Barth and associates (Abstract 25–15).

W.H. Hindle, M.D.

Ten-year Results Comparing Mastectomy to Excision and Radiation Therapy for Ductal Carcinoma *In Situ* of the Breast
Silverstein MJ, Barth A, Poller DN, et al (Univ of Bern, Switzerland; City Hosp, Nottingham, England; Breast Ctr, Van Nuys, Calif)
Eur J Cancer 31A:1425–1427, 1995   25–17

Background.—Despite the lack of convincing evidence, breast-conserving surgery (with or without radiation treatment) has become popular for the treatment of ductal carcinomas in situ (DCIS) of the breast. However, the long-term local recurrence rates range from 20% to 40%. Clinical, laboratory, and pathologic factors affecting local recurrence or survival have not yet been identified. The prognostic factors in 1 series of patients with DCIS were investigated.

Methods.—Three hundred patients with DCIS without microinvasion were followed up for 10 years. One hundred sixty-seven had undergone mastectomy, and 133, excision and radiation therapy.

Findings.—Ten-year disease-free survival differed significantly between groups. Ninety-eight percent of women treated with mastectomy were still alive at 10 years, compared with 81% treated with excision and radiation therapy (Fig 1). According to a multivariate analysis, nuclear grade was the only significant predictor of local recurrence or invasive local recurrence in the women treated with excision and radiation therapy (Table 2, Fig 2). The 2 groups did not differ significantly in overall survival or breast cancer–specific survival.

Conclusions.—Nuclear grade was the only significant predictor of local or invasive local recurrence in these women treated with excision and radiation therapy. Such patients had a 5-year local recurrence rate of 7% and a 10-year local recurrence rate of 19%, demonstrating the need for long-term follow-up for women with DCIS undergoing breast-conserving treatment.

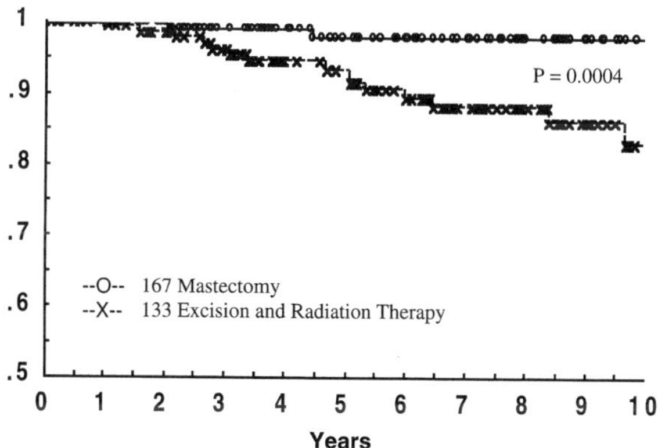

FIGURE 1.—Ten-year disease-free survival—mastectomy vs. excision and radiation therapy. (Courtesy of Silverstein MJ, Barth A, Poller DN, et al: Ten-year results comparing mastectomy to excision and radiation therapy for ductal carcinoma *in situ* of the breast. *Eur J Cancer* 31A:1425–1427, Copyright 1995, with kind permission from Elsevier Science Ltd, The Boulevard, Langford Lane, Kidlington 0X5 1GB, UK.)

TABLE 2.—Analysis of Prognostic Factors Influencing Local Recurrence After Excision and Radiation Therapy

	Univariate P-value	Multivariate P-value
Age	0.3	
Size	0.03	ns
Margins (involved versus clear)	0.05	ns
Histology (comedo versus non-comedo)	0.009	ns
Nuclear grade (1 versus 2 versus 3)	0.002	0.02
Presence of necrosis	0.003	ns
p53 (n = 58)	0.5	
HER-2/neu (n = 63)	0.09	

Abbreviation: ns, not significant.

(Courtesy of Silverstein MJ, Barth A, Poller DN, et al: Ten-year results comparing mastectomy to excision and radiation therapy for ductal carcinoma *in situ* of the breast. *Eur J Cancer* 31A:1425–1427, Copyright 1995, with kind permission from Elsevier Science Ltd, The Boulevard, Langford Lane, Kidlington 0X5 1GB, UK.)

▶ The number of patients and length of follow-up reported by Silverstein et al. are remarkable. However, because this is not a prospective, randomized clinical trial, selection bias (patient and physician) can influence the results. Nevertheless, the data are impressive. This study indicates that future evidence-based medical data (from multiple centers) may well demonstrate that overall survival is essentially the same for both methods of treatment. The individual patient's selection criteria for the options of DCIS treatment remain to be delineated and proved accurate.

W.H. Hindle, M.D.

Supplementary Paper

Page DL, Dupont WD, Rogers LW, et al: Continued local recurrence of carcinoma 15–25 years after a diagnosis of low grade ductal carcinoma in situ of the breast treated only by biopsy. *Cancer* 76: 1977–1200, 1995.

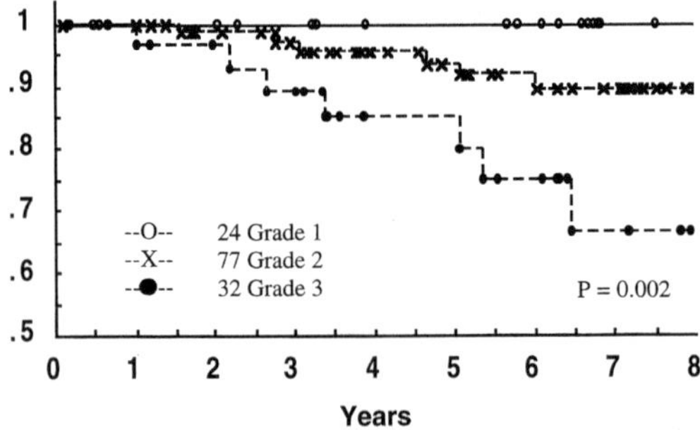

FIGURE 2.—Eight-year disease-free survival—Patients who had excision and radiation therapy stratified by nuclear grade. The recurrence rates were 0% for nuclear grade 1, 10% for grade 2, and 34% for grade 3. (Courtesy of Silverstein MJ, Barth A, Poller DN, et al: Ten-year results comparing mastectomy to excision and radiation therapy for ductal carcinoma *in situ* of the breast. *Eur J Cancer* 31A:1425–1427, Copyright 1995, with kind permission from Elsevier Science Ltd, The Boulevard, Langford Lane, Kidlington 0X5 1GB, UK.)

▶ Between 25% and 50% of women followed up for an average of 30 years after biopsy alone as therapy for small, noncomedo ductal carcinoma in situ had invasive carcinoma develop in the same site. Calculations revealed a 9-fold increased relative risk of invasive carcinoma over 30 years. Other published studies have demonstrated "virtually no recurrences" after careful wide excision with at least 4–8 years follow-up. Complete excision biopsy with generous clear surgical margins is essential for "cure" of these lesions.

W.H. Hindle, M.D.

Effect of Estrogen Replacement Therapy on the Specificity and Sensitivity of Screening Mammography

Laya MB, Larson EB, Taplin SH, et al (Univ of Washington, Seattle)
J Natl Cancer Inst 88:643–649, 1996   25–18

Background.—Mammographic breast density has been shown to be increased after estrogen replacement therapy (ERT) is begun. It is not known how this increase affects the specificity and sensitivity of screening mammography.

Methods and Findings.—A total of 8,779 postmenopausal women aged 50 years or older entered a breast screening program between 1988 and 1993. Mammographic specificity was lower among current ERT users than never or former users. When a positive reading was defined as any nonnormal finding, the adjusted relative risk (RR) of a false positive reading for current users vs. never users was 1.33. For former users compared with never users, the RR was 1. Adjusted mammographic specificity was 86% for never users, 86% for former users, and 82% for

---

TABLE 2.—Mammography Outcomes With 1 Year of Follow-Up in Never Users, Former Users, and Current Users of Estrogen Replacement Therapy

	Never used, n = 3826	Former users, n = 2853	*Current users,* n = 2100
True negatives	3228	2427	1720
False positives	564	410	367
True positives	32	15	9
False negatives	2	1	4
Cancer prevalance per 1000	8.8	5.6	6.2†
Specificity (95% confidence interval)	85% (84%–86%)	85% (84%–87%)†	82% (81%–84%)‡
Sensitivity (95% confidence interval)	94% (80%–99%)	94% (69%–99%)†	69% (38%–91%)

Note: Positive is defined as a reading of suspicious for cancer or indeterminate. Negative is defined as no evidence of cancer.

*Not statistically significant from former users or never users at the 0.05 level (normal theory method).

†Former users and never users not significantly different at the 0.05 level for sensitivity or specificity calculations.

‡2-sided $P = 0.006$ for current users vs. never users and 2-sided $P = 0.001$ for current users vs. former users (normal theory method).

§2-sided $P = 0.04$ for current users vs. never users and 2-sided $P > 0.05$ for current users vs. former users (exact method).

(Courtesy of Laya MB, Larson EB, Taplin SH, et al: Effect of estrogen replacement therapy on the specificity and sensitivity of screening mammography. *J Natl Cancer Inst* 88:643–649, 1996.)

TABLE 3.—False Positive Frequency Analysis: The Relationship of Estrogen Replacement Therapy to the Proportion of False Positive Mammograms Among Women Who Do Not Have Breast Cancer

ERT use category	Unadjusted risk ratio (95% confidence interval)	Adjusted* risk ratio (95% confidence interval)	Unadjusted specificity (95% confidence interval)	Adjusted* specificity (95% confidence interval)
Never used†	1.0	1.0	85% (84%–86%)	86% (84%–88%)
Former user	0.98 (0.85–1.12)‡	1.00 (0.87–1.15)‡	85% (84%–87%)§	86% (84%–87%)‡
Current user	1.22 (1.06–1.40)§	1.33 (1.15–1.54)‖	82% (81%–84%)	82% (80%–84%)‖

Notes: Positive is defined as any abnormal reading that is suspicious for cancer or indeterminate. N = 8,716.
*Adjusted for age, history of first-degree relative with breast cancer, history of a previous memmogram.
†Reference group.
‡Former and never users not significantly different at the 0.05 level.
§2-sided $P < 0.01$ for current users vs. never users and 2-sided $P < 0.001$ for current users vs. former users.
‖2-sided $P < 0.001$ for current users vs. never users and 2-sided $P = 0.001$ for current users vs. former users.
(Courtesy of Laya MB, Larson EB, Taplin SH, et al: Effect of estrogen replacement therapy on the specificity and sensitivity of screening mammography. *J Natl Cancer Inst* 88:643–649, 1996.)

current users. When a positive reading was defined as suspicious for cancer only, the adjusted RRs of false positive readings for current and former users compared with never users were 1.71 and 1.16, respectively. Mammography was also less sensitive in women currently receiving ERT. Current vs. never users had a 5.23 unadjusted RR of a false negative reading. For former vs. never users, this RR was 1.06. The unadjusted mammographic sensitivities were 94% for never users, 94% for former users, and 69% for current users (Tables 2, 3, and 6).

Conclusion.—Screening mammography has a lower specificity and sensitivity in women currently using ERT. This reduces the efficacy and cost effectiveness of breast cancer screening.

TABLE 6.—False Positive Frequency Analysis: The Relationship of Estrogen Replacement Therapy to the Proportion of False Positive Mammograms Among Women Who Do Not Have Breast Cancer

ERT use category	False positives	True negatives	Unadjusted risk ratio (95% confidence interval)	Adjusted risk ratio* (95% confidence interval)	Unadjusted specificity (95% confidence interval	Adjusted specificity* (95% confidence interval)
Never used†	187	3605	1.0	1.0	95% (94%–96%)	95% (94%–96%)
Former user	156	2681	1.12 (0.90–1.39)	1.16 (0.93–1.45)	95% (94%–96%)	94% (93%–96%)
Current user	163	1924	1.63 (1.31–2.03)‡	1.71 (1.37–2.14)§	92% (93%–94%)	91% (90%–94%)§

Notes: Positive is defined as a reading suspicious for cancer only. N = 8,716.
*Adjusted for age, history of first-degree relative with breast cancer, history of a previous mammogram.
†Reference group.
‡2-sided $P < 0.002$ for current users vs. never users (other intergroup comparisons not significant at the 0.05 level).
§2-sided $P < 0.001$ for current users vs. never users (other intergroup comparisons not significant at the 0.05 level).
(Courtesy of Laya MB, Larson EB, Taplin SH, et al: Effect of estrogen replacement therapy on the specificity and sensitivity of screening mammography. *J Natl Cancer Inst* 88:643–649, 1996.)

▶ This analysis from multiple university centers evaluated mammograms of women taken before hormone replacement therapy and those of the same women 1 year after beginning hormone replacement therapy. The mammographic densities increased 73% ($P = 0.003$) above the baseline studies taken prior to hormone replacement therapy. The authors state: "Multivariate analysis results indicated that the lower the tissue density percentage before treatment, the greater the increase in density percentage after treatment." It has been well documented elsewhere that increased mammographic density decreases the accuracy of lesion detection and mammographic diagnosis.

It is well known that many menstruating women have mammographically dense breasts which can adversely affect the accuracy and effectiveness with which suspicious mammographic lesions are perceived. Furthermore, all women, beginning at about age 25, have progressive fatty replacement of the glandular tissue of the breast with decreasing mammographic density as they grow older. This decrease in glandular tissue and mammographic density is most apparent in estrogen-deficient women, e.g., women more than 3 years postmenopausal.

However, there is marked individual variation in the mammographic density in women of all ages. Some young women have mammographically "clear" breasts and some postmenopausal women have mammographically dense breasts.

There is a general association of mammographic density and estrogen levels. In some women, changes in the mammographic density are apparent during different phases of the menstrual cycle. In about 25% of estrogen deficient women given ERT, there will be a noticeable increase in the mammographic density. In some women, these changes in the mammogram are striking.[1] Although hard data are not available, it seems that it takes several months of ERT to produce the maximum perceived increase in mammographic density and that it probably takes considerably longer for the ERT-associated increase in mammographic density to completely "clear" (decrease to the density seen before ERT) after ERT has been discontinued. Thus, mammographers and other physicians involved in the evaluation of the breast should have specific hormonal information as to the patient's past and current estrogen therapy, including oral contraceptive therapy and combined estrogen/progesterone therapy.

W.H. Hindle, M.D.

Reference

1. Cyrlak D, Wong CH: Mammographic changes in postmenopausal women undergoing hormonal replacement therapy. *AJR* 161:1177-1183, 1993.

SUPPLEMENTARY PAPER

Laya MB, Gallagher JC, Schreiman JS, et al: Effect of postmenopausal hormonal replacement therapy on mammographic density and parenchymal pattern. *Radiology* 196:433–437, 1995.

▶ This analysis from multiple university centers evaluated mammograms of women that were taken before hormone replacement therapy (HRT) and those taken 1 year after beginning HRT. The mammographic densities increased 73% ($P = 0.003$) above the baseline studies taken prior to HRT. The authors state that "multivariate analysis results indicated that the lower the tissue density percentage before treatment, the greater the increase in density percentage after treatment." It is well documented elsewhere that increased mammographic density decreases the accuracy of lesion detection and mammographic diagnosis. Clinicians should be aware of this mammographic density change in women who are on HRT. Patients should be given this information when the informed consent for HRT is obtained. Furthermore, the information that a woman has begun HRT, is continuing HRT, or has recently stopped HRT should be included in the clinical data given (usually written on the mammography request) to the mammographer.

W.H. Hindle, M.D.

The Cost-effectiveness of Mammographic Screening Strategies

Lindfors K, Rosenquist CJ (Univ of California, Davis, Sacramento)
JAMA 274:881–884, 1995

25–19

Background.—In an era where health care costs are a paramount concern, increased attention has been given to the cost-effectiveness of various medical procedures, including mammographic screening strategies. The cost-effectiveness of different mammographic screening strategies was

TABLE 6.—Cost-Effectiveness of Different Mammographic Screening Schedules

Age, y	Frequency of Mammography	Marginal Cost of Screening, $*	Marginal Effectiveness of Screening, y†	MCYLS, $‡
50–79	Biennial	1120	.0701	16 000
40–49	Annual			
		1915	.0950	20 200
50–79	Biennial			
40–64	Annual			
		2510	.1006	25 000
65–79	Biennial			
50–79	Annual	2212	.0863	25 600
40–79	Annual	2972	.1096	27 100
40–49	Biennial			
		2550	.0818	31 200
50–79	Annual			
40–49 (high risk)	Annual			
40–49 (normal risk)	Biennial	2583	.0809	31 900
50–79	Annual			

*Difference between total costs for screening and total costs for observation over the period of the model.

†Difference between years of life accumulated in the screened group and years of life accumulated in the observed group over the period of the model.

‡Marginal cost per year of life saved (*MCYLS*) is the marginal cost of screening divided by the marginal effectiveness of screening. Amounts rounded to the nearest $100.

(Courtesy of Lindfors K, Rosenquist CJ: The cost-effectiveness of mammographic screening strategies. *JAMA* 274:881–884, Copyright 1995, American Medical Association.)

TABLE 7.—Sensitivity of Cost-Effectiveness of Various Mammographic Screening Schedules to Changes in the Assumed Mortality Reduction Among Screened Women Aged 40–49 Years

| | | *MCYLS, $* | |
Assumed Mortality Reduction in Age 40–49 y, %	*Annual for Ages 40–79 y*	*Annual for Ages 40–49 y; Biennial for Ages 50–79 y*	*Biennial for Ages 40–49 y; Annual for Ages 50–79 y*
4	33 600	26 700	31 200†
8	31 900	25 000	29 300
12	30 400	23 500	27 700
16	29 100	22 200	26 300
20	27 900	21 000	25 000
23	27 100 (Baseline)	20 200 (Baseline)	

Note: Amounts are rounded to the nearest $100.
Abbreviations: MCYLS, marginal cost per year of life saved.
(Courtesy of Lindfors K, Rosenquist CJ: The cost-effectiveness of mammographic screening strategies *JAMA* 274:881–884, Copyright 1995, American Medical Association.)

compared and evaluated in an effort to help establish the optimal approach.

Methods.—Mammographic screening was compared with observation without screening using a computer simulation model. Cost-effectiveness was defined as marginal cost per year of life saved (MCYLS) and was determined for 7 different screening strategies. These included annual screening for ages 40–79 years; annual screening for ages 50–79 years; biennial screening for ages 50–79 years; annual screening for ages 40–49 years with biennial screening for ages 50–79 years; annual screening for ages 40–64 years with biennial screening for ages 65–79 years; biennial screening for ages 40–49 years with annual screening for ages 50–79 years; and annual screening for high-risk and biennial screening for normal-risk women aged 40–49 years with annual screening for ages 50–79 years. Previously published data or community experience were used to establish the probability and cost of all outcomes.

Results.—After calculating the MCYLS for each of the screening strategies in comparison to observation, biennial mammography for women aged 50–79 years was identified as the most cost-effective screening strategy, with an MCYLS of $16,000. When annual mammography for women aged 40–49 years was added, the MCYLS was increased to $20,200; however, this protocol was more cost-effective than other tested strategies that included women in their 40s (Table 6). Annual mammography for ages 40–49 years with biennial mammography for women aged 50–79 years also was more cost-effective when compared with annual mammography for ages 50–79 years. Because the extent of the reduction in breast cancer mortality among women aged 40–49 years is not clearly defined, the MCYLS also was calculated for a range of mortality reductions using 3 different screening strategies (Table 7). Discounting increased the MCYLS for all strategies, with the greatest effect noted for protocols including women in their 40s.

Conclusions.—Screening programs that include women in their 40s can be as effective as some that exclude this age group. Selection of a screening strategy should be based on available financial resources and the desired effectiveness of a mammographic screening program.

▶ Cost-effectiveness and the allocation of health care resources are critical economic issues and will continue to be important factors in what the third parties, including the federal and state governments, are willing to fund. These financial issues impact the suggested guidelines for screening mammography in various institutions, e.g., HMOs and managed care networks. Though it is prudent for physicians to be apprised of these economic issues, the fundamental responsibility of primary care physicians is the optimum health of each patient. Thus, appropriate medical advice to an individual woman may be at odds with institutional, organizational, or governmental screening mammography guidelines.

These computer-simulated, cost-effectiveness calculations by Lindfors and Rosenquist give mathematic insight with age-subset analysis into various screening mammography strategies. The "secondary cost" of screening and impact on patient anxiety, e.g., excision biopsies, are impressive. Each woman needs to be apprised of what is best for her personal health care. What third-party payers are willing to pay for is a distinct and separate issue. Unfortunately, physicians have limited influence on third-party payers. Nevertheless, though the process is time-consuming for the physician and requires sensitive counseling, individualized health care recommendations based on current medical data should be given to the patient.

W.H. Hindle, M.D.

Screening Mammography in Community Practice: Positive Predictive Value of Abnormal Findings and Yield of Follow-up Diagnostic Procedures
Brown ML, Houn F, Sickles EA, et al (Natl Cancer Inst, Bethesda, Md; Food and Drug Administration, Rockville, Md; Univ of California, San Francisco)
AJR 165:1373–1377, 1995   25–20

Introduction.—Although the benefits of screening mammography have been established, little is known about the induced costs of screening-,which are the financial costs and morbidity associated with follow-up diagnostic procedures. Therefore, data were collected on community-screening mammography and follow-up practices in 50 nationally representative mammography facilities participating in the National Survey of Mammography Facilities (NSMF). From these data, the positive predictive value of abnormal mammographic findings and the frequency and yield of follow-up diagnostic procedures were estimated.

Methods.—The NSMF selected a volume-stratified sample of 50 facilities in both metropolitan and nonmetropolitan areas. A total of 1,717 records of screening mammography examinations with abnormal results

TABLE 1.—Follow-up Procedures Performed in Comparison to Radiologic Recommendations

Recommendation (No. Recommended/ No. Performed	Procedure Was Done When Recommended	Different Procedure Was Done	No Procedure Was Done	% Unknown
	% in Which:			
Repeat standard (screening) views (610/635)	52	12	14	22
Additional mammographic views (785/707)	78	9	11	2
Sonography (400/345)	64	13	7	16
Clinical breast examination (196/116)	23	36	9	32
Open surgical biopsy (169/180)	40	30	7	23
Needle biopsy (20/49)	20	52	10	18
Needle aspiration (21/51)	67	33	0	0

(Courtesy of Brown ML, Houn F, Sickles EA, et al: Screening mammography in community practice: Positive predictive value of abnormal findings and yield of follow-up diagnostic procedures. AJR 165:1373–1377, 1995.)

were abstracted, including all clinical events following the abnormal mammographic findings. The frequency of specific follow-up recommendations, the procedures performed, and the outcomes were analyzed.

Results.—Overall, 87% of all mammography examinations performed were for screening purposes. There were abnormalities detected in 11% of all screening mammograms. The radiologists' recommendations included

TABLE 2.—Yield of Follow-up Procedure Performed (Cancers Detected per 100 Procedures)

Procedure	Of All Ages (n = 1551)	<50 Yr Old (n = 633)*	>50 Yr Old (n = 834)*	p Value For Difference in Means
	Mean (95% Confidence Interval) for Patients			
Examination showing abnormalities	3.49 (2.57–4.41)	1.98 (0.75–3.21)	4.65 (2.51–6.79)	<.05
Repeat standard (screening) views	0.59 (0.1–1.08)	0.26 (0.00–0.77)	0.82 (0.00–1.64)	NS
Additional mammographic views	2.80 (1.13–4.47)	1.91 (0.17–3.65)	3.80 (1.29–6.31)	NS
Sonography	2.09 (0.46–3.72)	0.36 (0.00–1.09)	4.43 (0.43–8.43)	<.05
Clinical breast examination	1.37 (0.00–3.41)	0.00	1.96 (0.00–5.72)	NS
Needle aspiration	7.05 (1.03–13.06)	3.57 (0.00–8.53)	11.76 (1.11–22.40)	NS
Needle biopsy	18.84 (7.86–29.82)	8.74 (0.00–20.59)	26.15 (11.02–41.28)	<.10
Open surgical biopsy	20.90 (12.90–28.90)	9.45 (3.45–15.45)	29.82 (16.08–43.56)	<.05

Note: Unweighted observations.
*Age data were missing for 84 individuals.
(Courtesy of Brown ML, Houn F, Sickles EA, et al: Screening mammography in community practice: Positive predictive value of abnormal findings and yield of follow-up diagnostic procedures. *AJR* 165:1373–1377, 1995.)

TABLE 3. University of California at San Francisco Database Yield of Procedures Performed per Cancers Detected (Cancers Detected per 100 Procedures)

	Mean (95% Confidence Interval) for Patients		
Procedure	Of All Ages (n = 65,792)	<50 Yr Old (n = 33,588)	>50 Yr Old (n = 32,204)
Examination showing abnormalities	9.52 (9.42–9.61)	5.30 (5.25–5.35)	14.40 (14.25–14.54)
Additional mammographic views only	19.31 (17.4–21.21)	10.69 (8.66–12.74)	29.42 (26.18–32.66)
Open surgical biopsy	33.97 (30.94–37.01)	22.62 (18.62–26.62)	43.22 (38.94–47.49)

Note: Differences in means by age groups were all statistically significant at $P < 0.001$.

(Courtesy of Brown ML, Houn F, Sickles EA, et al: Screening mammography in community practice: Positive predictive value of abnormal findings and yield of follow-up diagnostic procedures. *AJR* 165:1373–1377, 1995.)

additional mammographic views (most common), repeat standard views, sonography, clinical breast examination, open surgical biopsy, and needle biopsy or aspiration (least common) (Table 1). Compliance with these recommendations was highest for additional mammographic views and was lower for invasive procedures. The diagnostic yield of follow-up diagnostic procedures was highest for open surgical biopsy, with the yield for needle biopsy only slightly lower and the yield for noninvasive procedures relatively low (Table 2). Comparing these data with those from the University of California at San Francisco database revealed generally lower yields in the NSMF data, representing typical clinical practices, than in the University of California at San Francisco data (Table 3). Both studies showed increased diagnostic yield with increasing age.

Conclusions.—Typical community screening mammography practices and their follow-up show significant differences between the radiologists' recommendations for follow-up and the actual procedures performed. However, despite these variations, the correlation between diagnostic yield and advancing age is consistent with the increasing incidence of breast cancer associated with increasing age. These data will be useful in the documentation of screening and induced costs for mammographic services.

▶ What happens as a result of screening mammography? Is there a cascade of costly procedures? Do physicians follow the mammographers' recommendations? How efficient is this clinical avenue to the diagnosis of breast cancer? These nationwide data are keenly informative. Overall, 4 cancers were detected and diagnosed per 1,000 screening mammograms. This compares with the 6 per 1,000 reported on initial screening (mammography and breast examination) in the Breast Cancer Detection Demonstration Project, which showed a cancer detection rate of 3 per 1,000 on annual interval (follow-up) screening. Furthermore, in the NSMF analysis, it is of particular clinical interest that 40% of the mammographic abnormalities and 24% of the cancers were found in women under 50 years old. The impressive case numbers from the University of California at San Francisco indicate that increased effectiveness of cancers diagnosed per 1,000 procedures is obtainable, although selection of patients may influence these results. Hopefully, continuing analysis of similar national data will allow the formulation of practice guidelines for quality assurance within each mammography facility.

W.H. Hindle, M.D.

Diagnostic Outcome of Repeated Mammography Screening
Arnesson L-G, Vitak B, Månson J-C, et al (Univ Hosp, Linköping, Sweden)
World J Surg 19:372–378, 1995   25–21

Background.—A general mammography program was begun in Östergötland County, Sweden, in 1986 to screen all women aged 40 to 74 years. Diagnostic outcomes for 1987 to 1992, with a focus on repeated screening from 1989 to 1992, and the frequency of diagnostic surgery among groups were analyzed.

Methods and Findings.—Overall, the attendance rate was 82.8%. Three hundred sixty malignancies were diagnosed histologically between 1989 and 1992. Between 1989 and 1992, malignancy was detected in 2.6 of 1,000 women screened, yielding a positive predictive rate at surgery of 87.4% and an efficiency rate of 95.9%. Women 45 years of age and older had a positive predictive rate exceeding 94%. Fine-needle aspiration biopsy showed invasive disease in 84%. In another 15%, cancer was highly suspected. Sixty percent of the lesions were not palpable. For first-time screening from 1987 to 1988, the positive predictive rate was 86%, and the malignancy yield was 6.4 in 1,000. Only 1.6% of women 40 to 44 years of age were referred for surgery. However, the positive predictive rate at surgery was only 48.3%, indicating diagnostic problems in young women. The median size of all invasive cancers was 12 mm. Eighty-four percent were classified as pT1, and 23% showed lymph node involvement. Twenty-seven percent of all malignancies were classified as stage II disease.

Conclusions.—It is important to analyze diagnostic outcomes, especially focusing on a high positive predictive value at surgery. Regular analysis in mammographic screening programs should aid in keeping the number of diagnostic operations done for benign lesions to a minimum, thereby decreasing the patient's anxiety and health care costs while maintaining the expected benefits of screening.

▶ Patient compliance, validation of exact surgery, verification of precise pathology, and continuing follow-up make the Swedish mammography and breast cancer data unique and of paramount medical importance. The histopathologic types of breast cancers, axillary lymph node involvement, and tumor stage in this report are similar to those in other screening mammography breast cancer series. However, the positive predictive values obtained are outstanding, due to the routine use of fine-needle aspiration (FNA) cytology. The FNA was "digitally directed" (palpable lesion) in 40% of the mammographically suspect lesions. Is there a cost-effectiveness lesson to be learned here? It seems clear that there is. The high clinical "efficiency" of diagnosis obtained in this study is remarkable. Although the Swedish FNA experience continues to be about as accurate for nonpalpable lesions as for palpable lesions, in the United States, with nonpalpable lesions, tissue core needle biopsy with histologic diagnosis is more popular.

W.H. Hindle, M.D.

Neglected Aspects of False Positive Findings of Mammography in Breast Cancer Screening: Analysis of False Positive Cases From the Stockholm Trial

Lidbrink E, Elfving J, Frisell J, et al (South Hosp, Stockholm; Huddinge Univ, Stockholm)

BMJ 312:273–276, 1996

25–22

Background.—Some researchers have questioned whether the reduction in mortality resulting from mammographic screening outweighs the negative effects of screening, especially in women younger than 50 years in whom the incidence of breast cancer is less and the specificity and sensitivity of mammography is decreased. False positive findings may result in psychological problems and increased costs. The effects of false-positive mammographic findings were investigated.

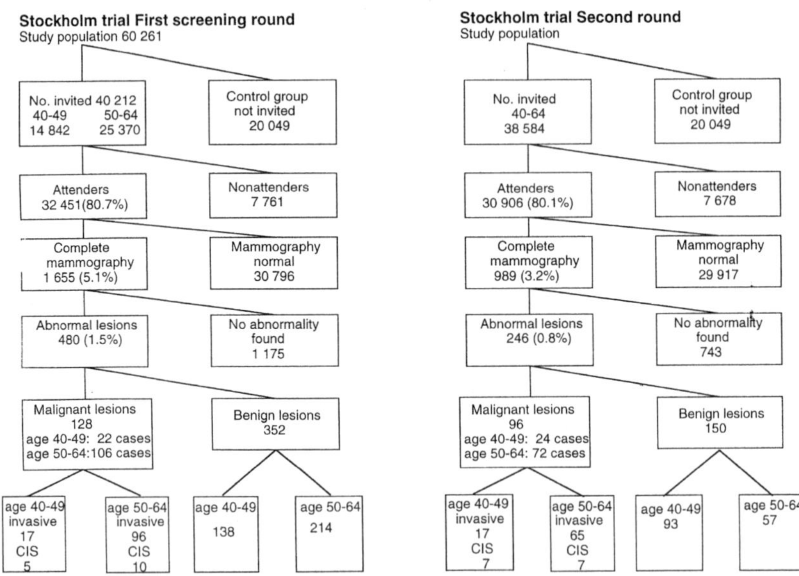

FIGURE 1.—Flow charts of first and second rounds of Stockholm mammography screening trial showing numbers of invited, screened, recalled, and referred women and numbers of cancer cases. Age groups represent age at entry. (Courtesy of Lidbrink E, Elfving J, Frisell J, et al: Neglected aspects of false positive findings of mammography in breast cancer screening: Analysis of false positive cases from the Stockholm trial. *BMJ* 312:273–276, 1996.)

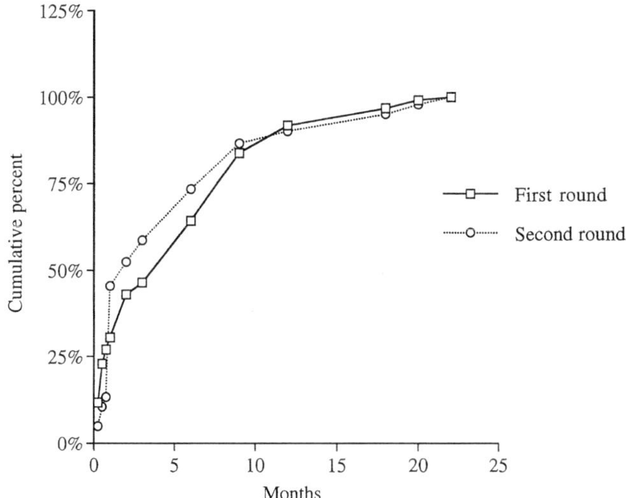

FIGURE 2.—Cumulative percentage of women with false positive findings in each screening round in relation to time (months) until they were declared cancer-free. Hospital records were missing for 10 women in the first round and seven women in second round. (Courtesy of Lidbrink E, Elfving J, Frisell J, et al: Neglected aspects of false positive findings of mammography in breast cancer screening: Analysis of false positive cases from the Stockholm trial. *BMJ* 312:273–276, 1996.)

Methods.—Women enrolled in the Stockholm mammography screening trial were included in the study. Three hundred fifty-two women with false positive findings in the first screening round and 150 women with false positive results in the second round were reviewed.

Findings.—In the first screening round, the patients with false positive findings had a total of 1,112 physician visits, 397 fine-needle aspiration biopsies, 187 mammograms, and 90 surgical biopsies before the diagnosis of cancer was definitively disproved. For 64% of the women, this process lasted 6 months. The women in the second screening round had a total of 427 physician visits, 145 fine-needle aspiration biopsies, 70 mammograms, and 28 surgical biopsies. After 6 months, 73% of this group were declared cancer free. The costs associated with follow-up in the first and second rounds were £250,000 and £84,000, respectively. Approximately 41% of these costs were accrued in the follow-up of women younger than 50 years (Figs 1 and 2; Tables 1 and 2).

Conclusions.—False positive mammographic findings entail lengthy follow-up, which is costly and stressful for patients. Almost half of the expense is incurred in following up women younger than 50 years.

▶ The number of participants and high levels of compliance in Swedish breast cancer screening programs are impressive. Studies such as this provide data for evidence-based medical decisions and patient counseling information. The cost data are especially valuable. Undoubtedly, the exact costs are different in every country and probably in each institution. However, the relativity of the cost should be accurate. To quote the authors, "In

TABLE 1.—Examinations and Costs of Positive Cases in Different Age Groups (Age Group at Entry) of Women at First and Second Screening Rounds Including 32, 451 and 30,906 Screened Women Respectively

| | Cost/ examination (Kr) | First screening round (352 women) | | | | Second screening round (150 women) | | | |
		Age 40–49 (n=138)		Age 50–64 (n=214)		Age 40–49 (n=93)		Age 50–64 (n=57)	
		No	Kr	No	Kr	No	Kr	No	Kr
Visits to physician		418		704		230		197	
First visit	735	135	99 225	207	152 145	93	68 355	50	36 750
Second or later visit	459	283	129 897	497	228 123	137	62 883	147	67 473
Fine needle aspiration biopsy (by palpation)	582	115	66 930	144	83 808	58	33 756	38	22 116
Fine needle aspiration (stereotaxic)	873	38	33 174	100	87 300	23	20 079	26	22 698
Mammography	526	62	32 612	125	65 750	30	15 780	40	21 040
Surgical conference	877	38	33 326	53	46 481	17	14 909	13	11 401
Blood sampling	Various	41	2 757	64	5 163	0	0	1	150
Excision biopsy	16 170	39	630 630	51	824 670	16	258 720	12	194 040
Lung radiography	525	9	4 725	33	17 325	0	0	2	1 050
Telephone calls						3	378	1	126
Total cost of investigations of false positive cases			1 033 276		1 510 765		474 860		376 844
Mean cost per woman with false positive findings			7 488		7 060		5 106		6 611
Cost of false positive cases per cancer discovered			46 967		14 252		19 786		5 234
No. of cancers (invasive and carcinoma in situ) discovered		22		106		24		72	

Cost of false positive cases per 1000 screened women aged 40–64: First round Kr78 400, second round Kr27 560.

Cost of screening programme (one view mammography plus complete mammography after recall): First round Kr6.7m, second round Kr6.1 m.

(Courtesy of Lidbrink E, Elfving J, Frisell J, et al: Neglected aspects of false positive findings of mammography in breast cancer screening: Analysis of false positive cases from the Stockholm trial. *BMJ* 312:273–276, 1996.)

TABLE 2.—Ratio of Benign to Malignant Breast Lesions Detected in Different Age Groups (Age at Entry) in First and Second Screening Rounds

Age (years)	First screening round			Second screening round		
	Benign	Malignant	Ratio	Benign	Malignant	Ratio
40–44	72	8	9–0	49	12	4–1
45–49	66	14	4–7	44	12	3–7
50–54	72	20	3–6	21	12	1–8
55–59	68	42	1–6	20	24	0–8
60–64	74	44	1–7	16	36	0–4
Total	352	128	2–8	150	96	1–6

(Courtesy of Lidbrink E, Elfving J, Frisell J, et al: Neglected aspects of false positive findings of mammography in breast cancer screening: Analysis of false positive cases from the Stockholm trial. 312:273–276, 1996.)

this series costs of following up women with false positive mammograms were almost one third of the cost of screening all women in the randomized Stockholm mammography trial." This presents a serious economic dilemma for breast cancer screening, particularly for those women younger than 50 years of age. In this era of seemingly universal "downsizing" and curtailment of health care resources, difficult economic decisions will have to be made by those responsible for financing health care. However, in clinical practice, physicians should differentiate between these economic considerations and their own medical advice to individual patients. Cost-effectiveness–based guidelines can conflict with what a physician would ordinarily recommend to a woman for her optimum health care.

W.H. Hindle, M.D.

Supplementary Papers

Liberman L, Giess CS, Dershaw DD, et al: Mammography of breast cancer in women under 30. *Breast J* 1:112–115, 1995.
▶ These clinical data from the Memorial Sloan-Kettering Cancer Center supplement the mathematic calculations of Lindfors and Rosenquist (see Abstract 25–19). The review covers 47 symptomatic breast cancers (94% palpable) of which 55% had a focal mammographic abnormality. The Wolfe[1,2] classification for mammographic density was DY (the most dense) in 57% and P2 in 43%. Although the mammographic sensitivity of malignant diagnosis is diminished in this age group, it is concluded that "a positive mammogram may hasten the diagnosis of carcinoma...."

W.H. Hindle, M.D.

References

1. Wolfe JN: A study of breast parenchyma by mammography in the normal woman and those with benign and malignant disease. *Radiology* 82:201–205, 1967.
2. Wolfe JN: Risk for breast cancer development determined by mammographic parenchymal pattern. *Cancer* 37:2486–2492, 1976.

U.S. Department of Health and Human Services: High-quality mammography: Information for referring providers: Quick reference guide of clinicians. *BMJ* 1:333–342, 1995.

▶ This Clinical Practice Guideline No. 13 by Bassett LW, et al., Agency for Health Care Policy Research (AHCPR) Publication No. 95-0632, is available from the AHCPR Publications Clearinghouse (phone: 800-358-9295) and is a clear, concise series of key points and graded recommendations for referring health care providers and mammographers. Obstetrician-gynecologists who order mammography should obtain a copy and share this valuable information with their consultant mammographers. Efficiency and effectiveness of patient care will result from following these guidelines. When utilized in conjunction with the American College of Radiology lexicon for mammography reports, BI-RADS,[1] prior confusion about and misunderstanding of breast imaging reports should be eliminated.

W.H. Hindle, M.D.

Reference

1. Kopans DB: Standardized mammography reporting. *Radiol Clin North Am* 30:257, 1992.

SUPPLEMENTARY PAPERS

Wald NJ, Murphy P, Major P, et al: UKCCCR multicentre randomized controlled trial of one and two view mammography in breast cancer screening. *BMJ* 311:1189–1193, 1995.
▶ These data from the United Kingdom on 40,163 women aged 50–64 years attending their first breast cancer screening documents that 2-view mammography detected 24% more breast cancers than did single-view mammography. Furthermore, the recall rate was less with 2 views, and the cost-effectiveness was improved. Two-view mammography is the standard in the United States.

W.H. Hindle, M.D.

Warren RML, Duffy SW: Comparison of single reading with double reading of mammograms, and change in effectiveness with experience. *Br J Radiol* 68:958–962, 1995.
▶ This report on data from 33,734 women screened by mammography in the United Kingdom confirms other reports that about 15% additional cancers (14% in this study) will be diagnosed by a second reading of the films by another trained and experienced mammographer. Furthermore, the recall rate was decreased from 6.9% to 4.2%, and the ratio of malignant to benign biopsies improved by this dual-reading technique. Double reading of mammograms is effective and efficient for health care providers and their patients. In addition, double reading is cost-effective when the total medical expenses are calculated.

W.H. Hindle, M.D.

Brown J, Bryan S, Warren R: Mammography screening: An incremental cost effectiveness analysis of double versus single reading of mammograms. *BMJ* 312:809–812, 1996.
▶ This study from the Health Economics Research Group in Middlesex, England, of 33,734 attendees to breast screening revealed that double reading of mammograms detected an additional 9 cancers per 10,000 women screened. With consensus of both mammographers, the decreased recall rate resulted in a

cost savings of £4,853 per 10,000 women screened. The authors advocate routine double reading and consensus recommendation for recall as the most effective and efficient method of mammographic screening.

W.H. Hindle, M.D.

Stereotactic Breast Biopsy as an Alternative to Open Excisional Biopsy
Cross MJ, Evans WP, Peters GN, et al (Baylor Univ, Dallas)
Ann Surg Oncol 2:195–200, 1995   25–23

Rationale.—In the search for less expensive diagnostic methods that do not sacrifice accuracy, stereotactic breast biopsy was considered as an alternative to open excision breast biopsy. More than a half million breast biopsies are done each year in the United States. About 80% of the lesions prove to be benign.

Objective and Methods.—The histologic findings were related to the degree of mammographic risk in 225 women who had a total of 250 stereotactic breast biopsies. A frozen-section sample was examined if malignancy was suspected. If microcalcifications were present, specimen radiography was performed. On screening mammography, the presence of a solitary irregular mass or any area of clustered calcifications was interpreted as suspicious of malignancy.

Results.—An average of 3.4 cores per lesion were obtained. Fifty-four lesions (22%) were considered to be suspicious on mammographic analysis, and 78% of those were found to be malignant. They included 41 invasive breast cancers, 5 in situ cancers, and 1 lymphoma. Three mammographically suspicious lesions were inadequately sampled.

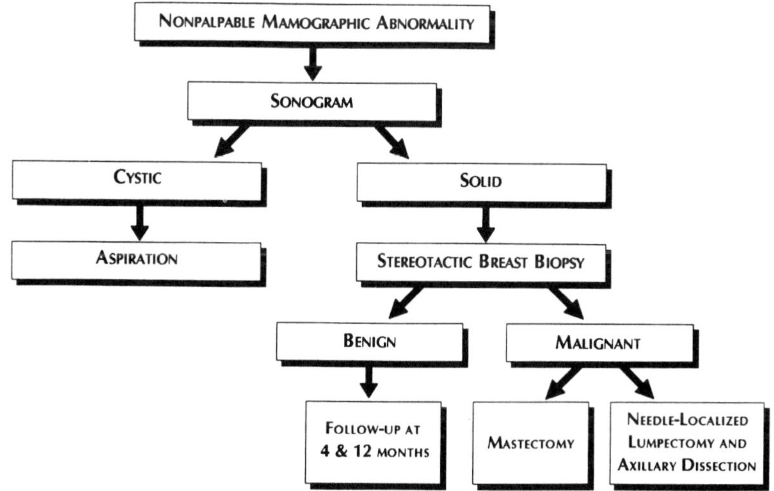

FIGURE 1.—Algorithm for nonpalpable mammographic abnormality. (Courtesy of Cross MJ, Evans WP, Peters GN, et al: *Ann Surg Oncol* 2:195–200, 1995.)

Costs.—Stereotactic breast biopsy cost approximately $1,200, including the radiologist's fee. If lumpectomy follows biopsy, an added cost of $1,200 is incurred. The average cost savings from stereotactic biopsy was $1,629 per lesion.

Discussion.—Stereotactic breast biopsy is an inexpensive alternative to open excision biopsy for diagnosing nonpalpable lesions detected by mammography. It should not be used solely to aspirate a cyst, because this is managed more easily and less expensively by sonography (Fig 1). The stereotactic technique may be used in women with breast implants. If a core sample exhibits in situ malignancy, open biopsy is necessary.

▶ Although the technique of mammographic stereotactic breast (fine-needle) biopsy has been in clinical use at the Karolinska Hospital, Stockholm, since 1976, it is only in recent years that the procedure has become widely available and popular in the United States. Tissue core needle biopsy with resultant histology is the preferred sampling method in the United States. This careful analysis of the Baylor (Dallas) experience adds to the data of multiple other published studies with similar results. It is of keen clinical interest that 2.5% of the "low-suspicion" mammographic lesions proved to be malignant. The multispecialty diagnostic (and treatment) team approach is essential for the optimum evaluation and treatment of women with abnormal mammograms. The idea in clinical practice is to diagnose breast cancer by mammography before a mass becomes palpable. Clinicians should be cognizant of the advantages, limitations, and cost-effectiveness of all diagnostic techniques and treatments of breast cancer. Women keenly appreciate continuing follow-up by the primary care physician throughout diagnosis, treatment, and thereafter.

W.H. Hindle, M.D.

Imaging-guided Core Biopsy of the Breast
McCombs MM, Bassett LW, Jahan R, et al (Univ of California, Los Angeles)
Breast J 1:9–16, 1995   25–24

Introduction.—Most excisional breast biopsy specimens after screening mammography reveal benign findings. However, these biopsies add significantly to the cost of screening and cause unnecessary morbidity and anxiety. Fine-needle aspiration cytology has been suggested as an alternative to excisional biopsy, but its usefulness is limited by the need for skilled cytopathologists, the high rates of insufficient samples, and the inability to differentiate between in situ and invasive carcinoma. Core needle biopsy (CNB), using a large-bore 16- or 14-gauge needle, can address many of these limitations and can be guided by mammography or ultrasound. Clinical experience with 304 imaging-guided core biopsies for breast abnormalities detected mammographically or ultrasonographically was reviewed.

TABLE 3.—Reported Results for Core Biopsy

Reference	# Cases	Needle gauge	Agreement with surgery (%)*	Sensitivity (%)	Specificity (%)	False negatives
Parker et al	6,152	14 g	—	99	100	15
Gisvold et al	160	14 g	90 [≥5] 80 [<5]	85	100	10
Parker et al	181†	14 g	—	100	100	0
Elvecrog et al	100	14 g	94	99	100	1
Dronkers et al	70	18 g	—	97	100	2
Dowlatshahi	250	20 g	88	71	96	13

Note: Numbers in brackets represent the number of core biopsy specimens taken per case.
*Includes only reported series in which all patients who had core needle biopsy also had excisional biopsy.
†All ultrasound-guided.
(Courtesy of McCombs MM, Bassett LW, Jahan R, et al: Imaging-guided core biopsy of the breast. *Breast J* 1:9–16, 1995. Reprinted by permission of Blackwell Science, Inc.)

Methods.—A total of 304 CNBs were performed in 277 patients, including 251 guided stereotactically and 53 guided ultrasonographically. Five specimens were obtained from masses and areas of asymmetric density or architectural distortion, and 5 to 10 specimens were obtained from

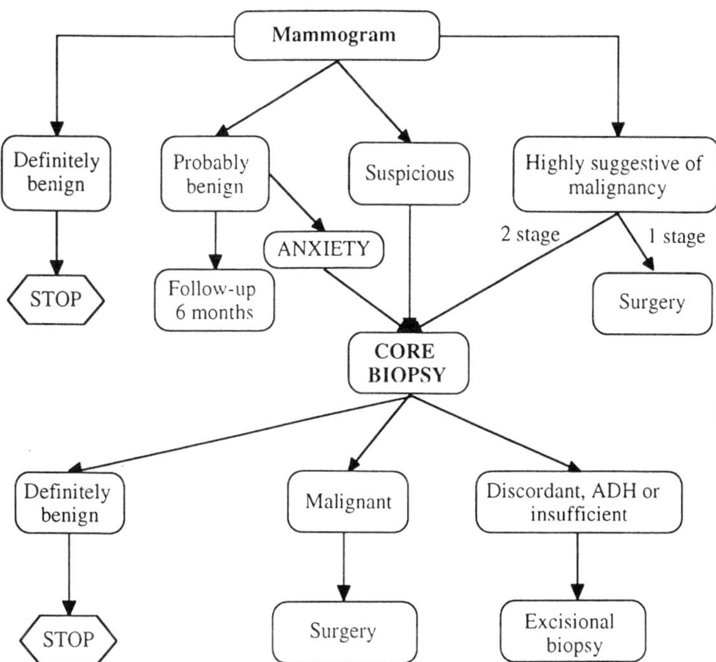

FIGURE 6.—Indications for core biopsy. (Courtesy of McCombs MM, Bassett LW, Jahan R, et al: Imaging-guided core biopsy of the breast. *Breast J* 1:9–16, 1995. Reprinted by permission of Blackwell Science, Inc.)

areas of calcification. Each specimen was sectioned at 3 levels for histologic analysis. The results were compared with those of excisional biopsy, if performed. Other patients were followed up to validate findings.

Results.—For the diagnosis of carcinoma, CNB had a sensitivity of 98%, a specificity of 99%, and a positive predictive value of 99%. Of the 304 biopsies, there were 3 false negative and 1 false positive diagnoses. The procedure resulted in few complications, none of which were serious.

Conclusions.—The results of CNB of nonpalpable lesions compared favorably with reported results of excisional biopsy (Table 3). Core needle biopsy could be performed quickly with minimal complications and reduced the limitations associated with fine-needle aspiration. Mammographic findings that are suspicious or highly suggestive of malignancy, as well as those that are probably benign in patients with anxiety, may be considered indications for performing CNBs (Fig 6). Further study of CNB is warranted.

▶ This report of the Iris Cantor Center for Breast Imaging, UCLA, experience with stereotactic mammography and ultrasound tissue CNB of nonpalpable breast lesions adds to numerous similar publications and presents a review of the current literature. With experience and ongoing quality assurance, these techniques are effective in diagnosing mammographically detected nonpalpable lesions. Which lesions are optimally approached by either stereotactic mammography or ultrasound is unresolved. However, both techniques seem to be effective for mass lesions. Asymmetric densities and clustered microcalcifications seem to be more difficult to resolve definitively. Sampling error (particularly the potential for missing an invasive component of ductal carcinoma in situ) is possible even when the usual 5 specimens are obtained. More work needs to be done, and the issue of the effectiveness of such techniques in a low-volume unit must be addressed. It seems clear that the indications for the accepted needle localization open surgical biopsy will be limited (even restricted) as these less traumatic techniques are proven to be accurate for diagnosis and effective for therapy.

W.H. Hindle, M.D.

Supplementary Papers

Morrow M: Clinical applications of stereotactic biopsy. *Breast J* 1:326–329, 1995.
▶ This is a balanced overview of the state of the art of stereotactic tissue core needle biopsy of nonpalpable breast lesions. Primary care providers for women will do well to read this article and develop a multidisciplinary approach for the diagnosis and treatment of those with breast problems. The role of the surgeon is no longer dominant in the care of breast lesions. With managed care and HMOs, primary care providers will appropriately manage breast complaints and benign conditions. Optimal cancer therapy requires a complex and coordinated multidisciplinary team approach. Even with women with breast cancer diagnosed, the primary care physician should continue to follow the patient and provide supportive care, counseling, and guidance throughout her treatment and continually thereafter. Women with breast cancer appreciate and are profoundly grateful for this continuing informative and compassionate care.

W.H. Hindle, M.D.

Doyle AJ, Murray KA, Nelson EW, et al: Selective use of image-guided large-core needle biopsy of the breast: Accuracy and cost-effectiveness. *AJR* 165:281–284, 1995.

▶ Using 5,772 screening mammograms taken from April 1992 to June 1994 compared with 5,039 taken from July 1990 to April 1992, this study compared the number of wire localization surgical biopsies and large-core needle biopsies for mammographically "indeterminate" nonpalpable lesions. During the 1992–1994 period, a strict protocol for intervention was followed. During this later period, the biopsy rate increased from 1:36 to 1:26. However, the cost of biopsy per cancer detected decreased 28%. Furthermore, the authors state that "the specificity of large-core needle biopsy was 98%; the sensitivity based on limited follow-up was 100%." These are remarkable results.

W.H. Hindle, M.D.

Liberman L, Dershaw DD, Rosen PP, et al: Stereotaxic core biopsy of impalpable spiculated breast masses. *AJR* 165:551–554, 1995.

▶ This report from the Memorial Sloan-Kettering Cancer Center reviews 43 nonpalpable spiculated (stellate) breast masses of which 93% proved to be invasive breast cancer by mammography-directed stereotactic tissue core needle biopsy: a remarkable sensitivity! This diagnostic approach to nonpalpable breast masses of all types is uniformly reported as reliably accurate.

W.H. Hindle, M.D.

Brenner RJ, Fajardo L, Fisher PR, et al: Percutaneous core biopsy of the breast: Effect of operator experience and number of samples on diagnostic accuracy. *AJR* 166:341–346, 1996.

▶ This compilation from 10 breast centers validated a 97% overall accuracy compared with immediate excision biopsy when 5 tissue core needle biopsy (TCNB) samples were taken in the evaluation of mammographically detected nonpalpable breast lesions. The lowest accuracy was 86% for architectural distortions. Five TCNB samples for histologic diagnosis of such mammographic lesions has become the standard of care.

W.H. Hindle, M.D.

Nath ME, Robinson TM, Tobon H, et al: Automated large-core needle biopsy of surgically removed breast lesions: Comparison of samples obtained with 14-, 16-, and 18-gauge needles. *Radiology* 197:739–742, 1995.

▶ This evaluation of the effect of needle size on the accuracy of diagnosis of palpable and nonpalpable surgically removed breast lesions ($n = 57$) found a 100% sensitivity for 14-gauge, 92% sensitivity for 16-gauge, and 65% sensitivity for 18-gauge needles used with a short-throw Biopty gun. The specificity for cancer was 100% for all 3 needle gauges. All 3 needle gauges accurately diagnosed all the benign lesions. This supports the findings of multiple other studies showing that the 14-gauge needle is the most reliable for accuracy of breast cancer diagnosis.

W.H. Hindle, M.D.

Analysis of Residual Cancer After Diagnostic Breast Biopsy: An Argument for Fine-needle Aspiration Cytology

Cox CE, Reintgen DS, Nicosia SV, et al (Univ of South Florida, Tampa)
Ann Surg Oncol 2:201–206, 1995   25–25

Background.—Technological advances and the range of treatment options have made breast biopsy a therapeutic challenge. For diagnostic breast biopsy, an effective strategy is needed to successfully treat the cancer by lumpectomy or mastectomy. Margin clearance is mandatory for local control. An analysis of residual cancer after diagnostic breast biopsy was reviewed.

Methods.—Eight hundred forty-four malignant diagnostic biopsy specimens were reviewed. Diagnostic breast biopsy was performed on all nonpalpable lesions, and fine-needle aspiration (FNA) was done on palpable lesions. Diagnostic biopsy was done when the FNA was equivocal. When diagnostic breast biopsy findings were positive, the biopsy cavity or FNA-positive mass was excised. Margins were confirmed using touch preparation cytology analysis and frozen section.

Findings.—Residual cancer was found at surgical excision in 52.3% of the 430 cases referred by outside institutions. At the study institution, 58% of the 169 nonpalpable lesions had residual tumor at resection (Fig 1). The 245 biopsies were done with FNA of palpable lesions. Five percent of these cases showed residual disease (Fig 2). Of 414 biopsies and FNA cytology done at the Moffitt Cancer Center, 111 (27%) of the specimens showed residual disease at the definitive procedure (Fig 3). Multifocal in situ

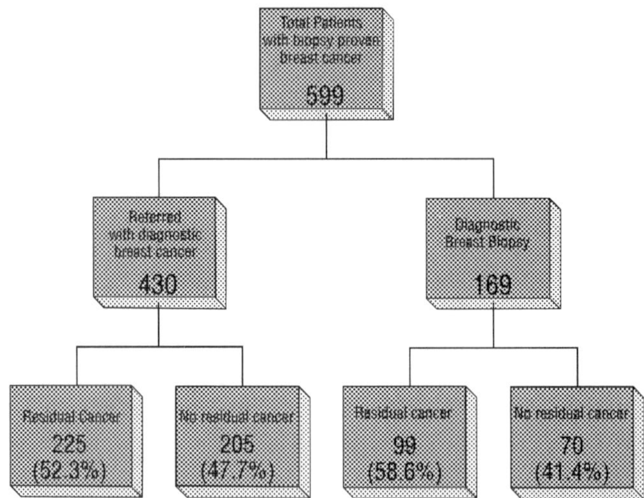

FIGURE 1.—Residual tumor after diagnostic breast biopsy, showing the number of patients who underwent diagnostic breast biopsies at referral institutions and at Moffitt Cancer Center. Represented are the number who had residual tumor at the time of definitive surgical excision. (Courtesy of Cox CE, Reintgen DS, Nicosia SV, et al: *Ann Surg Oncol* 2:201–206, 1995.)

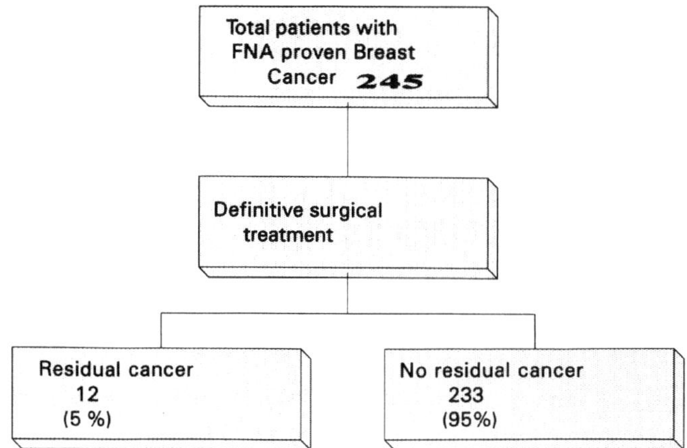

FIGURE 2.—Residual tumor after diagnostic fine-needle aspiration (*FNA*) cytology, demonstrating the number of patients who underwent diagnostic FNA who, on definitive surgical procedure, had residual tumor that required reexcision. (Courtesy of Cox CE, Reintgen DS, Nicosia SV, et al: *Ann Surg Oncol* 2:201–206, 1995.)

lesions and diffusely invasive carcinomas result in a more frequent incidence of residual disease left at the time of biopsy (Fig 4).

Conclusions.—More than half the patients undergoing diagnostic breast biopsy have residual breast cancer. Fine-needle aspiration should be done on all palpable masses. Diagnostic breast biopsy should be performed on

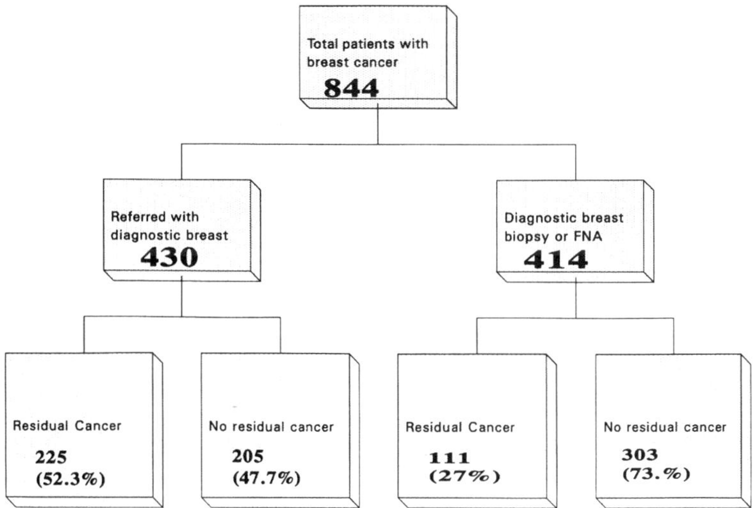

FIGURE 3.—Residual tumor after diagnostic fine-needle aspiration (*FNA*) and breast biopsy, showing the combined data from the entire series and representing all diagnostic procedures and their comparative rates of residual cancer at final operative intervention. (Courtesy of Cox, CE, Reintgen DS, Nicosia SV, et al: *Ann Surg Oncol* 2:201–206, 1995.)

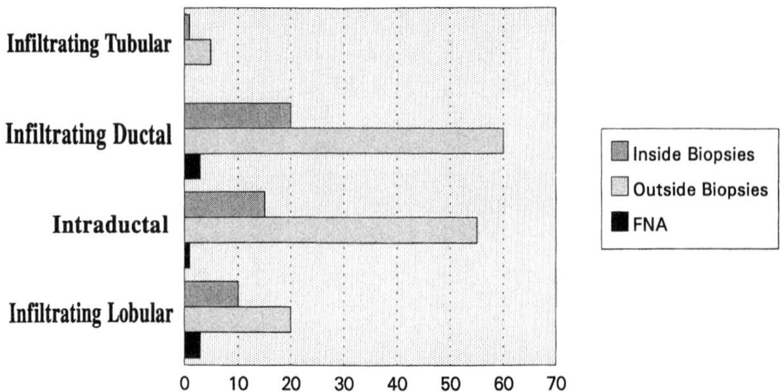

FIGURE 4.—Residual tumor: histologic comparison. Represented are the cases in which residual tumor was noted after biopsy and demonstrates that diffusely infiltrating or multifocal lesions result in a more frequent incidence of residual disease left behind at time of biopsy. *Abbreviation: FNA,* fine-needle aspiration. (Courtesy of Cox CE, Reintgen DS, Nicosia SV, et al: *Ann Surg Oncol* 2:201–206, 1995.)

nonpalpable masses. When cancer is diagnosed, surgical excision is indicated. When lumpectomy is an option, margins should be reexcised and assessed intraoperatively with touch preparation cytology analysis and frozen section when axillary dissection is done.

▶ In spite of precise protocols for lumpectomy as the excision biopsy procedure of choice, it is apparent from this report (and the experience of many breast centers) that less-than-optimal biopsies are often performed in clinical practice. Our policy at the Breast Diagnostic Center, Women's and Children's Hospital (Los Angeles) is to perform complete excision breast biopsies (lumpectomies) with grossly clear surgical margins and inking of the fresh tissue margins following the National Surgical Adjuvant Breast Project published surgical and pathologic protocol,[1] except when a specific cytologic diagnosis of fibroadenoma has been obtained by an adequate cellular sample of the mass obtained by FNA. If FNA cytology of the palpable breast mass is not available, then all excision breast biopsies should be performed in the same manner as lumpectomies for breast-conserving cancer therapy. Otherwise, a second breast operation for reexcision is necessary if the breast cancer patient desires breast-conserving therapy. In this day and age, incision biopsies are rarely, if ever, indicated, even for the histologic diagnosis of large (surgically unresectable) breast masses, when FNA and/or tissue core needle biopsy is readily available.

Wherever breast biopsies are performed, ongoing analysis and quality assurance, such as in this study, should be performed. All women with breast cancer deserve the acknowledged and appropriate diagnostic and therapeutic procedures.

W.H. Hindle, M.D.

Reference

1. Margolese R, Poisson R, Shibata H, et al: The technique of segmental mastectomy (lumpectomy) and axillary dissection: A syllabus from the National Surgical Adjuvant Breast Project workshops. *Surgery* 102:828–834, 1987.

Analysis of False Results in a Series of 835 Fine Needle Aspirates of Breast Lesions

Willis SL, Ramzy I (Baylor College of Medicine, Houston)
Acta Cytol 39:858–864, 1995   25–26

Background.—Although fine-needle aspiration (FNA) is cost-effective and highly accurate in the diagnosis of palpable breast lesions, it is also associated with a risk of erroneous diagnosis, especially false positive, which can lead to unnecessary mastectomy. The results of FNA of breast masses were reviewed in 1 series.

Methods.—The FNA results of 835 palpable breast lesions were reviewed. The reasons for false positive, false negative, and false suspicious diagnoses were determined. Five hundred forty-nine aspirates were negative, 174 were positive, and 66 were suspicious or atypical (Table 1). Tissue specimens from 286 patients were available for comparison. The cytologic/surgical pathology correlation and malignant cytodiagnosis data are shown in Tables 2 and 3, respectively.

Findings.—The cytologic diagnoses in these 286 cases were false positive in 0.8% and false negative in 13.2%. The 1 lesion erroneously diagnosed as positive was a case of fibrocystic change with hyperplasia, focal fat necrosis, and reparative atypia. Almost all 14 false negative cases involved sampling errors. Nine of these were infiltrating ductal carcinomas, 2 were ductal carcinomas in situ, 2 were infiltrating lobular carcinomas, and 1 was a tubular carcinoma. Thirty-five of the 50 suspicious and atypical lesions were found to be carcinomas (Table 4). The remaining 15 included 6 fibroadenomas; 4 cases of fibrocystic change; 2, gynecomastia; 2, adenosis; and 1, granulomatous mastitis.

Conclusions.—A positive FNA diagnosis of malignancy reliably establishes diagnosis and enables treatment planning in patients with breast lesions. In this study, the false positive rate was low. Most false negative diagnoses resulted from sampling difficulties rather than from interpretive problems.

▶ Continuing analysis of the sensitivity, specificity, and "false" reports of breast FNA cytology is essential quality assurance that should be performed by all cytology laboratories and institutions using FNA. Clinicians should be aware of the results of such continuing analyses both on the national level and at the particular cytology laboratory that processes and reports their FNAs. No diagnostic procedure is 100% reliable. Many of the "false negative" FNAs are related to slides with inadequate cellular material for cyto-

TABLE 1.—Distribution of Fine-Needle Aspiration (FNA)
Cytologic Diagnoses

	FNA cases (n = 835)	Tissue available (n = 286)
Positive	174	125
Suspicious	44	33
Atypical	22	18
Benign	549	92
Unsatisfactory	46	18

(Courtesy of Willis SL, Ramzy I: Analysis of false results in a series of 835 fine needle aspirates of breast lesion. *Acta Cytol* 39:858–864, 1995.)

TABLE 2.—Cytologic/Surgical Pathology Correlation

	Histologic diagnosis	
Cytodiagnosis	Malignant	Benign
Positive	124	1
Suspicious	26	7
Atypical	9	8
Benign	14	78
Unsatisfactory	4	14

(Courtesy of Willis SL, Ramzy I: Analysis of false results in a series of 835 fine needle aspirates of breast lesions. *Acta Cytol* 39:858–864, 1995.)

TABLE 3.—Malignant Cytodiagnosis

Diagnosis	No. of cases
Invasive ductal carcinoma	110
Mucinous carcinoma	4
Invasive lobular carcinomas	4
Papillary carcinomas	3
Ductal carcinoma in situ	2
Combined lobular/ductal carcinoma	1

(Courtesy of Willis SL, Ramzy I: Analysis of false results in a series of 835 fine needle aspirates of breast lesions. *Acta Cytol* 39:858–864, 1995.)

TABLE 4.—Histologic Diagnoses in Cases Cytologically Diagnosed
as Suspicious or Atypical

	Cytologic diagnosis	
Histologic diagnosis	Suspicious (n = 33)	Atypical (n = 17)
Carcinoma	26	9
Fibroadenoma	3	3
Gynecomastia	2	0
Sclerosing adenosis	1	1
Fibrocystic change	1	3
Granulomatous mastitis	0	1

(Courtesy of Willis SL, Ramzy I: Analysis of false results in a series of 835 fine needle aspirates of breast lesions. *Acta Cytol* 39:858–864, 1995.)

logic evaluation and clinicians should view "negative" reports as nondiagnostic. Furthermore, before making a tentative diagnosis and proceeding with further evaluation or treatment (including follow-up), clinicians should always consider the combined information gained from a breast-oriented history and the diagnostic triad of (1) clinical breast examination, (2) FNA, and (3) mammography.

W.H. Hindle, M.D.

A One-year Audit of Fine Needle Aspiration Cytology of Breast Lesions: Factors Affecting Adequacy and a Review of Delayed Carcinoma Diagnoses

Vural G, Hagmar B, Lilleng R (Norwegian Radium Hosp and Inst for Cancer Research, Oslo, Norway)
Acta Cytol 39:1233–1236, 1995   25–27

Background.—Fine-needle aspiration (FNA) cytology combined with clinical examination and imaging in triple-diagnosis breast clinics (TDBCs) increases the likelihood of an early diagnosis of cancer. However, several authors have reported significantly lower sensitivity when inexperienced or multiple aspirators obtain the aspirate, compared with cytopathologists or fully trained aspirators. The inadequacy rate of breast aspirates taken by cytopathologists was compared with that of aspirates taken by clinicians.

Methods.—A total of 2,923 specimens were reviewed, 1,515 of which were obtained in a TDBC. A cytologist aspirated palpable lesions, and a cytologist and radiologist aspirated nonpalpable lesions, using imaging techniques. The remaining specimens were aspirated by clinicians who sent them to the laboratory.

Findings.—The adequacy rate in the TDBC was 3.8%, compared with 14.8% mailed to the laboratory. Cancer was diagnosed in 395 women (13.5%). In 6 women, the diagnosis of carcinoma was delayed because of specimen inadequacy (Tables 1 and 2).

Conclusion.—The inadequacy rate of cytologic specimens obtained in a TDBC was lower than that of specimens mailed to the laboratory by

TABLE 1.—Number of Aspirations, According to Diagnosis

Diagnosis	No.	%
Benign	2,123	72.6
Suspicious	138	4.7
Malignant	395	13.5
Inadequate	267	9.1
Total	2,923	99.9

(Courtesy of Vural G, Hagmar B, Lilleng R: A one-year audit of fine needle aspiration cytology of breast lesions: Factors affecting adequacy and a review of delayed carcinoma diagnoses. *Acta Cytol* 39:1233–1236, 1995.)

TABLE 2.—Comparison of the Inadequacy Rate of Aspiration by Different Aspirators

Aspirator	Clinic	No. of aspirates	No. of inadequate specimens	%
Cytopathologist	TDBC	1,515	58	3.8
Surgeon	Private practice	543	45	8.2
Surgeon	Hospital	865	164	18.9
Total		2,923	267	9.3

(Courtesy of Vural G, Hagmar B, Lilleng R: A one-year audit of fine needle aspiration cytology of breast lesions: Factors affecting adequacy and a review of delayed carcinoma diagnoses. *Acta Cytol* 39:1233–1236, 1995.)

clinicians. Clinicians performing FNA cytology should be trained in aspiration technique and smear preparation to improve the detection rate of malignancies.

▶ This is a comparison of the application of the diagnostic triad—clinical breast examination, FNA, and mammography (herein called "triple diagnosis")—in a breast clinic with breast FNA specimens mailed in by multiple outside clinicians. Although the inadequacy rate of the outside FNA specimens was 14.8% compared with 3.8% in the breast clinic, the highest inadequacy rate (18.9%) was for hospital-based surgeons.

Taken alone, an inadequate FNA is nondiagnostic and does not defer further evaluation. The guiding principle of the clinical application of the diagnostic triad is the search for concordance of the findings of all 3 techniques. Such concordance can appropriately be the basis for clinical decisions and management. However, if the results of any 1 of the 3 techniques do not "fit" the clinical picture or if the physician or patient continues to be anxious about the conclusion of the diagnostic triad, then further diagnostic techniques—e.g., histologic diagnosis by tissue core needle biopsy or by surgical excision—are indicated and should be performed in a timely fashion (within 2 months but preferably sooner).

I prefer to emphasize that over 85% of the mailed-in FNA specimens were adequate and a cytologic diagnosis could be made. To me, FNA is a useful, efficient, and cost-effective diagnostic technique to have "at the examining table" where the woman with a palpable breast mass initially seeks medical care.

W.H. Hindle, M.D.

SUPPLEMENTARY PAPERS

Velanovich V: Fine-needle aspiration cytology in the diagnosis and management of ectopic breast tissue. *Am Surg* 61:277–278, 1995.
▶ A persistent dominant mass anywhere on the anatomical milk line can be ectopic breast tissue or a neoplasm. Fine-needle aspiration with an adequate cell sample gives a specific cytologic diagnosis for such a mass just as effectively and efficiently as fine-needle aspiration of a dominant mass within the breast. In this report, 63% of the fine-needle aspirations showed benign ductal epithelium consistent with ectopic breast tissue. All of the fine-needle aspirations showed

benign cellular material. There were no malignancies. The excision of the masses became elective after the reassurance of the reports. This was particularly helpful in the management of several women who were pregnant or lactating, time when elective breast surgery is best deferred.

W.H. Hindle, M.D.

Zalles C, Kimler BF, Kamel S, et al: Cytology patterns in random aspirates from women at high and low risk for breast cancer. *Breast J* 1:343–349, 1995.

▶ This study from the University of Kansas Cancer Center, which includes 263 women judged at high risk of developing breast cancer and 30 low-risk volunteers, represents an extension of the indications and use of breast fine-needle aspiration. For practicing clinicians, the indication for breast fine-needle aspiration is a persistent palpable dominant breast mass. However, in this report the random fine-needle aspirations of both breasts demonstrate the potential of fine-needle aspirations performed and analyzed in a dedicated cytopathology center. As with the histologic finding of atypical epithelial hyperplasia (with associated clinically meaningful increased risk of developing breast cancer) in tissue from a surgical breast biopsy specimen, the current recommendation continues to be routine periodic surveillance with clinical breast examination and mammography.

W.H. Hindle, M.D.

A Novel Diagnostic Index for Use in the Breast Clinic

Purasiri P, Abdalla M, Heys SD, et al (Univ of Aberdeen, Scotland)
J R Coll Surg Edinb 41:30–34, 1996   25–28

Background.—In specialist breast centers, benign and malignant lesions can be accurately diagnosed based on information from clinical assessments combined with mammography and/or fine-needle aspiration (FNA) cytology, obviating the need for formal biopsy and histologic evaluation. The diagnostic accuracy of "quadruple assessment"—clinical assessment, mammography, ultrasonography (US), and FNA cytology—was determined retrospectively in patients with solid breast lesions at the Professorial Breast Clinic at Aberdeen Royal Infirmary.

TABLE 1.—Diagnostic Accuracy of Each Modality

Tests	Sensitivity (%)	Specificity (%)	Prediction (%)
Examination (*n* =603)	76	86	81.6
Mammography (*n* = 516)	88	73	80.6
FNA cytology (*n* = 533)	87	98	92.6
Ultrasound (*n* = 123)	70	79	75.6

(Courtesy of Purasiri P, Abdalla M, Heys SD, et al: A novel diagnostic index for use in the breast clinic. *J R Coll Surg Edinb* 41:30–34, 1996. Publisher, Blackwell Science Ltd.)

Methods and Findings.—Six hundred three patients attended the clinic between January 1989 and September 1992. The highest overall prediction of malignancy—92.6%—was achieved with FNA cytology, with a sensitivity of 87% and a specificity of 98%. The lowest correct overall prediction, at 75.6%, was associated with US, with a sensitivity and specificity of 70% and 79%, respectively. A stepwise logistic discriminant analysis, including all available findings and patient age, was used to derive a mathematical equation to serve as a novel diagnostic index. Weighted scores derived from each variable in the equation predicted the likelihood of malignancy in more than 90% of patients of different ages. Discriminant analysis correctly predicted the diagnosis in 98% of women younger than 35 years.

Conclusion.—Clinical, mammographic, US, and FNA cytology findings can be used to establish the likely diagnosis in most women the same day they visit a breast clinic (Table 1). The diagnostic index, which is currently being studied prospectively, may further help establish a correct diagnosis.

▶ This report utilizes the diagnostic triad of clinical impression (by history and standardized examination), FNA, and mammographic impression with the subsequent addition of US impression. The authors call this "quadruple assessment." With the added datum of the patient's age, stepwise logistic discriminant analysis was applied and an age-related diagnostic index (probability score) produced.

As this was a retrospective study, the authors have now embarked on a prospective study of this diagnostic index. In their outpatient facility, this complete breast evaluation and diagnosis is performed during a single patient visit. Such a comprehensive breast evaluation is efficient, cost effective, and satisfying for both the clinician and the patient. This logistic (single visit) model is probably the ideal for optimum breast health care. Confirmation of the clinical reliability of the diagnostic index awaits further study and replication by similar breast centers.

W.H. Hindle, M.D.

Stereotactic Fine-needle Aspiration Biopsy for the Evaluation of Non-palpable Breast Lesions: Report of an Experience Based on 2,988 Cases
Mitnick JS, Vazquez MF, Pressman PI, et al (New York Univ; Beth Israel Med Ctr, New York)
Ann Surg Oncol 3:185–191, 1996   25–29

Background.—Stereotactic fine-needle aspiration biopsy (SFNB) appears to be a promising technique for the diagnosis of nonpalpable breast lesions detected by mammography. However, some reports question the diagnostic reliability of SFNB and its place in the integrated approach to diagnosis of clinically occult mammographic lesions. The reliability of SFNB was evaluated in a large series of patients with clinically occult breast lesions.

TABLE 1.—Mammographic Characteristics Evaluated by Stereotactic Fine-
Needle Aspiration Biopsy

Spiculated densities	477
Nodules	751
Focal asymmetric densities	603
Architectural distortion or	
prominent trabecular markings	694
Clustered microcalcifications	463

Note: N = 2,988
(Courtesy of Mitnick JS, Vazquez MF, Pressman PI, et al: Stereotactic fine-needle aspiration biopsy
for the evaluation of nonpalpable breast lesions: Report of an experience based on 2,988 cases. *Ann
Surg Oncol* 3:185–191, 1996.)

Methods.—The study included 2,988 consecutive patients with mammographically detected nonpalpable breast lesions (Table 1). All underwent SFNB by a previously described technique. If the cytologic results were malignant, suspicious, or atypical, surgical excision with definitive histologic diagnosis was performed. If the cytologic results were benign, the patients were managed with follow-up mammography or surgical biopsy.

Results.—Stereotactic fine-needle aspiration biopsy indicated malignancy in 295 lesions. In 99% of these cases, the diagnosis was confirmed by histopathologic examination (Table 2). Of 22 lesions diagnosed as suspicious on SFNB, all proved to be malignant. Seventy lesions were diagnosed as showing cytologic atypia on SFNB, 61% of which were histopathologically malignant. The correspondence of lesions diagnosed as benign by SFNB and histopathology is shown in Table 4. The rate of false negative aspirates was 0.6%. Sensitivity was 94.6%, specificity was 99.8%, and diagnostic efficiency was 99.3% (Table 8).

Conclusion.—The accuracy of SFNB in diagnosing carcinoma in mammographically detected, nonpalpable breast lesions was demonstrated. If the cytologic results indicate atypia, surgical biopsy is essential. Patients whose lesions are diagnosed as benign on SFNB must receive frequent mammographic follow-up. The high accuracy of SFNB can eliminate the

TABLE 2.—Correspondence of Malignant Suspicious and Atypical
Cytology With Histopathology

	Histopathology		
SFNB	Malignant	Benign	Total
Malignant	291	4	295
Suspicious	22	0	22
Atypical	43	27	70

Note: N = 387
Abbreviation: SFNB, stereotactic fine-needle aspiration biopsy.
(Courtesy of Mitnick JS, Vazquez MF, Pressman PI, et al: Stereotactic fine-needle aspiration biopsy
for the evaluation of nonpalpable breast lesions: Report of an experience based on 2,988 cases. *Ann
Surg Oncol* 3:185–191, 1996.)

TABLE 4.—Correspondence of Benign Cytology and Histopathology

| | Histopathology | | |
Immediate surgical biopsy	Benign	Malignant	Total
Mammographically suspicious	0	5	5
Patient/physician preference	661	0	661
Interval change	0	13	13
No change	—	—	1,922

Note: $N = 2,601$
(Courtesy of Mitnick JS, Vazquez MF, Pressman PI, et al: Stereotactic fine-needle aspiration biopsy for the evaluation of nonpalpable breast lesions: Report of an experience based on 2,988 cases. *Ann Surg Oncol* 3:185–191, 1996.)

need for excision of benign lesions in most cases, although it is essential to be aware of the potential pitfalls of this technique.

▶ In selected centers with a large volume of nonpalpable breast lesions and dedicated mammographers and cytopathologists working harmoniously together, SFNB has acceptable specificity and sensitivity with clinically reliable accuracy of the cytologic diagnoses compared with tissue histology diagnoses. This report is from such a center in New York. A few similar studies are reported from Europe. However, in the United States, tissue core needle biopsy (TCNB) of nonpalpable breast lesions has become more popular and is becoming the standard of care. With either diagnostic technique (SFNB or TCNB), ongoing quality assurance with comparison to the final histologic diagnosis is imperative. In addition, continuing surveillance and follow-up of every case investigated is essential.

Some authors think that even 1% false positive or false negative results are unacceptable. However, with all diagnostic techniques regarding biological processes—e.g., atypia or malignancy—there are occasional "failures" and exceptions. Particularly with breast lesions, comprehensive quality assurance programs and rigorous continuous follow-up are required. The application and continuation of diagnostic procedures (and treatment protocols) should be based on documented results and long-term outcome data.

W.H. Hindle, M.D.

TABLE 8.—Stereotactic Aspiration Biopsy of Nonpalpable Breast Lesions

$$\text{Sensitivity} \quad \frac{TP}{TP + FN} \times 100 = 94.6\%$$

$$\text{Specificity} \quad \frac{TN}{TN + FP} \times 100 = 99.8\%$$

$$\text{Efficiency} \quad \frac{TN + TP}{TP + FP + TN + FN} \times 100 = 99.3\%$$

Abbreviations: TP, true positive; *FN*, false negative; *FP*, false positive; *TN*, true negative.
(Courtesy of Mitnick JS, Vazquez MF, Pressman PI, et al: Stereotactic fine-needle aspiration biopsy for the evaluation of nonpalpable breast lesions: Report of an experience based on 2,988 cases. *Ann Surg Oncol* 3:185–191, 1996.)

Non-operative Management of Breast Masses Diagnosed as Fibroadenoma

Cant PJ, Madden MV, Coleman MG, et al (Univ of Cape Town, South Africa; Groote Schuur Hosp, Cape Town, South Africa)
Br J Surg 82:792–794, 1995   25–30

Introduction.—If benign disease is confirmed by cytologic examination, and strict clinical criteria are met, fibroadenomas of the breast in young women can be managed without surgery. The natural history of the outcome of this approach has been inconclusive. Patient satisfaction and the behavior of these lesions were reviewed.

Methods.—Ninety-nine women with 279 breast masses that were diagnosed as fibroadenomas were followed up for 7–9 years. Sixty-six of the patients elected to forego surgery because their benign masses were solid, well defined, painless, and mobile and the patients were younger than 25 years of age and had no family history of breast cancer.

Results.—Seventy-three masses were excised from 28 patients. The median duration of conservative treatment was 31 months. A total of 107 masses, 72% of those not lost to follow-up, resolved. The average time to resolution was 61 months. Masses persisted in 28% of those not lost to follow-up. The survival curve extrapolated to zero was about 15 years. Resolution occurred earlier in younger women. The probability of disappearance was 0.46 at 5 years and 0.69 at 9 years. The resolution rate was no different between single or multiple lesions or large and small lesions.

Conclusion.—Conservative management of fibroadenomas is a safe therapeutic direction. Nearly half the patients will experience resolution in 5 years.

▶ This study confirms the clinical conclusions of Sainsbury et al.,[1] Smallwood et al.,[2] and Wilkinson et al.[3] that breast fibroadenomas diagnosed by fine-needle aspiration cytology can be followed (or electively excised) and often diminish in size or even become nonpalpable. Careful surveillance and patient compliance are required for this "conservative" clinical approach. The clinician must be mindful of the possible confusion in cytologic diagnosis of fibroadenoma vs. phyllodes tumors and the rare occurrence of carcinoma within a fibroadenoma.[4] My clinical experience is similar to that of the authors in that many women, over time, decide to have "benign" breast lumps removed. However, they can do so at their convenience and without (or with limited) interval anxiety as to the possibility of cancer in that specific breast mass. Our policy at the Breast Diagnostic Center at Women's and Children's Hospital (Los Angeles) is to offer women with cytologically diagnosed fibroadenomas elective excision to be performed at a time of their convenience or, alternatively, 6 months of follow-up. In addition, the patient is instructed to perform regular monthly breast self-examinations and, if the mass under surveillance increases in size (or becomes otherwise symptomatic), to return for reevaluation as soon as possible.

W.H. Hindle, M.D.

References

1. Sainsbury JRC, Nicholson S, Needham GK, et al: Natural history of the benign breast lump. *Br J Surg* 75:1080–1082, 1988.
2. Smallwood JA, Roberts A, Guyer DP, et al: The natural history of fibroadenomas. *Br J Clin Pract* 56:86–87, 1988.
3. Wilkinson S, Anderson TJ, Rifkind E, et al: Fibroadenoma of the breast: A follow-up of conservative management. *Br J Surg* 76:390–391, 1989.
4. Yoshida Y, Takaoka M, Fukumoto M: Carcinoma arising in fibroadenomas. *J Surg Oncol* 29:132–140, 1985.

Assessment of the Acceptability of Conservative Management of Fibroadenoma of the Breast

Dixon JM, Dobie V, Lamb J, et al (Western Gen Hosp, Edinburgh, Scotland)
Br J Surg 83:264–265, 1996
25–31

Background.—Fibroadenomas, thought to be aberrations of normal development rather than true neoplasms, are benign breast lesions, that have traditionally been excised. However, such routine excision is being questioned. Conservative management would be appropriate if these lesions can be diagnosed accurately by noninvasive procedures, if their natural history is well defined, and if a conservative approach is acceptable to patients.

Patients and Findings.—Two hundred two women younger than 40 years of age with a total of 219 fibroadenomas were studied prospectively (Tables 1 and 2). A combination of clinical examination, ultrasonography, and fine-needle aspiration cytology was performed. Patients were asked to choose between excision and conservative management with regular ultrasound monitoring. Excision was chosen by 16 patients with 18 lesions, all of which were histologically confirmed as fibroadenomas. One hundred fifty-two patients with 163 lesions were observed for 2 years or more. Thirteen fibroadenomas in this group grew significantly. All these lesions were subsequently excised and histologically confirmed as fibroadenomas. Nineteen lesions significantly decreased in size, and another 42 lesions resolved. The other 89 lesions showed no size changes.

TABLE 1.—Age Distribution of Patients

Age (years)	Number of patients
< 20	25
20–29	116
30–39	53
> 39	8
Total	202

(Courtesy of Dixon JM, Dobie V, Lamb J, et al: Assessment of the acceptability of conservative management of fibroadenoma of the breast. *Br J Surg* 83:264–265, 1996.)

TABLE 2.—Maximum Clinical Size of Fibroadenoma

Size (cm)	Number of patients
< 1·0	22
1·0–1·9	116
2·0–2·9	66
3·0–4·0	15

(Courtesy of Dixon JM, Dobie V, Lamb J, et al: Assessment of the acceptability of conservative management of fibroadenoma of the breast. *Br J Surg* 83:264–265, 1996.)

Conclusions.—Conservative management of fibroadenomas in women younger than 40 years appears to be safe. During a 2-year period, less than 1 in 10 of all fibroadenomas grew, and more than one third became smaller or resolved. This approach is also acceptable to most patients.

▶ Our English colleagues have courageously followed up on diagnosed breast fibroadenomas and provided us with data about the biological behavior, natural history, and clinical course of these benign tumors. Serial mammography has demonstrated that many women have what appear to be nonpalpable fibroadenomas which, if followed up, tend to decrease in size in the later reproductive years of a woman's life. They often then eventually calcify into a characteristic "popcorn" pattern. In this study with a minimum 2-year follow-up, 8% of the fibroadenomas increased in size and were surgically excised with histologic confirmation of the diagnosis. The concurrence of the diagnostic triad of (1) clinical breast examination, (2) mammography (augmented by focused ultrasound evaluation in this study), and (3) fine-needle aspiration allows the conservative management (continuing follow-up) of breast fibroadenomas in clinical practice.

In my practice, over time, many patients with cytologically diagnosed fibroadenomas eventually elected to have surgical excision of their lesions at a time of their convenience and without undue worry as to the possibility of a breast cancer. Published data support the option of a choice of management for women with cytologically diagnosed (by fine-needle aspiration) breast fibroadenomas.

W.H. Hindle, M.D.

SUPPLEMENTARY PAPERS

Hunter TB, Roberts CC, Hunt R, et al: Occurrence of fibroadenomas in postmenopausal women referred for breast biopsy. *J Am Geriatr Soc* 44:61–64, 1996.
▶ This report from the University of Arizona Health Sciences Center (Tucson) is a retrospective review of 709 consecutive (1985–1990) breast biopsies, of which 100 proved to be fibroadenomas by histologic evaluation. Forty-four percent of the women with histologically diagnosed fibroadenomas were postmenopausal. Twenty percent of all the excised benign masses were fibroadenomas in postmenopausal women. Fibroadenomas constituted 12% of all the biopsied breast masses in postmenopausal women.

W.H. Hindle, M.D.

Silicone Breast Implants and the Risk of Connective-tissue Diseases and Symptoms

Sánchez-Guerrero J, Colditz GA, Karlson EW, et al (Harvard Med School, Boston; Brigham and Women's Hosp, Boston)
N Engl J Med 332:1666–1670, 1995   25–32

Introduction.—More than a million women in the United States have received silicone breast implants in the past 3 decades, either for reconstruction after removal of breast cancer or often prophylactic mastectomy, or for cosmetic reasons. Approximately 300 implant-bearing women with connective tissue disease or rheumatic disease have been reported in the English-language literature since 1982. In addition, numerous cases have been reported in abstract form.

Objective.—The relationship between silicone breast implants and connective tissue disease was examined in follow-up data from the Nurses' Health Study cohort, which included married female registered nurses 30 to 55 years of age.

Findings.—A definite diagnosis of connective tissue disease was made in 516 of 87,501 eligible women. Breast implants were present in 1,183 participants; most implants were filled with silicone gel (Table 1). Three women with implants had rheumatoid arthritis during an average follow-up of 10 years (Table 2). One each had a silicone gel–filled, a saline-

TABLE 1.—Breast Implant Surgery in 1,183 Women From the Nurses' Health Study

Variable	No. of Women (%)
Indication	
Cosmetic reasons	587 (50)
Cancer	387 (33)
Prophylaxis	138 (12)
Unknown	71 (6)
Type	
Silicone-gel-filled	876 (74)
Saline-filled	170 (14)
Double-lumen	67 (6)
Polyurethane-coated	14 (1)
Unknown	56 (5)
No. of operations*	
1	911
2	191
3	52
4	29
Side	
Unilateral	224 (19)
Right	112
Left	112
Bilateral	937 (79)
Unknown	22 (2)

*Each operation was counted as 1, irrespective of whether a bilateral operation was performed.
(Reprinted by permission of *The New England Journal of Medicine* from Sánchez-Guerrero J, Colditz GA, Karlson EW, et al: Silicone breast implants and the risk of connective-tissue diseases and symptoms. *N Engl J Med* 332:1666–1670, Copyright 1995, Massachusetts Medical Society.)

TABLE 2.—Age-Adjusted Relative Risk of Connective Tissue Disease Among Women With Breast Implants as Compared With Women Without Implants

| | | BREAST IMPLANT | |
| | NO IMPLANT | ANY TYPE | SILICONE-GEL-FILLED* |
CASE TYPE	(N=86.318)	(N = 1183)	(N = 876)
Self-reported connective-tissue disease			
No. of cases	5054	32	21
Age-adjusted relative risk	1.0	0.7	0.6
95% Confidence interval		0.5–1.0	0.4–0.9
Self-reported signs or symptoms of connective-tissue disease†			
No. of cases	1277	17	11
Age-adjusted relative risk	1.0	1.5	1.2
95% Confidence interval		0.94–0.24	0.7–2.2
Documented signs or symptoms of connective-tissue disease‡			
No. of cases	898	6	4
Age-adjusted relative risk	1.0	0.7	0.6
95% Confidence interval		0.3–1.6	0.2–1.6
Definitive Connective-tissue disease			
No. of cases	513	3	1
Age-adjusted relative risk	1.0	0.6	0.3
95% Confidence interval		0.2–2.0	0.0–1.9
Duration of implant			
Mean (±SD) yr		9.9±6.4	10.0±6.2
Range		1 mo–40.5 yr	1 mo–37.5 yr

*This category is a subgroup of "any type" of implant.

†The signs and symptoms are those included in the screening questionnaires on connective tissue disease.

‡Data were derived from the medical record review. Documented signs and symptoms included proximal weakness, high creatine kinase concentration, positive electromyogram, positive muscle biopsy, proximal scleroderma, sclerodactyly, digital scars, bibasilar lung fibrosis, malar or discoid rash, photosensitivity, nasopharyngeal ulcers, nonerosive arthritis, pleuritis, pericarditis, proteinuria, renal casts, seizures, psychosis, hemolytic anemia, leukopenia, lymphopenia, thrombocytopenia, positive test for lupus erythematosus, antibodies to double-stranded DNA, biological false positive serologic test for syphilis, positive test for anticardiolipin antibody, positive antinuclear-antibody test, Raynaud's phenomenon, morning stiffness for more than 1 hour, arthritis in 3 or more joint areas, arthritis in hand joints, rheumatoid nodules, positive rheumatoid-factor tests, radiographic changes characteristic of rheumatoid arthritis, keratoconjunctivitis, xerostomia, salivary-gland biopsy positive for Sjögren's syndrome, and anti-Ro, anti-La, anti-extractable-nuclear-antigen, and anti-U1-RNP antibodies.

(Reprinted by permission of *The New England Journal of Medicine* from Sánchez-Guerrero J, Colditz GA, Karlson EW, et al: Silicone breast implants and the risk of connective-tissue diseases and symptoms. *N Engl J Med* 332:1666–1670, Copyright 1995, Massachusetts Medical Society.)

filled, and a double-lumen implant. The age-adjusted relative risk of definite connective tissue disease being diagnosed in women with implants of any type was 0.6, and for those with silicone gel–filled implants, 0.3 (Table 3). When women with possible early, mild, or atypical connective tissue disease and those having any symptom or sign of such disease were considered, the age-adjusted relative risk for those with breast implants was 0.7.

Conclusion.—This large cohort gives no evidence of a significant association between silicone breast implants and connective tissue disease.

► With time and perspective, the specter of autoimmune diseases as a direct complication of silicone breast implants has faded and proved to be without valid scientific basis. This is not to say that a given woman may not have a particular sensitivity to silicone, either in the form of an intact breast

TABLE 3.—Incidence Rates of Connective Tissue Diseases in the Nurses' Health Study (1976 to 1990)

NURSES' HEALTH STUDY

DISEASE	NO. OF CASES	INCIDENCE RATE*	INCIDENCE RANGE IN OTHER STUDIES†
Rheumatoid arthritis	392	33.2	24–50
Systemic lupus erythematosus	96	8.1	1.8–7.6
Scleroderma	14	1.2	0.4–1.9
Polymyositis or dermatomyositis	12	1.0	0.5–1.1
Sjögren's syndrome	2	—	—
Mixed connective-tissue disease	0	—	—
Any connective-tissue disease	516	43.68	—

*Rates per 100,000 person-years.
†Range of incidence rates reported in 10 other studies.
(Reprinted by permission of *The New England Journal of Medicine* from Sánchez-Guerrero J, Colditz GA, Karlson EW, et al: Silicone breast implants and the risk of connective-tissue diseases and symptoms. *N Engl J Med* 332:1666–1670, Copyright 1995, Massachusetts Medical Society.)

prosthesis or leakage of silicone therefrom. These updated data from the statistically impressive Harvard Nurses' Health Study are reinforced by the findings of the United Kingdom's Department of Health's Medical Devices Agency and the Ministere des Affaires Sociales de la Sante et de la Ville (France) reports and actions. Both found no convincing medical evidence of increased risk of connective tissue disease associated with the use of silicone breast implants. Thus, the European Committee on Quality Assurance and Medical Devices in Plastic Surgery states that all moratoriums on the use of silicone-filled breast implants have been lifted and that silicone breast implants are now readily available throughout Europe. However, in all probability, the American legal courts (and involved attorneys) will continue their deliberations on the massive settlements (more than 4 billion dollars) currently being considered. Unfortunately, it is unlikely that the Food and Drug Administration will lift the restrictions on the use of silicone breast implants in the United States within the foreseeable future.

W.H. Hindle, M.D.

SUPPLEMENTAL PAPERS

Göksoy E, Düren M, Durgun V, et al: Tuberculosis of the breast. *Eur J Surg* 161:471–473, 1995.
▶ This additional report from Istanbul, Turkey, covers 9 women with tuberculosis of the breast who presented over a 20-year period. The presence of tubercle and central caseation was demonstrated in 8 of the 9 cases. Persistent sinuses and abscesses were the typical clinical manifestations. In Turkey, 4.9% of all mastitis is caused by tuberculosis. In this series, the patient typically had prior attempts of surgical drainage or sinus resection. When performed, fine-needle aspiration

revealed caseation with granuloma formation or necrotic debris. Except for 1 case that required mastectomy for eradication of the disease, after medical antituberculosis therapy, all cases responded to lumpectomy resection.

W.H. Hindle, M.D.

Shinde SR, Chandawarkar RY, Deshmukh SP: Tuberculosis of the breast masquerading as carcinoma: A study of 100 patients. *World J Surg* 19:379–381, 1995.
▶ This report from Bombay, India, highlights an entity that is now being seen in the United States border states and in areas where large numbers of immigrants seek medical care. The most common presentation in this study was a breast mass, with or without skin ulceration. One third of the patients had palpable axillary lymphadenopathy. Pretherapeutic pathologic confirmation was obtained by mammography (14%), fine-needle aspiration (12%), and excision biopsy (60%). Acid-fast bacilli were demonstrated in only 12% of the patients. Simple mastectomy was required for definitive therapy in 14% of the women. With a minimum of 2 years of follow-up, all treated patients remained free of disease. Tuberculosis of the breast can mimic fibroadenoma, carcinoma, or fibrocystic mastitis.

W.H. Hindle, M.D.

Solid Breast Nodules: Use of Sonography to Distinguish Between Benign and Malignant Lesions
Stavros AT, Thickman D, Rapp CL, et al (Radiology Imaging Associates, Englewood, Colo)
Radiology 196:123–134, 1995   25–33

Background.—The considerable overlap between the characteristics of benign and malignant breast lesions that was found in previous studies of sonography prompted some investigators to recommend sonography only for determining whether a lesion is cystic or solid or for needle guidance. Some have recommended that biopsies be performed on all solid nodules, regardless of their sonographic appearance. Since the publication of these initial sonographic studies, the near-field imaging ability of sonographic equipment has improved greatly. Thus, the questions of whether sonography could accurately distinguish benign solid breast nodules from indeterminate or malignant nodules and whether the findings were definite enough to obviate the need for biopsy were reexamined.

Methods.—Seven hundred fifty sonographically solid breast nodules were classified prospectively as benign, indeterminate, or malignant. Benign nodules had no malignant features. They had either intense homogenous hyperechogenicity or a thin echogenic pseudocapsule with an ellipsoid shape or fewer than 4 gentle lobulations. Sonographic determinations were compared with biopsy findings.

Results.—Eighty-three percent of the lesions had benign histologic features, and 17% had malignant histologic features. Four hundred twenty-four benign lesions had been prospectively classified as benign. At biopsy, 2 lesions classified as benign were found to be malignant. Thus, the negative predictive value of this classification scheme was 99.5%. Of 125 malignant lesions, 123 were classified correctly as indeterminate or malignant, for a sensitivity of 98.4%.

Conclusions.—Sonography is useful in characterizing some solid breast masses, improving the specificity of diagnosis for most malignant and benign solid breast nodules. These results were achieved through valid targeted indications, excellent sonographic technique, optimal machine and transducer characteristics, and strict adherence to the criteria, which rely on the absence of any malignant feature, for a benign lesion.

▶ Although the Europeans, particularly the French, have aggressively expanded the indications and use of breast ultrasound, the accepted role of ultrasound in the United States is as an adjunct to mammography. Ultrasound is as effective in the breast as in the ovary for discriminating a cyst from a solid mass. Ultrasound is also gaining popularity for tissue core needle ultrasound-directed biopsy of breast lesions, particularly mammographically detected nonpalpable lesions. This study extends the use of ultrasound to aid in distinguishing between benign and malignant solid breast lesions.

The reported risk of 1 "false negative" cancer per 212 ultrasonographically benign lesions ($r = 1{:}212$) is clinically acceptable. The alternative would be to biopsy all the mammographically detected lesions. In this age of managed care, cost-effectiveness alone would seem to preclude the latter alternative.

W.H. Hindle, M.D.

Influences of Percutaneous Administration of Estradiol and Progesterone on Human Breast Epithelial Cell Cycle In Vivo
Chang K-J, Fournier S, Lee TTY, et al (Natl Taiwan Univ, Taipei; Hopital Saint-Louis, Paris)
Fertil Steril 63:785–791, 1995   25–34

Objective.—A randomized, double-blind trial was carried out in 40 normally cycling premenopausal women 18–45 years of age who had not used estrogen or progestin in the past 2 months and who underwent removal of a suspicious breast lump. The goal was to compare the effects of estradiol (E_2) and progesterone (P) on the epithelial cell cycle of normal breast tissue in vivo.

Methods.—A hydroalcoholic gel containing placebo, 25 mg of P, 1.5 mg of E_2, or both hormones was applied daily to the breast to be operated on starting on the first day of a menstrual cycle and continuing for 11–13 days before surgery was performed.

Results.—Plasma P levels remained low in all treatment groups, but estrogen-treated patients had consistently higher plasma E_2 levels. Tissue levels of both hormones were higher in women treated with the respective hormones. Mitotic indices were significantly lower in P-treated patients than in placebo recipients and significantly higher in patients treated with

E_2. Analogous findings were obtained when estimating the proliferating cell nuclear antigen (cyclin) labeling index.

Implication.—Progesterone and related agents may help prevent hyperplastic changes in the breast epithelium through countering E_2-induced cell proliferation.

▶ The endocrinology of the human female breast is species- and site-specific. Studies of cellular hormonal responses in vitro and in vivo are variable and may not support the same conclusions. The responses of benign and malignant cells may be distinctly different. Furthermore, if the appealing concept is correct that carcinogenesis of the human female breast begins at puberty when the male and female breast tissues differentiate, short-term changes in hormonal status may have minimal, if any, impact on the long-term potential malignant transformation of the ductal epithelium. In addition, the slow growth of most human breast cancers over time, e.g., 7–10 years before the tumor is clinically evident, complicates the clinical application of short-term data.

In this study, the application of estrogen and/or P directly to the skin of the breast for fewer than 2 weeks resulted in measurable changes in the epithelial cell cycle and mitotic activity. The precise details of the methodology and techniques of such studies are critical to their evaluation. Standardized measurements for "normal" and malignant tissues are rarely available. The technology for making such measurements seems to change every year.

The results from this carefully structured study using current methodology appear to conflict with those from the work of Ferguson and Anderson,[1, 2] published in 1981 and 1982, which demonstrated the highest mitotic activity in the untreated human female breast glandular cells to be during the late luteal phase when P is "dominant" in the menstrual cycle. Even though the methodology and results of this new study appear valid, clinical application of the findings must await further research.

W.H. Hindle, M.D.

References

1. Ferguson DJP, Anderson TJ: Morphological evaluation of cell turnover in relation to menstrual cycle in the "resting" human breast. *Br J Cancer* 44:177–191, 1981.
2. Anderson TJ, Ferguson DJP, Rabb GM: Cell turnover in the "resting" human breast: Influence of parity, contraceptive pill, age and laterality. *Br J Cancer* 46:376–382, 1982.

Effects of Hormone Replacement Therapy on the Mammary Gland of Surgically Postmenopausal Cynomolgus Macaques

Cline JM, Soderqvist G, von Schoultz E, et al (Wake Forest Univ, Winston-Salem, NC; Karolinska Hosp, Stockholm)
Am J Obstet Gynecol 174:93–100, 1996   25–35

Background.—Research has shown that postmenopausal estrogen replacement prevents coronary heart disease and osteoporosis, but the public health benefits of such treatment have not been achieved. Concern about the risk of breast cancer is the main reason why American women do not use hormone replacement therapy. The mechanism underlying the increased risk of breast cancer in long-term current hormone replacement treatment users is unknown. The proliferative response and receptor status in the mammary glands of surgically postmenopausal macaques given hormone replacement therapy were investigated.

Methods.—Twenty-six macaques were given no treatment; 22, conjugated equine estrogens (CEE); and 21, combined CEE and medroxyprogesterone acetate (MPA).The drugs were given in doses equivalent on a caloric basis to 0.625 mg per woman per day for CEEs and 2.5 mg per woman per day for MPA. The trial lasted 30 months.

Findings.—Combined CEE and MPA treatment resulted in greater proliferation than CEE alone. In animals given combined treatment, the percentage of estrogen receptor–positive cells was reduced. Treatment with

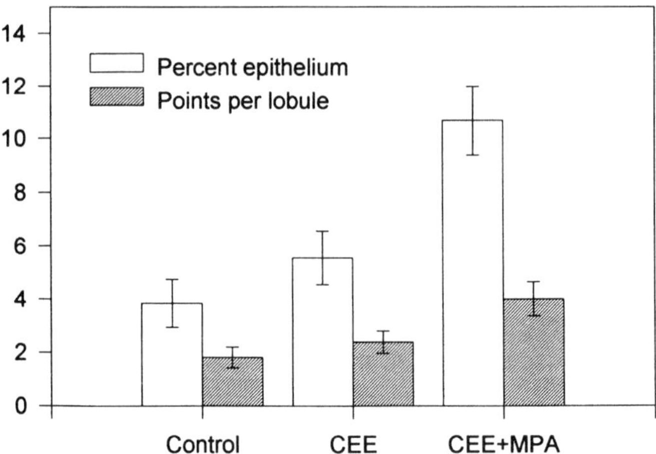

FIGURE 2.—Point-counting measurements of ± SEM of epithelium relative to stroma and number of points counted per lobule in the mammary gland of macaques. Both measures indicate glandular hyperplasia in the conjugated equine estrogens (*CEE*) plus medroxyprogesterone acetate (*MPA*) group. For percent epithelium, the CEE plus MPA group differs from the CEE group ($P < 0.05$) and from controls ($P < 0.0001$). For points per lobule, both CEE-treated ($P < 0.05$) and CEE plus MPA-treated animals ($P = 0.0007$) differed from controls respectively) but did not differ from each other. (Courtesy of Cline JM, Soderqvist G, von Schoultz E, et al: Effects of hormone replacement therapy on the mammary gland of surgically postmenopausal cynomolgus macaques. *Am J Obstet Gynecol* 174:93–100, 1996.)

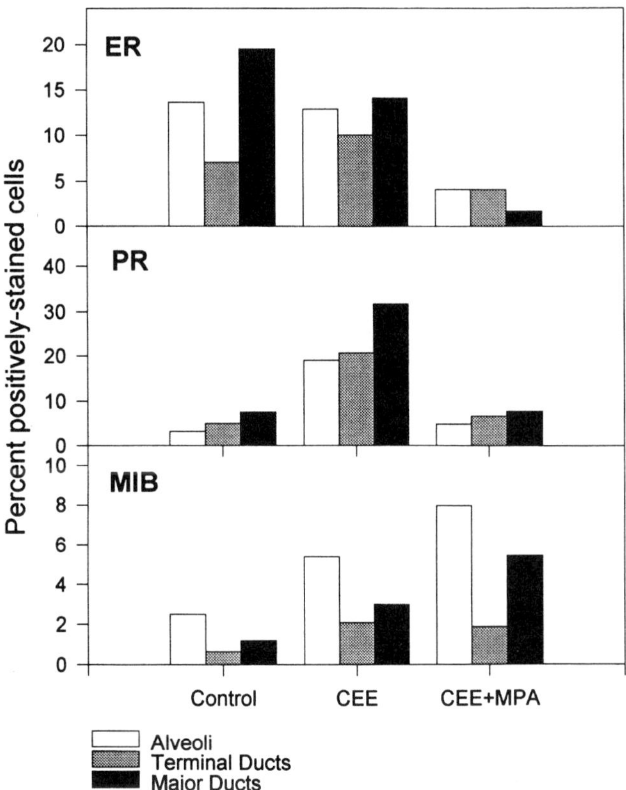

FIGURE 3.—Immunostaining of mammary epithelial cells. The MIB-1 labeling is increased in both treatment groups, most notably in the conjugated equine estrogens (*CEE*) plus medroxyprogesterone acetate (*MPA*) group. Estrogen receptor (*ER*) immunostaining is decreased in the CEE plus MPA group. Progesterone receptor (*PR*) immunostaining is significantly increased only in the group given CEE alone. (Courtesy of Cline JM, Soderqvist G, von Schoultz E, et al: Effects of hormone replacement therapy on the mammary gland of surgically postmenopausal cynomolgus macaques. *Am J Obstet Gynecol* 174:93–100, 1996.)

CEE alone increased the percentage of progesterone receptor–positive cells (Figs 2, 3, and 4).

Conclusions.—Mammary gland epithelium has a proliferative response to treatment with CEE and MPA combined in postmenopausal macaques. Thus, women receiving combined hormone replacement therapy may be at increased risk of the development of breast neoplasm.

▶ These well-designed and carefully controlled experimental data on monkeys are probably as close as any information will be about the human female breast under the influence of estrogen or progesterone or both. The results of this study are clear: the maximum breast epithelial proliferation occurred by treatment with both estrogen and progesterone. This finding is consistent with the published work of Ferguson and Anderson[1] and Anderson and Ferguson[2] utilizing breast biopsy (human female) tissue analysis.

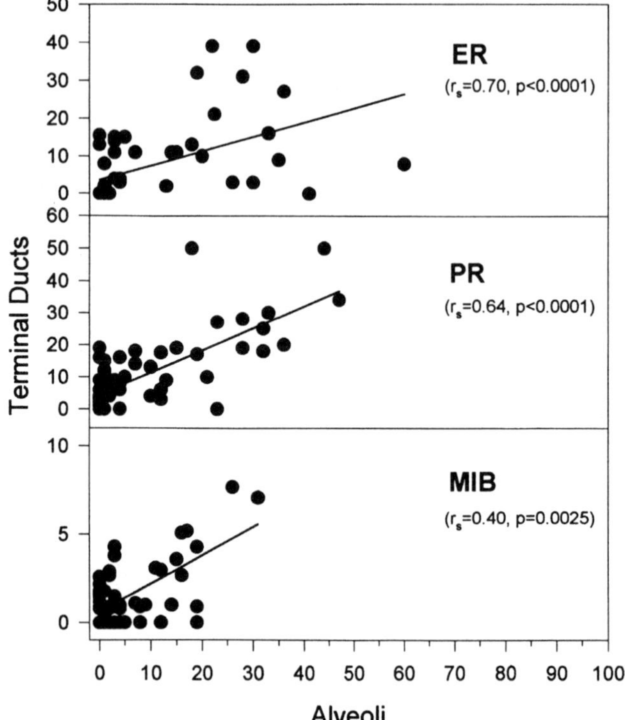

FIGURE 4.—Regression plots of correlations between immunostaining in alveoli and terminal ducts. Correlations are highly significant. *Abbreviations: ER,* estrogen receptor; *PR,* progesterone receptor. (Courtesy of Cline JM, Soderqvist G, von Schoultz E, et al: Effects of hormone replacement therapy on the mammary gland of surgically postmenopausal cynomolgus macaques. *Am J Obstet Gynecol* 174:93–100, 1996.)

However, it conflicts with the Chang et al.[3] data with short-term (10- to 13-day) percutaneous hormone treatment, which found that progesterone decreased the estrogen-induced proliferation of normal (human) breast epithelial cells in vivo. The Chang et al. study was double-blinded and randomized and included premenopausal women.

On balance, it seems prudent to withhold progestogen treatment for postmenopausal women who are receiving estrogen replacement therapy and who have had a hysterectomy. The known mitogenic effect of estrogen on the endometrium leaves unresolved for clinicians the question of how much of which hormones is optimal treatment for a postmenopausal woman with her uterus in situ.

W.H. Hindle, M.D.

References

1. Ferguson DJP, Anderson TJ: Morphological evaluation of cell turnover in relation to the menstrual cycle in the "resting" human breast. *Br J Cancer* 44:177–81, 1981.

2. Anderson TJ, Ferguson DJP: Cell turnover in the "resting" human breast: Influence of parity, contraceptive pill, age and laterality. *Br J Cancer* 46:376–382, 1982.
3. Chang K-J, Lee TTY, Linares-Cruz G, et al: Influence of percutaneous administration of estradiol and progesterone on human breast epithelium cell cycle in vivo. *Fertil Steril* 63:785–791, 1995.

Subject Index*

Author Index